Great Ormond Street Handbook of Paediatrics

Second Edition

Great Ormond Street Handbook of Paediatrics

Second Edition

Edited by

Stephan Strobel
MD, PhD, MRCP(Hon), FRCP, FRCPCH
Honorary Professor of Paediatrics and Clinical Immunology
University College London Institute of Child Health, London

Lewis Spitz
MBChB, PhD, MD(Hon), FRCS(Edin), FRCS(Eng), FAAP(Hon), FRCPCH, FACS(Hon)
Emeritus Nuffield Professor of Paediatric Surgery
Great Ormond Street Hospital for Children NHS Foundation Trust
and University College London Institute of Child Health, London

Stephen D. Marks
MD, MBChB, MSc, MRCP(UK), DCH, FRCPCH
Consultant Paediatric Nephrologist
Great Ormond Street Hospital for Children NHS Foundation Trust
and University College London Institute of Child Health, London

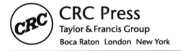

CRC Press
Taylor & Francis Group
Boca Raton London New York

CRC Press is an imprint of the
Taylor & Francis Group, an **informa** business

CRC Press
Taylor & Francis Group
6000 Broken Sound Parkway NW, Suite 300
Boca Raton, FL 33487-2742

Printed on acid-free paper
Version Date: 20151228

International Standard Book Number-13: 978-1-4822-2279-1 (Paperback)

Visit the Taylor & Francis Web site at
http://www.taylorandfrancis.com

and the CRC Press Web site at
http://www.crcpress.com

Contents

Contents

Contents

Foreword

My predecessor Sir Cyril Chantler wrote the foreword to the first edition and I am delighted to write the foreword to this new edition, in which three of the original authors have updated its contents, taking into account new developments in paediatrics since it was first published in 2007.

This book draws on the extraordinary knowledge and expertise of clinicians at Great Ormond Street Hospital. The hospital was founded by Dr Charles West, opening in 1852 with just 10 beds. It was the first children's hospital in the UK and it took its name from where it was located. After more than 160 years it is still in Great Ormond Street, but from small beginnings, it has been transformed into one of the great children's hospitals of the world, with an international reputation for work of the highest quality in the treatment of children with a wide range of serious conditions. There are now 55 surgical and medical specialties here, most of which are covered in this book.

To maintain and indeed enhance our reputation it is vital that we operate as a research hospital and not just as a hospital which does some research. With our academic partner the Institute of Child Health at University College London, we undertake ground-breaking research, which allows us to introduce innovation leading to better outcomes for the children we treat. Research here will be developed and expanded when our new Centre for Research on Rare Diseases in Children is opened in a brand new building with state of the art facilities. This book does not directly report research findings but indirectly it reflects discoveries made here on the genetic basis of many of the conditions it describes, and in the prognosis and treatment it sets out for each of the conditions it covers.

The illustrations are of the highest quality and are made possible through the excellent work done by the hospital's department of clinical photography and illustration. Few, if any, other paediatric text books can boast of such comprehensive pictures of the wide range of conditions that are described. Readers will find them invaluable in enhancing the knowledge they need to make informed accurate diagnoses.

What also distinguishes this book is the conciseness and the clarity of the writing. The way it is set out makes it wonderfully accessible. That quality as well as the comprehensive nature of its coverage makes it invaluable for those who treat sick children. They include general practitioners, paediatric nurses, community and general paediatricians as well as medical students. It is a superb reference book and it will not be a surprise to anyone who has used the first edition that it won the 2007 Royal Society of Medicine & Society of Authors Book Award.

I congratulate all the contributors, as well as the three authors who, in putting together this second edition, have undertaken the massive task of editing it. I hope it will be widely consulted not just in the UK but in many other countries too. It is a testament to the work of one of the greatest children's hospitals in the world.

Tessa Blackstone
Chairman
Great Ormond Street Hospital for Children
NHS Foundation Trust

Contributors

Huda Al-Ansari, Consultant in Paediatric Infectious Diseases, Salmaniya Hospital, Bahrain

Alice Armitage, Paediatric Academic Clinical Fellow, University College London Hospital, London, UK

C. Martin Bailey, Honorary Consultant Paediatric Otolaryngologist, Great Ormond Street Hospital for Children NHS Foundation Trust, London, UK

Jonathan A. Britto, Consultant Craniofacial/ Plastic Surgeon, Great Ormond Street Hospital for Children NHS Foundation Trust, London, UK

Penelope Brock, Honorary Consultant Paediatric Oncologist, Great Ormond Street Hospital for Children NHS Foundation Trust, London, UK

Paul Brogan, Honorary Consultant Paediatric Rheumatologist, Great Ormond Street Hospital for Children NHS Foundation Trust, London, UK

Alex Broomfield, Consultant in Metabolic Medicine, Willink Biochemical Genetics Unit, St. Mary's Hospital, Manchester, UK

Neil Bulstrode, Consultant Plastic Surgeon, Great Ormond Street Hospital for Children NHS Foundation Trust, London, UK

Michael Burch, Consultant Paediatric Cardiologist, Great Ormond Street Hospital for Children NHS Foundation Trust, London, UK

Tanzina Chowdhury, Consultant Paediatric Oncologist, Great Ormond Street Hospital for Children NHS Foundation Trust, London, UK

Joe Curry, Consultant Paediatric Surgeon, Great Ormond Street Hospital for Children NHS Foundation Trust, London, UK

Mehul Dattani, Professor and Honorary Consultant in Paediatric Endocrinologist, Institute of Child Health, University College London and Great Ormond Street Hospital for Children NHS Foundation Trust, London, UK

David Dunaway, Consultant Craniofacial Surgeon, Great Ormond Street Hospital for Children NHS Foundation Trust, London, UK

George Du Toit, Consultant in Paediatric Allergy, Guy's and St Thomas' NHS Foundation Trust, and Reader in Paediatric Allergy, Kings College London, London, UK

Deborah M. Eastwood, Consultant Paediatric Orthopaedic Surgeon, Great Ormond Street Hospital for Children and Royal National Orthopaedic Hospital NHS Foundation Trusts, London, UK

Adam Fox, Consultant in Paediatric Allergy, Guy's and St Thomas' NHS Foundation Trust, London, UK

Mark Gaze, Consultant Clinical Oncologist, Great Ormond Street Hospital for Children NHS Foundation Trust, London, UK

Stephanie Grünewald, Consultant in Metabolic Medicine and Honorary Senior Lecturer, Great Ormond Street Hospital for Children NHS Foundation Trust, London, UK

Ian Hann, Emeritus Professor of Haematology, University College London, London, UK

Darren Hargrave, Clinical Paediatric Oncologist, Great Ormond Street Hospital for Children NHS Foundation Trust, London, UK

John Harper, Emeritus Professor of Paediatric Dermatology and Honorary Consultant, Institute of Child Health, University College London and Great Ormond Street Hospital for Children NHS Foundation Trust, London, UK

Susan Hill, Consultant Paediatric Gastroenterologist, Great Ormond Street Hospital for Children NHS Foundation Trust, London, UK

Deborah Hodes, Consultant Community Paediatrician, Royal Free London NHS Foundation Trust, London, UK

Jane A. Hurst, Consultant Clinical Geneticist, NE Thames Genetics Service Great Ormond Street Hospital for Children NHS Foundation Trust, London, UK

David Inwald, Consultant in Paediatric Intensive Care, St Mary's Hospital, Imperial College Healthcare NHS Trust, London, UK

Chris Jephson, Consultant Paediatric Otolaryngologist, Great Ormond Street Hospital for Children NHS Foundation Trust, London, UK

Alison M. Jones, Consultant Paediatric Immunologist, Great Ormond Street Hospital for Children NHS Foundation Trust, London, UK

Loshan Kangesu, Consultant Plastic Surgeon, Great Ormond Street Hospital for Children NHS Foundation Trust, London, UK

Judith Kingston, Consultant Paediatric Oncologist, Great Ormond Street Hospital for Children NHS Foundation Trust, London, UK

Veronica Kinsler, Consultant Paediatric Dermatologist, Great Ormond Street Hospital for Children NHS Foundation Trust, London, UK

Fenella Kirkham, Professor of Paediatric Neurology, Institute of Child Health, University College London, London, UK

Helen Lachmann, Reader in Amyloidosis, University College London, London, UK

Gill A. Levitt, Honorary Consultant Paediatric Oncologist, Great Ormond Street Hospital for Children NHS Foundation Trust, London, UK

Keith Lindley, Consultant Paediatric Gastroenterologist, Great Ormond Street Hospital for Children NHS Foundation Trust, London, UK

Adnan Manzur, Consultant Paediatric Neurologist, Great Ormond Street Hospital for Children NHS Foundation Trust, London, UK

Stephen D. Marks, Consultant Paediatric Nephrologist, Great Ormond Street Hospital for Children NHS Foundation Trust and Institute of Child Health, University College London, London, UK

Antony Michalski, Consultant Paediatric Oncologist, Great Ormond Street Hospital for Children NHS Foundation Trust, London, UK

Paul Morris, Consultant Plastic Surgeon, Great Ormond Street Hospital for Children NHS Foundation Trust, London, UK

Ken K. Nischal, Professor and Director, Paediatric Ophthalmology, Strabismus and Adult Motility, Childrens' Hospital of Pittsburgh, UPMC School of Medicine of Pittsburgh, University of Pittsburgh, Philadelphia, USA

Kiran Nistala, Honorary Consultant Paediatric Rheumatologist, Great Ormond Street Hospital for Children NHS Foundation Trust, London, UK

Vas Novelli, Consultant in Paediatric Infectious Diseases, Great Ormond Street Hospital for Children NHS Foundation Trust, London, UK

Catherine Peters, Consultant Paediatric Endocrinologist, Great Ormond Street Hospital for Children NHS Foundation Trust, London, UK

Mark Peters, GOSHCC Professor of Paediatric Intensive Care, Institute of Child Health, University College London and Great Ormond Street Hospital for Children NHS Foundation Trust, London, UK

Clarissa Pilkington, Consultant Paediatric Rheumatologist, Great Ormond Street Hospital for Children NHS Foundation Trust, London, UK

Sian Pincott, Consultant General Paediatrician, Great Ormond Street Hospital for Children NHS Foundation Trust, London, UK

Stephanie Robb, Consultant Paediatric Neurologist, Great Ormond Street Hospital for Children NHS Foundation Trust, London, UK

Martina Ryan, Specialist Speech and Language Therapist, Great Ormond Street Hospital for Children NHS Foundation Trust, London, UK

Richard H. Scott, Consultant and Honorary Senior Lecturer in Clinical Genetics, Great Ormond Street Hospital for Children NHS Foundation Trust, London, UK

Delane Shingadia, Consultant in Paediatric Infectious Diseases, Great Ormond Street Hospital for Children NHS Foundation Trust, London, UK

Branavan Sivakumar, Consultant Hand, Plastic and Reconstructive Surgeon, Great Ormond Street Hospital for Children and Royal Free Hospital NHS Foundation Trusts, London, UK

Olga Slater, Consultant Paediatric Oncologist, Great Ormond Street Hospital for Children NHS Foundation Trust, London, UK

Naima Smeulders, Consultant Paediatric Urologist, Great Ormond Street Hospital for Children NHS Foundation Trust, London, UK

Gillian Smith, Consultant Plastic and Reconstructive Surgeon, Great Ormond Street Hospital for Children NHS Foundation Trust, London, UK

Owen P. Smith, Professor of Haematology, The University of Dublin, Trinity College Dublin, Ireland

Sam Sonnappa, Senior Lecturer and Honorary Consultant in Paediatric Respiratory Medicine, Institute of Child Health, University College London and Great Ormond Street Hospital for Children NHS Foundation Trust, London, UK

Helen Spencer, Consultant in Transplant and Respiratory Medicine, Great Ormond Street Hospital for Children NHS Foundation Trust, London, UK

Lewis Spitz, Emeritus Nuffield Professor of Paediatric Surgery, Institute of Child Health, University College London and Great Ormond Street Hospital for Children NHS Foundation Trust, London, UK

Stephan Strobel, Honorary Professor of Paediatrics and Clinical Immunology, Institute of Child Health, University College London, London, UK

Guy Thorburn, Consultant Plastic Surgeon, Great Ormond Street Hospital for Children NHS Foundation Trust, London, UK

Colin Wallis, Consultant in Respiratory Paediatrics, Great Ormond Street Hospital for Children NHS Foundation Trust, London, UK

Callum Wilson, Consultant in Metabolic Medicine, Starship Children's Hospital, Auckland, New Zealand

Abbreviations

17-OHP	17-hydroxyprogesterone	ALT	alanine aminotransferase
A&E	accident and emergency	AMKL	acute megakaryoblastic leukaemia
AAV	antineutrophil cytoplasmic antibody-associated vasculitides	AML	acute myeloid leukaemia
		(c)AMP	(cyclic) adenosine monophosphate
ACC	adenocortical carcinoma	AMN	adrenomyeloneuropathy
ACE	angiotensin converting enzyme	ANA	antinuclear antibody
ACHR	acetylcholine receptor	(p-)ANCA	(perinuclear) anticytoplasmic antibody
ACT	adrenocortical tumour		
ACTB	actin beta	AOM	acute otitis media
ACTH	adrenocorticotrophic hormone	AP	antero-posterior
AD	autosomal dominant (inheritance)	AP3B1	adaptor protein complex 3-beta-1 subunit
ADA	adenosine deaminase		
ADEM	acute demyelinating encephalomyelitis	APECED	autoimmune polyendocrinopathy ectodermal dysplasia
ADHD	attention deficit hyperactivity disorder	APL	acute promyelocytic leukaemia
		APLS	advanced paediatric life support
ADPKD	autosomal dominant polycystic kidney diseases	APT	atopy patch test
		AR	autosomal recessive (inheritance)
ADR	adverse drug reactions	ARDS	acute respiratory distress syndrome
AFB	acid-fast bacilli	ARPKD	autosomal recessive polycystic kidney disease
AFP	alpha-fetoprotein		
AGAT	arginine glycine amidinotransferase	ARVC	arrhythmogenic right ventricular cardiomyopathy
AID	activation-induced cytidine deaminase		
		AS	aortic stenosis
AIDS	acquired immunodeficiency syndrome	ASC	apoptosis-associated specklike protein with a caspase recruitment domain
AIP	aryl hydrocarbon interacting protein		
AIRE	autoimmune regulator	ASD	atrial septal defect
AIS	adolescent idiopathic scoliosis	ASOT	antistreptolysin o titre
AKI	acute kidney injury	AST	aspartate aminotransferase
ALCL	anaplastic large cell lymphoma	AT	ataxia telangiectasia
ALD	adrenoleukodystrophy	ATM	ataxia-telangiectasia mutated
ALI	acute lung injury	ATP	adenosine triphosphate
ALK	anaplastic lymphoma kinase	ATRA	all-trans retinoic acid
ALL	acute lymphoblastic leukaemia	AT/RT	atypical teratoid/rhabdoid tumour
ALPS	autoimmune lymphoproliferative syndrome	AVN	avascular necrosis
		AVSD	atrioventricular septal defect
ALS	acid labile subunit	BAL	bronchoalveolar lavage

BBS	Bardet–Biedl syndrome		CINCA	chronic infantile, neurological, cutaneous and articular syndrome
BCG	bacillus Calmette–Guérin		CK	creatine kinase
BDP	beclometasone		CKD	chronic kidney disease
β-HcG	beta-human choriogonadotrophin		CLD	chronic lung disease
BiPAP	biphasic positive airways pressure		CMC	chronic mucocutaneous candidiasis
BL	Burkitt lymphoma		CML	chronic myelogenous leukaemia
BLM	Bloom syndrome		CMN	congenital melanocytic naevi
BLNK	B-cell linker protein		CMP	cow's milk protein
BMD	Becker muscular dystrophy		CMS	congenital myasthenic syndromes
BMT	bone marrow transplantation		CMT	Charcot–Marie–Tooth disease
BOS	bronchiolitis obliterans syndrome		CMV	cytomegalovirus
BP	blood pressure		CNS	central nervous system
BPD	bronchopulmonary dysplasia		CoA	coarctation of the aorta
BPSU	British Paediatric Surveillance Unit		COCALD	childhood onset cerebral adrenoleukodystrophy
BSPGHAN	British Society of Paediatric Gastroenterology, Hepatology and Nutrition		CPAP	continuous positive airway pressure
BSS	Bernard–Soulier syndrome		CPEO	chronic progressive external ophthalmoplegia
BTK	Bruton tyrosine kinase		CPK	creatine phosphokinase
BTS	British Thoracic Society		CPP	cerebral perfusion pressure
C2TA	Class II transactivator		CPR	cardiopulmonary resuscitation
CAA	coronary artery aneurysm		CRH	corticotrophin releasing hormone
CAF	common assessment framework		CRIM	cross-reactive immunological material
CAH	congenital adrenal hyperplasia			
CALM	café-au-lait macule		CRMO	chronic recurrent multifocal osteomyelitis
CAKUT	congenital anomalies of the kidney and urinary tract		CRP	C-reactive protein
CAPS	cryopyrin-associated periodic syndrome		CSA	child sexual abuse
			CSD	cat-scratch disease
CARD	caspase recruitment domain		CSE	convulsive status epilepticus
CBS	cystathionine b-synthase		CSF	cerebrospinal fluid
CCAM	congenital cystic adenomatoid malformation		CSOM	chronic suppurative otitis media
			CSS	Churg–Strauss syndrome (now known as eosinophilic granulomatosis with polyangiitis [EGPA])
CCSK	clear cell sarcoma of the kidney			
CD	Crohn disease			
CD2BP1	CD2 binding protein 1			
CDG	congenital disorders of glycosylation		CSS	craniosynostosis
CEBPE CCAAT	(cytosine-cytosine-adenosine-adenosine-thymidine) enhancer-binding protein epsilon		CT	computed tomography
			CTD	connective tissue disease
			CTEV	congenital talipes equinovarus deformity
CEP	congenital erythropoietic porphyria			
CF	cystic fibrosis		CTRC	chymotrypsinogen C
CFH	complement factor H		CTSC	cathepsin C
CFTR	cystic fibrosis transmembrane conductance regulator (protein)		CTV	congenital vertical talus
			CTx	congenital toxoplasmosis
CGD	chronic granulomatous disease		CU	chronic urticaria
CGH	comparative genomic hybridisation		CVID	common variable immunodeficiency
CHH	cartilage hair hypoplasia		CVP	central venous pressure
CHI	congenital hyperinsulinism		CVS	cyclic vomiting syndrome
CHS	Chediak–Higashi syndrome		CXR	chest x-ray
CIAS1	cold-induced autoinflammatory syndrome 1		CYBA	cytochrome b alpha subunit
			CYBB	cytochrome b beta subunit
			CYP	cytochrome

DBPCFC	double-blind placebo controlled food challenge	EOS	early onset sarcoidosis
DC	dyskeratosis congenita	EPLS	European Paediatric Life Support
DCM	diffuse cutaneous mastocytosis	ERCP	endoscopic retrograde cholangiopancreatography
DCM	dilated cardiomyopathy	ERG	electroretinography
DDH	developmental dysplasia of the hip	ERT	enzyme replacement therapy
DEND	developmental delay, epilepsy and neonatal diabetes	ESPGHAN	European Society of Paediatric Gastroenterology, Hepatology and Nutrition
DEXA	dual energy x-ray absorptiometry	ESR	erythrocyte sedimentation rate
DHR	dihydrorhodamine	ESWL	extracorporeal shock wave lithotripsy
DI	diabetes inspidus	ETEC	enterotoxin producing *Escherichia coli*
DIC	disseminated intravascular coagulation	ETT	endotracheal tube
DIDMOAD	diabetes insipidus, diabetes mellitus, optic atrophy and deafness	EVER	epidermodysplasia verruciformis
DIOS	distal intestinal obstruction syndrome	FA	Fanconi anaemia
		FA	Friedreich ataxia
DIP	distal interphalangeal joint	FACS	fluorescence-activated cell sorting
DIPG	diffuse intrinsic pontine glioma	FAMA	fluorescent antibody to membrane antigen
DIRA	deficiency of IL-1 receptor antagonist	FAOD	fatty acid oxidation defect
		FAP	familial adenomatous polyposis
DKA	diabetic ketoacidosis	FAST	focused abdominal sonography in trauma
DMD	Duchenne muscular dystrophy		
DMSA	dimercaptosuccinic acid	FB	fructose 1,6 bisphosphatase
DNA	deoxyribonucleic acid	FBC	full blood count
DNMT3B	DNA (cytosine-5-)-methyltransferase 3-beta	FCAS	familial cold autoinflammatory syndrome
DOCK-8	dedicator of cytokinesis 8	FDA	food and drugs administration
DPG	diphosphoglycerate	FEV	forced expiratory volume
DS	Down syndrome	FEVR	familial exudative vitreoretinopathy
DSD	disorders of sex development	FFP	fresh frozen plasma
DVM	delayed visual maturation	FGD	familial glucocorticoid deficiency
EAEC	enteroaggregative *Escherichia coli*	FGFR	fibroblast growth factor receptor
EB	epidermolysis bullosa	FGM	female genital mutilation
EBV	Epstein–Barr virus	FH	familial hypercholesterolaemia
ECG	electrocardiography	FII	fabricated or induced illness
ECHO	echocardiography	FIPA	familial isolated pituitary adenoma
ECMO	extracorporeal membrane oxygenation	FISH	fluorescence *in situ* hybridisation
		FLG	filaggrin
EDA-ID	ectodermal dystrophy immune deficiency	FMF	familial Mediterranean fever
		FNAC	fine-needle aspiration cytology
EDC	eosinophilic disease of the colon	FOXN1	forkhead box N1
EDMD	Emery–Dreifuss muscular dystrophy	FOXP3	forkhead box protein 3
EEC	ectodermal dysplasia and cleft lip and palate syndrome	FPR1	formylpeptide receptor 1
		FSGS	focal segmental glomerulosclerosis
EEG	electroencephalogram	FSH	follicle stimulating hormone
EGG	electrogastrophy	FSHD	fascioscapulohumeral dystrophy
EHEC	enterohaemorrhagic *Escherichia coli*	FUCT1	fucose transporter 1
EIA	enzyme immune assay	FVC	forced vital capacity
EIEC	enteroinvasive *Escherichia coli*	G6PD	glucose-6-phosphate dehydrogenase
ELA2	elastase 2	GA	glutaric acidaemia
ELISA	enzyme linked immunosorbent assay	GAG	glycosaminoglycan
EM	erythema migrans	Gal-1-PUT	galactose-1-phosphate uridyltransferase
EMG	electromyography		

GAMT	guanidinoacetate methyltransferase		HPA	Health Protection Agency
Gb3	globotriaosylceramide		HPV	human papilloma virus
GBM	glomerular basement membrane		HRCT	high resolution computed tomography
GCS	Glasgow coma score		HS	hereditary spherocytosis
G-CSF	granulocyte colony stimulating factor		HSCT	haematopoetic stem cell transplantation
GEFS	generalised epilepsy febrile seizures		HSN	Henoch Schönlein nephritis
GFI1	growth factor independent 1		HSP	Henoch Schönlein purpura (now known as IgA vasculitis)
GFR	glomerular filtration rate			
(rh) GH	(recombinant human) growth hormone		HSV	herpes simplex virus
GHD	growth hormone deficiency		HUS	haemolytic uraemic syndrome
GHI	growth hormone insufficiency		IBD	inflammatory bowel disease
GHRH	growth hormone releasing hormone		ICOS	inducible costimulator
GI	gastrointestinal		ICP	intracranial pressure
GM	galactomannan		ICS	inhaled corticosteroids
GM-CSF	granulocyte monocyte colony stimulating factor		IDDM	insulin-dependent diabetes mellitus
GMFCS	gross motor function classification system		IDSA	Infectious Diseases Society of America
GnRH	gonadotrophin releasing hormone		IEF	isoelectric focusing
GORD	gastro-oesophageal reflux disease		IFA	immunofluorescence assay
GP	glycoprotein		IFN	interferon-gamma
GPA	granulomatosis with polyangiitis		IFNGR1	interferon-gamma receptor subunit 1
GSD	glycogen storage disease		IFNGR2	interferon-gamma receptor subunit 2
GTP	guanosine triphosphate		Ig(k)	immunoglobulin of k light-chain type
H&E	haematoxylin and eosin			
HAART	highly active antiretroviral therapy		IGF	insulin-like growth factor
HAX1	HLCS1-associated protein X1		IGRA	interferon-gamma release assay
hCG	human chorionic gonadotrophin		IH	infantile haemangioma
HCM	hypertrophic cardiomyopathy		IIF	indirect immunofluorescence
HCU	homocystinuria		IKBA	inhibitor of NF-kB alpha
HDM	house dust mite		IKBKG	inhibitory kappa B kinase gamma
HE	hereditary elliptocytosis		IM	infectious mononucleosis
HEPA	high-efficiency particulate arrestance		IL	(interleukin)
HES	hypereosinophilic syndrome		IL12B	interleukin-12 beta subunit
HFM	hemifacial microsomia		IL12RB1	interleukin-12 receptor beta-1
HFOV	high frequency oscillatory ventilation		ILD	interstitial lung disease
			INH	isoniazid
HI	harlequin ichthyosis		INO	internuclear ophthalmoplegia
HIDA	hepatobiliary iminodiacetic acid		INRG	International Neuroblastoma Risk Group
HIDS	hyperimmunoglobulin D and periodic fever syndrome		INSS	International Neuroblastoma Staging Study
HIES	hyper-IgE syndrome		IPEX	immune dysregulation, polyendocrinopathy, enteropathy, X-linked syndrome
HI/HA	hyperinsulinism/hyperammonaemia			
HL	Hodgkin lymphoma			
HLH	haemophagocytic lymphohistiocytosis		IQ	intelligence quotient
			IRAK4	interleukin-1 receptor associated kinase 4
HLH	hypoplastic left heart			
HLPP	hereditary liability to pressure palsies		IST	immunosuppressive therapy
HMG	CoA lyase 3-hydroxy-3-methylglutary-coenzyme A lyase		ITGB2	integrin beta-2
			ITP	immune or idiopathic thrombocytopenic purpura
HMG	CoA synthase 3-hydroxy-3-methylglutary-coenzyme A synthase			
			IVC	inferior vena cava

IVF	*in vitro* fertilisation	MFD	matched family donor
IVIg	intravenous immunoglobulin	MG	myasthenia gravis
IVP	intravenous pyelogram	MIBG	metaiodobenzylguanidine
IVU	intravenous urogram	MKD	mevalonate kinase deficiency
JAK3	janus-associated kinase 3	ML	myeloid leukaemia
JDM	juvenile dermatomyositis	MLD	metachromatic leukodystrophy
JIA	juvenile idiopathic arthritis	MLPA	multiplex ligation-dependent probe
JMML	juvenile myelomonocytic leukaemia		amplification
JNA	juvenile nasopharyngeal	MMA	methylmalonic acidemia
	angiofibroma	MMF	mycophenolate mofetil
JXG	juvenile xanthogranuloma	MMR	measles, mumps, rubella
KAFO	knee–ankle–foot orthosis	MODY	maturity onset diabetes of the young
KCS	keratoconjunctivitis sicca	MPA	microscopic polyangiitis
KD	Kawasaki disease	MPO	myeloperoxidase
KID	keratitis–ichthyosis–deafness	MPS	mucopolysaccharidoses
	syndrome	MRA	magnetic resonance angiography
L	lymphocytes	MRC	magnetic resonance cholangiography
LABA	long-acting β_2 agonist	MRC	Medical Research Council
LAD	leukocyte adhesion defects	MRI	magnetic resonance imaging
LAL	lysosomal acid lipase	MRS	magnetic resonance spectroscopy
LCH	Langerhans cell histiocytosis	MRU	magnetic resonance urography
LCT	long-chain triglyceride	MRV	magnetic resonance venography
LDH	lactate dehydrogenase	Mtx	methotrexate
LFT	liver function test	MWS	Muckle Wells syndrome
LGMD	limb girdle muscular dystrophy	MYD88	myeloid differentiation primary
LHON	Leber's hereditary optic neuropathy		response gene 88
LHRH	luteinising hormone releasing	NAAT	nucleic acid amplification test
	hormone	NBS1	Nijmegen breakage syndrome 1
LIP	lymphocytic interstitial pneumonitis	NBT	nitro-blue tetrazolium
LPN2	lipin-2	NCF1	neutrophil cytosolic factor 1
LS	Leigh syndrome	NCF2	neutrophil cytosolic factor 2
LYST	lysosomal trafficking regulator	NEC	necrotising enterocolitis
MAG3	mercapto-acetyltriglycine	NEMO	NF-kB essential modulator
MAPBPIP	MAPBP-interacting protein	NF1	neurofibromatosis types 1
MAPCA	major aortopulmonary collateral	NF-kB	nuclear factor-kB
	artery	NHEJ	non homologous end joining
m.c.&s.	microscopy, culture and sensitivity	NHL	non-Hodgkin lymphoma
MCAD	medium-chain acyl co-A	NICH	non-involuting congenital
	dehydrogenase		haemangioma
MCDK	multicystic dysplastic kidney	NICU	neonatal intensive care unit
MCM4	minichromosome maintenance-	NIV	non-invasive ventilation
	deficient 4	NK	natural killer (cell)
MCNS	minimal change nephrotic syndrome	NKH	non-ketotic hyperglycinaemia
MCP	metacarpophalangeal joint	NMDA(R)	N-methyl-D-aspartate (receptor)
MCT	medium-chain triglyceride	NNRTI	non-nucleoside reverse transcriptase
MCTD	mixed connective tissue disease		inhibitor
MCUG	micturating cystourethrogram	NNT	nicotinamide nucleotide
MD	meningococcal disease		transhydrogenase
MDS	myelodysplasia	NO	nitric oxide
MEFV	Mediterranean fever	NOMID	neonatal onset multi-system
MEN	multiple endocrine neoplasia		inflammatory disease
MERRF	mitochondrial encephalopathy with	NRAS	neuroblastoma Ras protein
	ragged red fibres	NRTI	nucleoside reverse transcriptase
MF	myelofibrosis		inhibitor

NS	nephrotic syndrome		PK	pyruvate kinase
NSAID	non-steroidal anti-inflammatory drug		PKD	polycystic kidney disease
			PKU	phenylketonuria
NSPCC	National Society for the Prevention of Cruelty to Children		PMBCL	primary mediastinal B-cell lymphoma
NTBC	nitisinone		PMI	phosphoisomerase
NTM	non-tuberculous mycobacterial infection		PML	promyelocytic leukaemia
			PMM	phosphomannomutase
NWTS	National Wilms Tumour System		PN	parenteral nutrition
OAS	oral allergy syndrome		PNH	paroxysmal nocturnal haemoglobinuria
OFC	oral food challenge			
OGTT	oral glucose tolerance test		PNMD	permanent neonatal diabetes mellitus
OME	otitis media with effusion			
ORS	oral rehydration solution		PNS	peripheral nervous system
OSA	obstructive sleep apnoea		POR	P450 oxidoreductase
OTC	ornithine transcarbamylase		PPAR	peroxisome proliferator activated receptor
PA	propionic acidaemia			
PALS	Paediatric Advanced Life Support		pPNET	peripheral primitive neuroectodermal tumour
PAN	polyarteritis nodosa			
PANDAS	paediatric autoimmune neuropsychiatric disorders associated with streptococcal infections		PPRF	paramedian pontine reticular formation
			PPV	positive predictive value
PAPA	pyogenic arthritis, pyoderma gangrenosum and acne		PR3	proteinase 3
			PRES	posterior reversible encephalopathy syndrome
PAS	projected adult size			
PBD	peroxisomal biogenesis disorders		PRF1	perforin 1
PCCL	percutaneous cystolithotomy		PROM	premature rupture of membranes
PCDAI	Paediatric Crohn Disease Activity Index		PS	pulmonary stenosis
			PSTPIP1	proline, serine, threonine phosphatase interacting protein 1
PCNL	percutaneous nephrolithotomy			
PCO(S)	polycystic ovary (syndrome)		PTH	parathyroid hormone
PCP	pneumocystis pneumonia		PTLD	post-transplant lymphoproliferative disorder
PCR	polymerase chain reaction			
PDA	patent ductus arteriosus		PTT	partial thromboplastin time
PDGFR	platelet derived growth factor receptor		PUJ	pelviureteric junction
			PUJA	pelviureteric junction anomaly
PDHC	pyruvate dehydrogenase complex		PUO	pyrexia of unknown origin
PEEP	positive end-expiratory pressure		PUV	posterior urethral valve
PEFR	peak expiratory flow rate		PWS	Prader–Willi syndrome
PEG	polyethylene glycol		RAD	reflex anal dilatation
PERT	pancreatic exocrine replacement therapy		RAEB	refractory anaemia with excess of blasts
PET	positron emission tomography		RAG	recombinase activating gene
PFAPA	periodic fever, aphthous stomatitis, pharyngitis and cervical adenitis		RAP27A	Ras-associated protein 27A
			RARα	retinoic acid receptor-alpha
PFFD	proximal femoral focal deficiency		RAST	radioabsorbent assay
PFO	patent foramen ovale		RBC	red blood cell
PHPV	persistent hyperplastic primary vitreous		RCAD	renal cysts and diabetes syndrome
			RCC	refractory cytopenia of childhood/renal cell carcinoma
PI	protease inhibitor			
PICU	paediatric intensive care unit		RDS	respiratory distress syndrome
PID	primary immunodeficiency syndrome		RDT	rapid diagnostic test
PIP	peak inspiratory pressure/proximal interphalangeal joint		RFC	reduced folate carrier
			RFX	regulatory factor X

RIA	radioimmunassay	TGFB	transforming growth factor-beta
RICH	rapidly-involuting congenital haemangioma	TIG	tetanus immune globulin
		TIR	toll and IL-1 receptor
RLD	radial longitudinal deficiency	TLESR	transient lower oesophageal sphincter relaxation
RMRP	RNA component of mitochondrial RNA processing endonuclease	T-LL	T-cell lymphoblastic lymphoma
RMS	rhabdomyosarcoma	TMD	transient myeloproliferative disorder
RNA	ribonucleic acid	TMJ	temperomandibular joint
ROP	retinopathy of prematurity	TNDM	transient neonatal diabetes mellitus
RPE	retinal pigment epithelial	TNF	tumour necrosis factor
RRP	recurrent respiratory papillomatosis	TNFRSF6	tumor necrosis factor receptor soluble factor 6
RSV	respiratory syncytial virus		
RTK	rhabdoid tumour of the kidney	TPMT	thiopurine methyltransferase
SAA	severe aplastic anaemia	TPN	total parenteral nutrition
SAPHO	synovitis, acne, pustulosis, hyperostosis and osteitis	TRAPS	TNF receptor-associated period syndrome
SBDS	Shwachman–Bodian–Diamond syndrome	TRH	thyrotrophin releasing hormone
		TSH	thyroid stimulating hormone
SCA	segmental chromosomal abnormalit	TSS	toxic shock syndrome
SCID	severe combined immunodeficiency	TST	tuberculin skin test
SCIg	subcutaneous immunoglobulin	tTg	tissue transglutaminase
SCT	stem cell transplantation	TTP	thrombotic thrombocytopenic purpura
SDF-1	stromal-derived factor 1	Tyk2	tyrosine kinase 2
SDS	standard deviation score	UC	ulcerative colitis
SGS	subglottic stenosis	UCD	urea cycle disorder
SH2D1A	SH2 domain protein 1A	UNCRC	United Nations Convention of the Rights of the Child
SHBG	sex hormone binding globulin		
SJS	Stevens–Johnson syndrome	UP	urticarial pigmentosa
SLE	systemic lupus erythematosus	UPD	uniparental disomy
SLO	Smith–Lemli–Opitz syndrome	URS	ureterorenoscopy
SM	solitary mastocytoma	UTI	urinary tract infection
SMA	spinal muscular atrophy/smooth muscle antibody	VCA	viral capsid antigen
		VEP	visual evoked potential
SMN	survival motor neuron	VL	visceral leishmaniasis
SPECT	single photon emission tomography	VLBW	very low birth weight
SPT	skin-prick test	VKH	Vogt–Koyanagi–Harada disease
SS	Sweet syndrome	VLCFA	very long-chain fatty acid
SSNS	steroid-sensitive nephrotic syndrome	V-P	ventriculoperitoneal
SSPE	subacute sclerosing panencephalitis	VSD	ventricular septal defect
STAT	signal transducer and activator of transcription	VUJA	vesicoureteric junction anomaly
		VUR	vesicoureteric reflux
STS	soft tissue sarcoma	vWD	von Willebrand disease
TA	Takayasu arteritis	vWF	von Willebrand factor
TAP	transporter associated with antigen processing	VZV	varicella zoster virus
		WCC	white cell count
TAPVD	total anomalous pulmonary venous drainage	WHO	World Health Organisation
		WT	Wilms tumour
TAR	thrombocytopenia absent radius	XIAP	X-linked inhibitor of apoptosis
TB	tuberculosis	XL	X-linked (inheritance)
TBM	tuberculous meningitis	XLA	X-linked agammaglobulinaemia
TC	transcobalamin	XLP	X-linked lymphoproliferative disease
TCR	T cell receptor	XLT	X-linked thrombocytopenia
TEN	toxic epidermal necrolysis		
TGA	transposition of the great arteries		

1

Emergency Medicine

David Inwald and Mark Peters

INTRODUCTION

A simple, structured approach to an acutely ill child has been the focus of Advanced Paediatric Life Support (APLS), Paediatric Advanced Life Support (PALS) and European Paediatric Life Support (EPLS) courses, with training recommended for all those involved in the care of acutely unwell children.

The advantages of this structured approach are clear: clinical problems are addressed in order of urgency and the chances of significant omissions are reduced. In all acutely ill children the A (airway), B (breathing) and C (circulation) should be assessed (and supported if inadequate) before a more detailed assessment is undertaken.

This chapter will outline the emergency management of the most common conditions requiring treatment in paediatric practice. In contrast to the APLS/EPLS approach, we include some details of ongoing care. This does not mean to distract from the vital importance of the initial assessment and resuscitation.

UPPER AIRWAY OBSTRUCTION

See also Chapter 4 Respiratory Medicine.

Stridor is an inspiratory noise related to obstruction of the extrathoracic airway. Dynamic intrathoracic airway obstruction can also result in expiratory stridor in conditions such as bronchomalacia or tracheomalacia. Obstruction of the extrathoracic airway is most commonly due to acute conditions such as viral laryngotracheitis (**Fig. 1.1**), bacterial tracheitis (**Fig. 1.2**), foreign body aspiration (**Figs 1.3–1.5**) and other conditions such as quinsy, retropharyngeal abscess (**Fig. 1.6**), epiglottitis (**Fig. 1.7**), inhalation of hot gases and angioneurotic oedema. Airway obstruction can also occur as a result of chronic lesions such as subglottic or tracheal stenosis (**Fig. 1.8**), vascular rings (**Fig. 1.9**), airway haemangiomata (**Fig. 1.10**) and polyps. These may present in the context of an intercurrent viral infection which may make the airway obstruction worse.

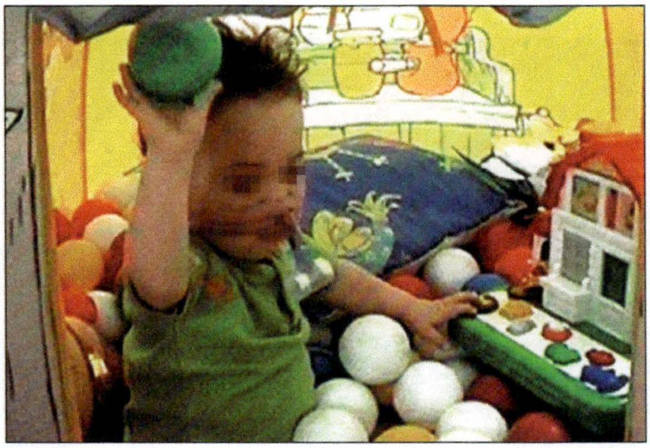

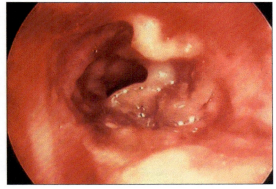

FIGURE 1.1 A 2-year-old child with viral tracheitis intubated in the ICU. As the lungs are unaffected he does not require mechanical ventilation. A humidification device is attached to the end of the tube to prevent secretions drying in the airway.

FIGURE 1.2 Bacterial tracheitis in an 18-month-old child who presented with a high pyrexia, shock and stridor.

1

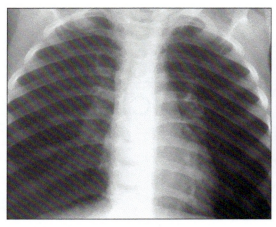

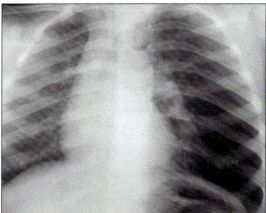

FIGURES 1.3, 1.4 Inspiratory (**1.3**) and expiratory (**1.4**) chest radiographs in a 4-year-old child with an inhaled peanut in the left main bronchus. Though foreign bodies usually cause occlusion of the entire airway lumen and distal collapse, in this case the peanut is causing a ball-valve effect and the left lung does not deflate on expiration.

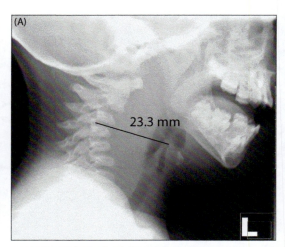

(A)

23.3 mm

L

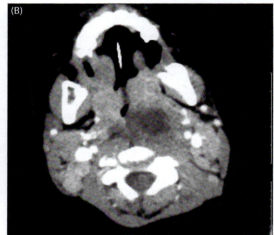

(B)

FIGURE 1.6 Retropharyngeal abscess demonstrated (A) on a lateral neck radiograph and (B) on CT scanning. Once the airway was secured, incision and drainage was necessary in addition to appropriate antibiotic therapy.

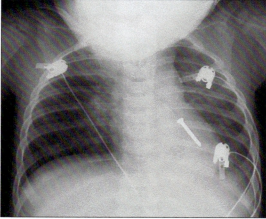

FIGURE 1.5 Nail in the left main bronchus. This will require removal with a rigid bronchoscope. Physiotherapy and flexible bronchoscopy are contraindicated, as both may cause the foreign body to slip further down the airway.

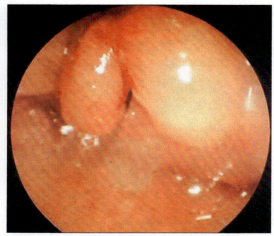

FIGURE 1.7 Acute inflammation of the epiglottis due to viral infection. The child required intubation.

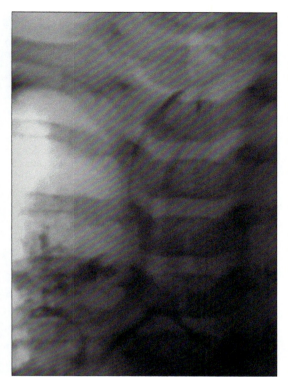

FIGURE 1.8 Congenital tracheal stenosis demonstrated by contrast bronchography. Surgical management was required.

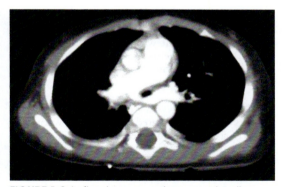

FIGURE 1.9 Left pulmonary artery vascular sling demonstrated by contrast CT scanning. The child presented with stridor.

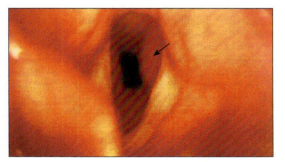

IMMEDIATE ASSESSMENT AND MANAGEMENT

Initial assessment should include rapid physical examination of the airway, breathing and circulation, with particular attention to the work of breathing (including respiratory rate, recession, use of accessory muscles) and pulse oximetry. Cyanosis, distress, exhaustion or oxygen saturations of <92% in air are all signs of severe obstruction and impending collapse. Children with these signs may require urgent intubation and ventilation. Intubation may be difficult and senior anaesthetic help should be summoned. Children with milder obstruction may require IV fluids in addition to more specific management (see below). The presence of a high fever in a toxic looking child should raise the possibility of bacterial tracheitis or epiglottitis. If the child is stable, a brief history should be taken with regard to recent coryzal illness (suggestive of viral tracheitis), foreign body aspiration and haemophilus influenza immunisation.

INVESTIGATIONS

Radiological investigations are not routinely required. Lateral neck x-rays are rarely helpful and immediate management (including intubation if necessary) is more important. Imaging, which may include a chest radiograph and CT neck and thorax, should only be performed when the child is stable. Laboratory investigations need only be performed if IV access is required.

FURTHER MANAGEMENT

Bacterial tracheitis and viral tracheitis

Children with mild or moderately severe viral tracheitis who do not require immediate intubation should be commenced on enteral dexamethasone, which has been shown to be of benefit in randomised controlled trials. However, children with bacterial tracheitis or severe viral tracheitis occasionally require intubation. An experienced anaesthetist should be called as the child will almost certainly require inhalational anaesthesia. Paralysing agents should be used with care in this setting as when muscle tone is lost the airway may completely obstruct. While waiting for assistance, nebulised adrenaline can be helpful in reducing airway oedema, but this should only be given in

FIGURE 1.10 An airway haemangioma in a 6-month-old child who presented with stridor. These lesions often present during viral lower respiratory tract infections when they are unmasked by additional airway swelling. The clue to the diagnosis may be the presence of haemangiomas elsewhere.

a high dependency area as reactive hyperaemia with worsening obstruction can occur when the nebuliser is completed. Children with suspected bacterial tracheitis (**Fig. 1.2**) may be septic and will require volume resuscitation prior to intubation. They should also have blood cultures sent and be commenced on antibiotics with good *Staphylococcus* and *Streptococcus* spp. cover.

Foreign body

Aspiration of a foreign body (**Figs 1.3–1.5**) may result in an asymptomatic child or cardiorespiratory collapse. Clearly, partial or complete obstruction at the level of the larynx or trachea may require urgent resuscitation. Again, senior anaesthetic help should be summoned. It may be possible to remove the foreign body at laryngoscopy with a Magill's forceps. If not, urgent tracheostomy may be required as an interim measure. A foreign body further down the airway may cause partial or complete obstruction of one or more major bronchi. A chest radiograph may demonstrate areas of hyperinflation or collapse, depending on the degree of airway obstruction. If in any doubt, inspiratory and expiratory films and the radiographic appearance of the pulmonary vascular tree will help to determine which lung is abnormal. These children need to be referred to a specialist centre where rigid bronchoscopy can be performed to remove the foreign body.

Other

Epiglottitis has become extremely rare since the introduction of *Haemophilus influenza* immunisation. If it is suspected, however, senior anaesthetic, ENT and paediatric advice should be sought. The airway will require securing, by tracheostomy if necessary, and the child will need volume resuscitation and antibiotic therapy with cefotaxime, which has good *Haemophilus* spp. cover. Quinsy (peritonsillar abscess) can often be seen on a lateral neck radiograph and will require incision and drainage, sometimes with a period of airway support while postoperative oedema settles. Anatomical lesions such as airway haemangiomata, vascular rings and tracheal stenosis may require specific surgical management.

ANAPHYLAXIS

Anaphylaxis is a type I hypersensitivity reaction triggered by cross-linking of IgE on mast cells. It occurs when enough antigen enters the systemic circulation to activate circulating basophils and tissue mast cells. This results in the release of inflammatory mediators, particularly histamine, prostaglandins and leukotrienes. These mediators cause massive peripheral vasodilation (cardiorespiratory arrest, shock), increased vascular permeability (angio-oedema, airway obstruction and urticaria), intense contraction of non-vascular smooth muscle (bronchoconstriction), abdominal pain, nausea, vomiting and tachycardia. Anaphylaxis may be due to drugs, insect stings (**Fig. 1.11**), foods, plants, chemicals or latex.

Anaphylaxis may progress slowly or rapidly and may range from a mild cutaneous reaction to circulatory arrest.

RECOGNITION

Clinical assessment should include rapid physical examination, with attention to airway, breathing and circulation, measurement of peak expiratory flow rate (PEFR) in children able to perform the technique and pulse oximetry. Children should be examined for generalised oedema, angio-oedema, erythematous rash and urticaria (**Fig. 1.12**) and a history taken for substance exposure (with particular reference to drugs or foodstuffs).

IMMEDIATE MANAGEMENT

Mild anaphylaxis

Mild reactions such as urticaria (**Fig. 1.12**) should respond to treatment with antihistamines and steroids. Drug treatment should be followed by a period of observation to ensure a more serious response does not occur.

Severe anaphylaxis

Patients should be treated with high-flow oxygen, and artificial ventilation if necessary. If stridor is present, airway angio-oedema is likely and senior anaesthetic assistance should be summoned to secure the airway. Intramuscular adrenaline should be administered as soon as possible in anaphylactic shock as per APLS guidelines. The IV route should be reserved for extreme emergency when there is doubt as to the adequacy of the circulation. However, when intramuscular injection might succeed, time should not be wasted seeking IV access. Adrenaline doses may be repeated at 5 minute intervals if necessary. Hypotension in anaphylaxis is due to vasodilatation and capillary leak and resuscitation with IV fluid is necessary to restore circulation. Corticosteroids and antihistamines should be given and an adrenaline infusion should be commenced if the patient's condition is not stable. Bronchospasm, if present, may respond to adrenaline and corticosteroids. If mechanical ventilation is necessary, a slow rate and long expiratory time should be used to allow full expiration to occur. Refractory bronchospasm should be treated as severe asthma (see also Chapter 4 Respiratory Medicine).

FOLLOW UP

The causative allergen may be identified by taking a careful history. Further investigation may include skin prick testing (SPT) and radioabsorbent assays (RAST) for specific IgE. The gold standard test for diagnosis of food allergy remains the food challenge. This should be carried out in a centre with adequate resuscitation facilities.

Any child who has had a serious reaction to peanuts should avoid all peanut products including oil. Peanuts are legumes and, although it is uncommon for patients to react to other legumes, cross-reactivity with tree nuts can occur. Peanut sensitive individuals should be introduced to these singly and with caution.

If there is evidence of a severe food or other allergy, the findings should be clearly documented and explained to the patient. Management primarily consists of avoidance. However, patients should also be instructed to carry a hand held summary and to wear a warning bracelet or necklace. Patients or parents of children at risk of anaphylactic reactions to foods, environmental allergens, chemicals or plants should carry injectable adrenaline at all times and know how to use it in an emergency.

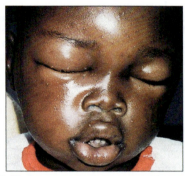

FIGURE 1.11 Severe anaphylaxis in a 11-month-old baby caused by bee stings with oedematous eyelids and lips, wheeze and shock.

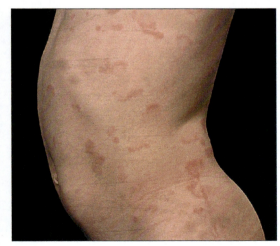

FIGURE 1.12 Urticarial rash in a child presenting with mild anaphylaxis caused by food allergy. If no other features are present this can be safely treated with antihistamines and allergen avoidance.

ASTHMA

See also Chapter 4 Respiratory Medicine, page 85.

Asthma is a chronic disease characterised by reversible airflow obstruction, particularly in the bronchi, with recurrent bouts of wheezing and breathlessness. However, all that wheezes is not asthma and important differential diagnoses of acute severe asthma include foreign body aspiration and bronchiolitis. Asthma has increased in prevalence over recent years and now affects 10–20% of children in the UK. Acute exacerbations of asthma represent 10–15% of all acute medical admissions in children. About 20 children and about 1600 adults die in the UK every year due to acute severe asthma. Common factors leading to acute exacerbations include viral respiratory infections, irritants, exercise and allergens.

RECOGNITION

Clinical assessment should include rapid physical examination, with attention to airway, breathing and circulation, measurement of PEFR and pulse oximetry (see Box below). Routine blood gas analysis is not recommended as arterial puncture is painful and may cause acute decompensation. Clinical assessment is more useful. Note severe tachypnoea is unusual in severe asthma and suggests either another diagnosis or toxic effects of bronchodilators. Work of breathing is a useful indicator. Assessment of pulsus paradoxus is no longer recommended.

IMMEDIATE MANAGEMENT

Severe asthma without life-threatening features should be treated with high-flow oxygen, nebulised salbutamol and ipratropium bromide, and oral corticosteroids. Salbutamol and ipratropium can safely be given continuously until improvement has occurred, when the dose frequency can be reduced. Oxygen should be given before, during and after administration of inhaled bronchodilators, to avoid hypoxaemia. The safest way to do this is via an oxygen driven nebuliser rather than a holding chamber.

If life-threatening features are present, senior help and an experienced anaesthetist should be summoned. In the meantime the airway should be maintained, oxygen should be administered by a rebreathing mask and IV access secured for administration of corticosteroids and bronchodilators. Proven effective IV bronchodilators include bolus salbutamol, aminophylline and magnesium sulphate. These should be given with cardiac monitoring, as salbutamol and aminophylline can cause arrhythmias.

INVESTIGATIONS

A chest radiograph should be obtained after initial stabilisation in any child with features of severe or life-threatening asthma, or with a first episode of wheeze, to exclude a foreign body, pneumothorax and mucus plugging (**Figs 1.13–1.15**). Routine chest radiographs in all cases of acute asthma are not necessary.

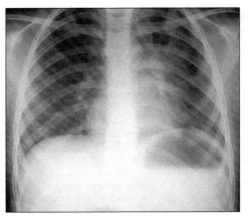

FIGURE 1.13 Plugging of the left lingular bronchus in acute severe asthma in an 8-year-old girl. The left heart border is indistinct but the left diaphragm is clearly seen.

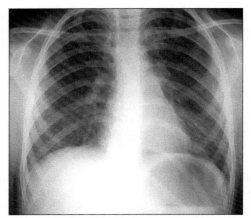

FIGURE 1.14 The plug seen in **1.13** was expectorated after bronchodilators were given.

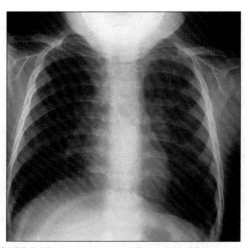

FIGURE 1.15 Acute severe asthma in a 13-year-old child. The lungs were grossly hyperinflated but there is no evidence of a pneumothorax. This child was ventilating at the top of his functional residual capacity and had little reserve.

INDICATIONS FOR VENTILATORY SUPPORT

- Patients who are tired.
- Those with a reduced conscious level.
- Those who continue to deteriorate despite maximal therapy.

Blood gas analysis is not a substitute for clinical assessment and the focus should remain on the clinical state of the patient.

Intubation

The patient should be pre-oxygenated and 10–20 ml/kg colloid given electively. Patients with acute severe asthma are often volume depleted and vasodilated. Ketamine (which has some bronchodilator activity) is a useful induction agent.

Ventilation strategies

High airway resistance may lead to a very prolonged expiratory phase during artificial ventilation, and slow ventilation rates may be required (10–15 breaths per min). Blood gases should not be normalised and very high $PaCO_2$ values may be tolerated without harm ('permissive hypercapnia') provided the pH remains >7.1 in the absence of other organ failure. Some positive end-expiratory pressure (PEEP) is necessary to counteract intrinsic PEEP. Neuromuscular paralysis should be discontinued as soon as possible as the combination of corticosteroids and paralysing agents is associated with an increased risk of critical illness neuropathy.

WHILE VENTILATED

Key in the management are generous humidification and physiotherapy to mobilise secretions and mucus plugs (**Figs 1.13, 1.14**). Drug treatment may include continued neuromuscular paralysis, ketamine by continuous infusion (for both sedative and bronchodilator effect), IV bronchodilators, corticosteroids and antibiotics. Heliox (a mixture of oxygen and helium with a lower density than air) has been used to ventilate patients with very high airway resistance but has not been widely adopted. Weaning from mechanical ventilation can be difficult. Any child requiring admission to a paediatric intensive care unit (PICU) for acute severe asthma should be referred to a paediatric respiratory specialist for outpatient follow up on hospital discharge.

BRONCHIOLITIS

See also Chapter 4 Respiratory Medicine, page 87.

Bronchiolitis is a clinical syndrome of infancy characterised by respiratory distress with both crepitations and wheezes on auscultation. It is often preceded by a coryzal illness and usually has a viral aetiology: respiratory syncytial virus (RSV), influenza, parainfluenza and adenovirus are common. Secondary bacterial infection is rare. Small airway obstruction leading to hyperinflation is typical, although many severe cases also have localised or diffuse atelectasis (**Fig. 1.16**).

RECOGNITION

Clinical assessment should include rapid physical examination, with attention to airway, breathing and circulation and pulse oximetry. In very sick infants, capillary or venous blood gases can help to guide treatment. However, clinical assessment is still more important than blood gas analysis.

IMMEDIATE MANAGEMENT

- Oxygen therapy. Humidified oxygen via headbox or nasal cannula should be given to maintain saturations >92%.
- IV fluids. Colloid may be given to maintain intravascular volume then crystalloid at 2/3 maintenance if the child is unable to feed. Beware hyponatraemia from reduced free water clearance. Orogastric feeding may be preferred in the acute phase as a nasal tube will increase airway resistance.
- Monitoring should include clinical assessment, pulse oximetry, apnoea monitoring and, in severe cases, blood gas analysis.
- Bronchodilators, including nebulised adrenaline, do not shorten the length of admission or alter outcome.
- Antibiotics are not routinely recommended.
- Ribavirin or corticosteroids treatment are not of benefit.
- Nebulised hypertonic saline may improve secretion clearance and lessen duration of symptoms.

INVESTIGATIONS

If severely unwell, alternative diagnoses such as pneumonia and empyema should be considered. This group of infants will require a chest radiograph. Further investigations should include a nasopharyngeal aspirate for viral immunofluorescence. A sweat test to exclude cystic fibrosis and investigation for immunodeficiency should be considered in those infants with severe or persistent symptoms.

INDICATIONS FOR VENTILATORY SUPPORT

Assisted ventilation is required in a small proportion of infants, who often fall into one of the high risk groups (see box below). Ventilatory support may be required in infants who are tired, who have a reduced conscious level or who continue to deteriorate with worsening respiratory failure with progressive hypoxaemia or hypercarbia. As with asthma, blood gas analysis is not a substitute for clinical assessment and the focus should remain on the clinical state of the patient.

Intubation

Ventilation is rarely required and is often accompanied by a transient worsening of gas exchange.

Ventilation strategies

Nasal continuous positive airway pressure (CPAP) may be all that is required. In more severe cases mechanical ventilation is required. In most cases a low tidal volume lung protective strategy can be adopted with tidal volumes of 4–7 ml/kg, peak inspiratory pressure (PIP) <30 cmH$_2$O, low respiratory rate, and permissive hypercapnia, allowing the pH to go down to 7.2. Moderate PEEP (6–8) helps to counteract intrinsic PEEP.

WHILE VENTILATED

There is no proven treatment for bronchiolitis other than good supportive care. Extracorporeal membrane oxygenation (ECMO) has been used in very severely affected infants with excellent results.

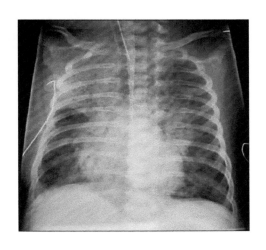

FIGURE 1.16 Respiratory syncitial virus infection with features of acute respiratory distress syndrome, showing generalised air space shadowing in addition to areas of collapse and hyperinflation.

CARDIAC EMERGENCIES

Cardiac emergencies in childhood are rare. Cyanosis in the neonatal period, pulmonary oedema, cardiogenic shock and arrhythmia are the common modes of presentation of previously undiagnosed disease.

CYANOSIS

Cyanosis in a newborn infant or baby should raise suspicion of a right to left shunt due to congenital heart disease (**Figs 1.17, 1.18**), but in a newborn can also be due to persistent pulmonary hypertension of the newborn. In later life it is possible, although now extremely rare, for children with missed congenital left to right shunts to develop pulmonary hypertension and for the shunt to reverse, causing cyanosis. This situation is known as Eisenmenger syndrome but is now almost unheard of in the developed world. Primary pulmonary hypertension can, however, can present with cyanosis in later childhood.

Any newborn child with persistent cyanosis that cannot be explained by a respiratory cause should be presumed to have a cardiac lesion. Prostaglandin E2 should be commenced to maintain ductal patency and the infant referred to a paediatric cardiology centre for further management. Prostaglandin E2 may cause apnoea and transfer may require the airway to be secured with an endotracheal tube.

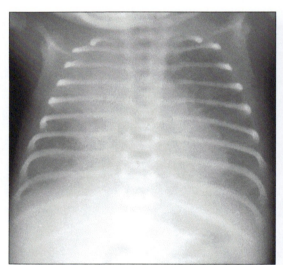

FIGURE 1.17 Chest radiograph of a neonate with total anomalous pulmonary venous drainage, showing the typical 'snowstorm' appearance. The baby presented with cyanosis on the first day of life.

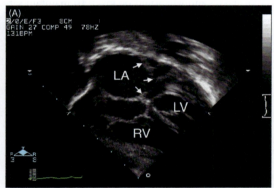

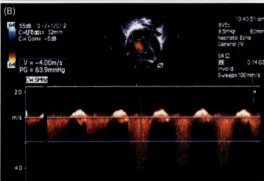

FIGURE 1.18 Echocardiography showing cor triatriatum with pulmonary hypertension. Figure (A) shows the abnormal left atrium (LA), which is obstructing pulmonary venous return; (B) shows a tricuspid regurgitant jet with a pressure gradient of 64 mmHg, indicating systemic right ventricular (RV) pressure due to pulmonary hypertension. The child was a 5-month-old baby who presented with respiratory failure, cyanosis and failure to thrive. LV, left ventricle.

CARDIOGENIC PULMONARY OEDEMA

Pulmonary oedema may occur in conditions associated with elevated left atrial pressure (e.g. mitral stenosis [**Fig. 1.19**]) or in the context of a left to right shunt with pulmonary overflow (e.g. atrial or ventricular septal defect [**Fig. 1.20**]). If cardiac output is preserved the clinical presentation may be as respiratory failure with or without a history of feeding difficulties and failure to thrive. The presence of viral or bacterial respiratory pathogens may further confuse the picture. A murmur or hepatic enlargement may give a clue to a cardiac diagnosis, as may the presence of cardiomegaly or pulmonary oedema on the chest radiograph. Echocardiography will be necessary to make an anatomical diagnosis.

Children should be treated as for 'acute lung injury/acute respiratory distress syndrome (ARDS)' with the caveat that high concentration inspired oxygen and normocapnea should be avoided to reduce pulmonary blood flow. Diuretics should be used if advised by a cardiac centre. Failure to wean from mechanical ventilation after any associated infection has resolved may be an indication for transfer to a cardiac centre for surgical repair.

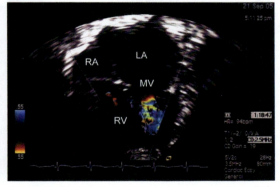

FIGURE 1.19 Echocardiogram showing congenital mitral stenosis. Note the enlarged left atrium (LA). MV, mitral valve; RA, right atrium; RV, right ventricle.

CARDIOGENIC SHOCK

Cardiogenic shock can occur in the newborn period, most commonly when the duct closes in duct-dependent lesions with left heart obstruction, for example hypoplastic left heart syndrome, coarctation of the aorta or critical aortic stenosis. An aberrant left coronary artery can have the same presentation, usually a few weeks later (**Fig. 1.21**). Cardiogenic shock may also occur secondary to acquired disease at any time, the most common of which in childhood is viral myocarditis or dilated cardiomyopathy (**Fig. 1.22**). However, coronary occlusion can occur in Kawasaki disease (see Chapter 3 Infectious Diseases, page 75 and Chapter 17 Rheumatology, page 518) and can have a similar presentation (**Figs 1.23, 1.24**). Arrhythmias may also present as cardiogenic shock (see below).

Infants presenting with cardiogenic shock in the newborn period should be presumed to have a duct-dependent circulation until proven otherwise and prostaglandin E2 should be commenced. The differential diagnosis includes sepsis, and infants should be commenced on broad-spectrum IV antibiotics after blood cultures have been taken. An enlarged liver is often a clue to a cardiac diagnosis. These infants are often profoundly acidotic and may require airway support, mechanical ventilation, fluids, bicarbonate and inotropes to maintain cardiac output. Central venous access and measurement of central venous pressure is useful to optimise filling pressures. If there is any suspicion of a hypoplastic left heart or a univentricular circulation, high concentrations of inspired oxygen should be avoided as the pulmonary vascular bed can become hyperperfused at the expense of systemic circulation. Older, previously well children presenting with cardiogenic shock will require similar management but without attention to the possibility of duct-dependent circulation or univentricular heart. Transfer to a paediatric cardiac centre should be arranged for ongoing supportive care, which may include mechanical cardiac support or cardiac transplantation.

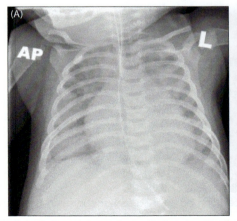
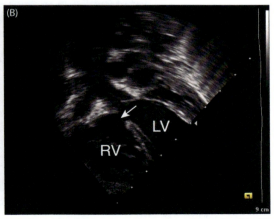

FIGURE 1.20 Chest radiograph (A) showing cardiomegaly and pulmonary oedema in a 4-month-old with a large ventricular septal defect (B). The presentation was with respiratory failure in association with viral infection. LV, left ventricle; RV, right ventricle.

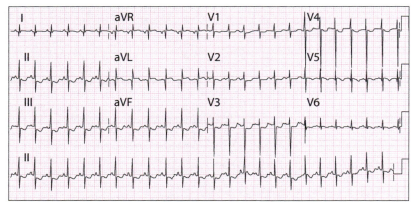

FIGURE 1.21 12-lead electrocardiograph of a 6-week-old infant with anomalous origin of the left coronary artery from the pulmonary artery (ALCAPA). The infant presented with poor feeding, lethargy and tachypnoea. Q waves are present in lead I and aVL, ST segment elevation in aVL and ST segment depression in II, III, and aVF and the anterior chest leads consistent with a full thickness anterior infarct.

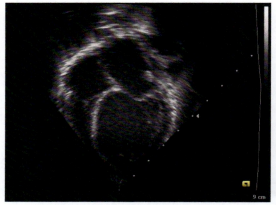

FIGURE 1.22 Echocardiogram showing severe left ventricular dilatation in an 8-month-old with cardiomyopathy due to vitamin D deficiency.

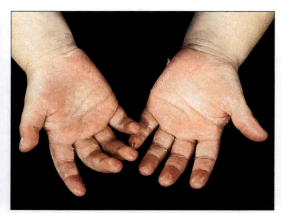

FIGURE 1.23 Desquamation of the hands in a 4-year-old with Kawasaki disease.

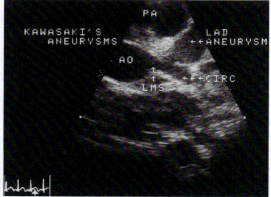

FIGURE 1.24 Echocardiograph showing left anterior descending coronary artery aneurysm in Kawasaki disease. Short axis view shown.
AO: aorta; LMS: left main stem; LAD: left anterior descending; CIRC: circumflex; PA: pulmonary artery.
(Courtesy of Dr Robert Yates.)

ARRHYTHMIAS

The commonest arrhythmias in the newborn period are congenital complete heart block (often secondary to maternal systemic lupus erythematosus [SLE] and transplacental carriage of anti-Ro antibodies) or supraventricular tachycardia due to an aberrant conduction pathway such as in Wolff–Parkinson–White syndrome (**Fig. 1.25**). In later life, supraventricular tachycardia is also the commonest arrhythmia (**Fig. 1.26**). Supraventricular tachycardia usually presents as cardiogenic shock in a young baby (see above) or as palpitations or syncope in an older child. Ventricular arrhythmias are extremely rare in childhood and may be due to cardiac (e.g. anomalous coronary artery, long QT syndrome, other channelopathy) or more commonly, a non-cardiac cause, (e.g. poisoning, hyperkalaemia or acidosis).

ACUTE ENCEPHALOPATHIC ILLNESS

CONVULSIVE STATUS EPILEPTICUS

Generalised convulsive (tonic–clonic) status epilepticus (CSE) is currently defined as a generalised convulsion lasting 30 minutes or longer, or repeated tonic–clonic convulsions occurring over a 30 minute period without recovery of consciousness between each convulsion. It is possible that in future the specified duration may be revised to 20, 10, or even 5 min of continuous seizure activity. CSE in childhood is a life-threatening condition with a serious risk of neurological sequelae. Although the outcome from an episode of CSE is mainly determined by its cause, duration is also important. In addition, the longer the duration of the episode, the more difficult it is to terminate.

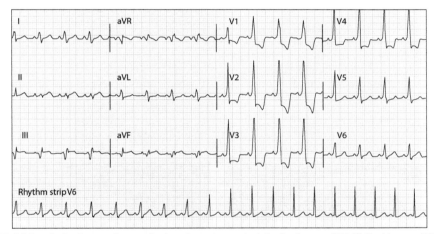

FIGURE 1.25 12-lead electrocardiograph showing characteristic features of Wolff–Parkinson–White syndrome with short PR interval, delta waves and ventricular repolarisation abnormalities.

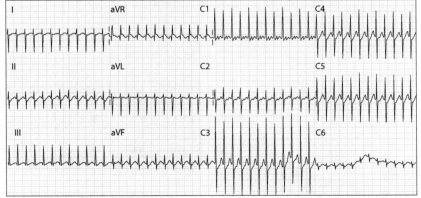

FIGURE 1.26 12-lead electrocardiograph showing AV re-entry tachycardia in a 6-month-old baby with an accessory AV pathway. The ventricular rate is about 200–250, P waves are absent and the QRS complexes are narrow with normal morphology.

From 0.4 to 0.8% of children will experience an episode of CSE before the age of 15 years, and 12% of children's first seizures are CSE. CSE in children has a mortality of approximately 4%. Neurological sequelae of CSE, such as epilepsy, motor deficits, learning difficulties, and behaviour problems, are rare but occur in a small minority of children.

OTHER ENCEPHALOPATHIC ILLNESS

Children presenting with non-convulsive acute encephalopathies may present with reduced conscious level, psychosis or confusion. These children may also be in non-convulsive status epilepticus. Structural and non-structural causes should be considered, including space occupying lesions, meningoencephalitis (**Fig. 1.27**), autoimmune disease such as acute demyelinating encephalomyelitis (ADEM) (**Fig. 1.28**), anti-N-methyl-D-aspartate (NMDA) receptor antibody encephalitis, cerebrovascular accidents, metabolic disorders and trauma including non-accidental injury.

RECOGNITION

Initial assessment and resuscitation should address, as always, the airway, breathing and circulation (A, B, C). High-flow oxygen should be given and bedside blood glucose level measured. A brief history and clinical examination should be undertaken to confirm genuine seizure activity.

Although the definition of CSE implies that the seizure should last 30 minutes, treatment should start within 10 minutes of continuous generalised tonic–clonic seizure activity. The times of drug administration in the guideline are from the time of hospital arrival. It has been assumed that the convulsion will have been continuing for at least 5 minutes prior to arrival.

IMMEDIATE MANAGEMENT OF CSE

If IV access is available, lorazepam should be given. Lorazepam is equally or more effective than diazepam and causes less respiratory depression. Lorazepam also has a longer duration of anti-seizure effect (12–24 hours) than diazepam (15–30 minutes). If after 10 minutes the convulsion has not stopped or another convulsion has begun, a second dose of lorazepam should be given, assuming IV access is established. An alternative to lorazepam is buccal midazolam followed by rectal diazepam.

If seizure activity continues for a further 10 minutes and in the unlikely event that IV access is still not possible, an intraosseous needle should be inserted. Continuing convulsive activity indicates a longer acting IV anticonvulsant is required. Phenytoin is recommended as it causes less respiratory depression than phenobarbitone. Heart rate, ECG and blood pressure monitoring during infusion are recommended as IV phenytoin can cause arrhythmias. In children already receiving phenytoin as a maintenance oral anticonvulsant, IV phenobarbitone should be given.

INVESTIGATIONS

If seizure activity is present, once it has ceased, a full examination including examination of the central nervous system and fundoscopy should be performed. Presentation with non-convulsive encephalopathy, new onset seizures, focal seizures or

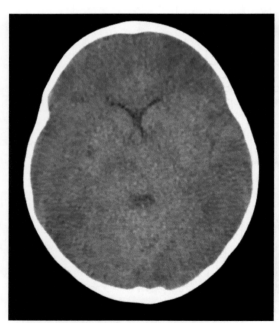

FIGURE 1.27 16 Generalised cerebral oedema with infarction in a child with pneumococcal meningoencephalitis.

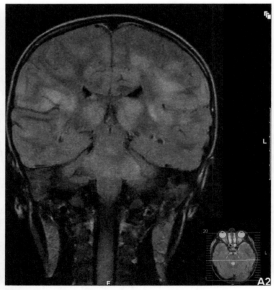

FIGURE 1.28 T2-weighted MRI scan in a an 8-year-old child with acute disseminated encephalomyelitis, showing multiple areas of increased signal in the white matter. The child presented in convulsive status epilepticus.

residual focal neurology suggest a structural cause and neuroimaging will be required. Fundoscopy may reveal retinal haemorrhages suggestive of non-accidental injury (see Chapter 2 Child Protection, page 35). Children with no previous history of a seizure disorder who remain encephalopathic should be presumed to have an infective aetiology until proven otherwise, particularly if a fever is present, and given aciclovir, cefotaxime and erythromycin.

When IV or intraosseous access is obtained, blood should be sent for a full blood count, urea and electrolytes, anticonvulsant, calcium and magnesium levels and blood glucose. Consideration should be given, particularly in infants, to sending metabolic investigations including lactate and serum ammonia,

acylcarnitine blood spots and plasma amino and urine organic acids. Appropriate specimens should also be sent for bacterial, viral and mycoplasma culture, serology and polymerase chain reaction (PCR). Lumbar puncture should be avoided until it is clear that intracranial pressure is not raised. Further investigation when the child is stable may include neuroimaging and neurophysiological investigation (**Figs 1.29–1.31**).

INDICATIONS FOR VENTILATORY SUPPORT

If the child remains in CSE or the airway is not protected because of reduced conscious level 20 minutes after IV phenytoin or phenobarbitone has commenced, then rapid sequence induction of

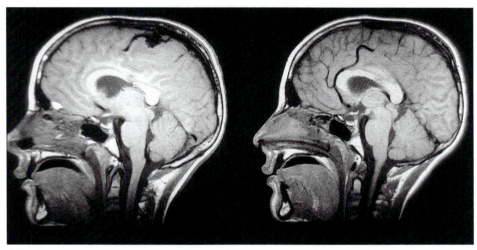

FIGURE 1.29 Tl-weighted magnetic resonance image in sagittal section of a 5-year-old who presented with intractable seizures. The diagnosis was an arteriovenous malformation (the tortuous black lesion seen arising anterior to the corpus callosum).

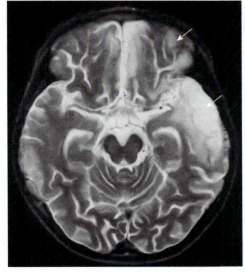

FIGURE 1.30 T2-weighted magnetic resonance image in transverse section of a 2-year-old with intractable seizures due to herpes simplex encephalitis. Increased signal, representing oedema, is seen in the left prefrontal and temporal lobes.

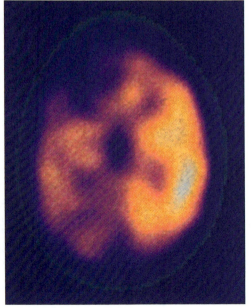

FIGURE 1.31 Perfusion scan from the same patient showing increased uptake in the same area.

anaesthesia should be performed using thiopentone. If neuromuscular paralysis is used, this should be short acting so as not to mask the clinical signs of the convulsion. Once ventilated, standard neuroprotective measures should be instituted including good oxygenation, avoidance of hyper or hypocapnia, maintenance of a good cerebral perfusion pressure, normothermia and adequate sedation. Mannitol or 3% saline should be considered if clinical signs of raised intracranial pressure (ICP) develop.

Children under 3 years of age with a prior history of chronic, active epilepsy who present with an episode of established CSE, following specialist advice may be treated with IV pyridoxine in case the seizures are pyridoxine-dependent or pyridoxine-responsive (**Figs 1.32–1.34**).

Once ventilated, the child will need to be transferred to a PICU. Advice on ongoing management should be sought from a paediatric neurologist.

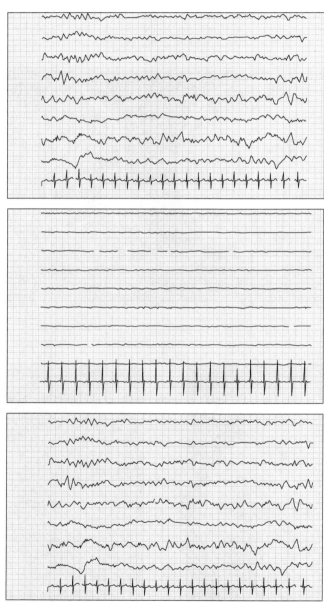

FIGURES 1.32-1.34 Electroencephalograms (EEGs) of a 5-month-old child with a history of neonatal seizures responding to phenobarbitone presented with increasingly severe and prolonged seizures with tonic–clonic and myoclonic elements. **1.32**: During status epilepticus, high amplitude (note the change in calibration) repetitive sharp waves are seen continuously. **1.33**: Following an injection of pyridoxine the EEG activity disappears, returning after 8–9 hours. **1.34**: An interictal EEG shows age appropriate activity. The child had pyridoxine-dependent seizures and was maintained fit-free on regular pyridoxine after the diagnosis was made. (Courtesy of Dr Stuart Boyd.)

DIABETIC KETOACIDOSIS

See also Chapter 13 Endocrinology.

Diabetic ketoacidosis (DKA) is the common presentation of insulin-dependent diabetes mellitus (IDDM) in childhood. The primary cause is insufficient endogenous or therapeutic insulin to allow adequate cellular uptake of glucose and inhibition of ketogenesis. This decompensation is frequently precipitated by an infective illness. The main clinical picture is of dehydration resulting from hyperglycaemia-induced osmotic diuresis, and a profound metabolic acidosis (with an increased anion gap) from the accumulation of acidic ketone bodies.

INITIAL ASSESSMENT AND RESUSCITATION

As with all acutely ill children the initial assessment of a child with DKA focuses on airway, breathing and circulation. Altered conscious level on presentation is an important poor prognostic factor and should trigger the early involvement of senior help. Children in DKA will be tachypnoeic as they attempt to compensate for metabolic acidosis by reducing $PaCO_2$. A low pH (<7.0) or low $PaCO_2$ (<2.5 kPa) indicate severe disease with a high risk of cerebral oedema. In the rare cases that require artificial ventilation for exhaustion or shock, the initial target $PaCO_2$ must be similar to the value that the patient was achieving. This will prevent worsening of acidosis and cerebral oedema. The heart rate, blood pressure and peripheral perfusion must be regularly assessed. Shock should be treated promptly with 10 ml/kg boluses up to 30 ml/kg of normal (0.9%) saline and the circulation reassessed. The possibility of a serious infection precipitating DKA must be considered.

Indications for referral to PICU include pH < 7.1, severe dehydration, shock, depressed sensorium and children <2 years. In particular, any significant reduction in conscious level should prompt discussion with anaesthetic and/or paediatric intensive care unit staff. Cerebral oedema in DKA is unpredictable but is associated with a low $PaCO_2$ on presentation, rapid changes in osmolarity and the use of bicarbonate solution. Treatment of cerebral oedema is essentially supportive as with raised ICP after head injury. Control of $PaCO_2$, support of the circulation and avoiding low plasma osmolarity are the main strategies. Invasive ICP monitoring should not be used in these cases.

INITIAL INVESTIGATIONS

These should include glucose, urea and electrolytes, bicarbonate, creatinine, plasma osmolality, liver and bone profile, FBC, electrolytes, arterial blood gas, urinalysis (for ketonuria and glycosuria) and partial septic screen (e.g. urine and blood cultures). Hourly blood glucose levels should be performed. Urea and electrolytes with at least venous blood gas should be performed 2–4 hourly for the first 12 hours, and then 6-hourly for the next 12 hours. Sudden changes in glucose, osmolarity, pH and potassium levels can therefore be addressed promptly.

FURTHER MANAGEMENT

If A, B, C are satisfactory, the child should be assessed as follows.

Although fluid resuscitation for shock should be undertaken promptly, there is no rush for rehydration, pH or electrolyte correction. Rehydration should be slow over 48 hours with regular checks of serum electrolytes and osmolarity. A urinary catheter should be placed in the presence of oliguria or reduced conscious level.

Once fluid replacement has commenced, the glucose level will start to reduce and a continuous infusion of rapid-acting soluble insulin must be started. The insulin infusion should not be commenced until IV fluids have been running for at least an hour as there is some evidence that cerebral oedema is more likely if insulin is started early. Once started, the insulin infusion should continue until resolution of ketoacidosis. To prevent a precipitous drop in plasma glucose, glucose should be added to the IV fluid when plasma glucose falls to about 14–17 mmol/l. Potassium replacement therapy should be started immediately if the patient is hypokalaemic. If the patient is hyperkalaemic, potassium replacement therapy should be deferred until there is urine output. Otherwise, potassium should be started with insulin therapy and should continue while the patient is on IV fluids. Bicarbonate administration is not necessary or justified in DKA. It has been associated with an increased risk of cerebral oedema. Anticoagulation should be considered in children with femoral central venous lines. A nasogastric tube should be considered in all cases with any reduction in conscious level or if there is a history of vomiting.

ACUTE RESPIRATORY DISTRESS SYNDROME

Acute respiratory distress syndrome (ARDS) is a life threatening respiratory condition characterised by hypoxaemia and stiff lungs. It is the consequence of the pulmonary response to a broad range of injuries occurring either directly to the lung or as the consequence of injury or inflammation at other sites in the body. Common causes of ARDS include:

- Sepsis.
- Pneumonia.
- Trauma.
- Aspiration/near drowning.
- Burns/inhalational injury.
- Massive blood transfusion.
- Transfusion-related acute lung injury.

Diagnostic criteria were developed for the syndrome in 1994 by an American–European Consensus Conference[1]. The criteria were updated in 2012 (the 'Berlin criteria') and a modification of the update was developed for paediatric intensive care in 2013[2].

DIAGNOSTIC CRITERIA

- Timing. Within 1 week of a known clinical insult or new or worsening respiratory symptoms.
- Chest x-rays or tomography scan. Bilateral opacities not fully explained by effusions, lobar/lung collapse, or nodules.
- Origin of oedema. Respiratory failure not fully explained by cardiac failure or fluid overload. Need objective assessment (e.g. echocardiography) to exclude hydrostatic oedema, if no ARDS risk factors are present.
- Oxygenation:
  - Mild: 200 mmHg < PaO_2/FIO_2 ≤ 300 mmHg with PEEP or CPAP ≥ 5 cm H_2O.
  - Moderate: 100 mmHg < PaO_2/FIO_2 ≤ 200 mmHg with PEEP ≥ 5 cm H_2O.
  - Severe: PaO_2/FIO_2 < 100 mmHg with PEEP 5 cm H_2O.

PATHOGENESIS

ARDS is characterised by widespread airway collapse, surfactant deficiency and reduced lung compliance. It is an inflammatory disorder with three phases: an exudative phase, a proliferative phase and a fibrotic phase (**Fig. 1.35**). The exudative phase lasts for the first week and is marked by alveolar oedema with hyaline membranes. In the proliferative phase, in the second 2 weeks and organisation of the inflammatory exudates occurs. In the fibrotic phase, which may occur from day 10, pulmonary fibrosis is seen. However, many studies show that survivors return to normal lung function, with complete resolution of pulmonary fibrosis. Although ARDS is a diffuse process, it is also a heterogeneous process, and not all lung units are affected equally. Normal and diseased tissue may exist side-by-side.

INITIAL ASSESSMENT

Assessment of the child with respiratory failure follows the standard ABC approach, with an emphasis on the work of breathing and on the effects of hypoxaemia on other organ systems, particularly the heart and brain. Once an initial assessment of severity has been made and supportive measures instituted, appropriate investigations should be arranged to determine the underlying cause so that specific therapy may be commenced. For example, infection requires appropriate antibiotic therapy and empyema, if present, should be drained (**Fig. 1.36**).

Indicators of respiratory distress
Moderate:

- Tachycardia.
- Tachypnoea.
- Nasal flaring.
- Use of accessory muscles.
- Recession.
- Head retraction.
- Unable to feed.

Severe:

- Cyanosis.
- Lethargy.
- Reduced conscious level.
- Saturation <92% despite O_2 therapy.
- Rising pCO_2.

SUPPORTIVE THERAPY

Supportive therapy ranges from oxygen by face mask, to non-invasive ventilation, endotracheal intubation and mechanical ventilation, nitric oxide (NO) and ECMO. Non-invasive ventilation refers to ventilatory support without endotracheal intubation. This includes CPAP or biphasic positive airways pressure (BiPAP) via face mask or nasal mask. Mechanical ventilation should be considered in any child who is tiring due to excessive work of breathing, or who has cardiovascular compromise or a reduced conscious level due to respiratory failure. While worsening hypoxaemia or worsening hypercarbia may confirm the imminent need for ventilation, as always, blood gas analysis is not a substitute for clinical assessment.

Ventilatory support
The goals of treating patients with ARDS are to maintain adequate gas exchange while avoiding ventilator-induced lung injury, to treat the underlying cause of the condition and to attenuate the inflammatory response.

Oxygenation
High concentration inspired oxygen should be avoided to limit the risk of direct cellular toxicity and to avoid reabsorption atelectasis. SaO_2 values of around 88–92% are commonly accepted. PEEP may improve oxygenation by encouraging movement of fluid from the alveolar to the interstitial space, recruiting collapsed alveoli, increasing in functional residual capacity and preventing cyclical alveolar collapse. A long inspiratory time may also improve lung recruitment.

Lung protective ventilation

Traditional mechanical ventilation, using high tidal volumes and low PEEP, is likely to induce lung injury in patients with ARDS. However, in ARDS, a 'lung protective strategy', optimising PEEP, using a tidal volume of <6 ml/kg, permissive hypercapnia, and pressure limited ventilation with PIP limited to <40 cmH$_2$O has been shown to improve outcome[3].

High frequency oscillatory ventilation

Although there are no trial data to support the use of high frequency oscillatory ventilation HFOV, it is still often used for patients with ARDS because it delivers small tidal volumes (typically 2 ml/kg) and may prevent 'atelectotrauma', keep the lungs open, improve alveolar recruitment and improve ventilation/perfusion matching.

Other therapies

Other therapies occasionally of benefit include prone positioning, inhaled NO, corticosteroids, exogenous surfactant and ECMO.

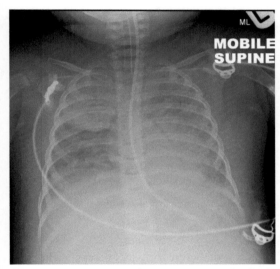

FIGURE 1.35 Severe ARDS in a 5-year-old with H1N1 influenza. The child did not survive.

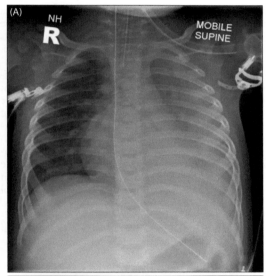

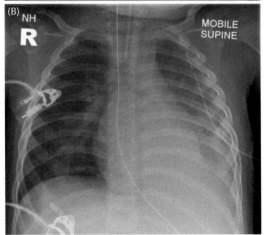

FIGURE 1.36 Empyema due to left lower lobe pneumococcal pneumonia in an 8-month-old before (A) and after (B) drainage. The child was ventilated, treated with antibiotics and intrapleural urokinase and made a full recovery.

SEPSIS

Sepsis is 'the systemic response to infection'. This is defined by changes in temperature, heart rate, respiratory rate and white cell count. 'Septic shock' is inadequate organ perfusion in addition to the above changes. The characteristic pattern of worsening cardiovascular, respiratory and subsequently other organ system dysfunction is termed 'multi-organ failure'. While the most extreme cases of severe sepsis are seen with gram-negative infections (classically *Neisseria meningitidis*) (**Fig. 1.37**) the pattern can be seen in response to many organisms, including viruses and fungi.

INITIAL ASSESSMENT AND RESUSCITATION

The immediate care of a child with suspected septic shock follows the principles of A, B, C, followed by specific therapy for the probable causative organism. Depressed conscious level (Glasgow coma score [GCS] ≤8), poor airway reflexes, tachypnoea and requirement for supplemental oxygen indicate impending need for assisted ventilation. Such signs will usually be accompanied by significant shock and so induction of anaesthesia presents a significant risk. This can be minimised by: aggressive volume replacement, pre-oxygenation, and selection of a cardiostable anaesthetic agent. An adrenaline bolus should be prepared and available. A range of endotracheal tube (ETT) sizes should also be prepared (a good fit with a cuff may be necessary to ensure adequate ventilation in the face of pulmonary oedema). Optimal drugs for induction include fentanyl and/or ketamine. Myocardial depression agents such as thiopentone, midazolam or propofol are not good choices in children with septic shock. Intubation should be performed by the most experienced staff available. Children with meningococcal disease should be orally intubated unless a coagulopathy has been excluded.

If the child is in shock peripheral (or central) venous access should not be attempted for more than 90 seconds. Initial resuscitation via an anterior tibial intraosseous needle is easy and effective. Cardiovascular decompensation should be immediately treated with 20 ml/kg of IV fluid (e.g. 4.5% human albumin solution or 0.9% sodium chloride), which can be safely repeated while management is continuing. Intubation should be considered after 40–60 ml/kg because of evolving pulmonary oedema.

INVESTIGATIONS

These should include full blood count, coagulation screen (including fibrinogen and d-dimers or fibrin degradation products to look for evidence of disseminated intravascular coagulopathy), urea and electrolytes, calcium, magnesium, phosphate, liver function tests, blood and urine for culture and rapid antigen screening and/or PCR where available. Lumbar puncture should not be performed in children with coagulopathy or with a reduced conscious level.

FURTHER MANAGEMENT

Antibiotics

Appropriate antibiotic therapy should be commenced as soon as possible, ideally after taking blood and urine for culture. The only exception to this is in meningococcal disease, where the primary care provider may have already administered parenteral benzylpenicillin.

Circulatory support

Some children require vast amounts of fluid resuscitation: 100–200 ml/kg. Ideal subsequent management will involve the siting of central venous access to titrate fluids to maintain right heart filling pressures (usually 8–12 cm H_2O) to avoid pulmonary oedema. If pulmonary oedema is present it should be managed with ventilation and high end expiratory pressure rather than diuretics initially. The use of fresh frozen plasma (FFP) or packed cells as volume should be considered to correct coagulopathy and to maintain haematocrit. In the presence of persistent hypotension despite adequate filling, inotropic support should be initiated. The choice of inotropic agent varies but a reasonable starting regimen would be dopamine, followed by adrenaline for cold shock (low cardiac output state) or noradrenaline for warm shock (high cardiac output state). Adrenaline and dopamine may be given peripherally if necessary.

Coagulopathy

Profound coagulopathies should be treated with FFP. Low fibrinogen concentrations suggesting disseminated intravascular coagulation (DIC) can be replaced with cryoprecipitate. Thrombocytopenia in the absence of clinical bleeding should not be supplemented.

Other

Children with severe sepsis may develop multi-organ failure and require multiple supportive treatments, including ventilation, inotropes, renal support and even ECMO (**Fig. 1.38**). These should be continued while specific measures are taken to treat the infection, including antibiotic therapy and surgical source control, if necessary. Some children with severe infection develop limb compartment syndrome in the acute phase or skin and limb necrosis and gangrene in the recovery phase. These may require specialist management including plastic, orthopaedic and vascular surgery.

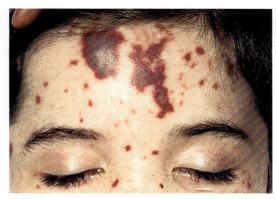

FIGURE 1.37 Rash of meningococcal disease with purpura and petechiae.

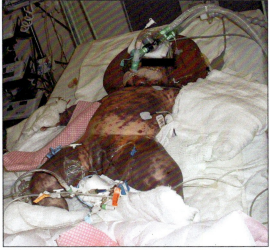

FIGURE 1.38 Infant with meningococcal sepsis in multi-organ failure.

TRAUMATIC BRAIN INJURY

Head injury is the major cause of death in children after infancy. The majority of cases in this age group are the result of blunt trauma, with road traffic collisions and falls responsible for most. In infancy, most serious head injuries are non-accidental, resulting from shaking with or without an impact against a hard surface (see Chapter 2 Child Protection, page 35). Such mechanisms are relatively rare after 12 months of age. Penetrating injuries are very rare. The majority of head injuries seen in emergency departments are minor. The probability of a serious injury is increased by a violent mechanism of injury (e.g. pedestrian versus car, fall from a height), reduced conscious level – either on history or still present on examination, any focal neurological signs and penetrating injury. A combination of these factors makes a serious injury very likely (**Figs 1.39–1.42**).

INITIAL ASSESSMENT AND RESUSCITATION

The initial assessment and management of the severely injured child follows the routine of <C>, catastrophic haemorrhage, A (and cervical spine), B, C. Catastrophic haemorrhage should be controlled by compression or surgery as appropriate. Direct airway trauma is rare but loss of the airway due to reduced conscious level and absent cough and gag reflexes is common. The child's conscious level must be assessed and any concern about the ability to protect the airway should be aggressively managed with elective intubation and ventilation to avoid hypoxaemia

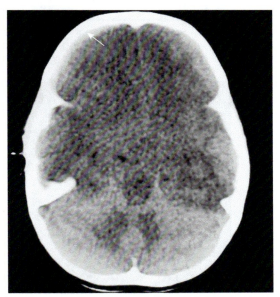

FIGURE 1.39 Severe non-accidental injury in a 2-year-old child. There is a right subdural haematoma and severe cerebral oedema.

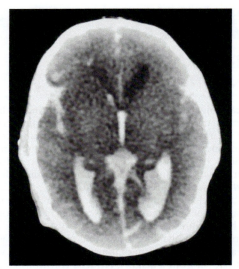

FIGURE 1.40 Traumatic brain injury with intraventricular and subarachnoid blood. Generalised cerebral oedema is also present.

or hypercarbia. The airway reflexes should be assessed in all cases in which there is evidence of a reduced conscious level. All children with serious head injuries should be considered to have sustained a cervical spine injury, even in the presence of a normal lateral neck x-ray (because of the relatively high risk of ligamentous injury in childhood). Current recommendations are to perform a CT scan of the cervical spine at the same time as the brain. A normal CT cervical spine is now accepted as adequate for exclusion of significant cervical spine injury.

Retinal haemorrhages are more common in non-accidental than accidental head injury. If there is uncertainty about mechanism, formal ophthalmological assessment with retinal photography should be undertaken as soon as possible (**Fig. 1.43**).

Hypoventilation raises arterial carbon dioxide levels leading to cerebral vasodilatation and increased ICP. The aim of respiratory support in severe head injury is to avoid hypercarbia and maintain $PaCO_2$ in the normal range (4.5–5.3 kPa). Lower levels are detrimental and may contribute to cerebral ischaemia via excessive cerebral vasoconstriction. Hypotension

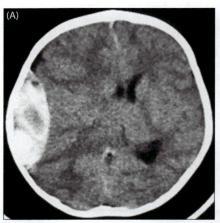

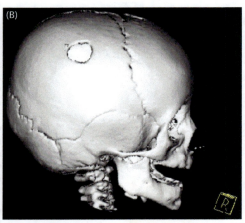

FIGURE 1.41 CT scan (A) showing right sided acute extradural haemorrhage with mass effect in a 7-month-old who rolled off the changing mat onto a hard floor. The baby required a craniotomy (B) and made a full recovery.

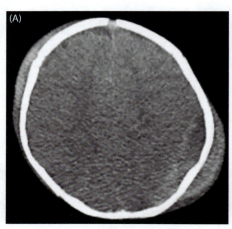

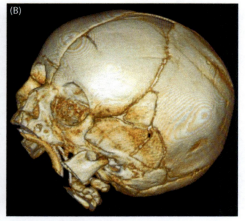

FIGURE 1.42 CT scan (A) showing left sided acute subdural haemorrhage with cerebral oedema in a 3-month-old who was dropped to the floor and sustained multiple skull fractures (B). The haemorrahge was drained and the child made a full recovery after a period of neurointensive care.

must be avoided in order to maintain cerebral perfusion. Fluid resuscitation may be required, but in cases with severe cerebral oedema, inotrope or vasopressor treatment may be essential to maintain cerebral perfusion pressure (CPP). A child who has been ventilated with a severe head injury must receive both sedation and analgesia to assist in the control of raised ICP.

MANAGEMENT AFTER INITIAL STABILISATION

Primary brain injury occurs on impact and is, as yet, untreatable. The care of the child with head injury is aimed at avoiding secondary brain injury. This can be summarised as providing a 'well-perfused and well-oxygenated brain'. Three principal mechanisms lead to the generation of secondary brain injuries: hypoxaemia, reduced cerebral perfusion and metabolic disturbances (e.g. hypoglycaemia, hyponatraemia). Raised ICP may occur due to a rapidly expanding intracranial haematoma or acute hydrocephalus resulting in a decrease in cerebral perfusion, which is a neurosurgical emergency. However, raised ICP is more commonly the result of diffuse cerebral oedema in children. In this scenario, the circulation must be supported to maintain cerebral blood flow.

Although there is consensus on the ongoing intensive care management of head-injured children, there is a very limited evidence base on which to support current practice. Treatments commonly employed include head up 30° tilt, midline head position, sedation, analgesia and ICP monitoring with circulation support (fluid and vasopressors) to maintaining CPP. Mannitol or 3% sodium chloride may be useful to decrease ICP prior to emergency neurosurgical intervention. Some centres used phenytoin as seizure prophylaxis. Hyperventilation can be harmful as it reduces cerebral perfusion and is no longer recommended. Hypothermia and steroids are not of benefit.

THE CHILD WITH MULTIPLE INJURIES

Few paediatricians will be regularly involved with the resuscitation of children with multiple injuries. Such cases must be approached in a structured way (<C> (Catastrophic haemorrhage) A, B, C (Airway/cervical spine, Breathing, Circulation)), including focused abdominal sonography in trauma (FAST) scanning, in order to identify and treat life-threatening injuries. The care of a child with multiple injuries requires careful organisation and can be best achieved in large centres with all the relevant specialities available onsite (e.g. anaesthesia/ICU, radiology, orthopaedics, neurology, general, cardiothoracic, maxillofacial and plastic surgery).

INITIAL ASSESSMENT AND RESUSCITATION

This is identical to that already described for the head-injured child. As before the patient should be considered to have a cervical spine injury until they are awake and able to demonstrate normal neurology in the absence of neck pain and with appropriate imaging if necessary. Airway assessment must include an assessment of the airway reflexes and conscious level as well as the effects of any direct trauma or foreign body (**Fig. 1.44**).

Haemorrhagic shock is the main threat to the circulation in multiple trauma. The priority is early control of haemorrhage and fluid resuscitation, ideally with a combination of packed cells, FFP and platelets. Secure IV or intraosseous access will be required (ideally away from the site of obvious injuries) and fluid resuscitation of 5–10 ml/kg should be given, repeated as necessary, until haemorrhage control is achieved. Acute tension

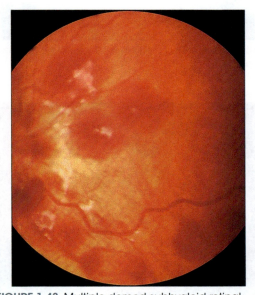

FIGURE 1.43 Multiple domed subhyaloid retinal haemorrhages in a case of non-accidental injury caused by shaking. The white spots in the centre of the haemorrhages are light reflexes. Fundoscopy should be performed in all infants presenting with significant head injuries.

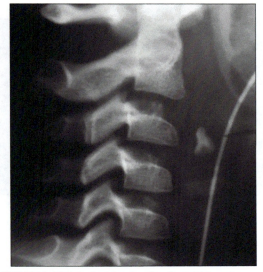

FIGURE 1.44 Inhaled tooth after facial trauma.

pneumo- or haemopneumothorax may require emergency aspiration and drainage. Cardiac injuries should be considered and treated if present (**Fig. 1.45**). Blood samples for FBC, coagulation screen, grouping and cross-matching should be taken as early as possible. Resuscitation must continue while sites of potential blood loss are assessed and treated.

MANAGEMENT AFTER INITIAL STABILISATION

After immediately life-threatening <C>ABC problems have been addressed, a careful examination to detail all injuries must be undertaken, including log-rolling to examine the back and thoracolumbar spine. It is at this stage that imaging (that must include a chest x-ray and lateral neck film) appropriate to the injures (e.g. CT cranial, thorax and abdomen) should be performed if haemodynamic stability can be obtained. If stability cannot be achieved, 'damage control' surgery by appropriate surgical teams will be required prior to imaging. The purpose of such surgery is to mitigate any immediately life-threatening injuries and to regain physiological stability rather than to provide definitive treatment for all injuries. The management of injuries that are not immediately life threatening, may be deferred and should be planned with the relevant surgical teams.

Blood loss from fractures (especially to the pelvis or femora) is easily underestimated and often requires early fixation. Hepatic, renal, splenic and other vascular injuries are all sites of potentially lethal haemorrhage although many such injuries, particularly those caused by blunt trauma, can be managed without surgical intervention in children (**Fig. 1.46**). Some will, however, require interventional radiology or surgery (**Fig. 1.47**).

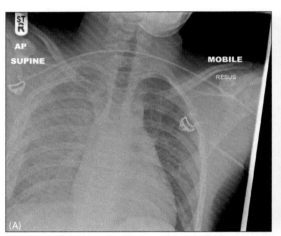
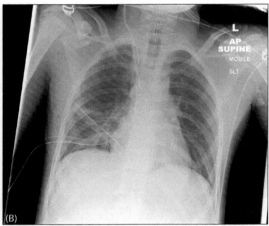

FIGURE 1.45 Right sided haemothorax in association with cardiac tamponade in a 15-year-old after penetrating thoracic injury before (A) and after (B) thoracotomy.

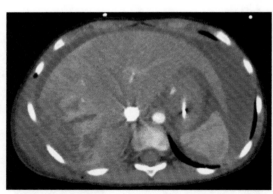

FIGURE 1.46 Liver maceration with intraperitoneal blood in a 3-year-old with blunt abdominal and thoracic trauma. The child made a full recovery with non-operative management.

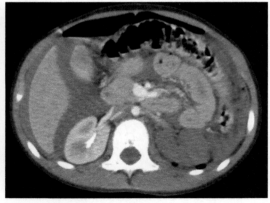

FIGURE 1.47 Intraperitoneal air due to perforation of a viscus, infarction of the left kidney and pancreatic haemorrhage and intraperitoneal blood in a 7-year-old after a crush injury to the abdomen. Laparotomy is mandatory in the context of perforation.

BURNS

The initial management of a child with severe burns can be summarised as 'forget about the burn'. The priorities remain A, B, C. If the mechanism of burn is unclear or there is coexistent trauma then cervical spine precautions must be observed. Analgesia must also be addressed urgently.

GENERAL APPROACH TO THE CHILD WITH BURNS

Reduced conscious level and airway obstruction from facial (**Fig. 1.48**) or inhalational burn injury are the major causes of airway obstruction in burns. A child with facial or airway burns should be assessed for early intubation because of the high risk of swelling tissue.

Smoke inhalation or reduced chest wall movement from circumferential burns must be considered. High-flow oxygen should be administered to cases in which smoke inhalation is possible (to limit the effects of carbon monoxide poisoning). Large fluid losses will occur through areas of burned skin in proportion to the area affected (**Figs 1.49, 1.50**). Complex formulae exist for calculating fluid replacement required but this should not confuse the initial management. Immediate circulation support should be as for shock from any cause, with 20 ml/kg of colloid/crystalloid. If shock is present it should not be ascribed to fluid losses through the burn without considering the possibility of associated fractures, abdominal and thoracic injuries.

After the initial resuscitation, ongoing care including fluid management should be undertaken in combination with the specialist burns centre and/or PICU.

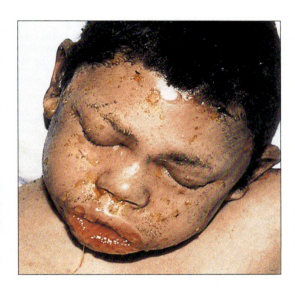

FIGURE 1.48 Facial oedema with eyelid and lip swelling caused by a flash burn. Swelling occurs up to 24 hours after the injury and the airway must be secured with an endotracheal tube.

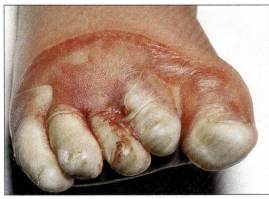

FIGURE 1.49 Full thickness electrical burn of the foot. An entry point is clearly visible between the second and third toes. Respiratory failure and cardiac dysrhythmias may require immediate treatment. Urgent exploration and debridement is usually required.

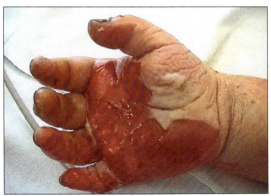

FIGURE 1.50 Partial thickness burn of the palm of the hand caused by grasping a hot object. This sort of injury, sustained during exploration of the environment, is likely to be accidental.

POISONING

Suspected poisoning in children results in 40,000 visits to Accident and Emergency departments in England and Wales every year and 15–20 deaths. Poisoning may occur accidentally in a young child or toddler, intentionally in teenagers or deliberately in some cases of child abuse (see Chapter 2 Child Protection, page 29).

RECOGNITION AND ASSESSMENT

Primary assessment should be directed to airway patency, adequacy of breathing and circulation and neurological status. Acidotic breathing is seen in salicylate or ethylene glycol poisoning. QRS prolongation and ventricular tachycardia are seen in tricyclic antidepressant poisoning. A depressed conscious level suggests poisoning with opiates, sedatives, antihistamines or hypoglycaemic agents. Small pupils suggest opiate poisoning but large pupils suggest amphetamines, atropine or tricyclic poisoning. Convulsions are associated with many drugs, particularly tricyclic antidepressants.

IMMEDIATE MANAGEMENT

Airway patency should be maintained, with intubation if necessary (**Fig. 1.51**). Children with cardiorespiratory failure or a decreased conscious level should receive high-flow oxygen through a face mask with reservoir if the airway is patent. Shock should be treated with fluid boluses rather than inotropes as inotropes can cause arrhythmias in combination with some toxins. Cardiac dysrhythmias caused by poisons need specific treatment, which should be discussed with a poisons centre. Hypoglycaemia should be treated with IV 10% dextrose and convulsions treated with diazepam, midazolam or lorazepam. Naloxone should be given if the pupils are very constricted or there is a history of opiate poisoning.

INVESTIGATIONS

When IV access is obtained, blood should be sent for a FBC, urea and electrolytes, paracetomol and salicylate levels, toxicology and blood glucose. Urine specimens should be collected and sent to the laboratory. Monitoring should include ECG, blood pressure, pulse oximetry, core temperature, blood glucose and sometimes blood gases.

FURTHER MANAGEMENT

Gut decontamination

Syrup of ipecacuanha, an emetic, is no longer recommended. Activated charcoal can be given as a single dose up to 1 hour after ingestion of toxin. Beyond this time adsorption is reduced. Charcoal should not be given if the airway cannot be protected because of the risk of aspiration pneumonia. Gastric lavage is rarely required as benefit rarely outweighs risk; advice should be sought from the National Poisons Information Service, particularly following ingestion of iron or lithium, which are not adsorbed to activated charcoal. Whole gut irrigation with polyethylene glycol may also be considered when patients have ingested potentially lethal substances or sustained release or enteric coated preparations.

Paracetamol poisoning

N-acetyl cysteine should be given as soon as possible after a large overdose of paracetamol or if levels are toxic 4 hours after ingestion. The management of patients presenting 15 hours or more after ingestion or patients taking staggered overdoses of more than 150 mg/kg/day or 12 g for a child over 12 is controversial. Advice should be taken from the National Poisons Information Service and a liver transplant unit.

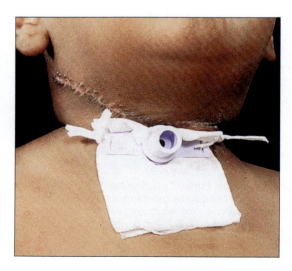

FIGURE 1.51 Tracheostomy in a 2-year-old child after ingestion of caustic soda. Caustic soda causes severe burns and scarring to the oropharynx, oesphagus and stomach, which, in this case, has required surgical debridement and eventually resulted in airway obstruction necessitating a tracheostomy.

Other

Management for other poisons should be guided by advice from a poisons centre (**Figs 1.52, 1.53**) and may include chelating agents, antidotes and active elimination techniques such as haemofiltration.

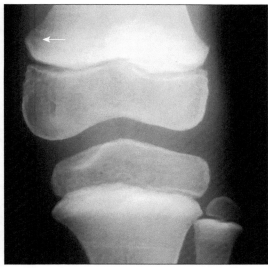

FIGURE 1.52 Lead poisoning causing a dense metaphyseal line at the growing ends of long bones. Chelation can be effected with dimercaprol, edetate calcium disodium and 2,3 dimercaptosuccinic acid. Management should be undertaken in conjunction with the local poisons unit.

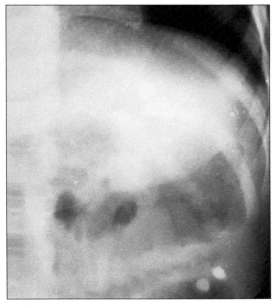

FIGURE 1.53 Multiple dense opacities seen in the stomach and left flank in a 2-year-old boy who had ingested his mother's iron tablets. He was treated with desferrioxamine and made a full recovery.

REFERENCES/FURTHER READING

1 Bernard GR, Artigas A, Brigham KL. The American-European Consensus Conference on ARDS. Definitions, mechanisms, relevant outcomes, and clinical trial coordination. *Am J Respir Crit Care Med* 1994;149:818–24.
2 De Luca D, Plastra M, Chidini G, *et al.* The use of the Berlin definition for acute respiratory distress syndrome during infancy and early childhood: multicenter evaluation and expert consensus. *Intensive Care Med* 2013;39:2083–91.
3 Briel M, Meade M, Mercat A, *et al.* Higher vs lower positive end-expiratory pressure in patients with acute lung injury and acute respiratory distress syndrome; systematic review and meta-analysis. *J Am Med Assoc* 2010;303:865–873.

Brierley J, Carcillo JA, Choong K. Clinical practice parameters for hemodynamic support of pediatric and neonatal septic shock: 2007 update from the American College of Critical Care Medicine. *Crit Care Med* 2009;37:666–88.
British Society for Paediatric Endocrinology and Diabetes. Recommended DKA Guidelines. 2009.
Guidelines for the acute medical management of severe traumatic brain injury in infants, children, and adolescents. *Ped Crit Care Med* 2012;13(Suppl 1):S1–S82.
Hodgetts TJ, Mahoney PF, Russell MQ, Byers M. ABC to <C>ABC: redefining the military trauma paradigm. *Emerg Med J* 2006;23:745–6.
International Society of Paediatric and Adolescent Diabetes. Clinical Practice Consensus Guidelines 2006–2007. Diabetic ketoacidosis. *Pediatr Diabetes* 2007;8:28–43. Available at http://www.ispad.org/FileCenter/10-Wolfsdorf_Ped_Diab_2007,8.28-43.pdf
Mahoney PF, Russell RJ, Russell MQ, Hodgetts TJ. Novel haemostatic techniques in military medicine. *J R Army Med Corps* 2005;151:139–141.
NICE Clinical Guideline. Bacterial meningitis and meningococcal septicaemia. June 2010.
NICE Clinical Guideline. Epilepsy in adults and children: full guideline, appendix C (corrected). Available from http://www.nice.org.uk. 2004.
NICE Clinical Guideline: Feverish illness in children: assessment and initial management in children younger than 5 years. May 2007.
Samuels M, Wieteska S (eds). *Advanced Paediatric Life Support*, 5th edn. London: BMJ Books, 2011.
Scottish Intercollegiate Guideline Network and British Thoracic Society. British Guideline on the Management of Asthma. May 2008.
Scottish Intercollegiate Guideline Network. Bronchiolitis in children. November 2006.

2

Child Protection

Alice Armitage and Deborah Hodes

INTRODUCTION

Child abuse exists in all cultures across the world. In the modern era there is general international agreement that child maltreatment is morally wrong, requiring active prevention and punitive measures by governments. This stance has been enshrined in article 19 of The United Nations Convention of the Rights of the Child (UNCRC) that states:

> *"Parties shall take all appropriate legislative, administrative, social and educational measures to protect the child from all forms of physical or mental violence, injury or abuse, neglect or negligent treatment, maltreatment or exploitation, including sexual abuse, while in the care of parent(s), legal guardian(s) or any other person who has the care of the child."*

Currently 193 countries are party to the UNCRC and once a country has ratified the treaty they are bound to its terms by international law.

MALTREATMENT WORLD-WIDE

Clearly there is international condemnation of child maltreatment, but it remains a universal problem that is defined by culture and tradition. The lack of standardised statistics and variation in definitions of child maltreatment make world-wide conclusions and comparisons difficult to draw. The UN secretary General's report on violence against children estimates that in 2002 almost 53,000 children were murdered world-wide. The report also highlights the lack of governance and funding in poverty-stricken, fragile countries that provide the setting for widespread and serious forms of abuse and exploitation. Hundreds of millions of children are subject to child labour, sexual exploitation, female genital mutilation (FGM), 'honour'-based violence and trafficking. Other abuses include child soldiers, feticide, abandonment, begging and orphans who are often institutionalised. A global action plan will address the determinants of abuse that include poverty, family violence, culture and tradition, institutional care, discipline, armed conflict and treatment of girls.

MALTREATMENT NORTH AMERICA AND AUSTRALIA

The USA has one of the highest recorded rates world-wide of child deaths from maltreatment at approximately 2.2 children per 100,000 (5 children dying every day). The maltreatment of 6 million children is reported yearly, with neglect representing 80% of this. Proposed reasons for the high rates include social problems such as high-school drop-out rates, violence, teenage pregnancy, poverty and imprisonment, all known to be linked to abuse, in addition to lack of appropriate health coverage. The USA also have mandatory reporting of abuse when professionals working with children have 'a reasonable cause to know or suspect child abuse or neglect', unlike the UK where referral to safeguard the child is a professional duty (GMC guidelines) with only FGM (female genital mutilation) being mandatory. Canada and Australia similarly practice mandatory reporting. They have child death rates of 0.7 per 100,000 children.

MALTREATMENT ENGLAND

In England a series of high profile child deaths have shaped attitudes and legislature towards child protection. Two particular cases were the tragic deaths of Jasmine Beckford and Victoria Climbié. Jasmine Beckford's death in 1984 shocked the nation, and led to the Children's Act of 1989. This established the principle that the welfare of the child (as opposed to the rights of the parents) is the paramount consideration in decisions made regarding their upbringing, and replaced the concept of parental rights with parental responsibility. Victoria Climbié's death in 2000 resulted in the Children's Act 2004, which recommended integration of local services focused on the needs of the child.

Jasmine Beckford 1984

Jasmine died aged 4 years, desperately underweight and following a catalogue of abuse at the hands of her stepfather. In the weeks building up to her death she had been left chained to a bed with multiple injuries including a broken leg.

Of approximately 11 million children across the UK, professional efforts are directed towards those subject to a child protection plan and 'looked after children'. As shown in **Fig. 2.1**, this represents only a small proportion of the children 'in need' and those vulnerable, which includes those disabled and others living in poverty. Sadly high-profile cases continue with Peter Connolly in 2007 and Daniel Pelka in 2012, representing two of approximately 85 child deaths per year (a rate of 0.4 per 100,000 children).

Daniel Pelka 2013

Described as 'invisible' to the professionals around him, Daniel died of a blow to the head following starvation, neglect and beatings. Teachers at school had reported he was so hungry that he scavenged for food in the bins.

In child protection today there is an emphasis on the importance of multi-agency information sharing and communication along with early intervention. According to the multi-agency document *Working together 2015*, the approach to child protection should be underpinned by two key principles:

- Safeguarding is everyone's responsibility.
- A child-centred approach.

WHY IS RECOGNITION AND RESPONSE IMPORTANT?

The terrible consequence with which we are all familiar is the child who dies as a result of abuse. Less well recognised, but key, are the long-term sequelae in adulthood, which spare only the resilient minority; they include poor physical and mental health, lower educational attainment and perpetuating of the abusive cycle. There is accumulating evidence that child maltreatment has long-term adverse effects on children's development. During the phase of brain development, especially during the first 2 years of life, it may lead to disruption of neuroendocrine systems.

Surprisingly, maltreatment is more common than many other medical conditions, (see **Table 2.1**),

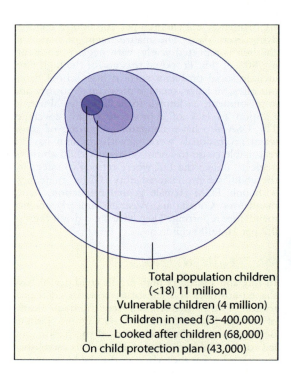

Total population children (<18) 11 million
Vulnerable children (4 million)
Children in need (3–400,000)
Looked after children (68,000)
On child protection plan (43,000)

FIGURE 2.1 Representation of extent of children 'in need' in England at any one time. (From National Statistics 2012–2013, available at https://www.gov.uk/government)

TABLE 2.1 Rates of childhood conditions

Childhood condition	Rates per 10,000
Human immunodeficiency virus	0.15
Cerebral palsy	20
Sensorineural hearing loss	30
Subject to a child protection plan	38
Children in need	332

TABLE 2.2 Numbers of children subject to a child protection plan

Category of abuse	1999	2008	2013 (%)
Neglect	13,400 (38)	13,400 (46)	17,930 (41)
Physical abuse	9,100 (26)	3,400 (12)	4,670 (11)
Sexual abuse	6,600 (19)	2,000 (7)	2,030 (5)
Emotional abuse	5,400 (15)	7,900 (27)	13,640 (32)
Multiple	–	2,500 (8)	4,870 (11)
Total	**34,500 (100)**	**29,200 (100)**	**43,140 (100)**

(From National Statistics 2012–2013, available at https://www.gov.uk/government)

but even these numbers are likely to be significant underestimates of the true prevalence. From interviewing adults, a National Society for the Prevention of Cruelty to Children (NSPCC) study found that 25% had been subject to severe maltreatment in childhood.

The relationship between medical conditions and abuse is complex. Medical problems coexist with abuse, may be caused by abuse and may put a child at risk of abuse. Recent studies found that as many as 30% of maltreated children will have a coexisting medical condition. Therefore, as many abused children will be seen either routinely or for a medical condition, it should be part of the differential diagnosis for any childhood presentation. The Department of Health statistics show the increasing numbers of children subject to a child protection plan over the last 13 years. There has been a decrease in physical abuse and sexual abuse with an increased recognition of emotional abuse (**Table 2.2**).

WHY IS RECOGNITION AND RESPONSE DIFFICULT?

Historically child protection has been taught as a separate topic in paediatrics, but no such separation exists. Child maltreatment is a differential diagnosis for many medical conditions discussed in this textbook. Protecting children requires thinking of the possibility of maltreatment in any child who presents. Serious case reviews highlight the failure to 'think the unthinkable' when professionals accept parents' explanations too readily.

Although easy in theory, there are many barriers that prevent the professional from recognising the possibility of abuse, including:

- Busy looking for rare medical condition to explain the symptoms.
- Opening 'a can of worms'.
- Fear of being reported to the General Medical Council.
- Fear of being wrong and missing a medical cause.
- Reluctance to consider abuse – it's too hard.
- Fear of parent's reaction to the possibility.
- Loss of relationship with parents or carers.

TYPES OF ABUSE AND NEGLECT

The commonly used categories of abuse in the UK are defined in the document *Working together 2015*. Although a useful framework, in practice there is usually coexistence and overlap between the types of abuse.

- Physical abuse: a form of abuse that may involve hitting, shaking, throwing, poisoning, burning or scalding, drowning, suffocating or otherwise causing physical harm to a child. Fabricated or induced illness can be a form of physical abuse.
- Emotional abuse: the persistent emotional maltreatment of a child such as to cause severe and persistent adverse effects on the child's emotional development.
- Neglect: the persistent failure to meet a child's basic physical and/or psychological needs, likely to result in the serious impairment of the child's health or development.
- Sexual abuse: involves forcing or enticing a child or young person to take part in sexual activities, whether or not the child is aware of what is happening.

These types of abuse, typically perpetrated by the parents or main carer, have been well understood for some time. However, particularly as children get older, the categories and perpetrators of abuse become less clear-cut. Teenagers may be at risk due to their own risk-taking behaviours, involvement in gangs, self-harm or sexual exploitation. There also starts to be overlap between victims and perpetrators. These complex child protection issues are discussed in more detail later in the chapter.

It is important to note that the World Health Organisation (WHO) defines exploitation as the fifth category of abuse, incorporating slavery and child labour recognising sexual exploitation as an important child protection issue.

Case example

A baby is found to have bruises suspicious for physical abuse. On questioning, the mother is a teenager, still subject to a child protection plan herself for neglect and physical abuse.

RISK, VULNERABILITY, RESILIENCE

We know that there are factors that impact on the likelihood of abuse occurring. However, none of these factors have a causal link and there will be families who provide excellent parenting despite very difficult circumstances. It is therefore helpful to consider the risks, vulnerability and resilience factors in a non-judgemental fashion.

The common assessment framework (CAF) is a tool used by all practitioners working with children (**Fig. 2.2**). It offers a useful basis for assessing which children and young people may be more vulnerable and what support can be offered. Vulnerability to abuse and neglect and resilience will be elicited in full history taking.

- Child's developmental needs:
  - Premature and low birth weight.
  - Separated from mother/primary caregiver.
  - Disabled and/or have chronic ill health, including physical and mental health.
  - Unwanted/unplanned or different to expectations, for example the 'wrong' sex.
- Parenting capacity:
  - Drug and alcohol misuse.
  - Domestic violence.
  - Mental health problems.
  - Learning disability.
  - Personal history of abuse and neglect.
- Family and environmental factors:
  - Frequent moves, homelessness.
  - Social isolation, weak supportive networks of family and friends.
  - Socio-economic problems, such as poverty and unemployment.
  - Strong cultural beliefs leading to:
    - FGM.
    - Forced marriage.
    - 'Honour' killing.

Resilience

As well as factors that make children vulnerable to abuse, there are similarly factors that are generally protective. A child may be resilient against abuse taking place, and when children are abused, some will have more resilience in terms of the outcomes. A strong relationship with a parent, an easy temperament and high cognitive ability are a few examples.

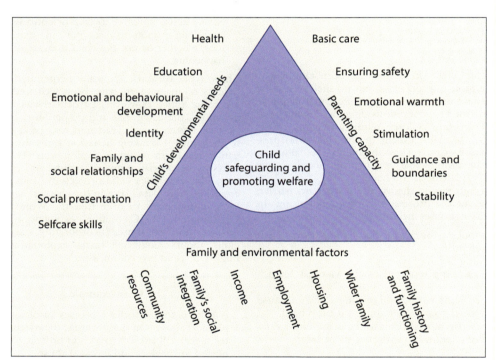

FIGURE 2.2 Common assessment framework triangle. (From https://www.gov.uk/government/uploads/system/uploads/attachment_data/file/190604/DFES-04320-2006-ChildAbuse.pdf, with permission under the Open Government Licence.)

PAEDIATRIC ASSESSMENT OF A CHILD WITH SUSPICION OF MALTREATMENT

GENERAL APPROACH

It is important to assess the child in a rigorous and systematic way irrespective of whether there is an allegation of abuse, unexplained injury or the incidental discovery of abuse and/or neglect during any medical consultation. The only difference from the diagnostic process in any other disorder is that when maltreatment is diagnosed or suspected the management occurs within a multi-agency context of assessment and planning for the child.

DOCUMENTATION

It is vital to document findings fully as any consultation can be subject to legal scrutiny; make clear, precise and contemporaneous notes and sign them. Body maps or drawn diagrams should be used, whether accidental injury, non-accidental or uncertain, and site, size, colour, stage of healing (although difficult to do with accuracy), cause of each lesion/injury as given by child and/or parent should be commented on and notes signed. Birthmarks and scars should be included. Increasingly there is a role for photography to supplement the notes. Quotations and explicit descriptions should be used when possible and the history, observations, suspicions and interpretations should be distinguished. Additional care should be taken in documenting time, place and people present and from whom the history was taken, including the child.

CONSENT

Ideally, every child should be seen with a parent, unless considered a danger to the child. If the child is brought without the parent, consent must be obtained from someone with parental responsibility; this is usually the parent but rarely parental responsibility will have been transferred over to the local authority.

HISTORY TAKING

Ideally a parent or long-term carer will be present and able to provide details of the pregnancy, birth, neonatal period and past medical history. When taking the history of any alleged abuse, if possible the child should be spoken with alone, unless this has already been done by other professional colleagues who can relay it. It may be easier to do this later in the consultation when a rapport has been established with the child and carer. When taking the family and social history these should be focused to the medical complaint. Risk factors and vulnerabilities for abuse (see above) should be noted in the history,

remembering that cycles of abuse and neglect often repeat themselves through generations.

Case examples

Victoria Climbié at the age of 7 years was not enrolled in school.

A 6-year-old boy with coeliac disease presents with weight falling through the centiles. On questioning he is not eating correctly because there is sudden loss of income from redundancy.

A 7-year-old girl presents with nocturnal enuresis. It emerges that she is wetting because she is frightened to go to the shared toilet in the bed and breakfast accommodation.

It is important to establish whether the child may have unmet health needs such as outstanding immunisations, dental caries or chronic urinary tract infections, which could indicate medical neglect. Behavioural and emotional problems, including symptoms of post-traumatic stress maybe a consequence of maltreatment.

EXAMINATION

A thorough general physical examination should be conducted, to include height, weight and head circumference plotted on growth charts. Respiratory, cardiovascular and abdominal examinations should be conducted, with any additional systems as indicated. The whole body should be examined, including hair, nails, mouth, teeth, ears, nose, head, skin and hidden areas – behind the ears and neck.

The child's demeanour, response to carer, play, attention and behaviour should be evaluated during the examination and whether or not the child was able to co-operate recorded. If the examination is incomplete, it should be explained how and why. Developmental milestones, cognitive ability and school attainment (and attendance) should be commented on, all of which can be relevant to the diagnosis. The pubertal stage should be noted.

With the child's permission, it is important to examine the buttocks and genitalia of all children whether or not there is a suspicion of sexual abuse; in 1 in 7 physically abused children there is associated sexual abuse. The child or young person should have a clear explanation of the process and that it is part of a thorough paediatric assessment.

Initially the buttocks, anus and external genitalia are viewed. In boys, injury to the urethra, penis and scrotum should be looked for, state of the testes and presence of circumcision commented on. In girls, any injuries to the external genitalia (including FGM) and any vaginal discharge should be noted. The anus and surrounding area should be examined for any injury including fissures or scars.

If sexual abuse is suspected, a more detailed examination of the anogenital area with a colposcope should be undertaken by an expert (see below for more details).

INVESTIGATIONS

The need for medical investigations will be indicated by examination findings and any allegations.

DIAGNOSIS/OPINION

An opinion on whether the findings are consistent with the history given is important to note. If there is uncertainty and/or no diagnosis, this should be reported and the next steps indicated, i.e. investigations, further referrals, and so on. Other findings from history and examination, such as growth or language development, medical comorbidities or unmet medical needs should also be commented on.

MANAGEMENT

Clear information (with an opinion) should be given to parents, police and social care. The immediate safety of the child and any siblings should be considered. In complex cases ongoing responsibilities include obtaining past records and completing a medical chronology. Follow-up and/or referrals such as to child and adolescent mental health services should be considered. Staff should undertake to write reports and participate in strategy meetings, child protection conferences and, if needed, care proceedings. Sometimes witness statements and attending criminal court is required.

PHYSICAL ABUSE

INTRODUCTION

Evidence is increasingly moving away from the idea of certain injuries being classical or pathognomic of child abuse. Instead, child maltreatment should be part of the differential in any child presenting to medical services. It is important to remember that an abused child can have a normal physical examination at any given time.

Where physical signs are present, certain characteristics in the history should promote suspicion of child abuse. These include:

- Inconsistent or changing story.
- Unclear mechanism of injury.
- Delay in presentation.
- Abnormal interaction between child and carer.
- Aggression of parents/caregivers towards each other, staff or the child.
- Injury in a non-ambulant child is always suspicious for abuse.

Case example

A 2-year-old is brought to A&E with a burn to his right foot. His father claims that he stood on one leg and placed his foot in a bucket of hot water – this is developmentally impossible!

BRUISING

Bruising is a very common finding in children. A recent systematic review into patterns of bruising showed that the majority of school-aged children will have bruising at any given time, with accidental bruising tending to be over bony prominences and on the front of the body. The distribution of accidental bruising varies with the developmental age of the child: crawling babies typically injure their chin, nose and forehead, while older children have bruises to their knees and shins (**Fig. 2.3**).

Abusive bruising can occur anywhere and is commonly found on soft tissues areas and on the head, face, neck, eyes, ears, trunk, arms, buttocks and hands (**Fig. 2.4**). Multiple bruises or bruises in clusters are suspicious, as is any bruising in a non-ambulant child. Bruises inflicted with significant force may have surrounding petechiae and this finding is strongly correlated with abuse. Inflicted bruises may bear the imprint of a hand or implement, which can be correlated with allegations.

Ageing of bruises

Paediatricians are often asked to comment on the age of a bruise. Recent evidence suggests that bruises cannot be aged with any certainty and recommendations are now that this should not be commented on as part of a child protection proceedings. However, multiple bruises of different size and colour may indicate multiple episodes of trauma and are suggestive of physical abuse (**Figs 2.5, 2.6**).

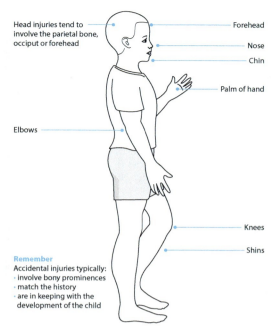

Head injuries tend to involve the parietal bone, occiput or forehead

Forehead
Nose
Chin
Palm of hand

Elbows

Knees
Shins

Remember
Accidental injuries typically:
· involve bony prominences
· match the history
· are in keeping with the development of the child

FIGURE 2.3 Typical sites of accidental injury. (With permission, Harris J, Sidebotham P, Welbury R *et al. Child Protection and the Dental Team: an introduction to safeguarding children in dental practice.* COPDEND: Sheffield, 2006: www.cpdt.org.uk.)

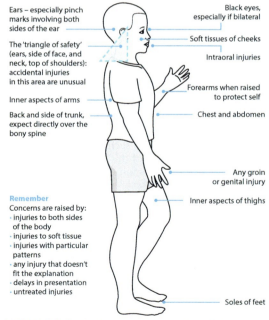

Ears – especially pinch marks involving both sides of the ear

The 'triangle of safety' (ears, side of face, and neck, top of shoulders): accidental injuries in this area are unusual

Inner aspects of arms

Back and side of trunk, expect directly over the bony spine

Black eyes, especially if bilateral
Soft tissues of cheeks
Intraoral injuries
Forearms when raised to protect self
Chest and abdomen
Any groin or genital injury
Inner aspects of thighs
Soles of feet

Remember
Concerns are raised by:
· injuries to both sides of the body
· injuries to soft tissue
· injuries with particular patterns
· any injury that doesn't fit the explanation
· delays in presentation
· untreated injuries

FIGURE 2.4 Typical sites of non-accidental injury. (With permission, Harris J, Sidebotham P, Welbury R *et al. Child Protection and the Dental Team: an introduction to safeguarding children in dental practice.* COPDEND: Sheffield, 2006: www.cpdt.org.uk.)

Investigations

There are rare medical causes for bruising and bleeding that may need to be excluded before a diagnosis of non-accidental injury is made. A thorough medical history and baseline blood tests including a full blood count (FBC) and clotting studies can exclude rare bleeding disorders such as von Willebrand disease or immune thrombocytopenic purpura (ITP).

BITE MARKS

A human bite mark is always an inflicted injury and is therefore highly suspicious for abuse (**Fig. 2.7**). It can be helpful to refer bite marks and possible bite marks to a dentist or forensic odontologist who may be able to gather dental imprints and DNA. They are also able to give expert advice distinguishing child bites, adult bites and animal bites.

BURNS AND SCALDS

Burns are a common cause of emergency presentations in children and can be associated with abuse

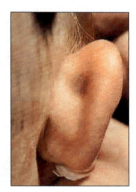

FIGURE 2.5 Bruising to the pinna suggestive of excessive pinching.

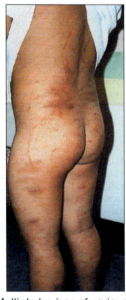

FIGURE 2.6 Multiple bruises of various colours and shapes suggestive of physical abuse.

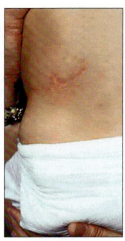

FIGURE 2.7 Bite marks on the back of an 8-month-old girl.

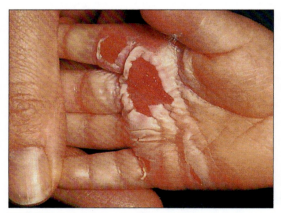

FIGURE 2.8 Burn caused by grabbing curling tongs.

of all types. Assessing the likelihood that the burn is non-accidental should take into account the alleged mechanism of injury and developmental stage of the child. Evidence shows the most common type of intentional burn is an immersion injury in hot water. These burns typically have clear margins and a symmetrical distribution. They may show a 'glove and stocking' distribution or skin sparing in buttock creases (the 'hole in doughnut' effect). They are more frequently found on the buttocks and lower extremities. Features that should increase suspicion include coexistent unrelated fractures or injuries, a history of previous abuse or domestic violence and a quiet or withdrawn child. The history may be inconsistent with the findings; for example, a history of a burn from flowing water when the examination findings indicate immersion, and a sibling may be blamed for the burn.

Accidental burns are more commonly from flowing water or spills. They are characteristically asymmetrical and more likely to involve the head, neck, trunk and upper extremities. Burns caused by grabbing of hot objects tend to involve the fingertips and the palm of the hand (Fig. 2.8). Although not

usually inflicted, these may indicate a lack of supervision and safety measures.

Inflicted burns may show the imprint of whatever is used, e.g. an iron. Intentional cigarette burns cause symmetrical round, well-demarcated burns of uniform thickness. Accidental burns of this nature occur after a brief contact and have an elliptical shape with a tail.

FRACTURES

Fractures may present with pain, swelling and bruising, but some of the fractures caused by abuse may be clinically silent, or a loss of function may be the only indicator in a younger child.

Patterns of fractures

As with other injuries, the characteristics of a fracture alone cannot be used to distinguish between accidental and non-accidental injury. The evidence increasingly suggests that many types of fractures classically associated with child abuse can also result from accidental injury; therefore the history taking and developmental age of child are again key to making a diagnosis.

The recent UK systematic review compares characteristics of accidental and abusive fractures. In general there is an inverse correlation between the age of a child and the probability of a fracture being the result of abuse, with any fracture in a child less than 18 months of age highly suspicious for abuse. The majority of accidental fractures have been shown to occur in children over 5 years.

Of all fractures presentations, children presenting with rib fractures are the most likely to have been abused (more likely than not in the absence of significant accidental trauma), particularly if multiple or posterior rib fractures are present (Fig. 2.9). Evidence suggests that CPR very rarely causes rib fractures, and the only fractures found were multiple, anterior or anterolateral.

Humeral fractures may be seen as a result of abuse, with midshaft fractures being more suspicious than supracondylar fractures (that are more likely to be accidental) (Fig. 2.10). A spiral fracture of the humerus may result from an applied twisting force and is therefore suspicious for abuse, particularly in the non-ambulant child. Fractures of the leg including the femur can occur in significant trauma, such as a road traffic accident, and in the absence of this history are suspicious for abuse. The most common type of femur fractures are midshaft; however, type of fracture (oblique, transverse, spiral) is not correlated with abuse. Multiple fractures are significantly more likely to be result of abuse than single fractures. Metaphyseal fractures in children under the age of 2 years are suspicious for abuse. They are easily missed on radiographs and require an experienced radiologist's opinion.

Case example

Daniel Pelka was brought to A&E 1 year prior to his death with a spiral fracture of his humerus. Although doctors at the time were concerned about abuse the medical evidence was felt to be inconclusive.

Non-accidental head injury

Injury to the head is the most common cause of death in abused children, as well as having serious long-term consequences in children who survive. 'Shaken baby syndrome', first described in the 1970s, is characterised by intracranial and intraocular bleeding in the abused child, resulting in long-term brain damage. Intracranial injury can be caused by impact, shaking or a combination of both. Presentation may be as a result of the identification of an overlying soft, boggy swelling or obvious bruising; trauma to the head should also be part of the differential diagnosis in any child presenting with a low Glasgow coma score (GCS), new onset of seizures or unexplained drowsiness or irritability. In the baby with an open fontanelle the signs may be less obvious and an abusive parent may only report poor feeding or excessive crying.

Distinguishing inflicted from non-inflicted brain injury remains a challenge, but the recent Welsh systematic review provides the best framework to assess this probability. The presence of apnoea in the child with brain injury is highly correlated with inflicted injury, a fact that has only recently been realised. As such the presence or absence of apnoea should be recorded in every child with brain injury. The presence of retinal haemorrhages is strongly associated with inflicted brain injury. Other features that should increase suspicion of abuse include rib fractures, long bone fractures and bruising to the head and neck. Appearance on neuroimaging is poorly correlated with the probability of abuse.

Skull fractures

The commonest skull fracture is that of a single, linear, hairline parietal fracture which may be seen either as a result of accidental or non-accidental injury. **Fig. 2.11** shows a branched pattern. Accidental skull fractures need an appropriate history of a significant incident, usually of a fall from several feet onto a firm or hard surface, to account for them. Fractures resulting from accidental domestic falls rarely result in intracranial injuries. Skull fractures do not heal by developing callus and cannot be dated from the radiographic appearances. If soft tissue swelling is present overlying the fracture it is likely to have occurred within the previous 7 days.

Investigations

In a child under 2 years with an injury thought to be abusive, or with an abused sibling, investigations should be considered to detect any occult injuries. These should include a skeletal survey with repeat films, neuroimaging and ophthalmology to look for retinal haemorrhages. It is important to consider intracranial and intra-abdominal injuries and make a decision regarding the need for further investigations.

In a child with a fracture, it is important to exclude any predisposing skeletal disorder such as osteogenesis imperfecta or osteopenia of prematurity. Baseline blood tests should be done including a bone profile and vitamin D levels.

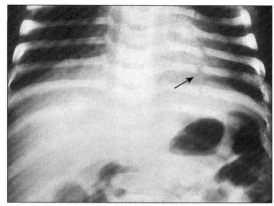

FIGURE 2.9 Posterior rib fractures.

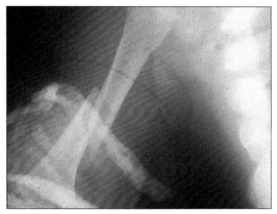

FIGURE 2.10 Fracture of the humeral shaft.

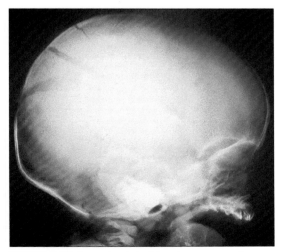

FIGURE 2.11 Branched skull fracture emanating from the occipital bone.

Ageing of fractures

Delayed images after a few days or weeks may help in dating fractures, as can a radionuclide scan. The evidence suggests that dating of fractures is crude and can be confounded by further injuries or immobilisation. Advice from a paediatric radiologist should be sought and statements about dating of fractures should be made in terms of weeks rather than days.

FABRICATED OR INDUCED ILLNESS (FII)

Fabricated or induced illness (FII) is a spectrum from the normally anxious parent, keen to get the best help for their child, to the abusive parent intentionally fabricating symptoms in their child (Munchausen's-by-proxy), which is a form of physical abuse. It is often suspected and later confirmed when reported or observed symptoms do not have a medical explanation. Management of these children and families can be challenging and it is important to avoid multiple referrals and best to have one paediatrician working closely with the general practitioner. Thorough history taking is paramount and it may be appropriate to perform some baseline investigations to exclude common causes of reported symptoms. In general the approach should be one of transparency and reassurance while trying to avoid iatrogenic harm with unnecessary investigations; there may be improvement following reassurance that a medical cause is not present and only a minority will need consideration of child protection proceedings.

NEGLECT

INTRODUCTION

Neglect is the persistent failure of the parent to meet the child's basic needs. Unlike the other forms of abuse it is the result of an omission rather than an act.

Neglect is increasingly used as a category for placing children on the child protection register; however, actual incidence is difficult to measure and neglect frequently coexists with other forms of abuse. A series of serious case reviews have highlighted the prevalence of neglect where severe maltreatment is present; neglect is harmful and can be life threatening, it needs to be taken as seriously as the other types of abuse.

CLINICAL FEATURES

It is possible to categorise the types of neglect in various ways. These are not fixed but can be a helpful framework within which to consider presenting features and extra considerations.

- Emotional neglect (emotional neglect is often described with emotional abuse and will be discussed later in this chapter).
- Abandonment; e.g. child found unattended in the home by a social worker.
- Medical neglect; e.g. failure of immunisation, missed clinic appointments, poor dentition.
- Nutritional neglect; e.g. inadequate growth.
- Educational neglect; e.g. poor school attendance.
- Physical neglect; e.g. unkempt and dirty appearance.
- Failure to provide supervision and guidance; e.g. recurrent accidents (falls, scalds, road traffic accidents).

Case example

Fig. 2.12 shows Daniel Pelka's growth chart (plotted from weight information documented in the Serious Case Review).

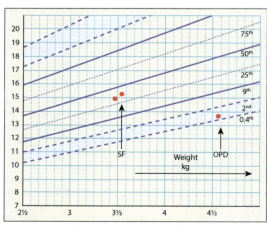

FIGURE 2.12 Daniel Pelka's growth chart (plotted from weight information documented in the Serious Case Review). OPD: outpatient department appointment; SF: spiral fracture.

In assessing these children a detailed history including social and family history is paramount. Consider risk factors for neglect, which include poverty, parent's mental health problems and history of domestic violence. The child's educational attainment and school attendance must be asked about in the history.

Examination of these children should specifically look for evidence of poor clothing, dirty hair and skin, poor dentition and recurrent skin infections (including nappy rash in babies). There may be evidence of poor growth when reviewing the centile charts and general muscle bulk may be reduced, in particular subscapular skin thickness. Signs of physical and sexual abuse should be looked for in the examination, as the different types of abuse frequently coexist.

EMOTIONAL ABUSE AND NEGLECT

Both emotional abuse and neglect are forms of psychological maltreatment of children and represent the biggest challenge for professionals in terms of recognition. Persistent psychological maltreatment, particularly in early infancy, is extremely harmful and is associated with aggression, depression and antisocial behaviour later in life. There is strong correlation with maternal depression, which should be considered the strongest risk factor for this type of abuse.

Evidence suggests that there are characteristics of the interaction between child and caregiver that are indictors of emotional abuse and neglect. These will vary with the age of the child.

In babies under 12 months:

- Mother not being emotionally engaged with the child's needs.
- Not speaking to the child, or speaking very little.
- Mother describes baby as irritating and demanding.

Toddlers (aged 1–3 years):

- Parent/caregiver is unresponsive to the child and fails to respond to them appropriately.
- They are critical of the child or verbally aggressive and often have developmentally unrealistic expectations.
- They do not show affection towards the child and are not upset by the child being in distress.

Older children (aged 3–6 years):

- Parent/caregiver does not play with the child.
- No praise or positive reinforcement is given.
- They exhibit negative beliefs about the child, 'scape-goating'.
- Neglectful mothers are more likely to use physical chastisement.

Independent from the caregiver there are signs that may be observed in the child as a result of emotional neglect and abuse. The child may show abnormal behaviour in terms of attachment to their mother, for example, being unnaturally passive, poor feeding, sleeping problems and developmental delay. Toddlers start to have behavioural problems with aggression and hostility towards other children.

Speech and language delay is more common. Older children may have problems interacting with their peers; they may be socially isolated and quick to anger. Various labels such as 'autistic spectrum disorder' or 'attention deficit hyperactivity disorder (ADHD)' may be used erroneously. As adolescents they may be depressed and self-harm, employ substance abuse and show delinquent behaviours.

SEXUAL ABUSE

Sexual abuse involves forcing or enticing a child or young person to take part in sexual activities, not necessarily involving physical contact whether or not the child is aware of what is happening.

INCIDENCE

Although sexual abuse accounts for a minority of child protection registrations in the UK, it is often unrecognised and therefore frequently missed. 4% of all children in the UK are subject to sexual abuse at some time, most commonly perpetrated by those close to the child. This figure is in contrast to the NSPCC survey of 11–17-year-olds, where 9.4% considered they had been sexually abused.

Sexually abused children may not manifest any signs or symptoms, and may not allege it is happening for fear of not being believed. These children are more likely to grow up into adults who have are more vulnerable to further sexual abuse, are promiscuous, more likely to have a teenage pregnancy, suffer with mental ill health, drug misuse and difficulties with relationships and protecting their own children.

Child sexual abuse (CSA) may present in a variety of ways:

- Allegation: this may be in the acute period when forensic evidence may be gathered, or more commonly the child will allege chronic or historic abuse.
- Physical symptoms: a wide range of physical symptoms may be linked to CSA, some may be detected incidentally by a carer, some may be reported by the child and some may be found on examination. A benign medical cause may explain the symptoms but sexual abuse should be considered. Symptoms include: constipation, dysuria, enuresis and recurrent urinary tract infections; vaginal discharge or vulvovaginitis; recurrent itching or soreness (consider lichen sclerosus et atrophicus); rectal fissures; bleeding – distinguish vaginal from rectal.
- Emotional/behavioural: sudden changes in behaviour maybe a pointer especially if associated with other changes such as a new stepfather moving in and mother on night shift. It is always important to ask the child if there is anything worrying or if they have a bad secret.

Other non-specific symptoms include:

- Sleep disturbance or nightmares.
- Anxiety, depression, withdrawal.
- Aggression, attention seeking and/or poor concentration.

- Sexualised behaviour – repeated, coercive or persistent.
- Encopresis (soiling).

Older children/adolescents:

- Self-harm.
- Suicidal ideation.
- Running away.
- Psychosomatic: recurrent headaches, abdominal pains and anorexia.

Case examples

A 7-year-old at school starts to lose concentration. On questioning, her mother says her new boyfriend has just moved in and is very helpful because he bathes the child and looks after her when she goes to work. On talking to the child alone she says he gets onto her bed at night and 'white stuff' goes on her leg.

A mother saw her husband inappropriately touching her 10-year-old daughter on viewing them through the reflection in the window. On questioning the daughter confirmed he had been touching her 'privates'. Urine NAAT was positive for *Chlamydia* infection; she was asymptomatic. He was convicted in the criminal court.

ACHIEVING BEST EVIDENCE (ABE) INTERVIEW

Following an allegation, the child is interviewed by a trained police officer and social worker in a purpose-built suite with videotape. On occasion this will occur after urgent medical examination, in which case the health professionals should only ask questions important for the examination and not ask about the allegations.

RAPE AND SEXUAL ASSAULT

Teenagers and children represent 35% of reported accounts of rape and sexual assault. Any acute injuries need to be managed promptly and should be followed by the collection of forensic evidence, including intimate body swabs, and detailed medical evaluation for signs of trauma, the risk of pregnancy and infection. Evidence is more commonly found on the clothes and bedding than from the intimate body swabs, especially in children. Immediate and later psychological assessment and treatment should be offered for this vulnerable group.

EXAMINATION

The child and care giver's permission should be obtained and the child reminded of how to keep safe.

Following a thorough physical examination, an experienced senior doctor should carry out the examination of the anogenital area using the colposcope. This enables detailed examination of the hymen and anus with photo-documentation (the descriptions of markings around the hymen and anus

are likened to that of a clock face). There is much variation in normal anatomy (**Fig. 2.13**). The size and appearance of the hymen changes with the onset of puberty when the hymen becomes fleshy, pale, and oestrogenised.

Acute genital or anal injury can cause erythema, bruising or lacerations. Vaginal penetration classically results in a laceration to the hymen and posterior fourchette (between 3 and 9 o'clock). In non-acute allegations of penetration, notches in the hymen are found in only a small percent. Transections (healed lacerations) can be demonstrated with a swab. **Fig. 2.14** shows a transection at '5 o'clock'. The young girl had alleged penile vaginal penetration causing pain on five occasions.

Anal penetration also presents acutely with erythema, bruising or lacerations.

Following an acute allegation there may be other injuries to the body such as bruising, scratches or bite marks.

The anus is examined in the left lateral position and anal dilatation occurs when the anus dilates to

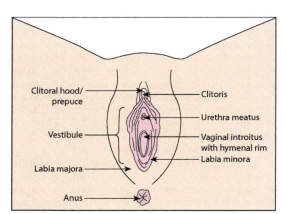

FIGURE 2.13 Female genitalia. (With permission, Simpson J, Robinson K, Creighton SM, Hodes D. Female genital mutilation: the role of health professionals in prevention, assessment, and management. *BMJ* 2012;344:e1361.)

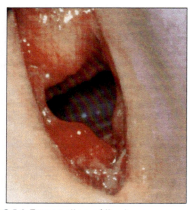

FIGURE 2.14 Transection of the hymen.

reveal the rectum after separating the buttocks for up to 30 seconds. This occurs in a small percentage of those alleging sexual abuse; however, this sign has been found in non-abused children with constipation and other children who may have poor anal tone.

At the conclusion, it is essential to draw the findings on a body map. The DVD recording is part of the medical records and is taken to peer review. Approximately 90% of children alleging historic abuse have normal physical findings. This does not refute the allegation but explanation of this to the child and parents is necessary and always a great relief.

OTHER CONSIDERATIONS IN CHILD PROTECTION

ADOLESCENCE

A good understanding of the unique needs of the adolescent is integral to the practice of paediatrics. The second most dangerous period of childhood after the neonatal period in England is the adolescent years but the needs of adolescents are frequently ignored or marginalised in our society. Many adolescents are abused or at risk of abuse but this is far less likely to be recognised or managed than in a younger child. Each patient should be considered as an individual with experiences, medical needs and rights appropriate to their age and stage of development. Capacity should be assessed without prejudice and remembering that it is decision-relative.

When taking a history from an adolescent patient it may be appropriate to speak to them alone without a parent or carer present. The routine history covers:

- School, college or work.
- Relationships with peers, boyfriends and girlfriends.
- Depression, self-harm and suicide risk.
- Drugs and alcohol.
- Home environment.

SELF-HARM

A common presentation in teenagers will be self-harm. Although not maltreatment itself this is often a symptom of maltreatment, for example undisclosed sexual assault, emotional abuse or bullying. In assessing and managing these children it is important that their wider needs are considered. Most children who present with acute self-harm will need admission to hospital, referral to social care and assessment by mental health teams.

BULLYING

According to an NPSCC study almost half of all children (46%) of children have been bullied at some point in their lives; as such it represents a huge cause of child maltreatment with wide-ranging consequences to children's emotional and physical well-being. Bullying can take many forms including verbal, non-verbal, exclusion, racial and sexual bullying, cyberbullying or physical abuse by a peer or sibling.

Children who are bullied may show a range of symptoms and, at worst, may present to health services following physical assault or self-harm. Bullying should be part of the differential diagnosis in any school-age child seen. It may be worth asking specifically about cyberbullying, including texting and use of social networking sites, and sexual bullying, which represents an increasing problem.

SEXUAL EXPLOITATION

We are only starting to have an awareness of sexual exploitation in the UK and elsewhere and it remains a largely hidden problem. It can involve a range of practices where a person or persons use a position of power over a child to coerce the child into sexual activities. Both boys and girls are at risk and many children are unaware that abuse is taking place. They are tricked into thinking they are in a loving relationship and feel unable to speak out against their abusers.

A recent report into sexual exploitation highlighted the confused attitudes to consent even among professionals. A child under 13 years is not legally capable of consenting to sexual activity and it is classified as statutory rape. Sexual activity with a young person over 13 but under 16 is also an offence but the imperative is to ascertain it is consensual and whether there is sexual exploitation if it is consensual. No child under 18 is able to consent to an abusive relationship.

Sexual exploitation of a child may start with a grooming period where the abuser forms a relationship with the child, often supplying them with drugs and alcohol prior to the abuse starting. Suspicions that a child is being sexually exploited include relationships with older men, behavioural changes, going missing and self-harm.

Case example

A young woman has disclosed that she was sexually exploited from the age of 11 to 13 by a local street gang; although this is statutory rape her former friends thought that she had given consent and labelled her a 'slag'.

FEMALE GENITAL MUTILATION (FGM)

FGM is a cultural practice involving cutting or removal of parts of the female genitals practiced on millions of women world-wide. With an increasingly multicultural patient population FGM needs to be considered and understood by all UK health professionals, particularly those working with children.

Currently very few health professionals ask about FGM and therefore it is rarely picked up. There may be specific medical features that raise suspicion, such as enuresis, abdominal pain or recurrent UTIs; or behavioural indicators such as becoming withdrawn and quiet, signs of post-traumatic stress or self-harm. However, it should be routine in any paediatric history taking that consideration is given to asking whether the family comes from a community where FGM ('cutting' or 'female circumcision') is practiced.

FGM, as any other child protection concern, must lead to involvement of social care and mandatory reporting to the police, who will need to consider whether a (recent) crime has been committed. Physical findings may vary from a small ceremonial cut or prick (which may have no scar) to total excision of the external genitalia and sewing up of the orifice (infibulation).

UNACCOMPANIED ASYLUM SEEKERS

Immigrants to the UK on their own who are thought to be under the age of 18 are the responsibility of the state. Many of these children will have had traumatic experiences in their past and they may well have unmet health needs. A thorough paediatric assessment should be undertaken considering failure of immunisations, possibility of post-traumatic stress disorder, behavioural problems or signs of chronic disease.

WHAT TO DO WHEN ABUSE IS SUSPECTED

THE ROLE OF SOCIAL CARE

In the UK, when there is suspicion of abuse or neglect social care are responsible for assessment of risk, deciding if the child is 'in need' or 'suffering significant harm', providing support for the child and family and the ultimate decision whether to keep a child with their family. In reaching this decision social care work closely with other agencies and professionals.

If there are concerns that a child is at risk of abuse or has been abused then staff should discuss this with their immediate manager, and if still concerned, with the named or designated doctor or nurse for safeguarding in the Trust. If a referral to social care is required, there is a multi-agency framework (the common assessment framework, CAF) for doing so.

The flow-chart shown in **Fig. 2.15** can be used by any professional working with children.

WHAT HAPPENS NEXT?

After receiving a referral social care will make a decision as to the response required; this will include a decision about whether immediate action is needed, for example removing the child under an emergency protection order. When there are concerns that a child may be 'in need' or at risk of 'significant harm' then social care can initiate an assessment under Section 17 or Section 47 of the Children's Act respectively. Further details of social care proceedings can be found in the multi-agency document *Working Together 2015*.

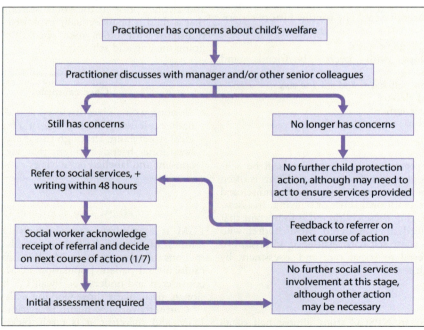

FIGURE 2.15 What to do if you're worried a child is being abused. (Reproduced from https://www.gov.uk/government/uploads/system/uploads/attachment_data/file/190604/DFES-04320-2006-ChildAbuse.pdf, with permission under the Open Government Licence.)

THE ROLE OF HEALTH PROFESSIONALS

Although the ultimate decision-making responsibility rests with social care, the health professionals have an increasingly important role including:

- Recognising and referring children at risk of significant harm.
- Providing a chronology with explanation of the medical findings that is understood by a non-medical professional or parent/carer.
- Contributing to enquiries about a child and family.
- Participating in the child protection case conference.
- Playing a part – through the child protection plan – in safeguarding children from significant harm for example by referral for early intervention.
- Providing therapeutic help to abused children.
- Writing reports for court and appearing as a witness when called.

CONCLUSION

Child safeguarding is everyone's business. Given its high incidence in society, it must by definition come to the attention of all paediatricians at some point and so thorough knowledge and an understanding of appropriate action when there is a suspicion is of vital importance. Safeguarding procedures may vary from country to country and health professionals should be aware of local procedures.

FURTHER READING

Barker J, Hodes D. *The Child in Mind: A Child Protection Handbook*. Taylor Francis, 2007.

Bass C, Glaser D. Early recognition and management of fabricated or induced illness in children. *Lancet* 2014;383:1412–21.

Cardiff Child Protection Systematic Reviews – CORE INFO (A collaboration between the National Society for the Prevention of Cruelty to Children (NSPCC) and the Early Years research section of the Cochrane Institute of Primary Care and Public Health, Department of Child Health, School of Medicine, Cardiff University), available at www.core-info.cardiff.ac.uk

Children Act 1989 and 2003.

Convention on the Rights of the Child, United Nations 1989, Office of the High Commissioner for Human Rights.

Department of Education, Collections: Statistics: children in need and Statistics: child protection, England March 2013, available at www.gov.uk

Jütte S, Bentley H, Miller P, Jetha N. *How Safe are our Children?* London: NSPCC, 2014.

NICE guidelines. *When to Suspect Child Maltreatment*. (CG89), 2009.

Royal College of Paediatrics and Child Health. *Child Protection Companion*, 2013.

United Nations Secretary-General. *Report on Violence against Children*, 2006.

Working Together to Safeguard Children: A guide to inter-agency working to safeguard and promote the welfare of children, March 2015.

www.childwelfare.gov (US Department of Health and Human Services)

www.Transmonee.org (monitoring the situation of the women and children in Central and Eastern Europe and the Commonwealth of Independent States)

3

Infectious Diseases

Vas Novelli, Delane Shingadia and Huda Al-Ansari

BACTERIA

DIPHTHERIA

INCIDENCE

The disease is endemic in most less developed countries. Infection is acquired via droplet inhalation or via direct contact with respiratory secretions or exudates from skin lesions. Epidemics have been caused by contaminated milk. Cases in most developed countries are usually imported. There has been a significant resurgence of diphtheria in Eastern Europe; the numbers have declined after reaching a peak in the mid-1990s, but the disease remains endemic in these countries.

AETIOLOGY/PATHOGENESIS

Corynebacterium diphtheriae is a gram-positive, non-motile, pleomorphic bacillus. Three colony types are recognised (mitis, gravis and intermedius). Humans are the only known reservoir of *C diphtheriae*. Following transmission of *C diphtheriae* to a susceptible contact, the bacilli tend to remain localised at mucosal surfaces of the nose and upper respiratory tract. They initiate an inflammatory response with local tissue necrosis and eventually the formation of an adherent greyish 'pseudo-membrane' that may cause respiratory obstruction. Exotoxin production by *C diphtheria* depends on the presence of a lysogenic bacteriophage, which carries the gene encoding for the toxin. Myocarditis and neuritis are the result of systemic absorption of the toxin and end-organ damage.

CLINICAL PRESENTATION

The initial clinical presentation depends on the anatomic location of the infection and diphtheric membrane (nasal, tonsillopharyngeal, laryngeal, conjunctival, skin and genital). Infection involving the tonsils or pharynx is the most common site, followed by the nose and larynx. Nasal diphtheria (**Fig. 3.1**) is mainly seen in infants who usually present with a foul smelling, profuse, mucopurulent nasal discharge leading to excoriation of the nose and lips. Tonsillo-pharyngeal diphtheria is a more severe form of the disease. Initially there is anorexia, malaise, low-grade fever and pharyngitis, followed in 1–2 days by the appearance of a white-grey adherent membrane covering the tonsils, uvula, pharynx and larynx. Cervical adenitis is sometimes noted with tissue oedema (bull neck) (**Fig. 3.2**). Laryngeal diphtheria may present as a croup-like illness. Complications of diphtheria include respiratory obstruction, myocarditis (second week of illness), thrombocytopenia and neuritis (vocal cord palsy, Guillain-Barré syndrome), which occurs after several weeks.

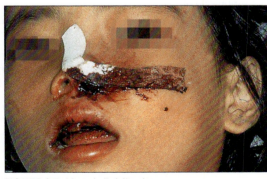

FIGURE 3.1 Nasal diphtheria.

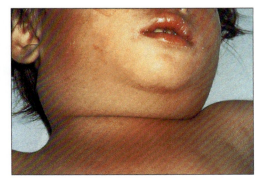

FIGURE 3.2 Diphtheria, showing bull neck.

Diphtheria

43

DIAGNOSIS

Definitive diagnosis depends on isolation of the organism. Loeffler's media is an effective enrichment media that is often used. Cultures should be obtained from the nose and throat (from beneath the membrane). Strains should then be tested for toxigenicity, i.e. production of diphtheria toxin by the use of antitoxin membrane immunoprecipitin technique (Elek test).

TREATMENT

Equine diphtheria antitoxin should be given as soon as possible. The dose prescribed depends on the site and size of the diphtheric membrane, degree of toxicity and duration of the illness (severe disease – 80,000 U). The preferred route of administration is IV; however, before this is given, tests for sensitivity to horse serum should be performed. Penicillin or erythromycin is also given for 14 days to eradicate the organism, stop toxin production and to prevent transmission, but it is not a substitute for antitoxin. General supportive measures are also important (bed rest, hydration, serial ECG, suction of secretions).

PROGNOSIS

Overall mortality is around 10% (mainly in resource poor countries). The more extensive the diphtheric membrane, the more severe the disease. Delayed treatment is also associated with an increased mortality.

PREVENTION

Prevention is carried out by active immunisation. Booster doses of toxoid should be given every 10 years. Patients recovering from the disease should be vaccinated.

TETANUS

INCIDENCE

Tetanus is an acute, spastic paralytic illness historically called lockjaw that is caused by the neurotoxin produced by *Clostridium tetani*. The disease occurs world-wide but is more frequent in resource poor countries and in hot climates. In developed countries, tetanus is usually seen in older individuals (>60 years), following waning of immunity. A high incidence of neonatal tetanus occurs in those countries with low immunisation rates and no vaccination programmes of pregnant women.

AETIOLOGY/PATHOGENESIS

C tetani is a gram-positive, motile rod which under certain environmental conditions forms spores that remain in soil for years. In the presence of tissue injury and low oxygen tension, contaminating spores change into vegetative forms. They multiply and produce a specific toxin (tetanospasmin) that affects the motor nerve endings, spinal cord, brain and sympathetic nervous system. This results in the onset of spasms and sympathetic dysfunction.

CLINICAL PRESENTATION

Tetanus is seen in two forms, generalised or local. The most common presentation is the generalised form, which manifests as trismus (tonic spasms of the masseter muscles/risus sardonicus) (**Fig. 3.3**) in over 50% of the cases. Other manifestations may include irritability, difficulty in swallowing and rigidity of abdominal muscles. Slight external stimuli may precipitate a sudden burst of painful tonic contractions of all groups of muscles leading to the characteristic opisthotonus posture.

Local tetanus is a generally mild disease, characterised by painful rigidity of groups of muscles near the site of entry of *C tetani*. It may be an antecedent of generalised tetanus. Cephalic tetanus is a form of local tetanus that occurs following injuries to the face, scalp, neck or eye. It may also follow otitis media and tonsillectomy. Cranial nerve palsies (III, IV, VII, IX, X, XII) are commonly seen. Neonatal tetanus (**Fig. 3.4**) is a major cause of mortality in less developed countries. The disease is related to unhygienic practices carried out on the umbilical cord at birth, as well as the use of unclean instruments to cut the umbilical cord.

DIAGNOSIS

There is no specific laboratory test, although any wound should be cultured. Isolation of *C tetani* occurs in about 30% of cases. The diagnosis is usually established clinically and depends on maintaining a high index of suspicion in patients with a history of injury, signs of muscle spasm and a clear sensorium.

TREATMENT

Human tetanus immune globulin (TIG) 3000–6000 units is given as soon as possible to neutralise the effect of the toxin. Penicillin G is administered intravenously for 10 days to eradicate the toxin producing organisms. All wounds should be debrided. Supportive care includes the use of diazepam to control spasms, endotracheal intubation and ventilation and, if necessary, tracheostomy to stabilise the airways. Tetanus toxoid should be given later.

PROGNOSIS

The most important factor that influences prognosis is the quality of the supportive care. Mortality is highest in the very young and the very old. A poor outcome is associated with the onset of trismus <7 days after injury, and with onset of generalised tetanic spasms <3 days after the onset of trismus. Case fatality rates for neonatal tetanus range from <10% with intensive care facilities to >75% without it.

PREVENTION

Following the administration of a primary vaccination course, booster doses should be given every 10 years. Vaccinating unimmunised pregnant women with two doses of toxoid is highly protective against tetanus neonatorum. Tetanus prone wounds (i.e. contaminated with dirt, faeces, etc.) should be cleaned and debrided. Tetanus toxoid +/– TIG should also be administered.

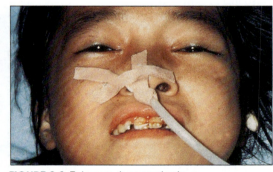

FIGURE 3.3 Tetanus: risus sardonicus.

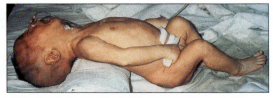

FIGURE 3.4 Neonatal tetanus.

MENINGOCOCCAL INFECTIONS

INCIDENCE

In England and Wales there were around 1800 cases of invasive meningococcal infections in 2011, with peak incidence occurring in children younger than 2 years. The case fatality rate was 10%. Meningococcal disease (MD) most commonly presents as bacterial meningitis (15% of cases), septicaemia (25% of cases) or as a combination of both (60% of cases). The disease tends to be sporadic with very occasional small outbreaks. In sub-Saharan Africa, there are regular epidemic outbreaks of disease (serogroup A), which tend to abate with the coming of the rainy season. (See, for example, http://www.cdc.gov/vaccines/pubs/pinkbook/downloads/mening.pdf.)

AETIOLOGY/PATHOGENESIS

Neisseria meningitidis is a gram-negative diplococcus. Thirteen serogroups are recognised by their different capsular polysaccharide antigen. Most disease is caused by serogroups A,B,C,Y and W-135. In the UK, due to the introduction of group C conjugate vaccine in 1999, serogroup B strains are responsible for the majority of cases of MD.

Asymptomatic carriage of meningococci in the upper respiratory tract may occur in 5–15% of the population. Humans are the only natural hosts. Transmission of meningococci occurs from person to person via respiratory droplet spread. In some individuals, meningococci are able to invade the circulation (also the meninges), with resultant release of bacterial products, including endotoxin, thereby initiating an inflammatory process. The end result is vascular endothelial damage that results in capillary leak syndrome (responsible for severe hypovolemia), and intravascular thrombosis with consequent vascular occlusion leading to extensive organ damage.

CLINICAL PRESENTATION

These may present as either meningococcaemia and/or meningitis. Meningococcaemia is usually manifested by an abrupt onset of fever, malaise and a characteristic petechial rash (**Fig. 3.5**) that may initially be maculopapular. In its most devastating form, large ecchymotic areas develop (purpura fulminans) (**Fig. 3.6**), with disseminated intravascular coagulation (DIC), shock and coma, which lead to a rapidly fatal outcome, despite appropriate therapy. The presentation of meningococcal meningitis is much the same as other forms of meningitis with fever, headache, vomiting and neck stiffness. Complications of invasive meningococcal disease include arthritis, pericarditis, endophthalmitis and pneumonia.

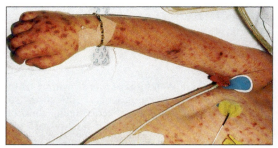

FIGURE 3.5 Meningococcal infections demonstrating petechial rash.

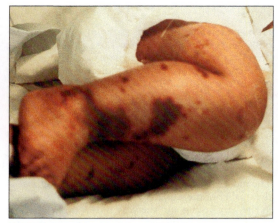

FIGURE 3.6 Meningococcal infection with disseminated intravascular coagulation.

DIAGNOSIS

A clinical diagnosis should be made. Blood and/or CSF cultures may be positive: blood cultures tend to be positive in 50% of cases, while CSF cultures are positive in 70%. Whole blood polymerase chain reaction (PCR) test for *N meningitidis* should also be obtained; this is a very sensitive test, especially in cases where antibiotics have been given. Cultures of petechial scrapings do not add anything to obtaining blood culture and a PCR test. Sensitivity is a problem with latex agglutination tests to detect antigen in CSF, serum and urine.

TREATMENT

Early recognition, initiation of antibiotic therapy (intramuscular or IV benzylpenicillin 1200 mg for children >10 years of age, 600 mg for those aged from 1–9 years, and 300 mg for those younger than 1 year) and prompt referral to hospital is essential for a good outcome. Inpatient treatment consists of initial empiric therapy with IV cefotaxime or ceftriaxone, until confirmation of the aetiology of the invasive disease; these antibiotics can be continued for the full course of treatment (7 days). Patients should be admitted to the Paediatric Intensive Care Unit (PICU), and elective ventilation may be required for severely ill patients. Hypovolaemic shock, manifested by cold peripheries, poor capillary refill, tachycardia and oliguria should be corrected promptly with boluses of IV fluid (colloids or crystalloids). Treat any raised intracranial pressure. Correction of DIC and maintenance of the circulation are also priorities.

PROGNOSIS

Mortality has fallen in recent years, but is higher in patients with shock.

PREVENTION

All household contacts (apart from pregnant women) should receive rifampicin 10 mg/kg twice daily for 2 days. Day-care contacts and healthcare personnel in close contact with an index case should also be considered for rifampin prophylaxis. Other antibiotics used for chemoprophylaxis include ceftriaxone and ciprofloxacin.

The specific serogroup vaccine has also been administered to control outbreaks of serogroup A and C strains (i.e. Group A + C vaccine, and the Group A,C,Y,W-135 combined vaccine). Travellers to epidemic areas in Africa/Asia should be vaccinated with one of the combined meningococcal vaccines prior to departure. As of November 1999, a meningococcal group C conjugate vaccine has been introduced into the immunisation schedule in the UK with spectacular success. Meningococcal group B vaccines have now been released.

TUBERCULOSIS

INCIDENCE

There has been a dramatic resurgence of tuberculosis (TB) worldwide. In developed countries, this increase is strongly associated with poverty, homelessness, urban overcrowding, the AIDS pandemic, the breakdown in TB control programmes and the increase in the number of immigrants from areas of high endemicity. In the UK there are currently 8,000 cases notified annually, with around 500 paediatric cases per year.

AETIOLOGY/PATHOGENESIS

Mycobacterium tuberculosis, an acid-fast bacillus, is the major cause of human TB. Transmission occurs via inhalation of droplet particles, usually from an adult with 'open' pulmonary TB (cavitary TB). The inhaled organisms multiply in alveolar macrophages and spread via lymphatics to regional lymph nodes. The primary complex (Ghon) consists of local disease at the portal of entry and the involved regional lymph nodes.

While this is developing, some tubercle bacilli spread via the bloodstream to establish metastatic infection in the lungs, reticuloendothelial system and various other organs. After 6–8 weeks, cell-mediated immunity develops (skin test conversion), and is usually followed by progressive healing of infected foci. In a small proportion of patients, symptomatic disease will develop at the time of primary infection. In general, complications in children occur commonly within 6–12 months after initial infection.

CLINICAL PRESENTATION

Most children infected with *M tuberculosis* are asymptomatic. Clinical manifestations of tuberculous disease may occur 1–6 months after infection. Patients may present with radiographic abnormalities consistent with hilar or mediastinal lymphadenopathy, cervical adenitis, pulmonary involvement (atelectasis, consolidation, pleural effusion) (**Figs 3.7, 3.8**), miliary disease (**Fig. 3.9**) or meningitis. Later manifestations may include bone and joint involvement, renal and cutaneous disease. The classic symptoms of TB of fever, night sweats, and loss of weight are rare in young children. Extrapulmonary disease occurs in around 25% of patients.

DIAGNOSIS

Definitive diagnosis is made via the identification and isolation of *M tuberculosis* from early morning gastric aspirates or from other normally sterile body fluids (CSF, pleural fluid, urine, sputum). Recovery of organisms may take up to 10 weeks by conventional methods; using the BACTEC radiometric system, this can be reduced to 2 weeks. Newer more rapid methods of diagnosis, including PCR and the use of DNA probes, are available. A positive tuberculin skin test (Mantoux reaction >10 mm induration) is suggestive of either infection in an asymptomatic individual, or disease in a symptomatic patient.

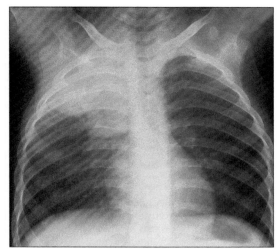

FIGURE 3.7 Tuberculosis: pulmonary involvement.

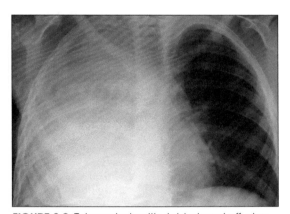

FIGURE 3.8 Tuberculosis with right pleural effusion.

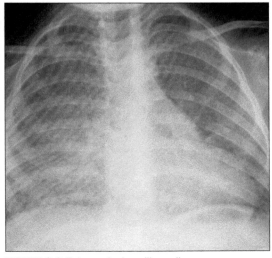

FIGURE 3.9 Tuberculosis; miliary disease.

Interferon-gamma release assays (IGRAs) are also being increasingly used and measure interferon-gamma production from T-lymphocytes in response to stimulation from antigens that are fairly specific for *M tuberculosis* complex. Thus they have been mainly introduced to either replace tuberculin skin tests (TST), or to exclude false-positive TST due to BCG or non-tuberculous mycobacteria.

TREATMENT

It is important to differentiate between infection and disease. Asymptomatic tuberculin positive cases with normal chest x-rays (infection) are treated with isoniazid (INH) 10 mg/kg for 6–9 months (chemoprophylaxis). Some authorities recommend 3 months of INH and rifampicin as chemoprophylaxis. Pulmonary disease, including TB adenitis, requires short-course chemotherapy which consists of a 2-month course of INH (10 mg/kg), rifampicin (15 mg/kg) and pyrazinamide (30 mg/kg) and ethambutol (15 mg/kg), followed by INH and rifampicin for a further 4 months. Miliary TB and TB meningitis are treated for a total of 12 months (2 months with 4 drugs, 10 months with 2 drugs).

PROGNOSIS

Although overall some 10% of patients infected with *M tuberculosis* will develop disease, this is more likely to occur in young infants. 45% of infected infants younger than 1 year will develop disease, 25% of those aged 1–5 years, and 15% of those aged 11–15 years. Mortality rates in children are around 0.6%.

PREVENTION

In some trials, vaccination with BCG has been thought to reduce the risk of childhood infection and disseminated disease (miliary and TB meningitis) by up to 60%. Screening the contacts of TB-infected patients is an essential public health measure. A baseline chest x-ray and TST (or IGRA) are performed, and in patients with a high risk of developing disease (e.g. an immunocompromised host or young infant) preventive therapy with INH is started. Chest x-rays and TST (or IGRA) tests are repeated after 3 months and, if there is no evidence of infection, INH is stopped.

TUBERCULOUS MENINGITIS

INCIDENCE

Tuberculous meningitis (TBM) constitutes 2–3 % of total TB cases. It is characteristically a disease of infants and children. The disease usually develops within 3–6 months of the primary infection. There is often a history of recent contact with an adult who has active TB.

AETIOLOGY/PATHOGENESIS

The organism is *M tuberculosis*, an acid-fast bacillus. Central nervous system (CNS) infection occurs following haematogenous spread from a primary focus in the lungs. Metastatic caseous lesions develop in cerebral tissue or in the meninges. These subsequently 'discharge' tubercle bacilli into the subarachnoid space resulting in meningitis and characterised by the formation of a thick gelatinous exudate at the base of the brain. In severe cases this invariably leads to obstructive hydrocephalus, generalised thrombophlebitis and infarction. Meningitis may also occur as part of a disseminated miliary TB and is found in 30–50% of such cases.

CLINICAL PRESENTATION

Presentation is usually subacute over a number of weeks with weight loss, anorexia, pallor, night sweats and low-grade fever, the non-specific early symptoms. These are subsequently followed by the appearance of CNS manifestations: headache, vomiting, neck stiffness, seizures and deterioration of conscious level. Focal neurological signs may be present and usually involve cranial nerves, III, IV and VII, as well as the appearance of pyramidal tract signs. The MRC has proposed a classification of disease on presentation which is related to prognosis:

- Stage I: conscious, non-specific symptoms.
- Stage II: some depression of conscious state.
- Stage III: coma, focal neurological signs.

DIAGNOSIS

Cerebrospinal fluid (CSF) changes include a pleocytosis with predominant lymphocytosis, low CSF sugar and high protein. CSF culture for acid-fast bacilli (AFB) is positive in 50% of cases. Commercial PCR tests to demonstrate specific DNA sequences of *M tuberculosis* may be helpful. CT scans of the brain invariably show hydrocephalus (**Fig. 3.10**), basilar enhancement or tuberculoma formation (**Fig. 3.11**). The chest x-ray may show abnormalities in half of the cases, while the Mantoux test may only be positive in 30% of cases.

TREATMENT

INH 10 mg/kg/day and rifampicin 10–15 mg/kg/day are given for a total of 1 year. Pyrazinamide 30 mg/kg/day and ethambutol 15 mg/kg/day (streptomycin may be given instead) are also given for the first 2 months. There is some evidence that steroids are beneficial and these should be administered for the first 4–6 weeks. Early surgical intervention, in the form of placement of a ventriculoperitoneal (V-P) shunt or external ventricular drain, may be required for management of hydrocephalus and severe disease.

PROGNOSIS

The outcome is better when treatment is initiated early in the disease. Before the advent of anti-TB therapy, TBM was uniformly fatal. Morbidity and mortality are worst for Stage III patients, among whom there is approximately 50% mortality with 60–70% having neurological sequelae.

Stage II patients have a cure rate of around 85%, with some 50% of survivors having some sequelae. For Stage I patients, cure rates are high, with relatively little in the way of sequelae.

PREVENTION

BCG vaccination is helpful in reducing the risk of this serious complication of TB.

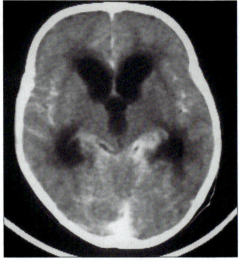

FIGURE 3.10 Tuberculous meningitis. CT scan showing hydrocephalus.

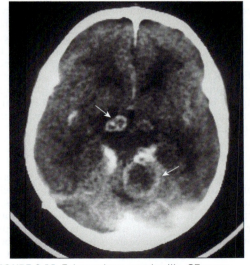

FIGURE 3.11 Tuberculous meningitis. CT scan showing tuberculoma formation.

NON-TUBERCULOUS MYCOBACTERIAL INFECTIONS

INCIDENCE

More than 50 species of non-tuberculous myco-bacterial (NTM) infections have been implicated in human disease. There is marked variation of disease incidence in different geographical regions. In developed countries, NTMs are more common, than infection due to *M tuberculosis*. In less developed countries, chronic cervical adenitis is most often due to *M tuberculosis*.

AETIOLOGY/PATHOGENESIS

Non-tuberculous mycobacteria are acid fast bacilli (AFB), the most common species in children being *M avium-intracellulare*, *M marinum* and *M scrofulaceum*. The organisms are ubiquitous and are found in soil, food and water. Transmission results from environmental acquisition by inhalation or ingestion (lymphadenitis and pulmonary diseases) or direct contact (cutaneous and soft tissue diseases) from a contaminated source. There is no person-to-person spread. The disease causes a granulomatous reaction and subsequent symptoms at the portal of entry or in regional lymph nodes.

CLINICAL PRESENTATION

The most common presentation is the development of chronic localised lymphadenopathy, usually unilateral, and in the form of a neck lump. Affected nodes tend to be in the anterior cervical chain and submandibular area (less commonly there is involvement of the pre-auricular, postauricular and submental lymph nodes). The affected nodes are usually firm, painless and may be fixed to underlying tissues. They often develop an overlying, superficial, dark reddish or purplish hue (**Fig. 3.12**). The natural history is for fluctuance to develop with eventual chronic discharging sinus formation and scarring. Occasional low-grade fever may be present but no other constitutional symptoms are usually seen. Some children may present with either bony involvement, cutaneous disease or lung disease. Disseminated disease, characterised by multiple

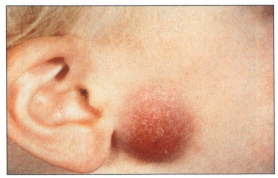

FIGURE 3.12 Non-tuberculous mycobacterial infection with lymphadenopathy.

49

organ (lung, liver and spleen) and bony involvement, persistent fever and failure to thrive, may be seen in immunocompromised patients (**Fig. 3.13**), including patients infected with human immunodeficiency virus (HIV).

DIAGNOSIS

Isolation and identification of non-tuberculous AFB from specimens taken from sterile sites such as blood, CSF, bone marrow or lymph node aspirate is required for a definitive diagnosis. A positive Mantoux test of less than 10 mm of induration is suggestive of NTM in a child with a negative chest x-ray and negative family history of TB. Cases with disseminated disease should be evaluated for immunodeficiency.

TREATMENT

Complete surgical excision of involved lymph nodes is the definitive treatment for non-tuberculous lymphadenitis. If this is not possible, then a period of antituberculous chemotherapy may be necessary (up to 6 months usually). Pending results of sensitivity testing, a regimen of clarithromycin 15 mg/kg/day and rifampicin 10 mg/kg/day, with or without ethambutol 15 mg/kg/day, is often used.

Management of cutaneous disease and disease at other sites may also require both chemotherapy and surgical debridement. Triple or quadruple antituberculous therapy (macrolide, rifampicin, ethambutol, quinolone +/– amikacin) is generally indicated for disseminated disease in immunocompromised patients.

PREVENTION

Human-to-human transmission does not occur, hence no isolation precautions are necessary. Patients with HIV and low CD4 counts may benefit from long-term clarithromycin prophylaxis. All patients with severe immunodeficiency may also benefit from the use of sterilised/boiled water, as water-borne transmission of organisms may occur.

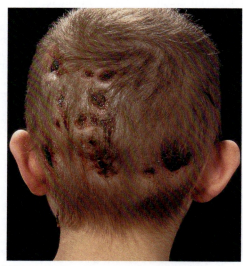

FIGURE 3.13 Non-tuberculous mycobacterial infection affecting the skull.

PROGNOSIS

Most infections involving lymph nodes, even if untreated, eventually resolve, although with disfiguring scarring. Disseminated disease in immunocompromised patients may be fatal if not treated with combination chemotherapeutic agents.

CAT-SCRATCH DISEASE

INCIDENCE

Cat-scratch disease (CSD) tends to occur over the autumn and winter periods. There are about 100 confirmed cases/year in the UK, but this is an underestimate of the true incidence of the disease. It mainly occurs in children and adolescents, and is a common cause of benign regional lymphadenopathy.

AETIOLOGY/PATHOGENESIS

Bartonella henselae is the causative organism causing CSD. It is a fastidious, slow-growing, pleomorphic, gram-negative bacillus. It can also cause bacillary angiomatosis and bacillary peliosis, occurring mainly in HIV patients. Cats are the natural reservoir for the bacillus, and in 90% of cases of CSD there is a history of close contact with cats or kittens.

Cat-to-cat transmission occurs via cat fleas. There is no evidence of person-to-person transmission

CLINICAL PRESENTATION

A cat scratch inoculates the bacteria into the skin. After about 10 days, a small papule (**Fig. 3.14**) appears at the site of the scratch. Localised lymphadenopathy (**Fig. 3.15**) then appears some 2 weeks after the primary lesion. Scratches generally occur over the hands, arms or legs, and subsequent involvement of the axillary, cervical, epitrochlear or inguinal nodes may occur. The area over the enlarged nodes is generally warm, red and tender. Around 30% of patients have systemic symptoms which may include fever, malaise, headaches and anorexia. CSD can present as a fever of unknown origin, and there may be granulomatous involvement of the liver and spleen (**Fig. 3.16**). Complications can also include the development of an encephalopathy, aseptic meningitis, optic neuritis, osteomyelitis and Parinaud syndrome (granulomatous conjunctivitis with ipsilateral adenopathy).

DIAGNOSIS

A lymph node biopsy, early in the disease, classically shows lymphocytic infiltration with epithelioid granuloma formation(**Fig. 3.17**); later this is replaced with neutrophilic infiltrates, and necrotic granulomas. *B henselae* may be seen in the biopsy specimen on Warthin–Starry silver stain. Antibody tests (IFA) are useful for diagnosing CSD. PCR assays are available for testing pleural and CSF samples.

TREATMENT

Most children require no treatment and get better over a period of time (2–4 months). Some authorities recommend a 5-day course of azithromycin.

Patients with systemic symptoms, especially patients with hepatosplenic involvement, or immunocompromised patients are treated with antibiotics. Macrolides, ciprofloxacin, septrin, rifampcin and parenteral gentamicin have all been used and are reasonably effective. The optimal duration of therapy is not known; however in immunocompromised patients treatment may be required for several months to prevent relapses.

PROGNOSIS

Complete recovery usually occurs in 2–4 months. The disease tends to be more severe in immunocompromised patients, and treatment with antibiotics is required; patients usually experience full resolution of disease.

PREVENTION

Immunocompromised patients should avoid close contact with cats. Cat scratches should be immediately washed. After playing with a cat, hands should be washed thoroughly. It is important that care of cats should include flea control.

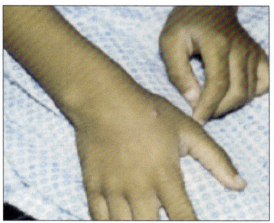

FIGURE 3.14 Cat-scratch disease with a papule at the site of the scratch.

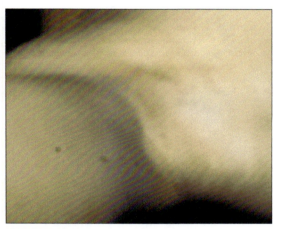

FIGURE 3.15 Cat-scratch disease with axillary lymphadenopathy.

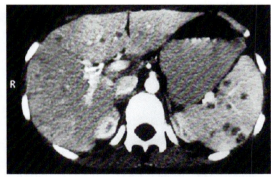

FIGURE 3.16 Cat-scratch disease with granulomas of liver and spleen.

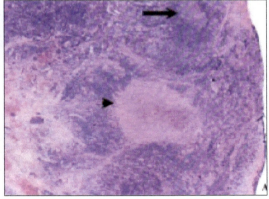

FIGURE 3.17 Cat-scratch disease. Biopsy showing epithelioid granuloma formation.

LYME DISEASE

INCIDENCE

In England and Wales, Lyme disease is the commonest vector-borne human infection and in 2010 there were 905 cases identified (incidence of 1.64/100000 population). The cases reported were most commonly in the summer and early autumn. About 18% of cases reported had a history of overseas travel; most were holidaymakers who presented with symptoms after visiting North America (15%) and countries in continental Europe (85%), many of which have considerably higher local incidence rates than are found in England and Wales.

AETIOLOGY/PATHOGENESIS

Lyme disease is caused by the spirochaete *Borrelia burgdorferi*. Transmission usually occurs from tick vectors (usually *Ixodes* species in Northern Europe). Tick bites usually need to be longer than 24 hours for human infection to occur. The incubation period is 3–20 days with a median of 12 days.

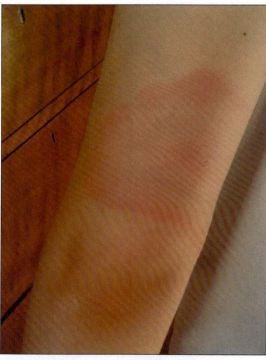

FIGURE 3.18 Lyme disease with erythema migrans rash.

CLINICAL PRESENTATION

The clinical presentations of Lyme borreliosis vary widely and are often divided into different stages, namely early localised, early disseminated and late disease. Early localised disease usually has a distinctive rash called erythema migrans (EM) occurring at the site of a recent tick bite. The typical EM lesion begins as a red macule at the site of the tick bite with a slow expansion over weeks with central clearing **(Fig. 3.18)**. Other features that may accompany the rash include fever, malaise, headache, neck stiffness, myalgia and arthalgia. Early disseminated disease is characterised by multiple erythematous skin lesions usually accompanied by other features including cranial nerve palsies, lymphocytic meningitis and conjunctivitis. Late disease is characterised by relapsing arthritis, most commonly pauciarticular and affecting the large joints.

DIAGNOSIS

Serological testing is the most useful diagnostic test, although these tests may be negative in the first few weeks of infection.

In the UK, the Lyme Borreliosis Unit of Public Health England uses a two-stage procedure, the first being an enzyme immune assay (EIA) screen followed by an immunoblot or western blot to confirm antibodies.

TREATMENT

Early localised disease and early disseminated disease can usually be treated with doxycycline (in children >12 years) or amoxicillin orally for 14–21 days. Clarithromycin can be used where there is a definite history of penicillin allergy. IV ceftriaxone is recommended for CNS involvement for 2–4 weeks duration.

PROGNOSIS

The majority of children make a full recovery with no long-term sequelae.

PREVENTION

Tick bite prevention by wearing long trousers and shirts and insect repellents are recommended when walking in the woods in endemic areas. Prompt and appropriate removal of ticks using tweezers is also recommended. Prophylactic antibiotics after tick bites are not routinely indicated and depend on local epidemiological factors.

Infectious diseases

PYOGENIC LIVER ABSCESS

INCIDENCE

Although rare in childhood, pyogenic liver abscess tends to occur in younger children and in those with underlying disease (e.g. immunodeficiency, biliary atresia, chronic inflammatory bowel disease and haemoglobinopathies). In one autopsy series, the incidence was 38 per 1000 in children under 15 years of age. Retrospective hospital series suggest lower incidences of 3 per 100,000.

AETIOLOGY/PATHOGENESIS

In around 50% of cases, the aetiology is polymicrobial with gram-positive cocci (*Staphylococcus aureus*, streptococci, 33% of isolates), enteric gram-negative bacilli (33%), and anaerobes as the predominant agents.

Most cases in children follow systemic haematogenous spread (80%), and usually occur in those with abnormalities of host defence. About 10–15% occur following portal vein inflammation and bacteraemia, secondary to appendicitis/peritonitis or chronic inflammatory bowel disease. A small number either follow extension of infection from contiguous structures (e.g. from biliary tract as in ascending cholangitis), or are cryptogenic in origin.

CLINICAL PRESENTATION

Often presents with non-specific manifestations such as fever, nausea, vomiting, anorexia, malaise and abdominal pain. A pyrexia of unknown origin (PUO) with abdominal pain should alert the practitioner to the possibility of a liver abscess, especially in an immunocompromised patient (e.g. chronic granulomatous disease). Hepatomegaly is present in more than half the patients although jaundice is uncommon.

DIAGNOSIS

Ultrasound and CT scanning are used initially as non-invasive diagnostic techniques. On CT scan, liver abscesses appear as areas of low attenuation (**Fig. 3.19**), and should differentiate from hydatid cysts. Amoebic liver abscesses are an important differential diagnosis (although they tend to be a single, solitary abscess) and need to be excluded by obtaining serum antibody titres to *Entamoeba histolytica*.

A microbiological diagnosis is made, following culture of fluid/pus obtained from either needle aspiration (for multiple abscesses) (**Fig. 3.20**) or percutaneous drainage in the case of a single solitary abscess. Blood cultures may be positive in some cases. Other laboratory features include an elevated white cell count, anaemia, and a raised ESR; abnormal LFTs are unusual.

TREATMENT

For the single solitary liver abscess, percutaneous needle aspiration and drainage (pigtail catheter placed into the abscess cavity under CT scan guidance) and antibiotic therapy for 6 weeks is the treatment of choice. Multiple liver abscesses are more difficult to treat as drainage is not possible; diagnostic aspiration, however, is often performed and prolonged antibiotic therapy (intravenously for 2–4 weeks) for 3–4 months is necessary, as well as the treatment of any underlying disease. Initial antibiotic combinations used for liver abscesses include:

- Piptazobactam/amikacin.
- Penicillin/gentamicin/metronidazole.
- Clindamycin/gentamicin.

PROGNOSIS

Mortality from undrained and untreated lesions tends to be high (up to 100%). However, since the introduction of percutaneous aspiration and drainage techniques, mortality in some adult series has fallen appreciably (around 20%). Complications that may occur include peritoneal spillage, haemorrhage and spread to other organs (e.g. empyema).

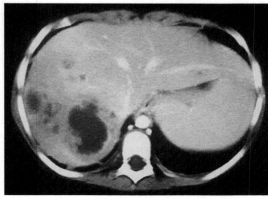

FIGURE 3.19 Pyogenic liver abscess. Appearance on CT scanning.

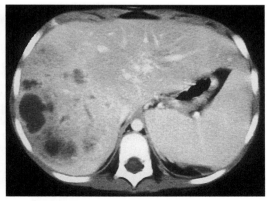

FIGURE 3.20 Appearance of CT scan of the patient in **3.19** after contrast enhancement, showing multiple liver abscesses.

STAPHYLOCOCCAL TOXIC SHOCK SYNDROME

INCIDENCE

Although initially described in children in the USA, most cases of staphylococcal toxic shock syndrome (TSS) occurred in young menstruating women using tampons. Over the last two decades, the number of cases of menstrual TSS has steadily declined; 50% of cases of TSS are not associated with menstruation. Non-menstrual cases have been associated with cutaneous or subcutaneous lesions, surgical wound infections, and other focal staphylococcal infection.

AETIOLOGY/PATHOGENESIS

The most common aetiologic agent is toxic shock syndrome toxin-1 (TSST-1)- producing strains of *S aureus*. Often the *S aureus* is merely a coloniser of a body site and does not cause a focal infection. The toxin produced has superantigen properties and is able to cause widespread activation of the immune system with consequent endothelial damage. This results in multi-system organ damage secondary to capillary leak syndrome, loss of intravascular volume and tone, and interstitial oedema.

CLINICAL PRESENTATION

An acute febrile illness characterised by the onset of a diffuse macular rash, mucositis (**Fig. 3.21**), myalgia, gastrointestinal symptoms, hypotension and often multi-organ system dysfunction including renal failure. A flaky desquamation of the trunk (**Fig. 3.22**) begins after 7 days, followed by involvement of the palms and soles.

DIAGNOSIS

Diagnosis is based on established clinical criteria. Typically, fever, rash, myalgia, headache, diarrhoea and vomiting, along with hypotension, occur on day 1. These signs and symptoms are followed on days 2–3 by mucositis and mental confusion, and later by skin desquamation. Laboratory abnormalities usually include anaemia, clotting derangements, thrombocytopenia, elevated creatinine phosphokinase (CPK), and in some patients evidence of liver and/or kidney damage. Isolates of *S aureus* (from superficial and potential infected sites) should be examined for their ability to produce TSST-1.

TREATMENT

This consists of management of the multi-system organ failure, antibiotic therapy with an antistaphylococcal agent, and eradicating the source of toxin production (removal of any foreign body and/or irrigation of wound). Due to the severe capillary leak, fluid replacement in excess of 150–200 ml/kg may be required to restore intravascular volume. The addition of clindamycin may be useful, as it may have an effect on decreasing toxin production. There is a role for IV immunoglobulin and this agent should be considered in any severely ill patient. Steroids are of uncertain value.

PROGNOSIS

TSS can be a serious and even fatal disorder. With treatment, the mortality is in the order of 3%. Death is usually due to myocardial or pulmonary failure.

PREVENTION

To lower the risk of menstrual TSS, changing tampons at least every 8 hours is recommended. Localised staphylococcal infections should be treated.

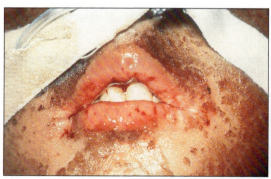

FIGURE 3.21 Staphylococcal toxic shock syndrome with mucositis.

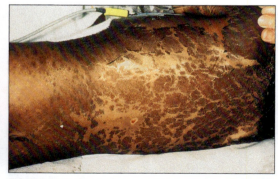

FIGURE 3.22 Staphylococcal toxic shock syndrome with flaky desquamation of the trunk.

TULARAEMIA

INCIDENCE

Tularaemia does not naturally occur in the UK, but can be found in several countries in Europe and in North America.

AETIOLOGY/PATHOGENESIS

Tularaemia is a zoonosis caused by the bacterium *Francisella tularensis*, a gram-negative pleomorphic coccobacillus. The source of the organism is usually wild animals (e.g. rabbits, hares, rats, voles and other rodents), some domestic animals (e.g. sheep, cattle), blood-sucking arthropods that bite these animals (e.g. ticks) and water and soil contaminated by infected animals. People at greatest risk of infection are those with occupational or recreational exposure to infected animals or their habitats.

The incubation period is usually 3–5 days, with a range of 1–21 days. Organisms may be present in blood during the first 2 weeks of disease and in cutaneous lesions for as long as 1 month if not treated. Person-to-person transmission does not occur.

CLINICAL PRESENTATION

Most patients with tularaemia present with fever, chills, myalgia and headache. The commonest presentation is the ulceroglandular syndrome (maculopapular lesion at site of entry with subsequent ulceration and painful regional lymphnodes). The glandular syndrome (regional lymphadenopathy with no ulcer) can also occur **(Fig. 3.23)**. Other clinical syndromes that may occur less commonly include oculoglandular (severe conjuncitivitis and lymphadenopathy), oropharyngeal (severe stomatitis, phayringitis or tonsillitis), vesicular skin lesions (often mistake for herpes simplex or varicella zoster infection), typhoidal, intestinal and pneumonic.

DIAGNOSIS

Diagnosis is established through serological testing. A single serum antibody titre of 1:128 or greater by microagglutination (or 1:160 by tube agglutination) is consistent with recent or past infection. Confirmation by serological testing requires a fourfold or greater titre change between two serum samples at least 2 weeks apart.

Identification of the organism directly from ulcers or exudate using direct fluorescent antibody or PCR assays has also been used. *F tularensis* may also be isolated on culture (usually cysteine-enriched media) from specimens of blood, skin, ulcers, lymph node drainage or respiratory secretions.

TREATMENT

Antibiotic therapy with an aminoglycoside (streptomycin, gentamicin or amikacin) for 10 days is usually recommended. Longer courses of treatment may be needed for severe disease. Alternative drugs for less severe disease include ciprofloxacin, doxycycline (children >12 years) or chloramphenicaol. These drugs are associated with a prompt clinical response, but relapses may occur especially with tetracyclines.

PROGNOSIS

Usually good prognosis with prompt antibiotic therapy.

PREVENTION

Bite and contact prevention recommended, particularly for those at high risk of exposure.

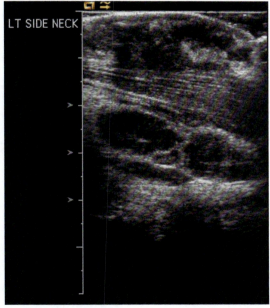

FIGURE 3.23 Tularaemia. Ultrasound of the neck showing glandular syndrome.

VIRUSES

HIV INFECTION AND AIDS

AETIOLOGY/PATHOGENESIS

HIV infection is due to a human RNA retrovirus (usually HIV-1, less commonly HIV-2), which is trophic for CD4 T-lymphocytes. Transmission is via one of three routes:

- Perinatal infection.
- Transfusion of infected blood products.
- Sexual transmission.

The virus is able to integrate its genome into the host's genome (mainly in CD4 cells) through the action of reverse transcriptase enzyme. There follows a long incubation period (around 10 years in adults) prior to the development of symptoms. It is now known that viral expression and replication are occurring continuously during this period; hence there is also a large turnover of CD4 cells to compensate. The eventual consequences of infection are a gradual CD4 T-cell depletion and a mainly cell-mediated immunodeficiency. With the occurrence of a major opportunistic infection or cancer (AIDS-defining illness), the diagnosis is then one of AIDS.

INCIDENCE

The WHO estimates that in 2011, 34 million people world-wide were living with HIV (3.4 million children), the majority being in sub-Saharan Africa. In the UK, as of 2011, more than 1,600 children were known to have been infected with HIV. In the Inner London area, it has been estimated that 1 in 250 pregnant women are HIV-infected. The perinatal transmission rate varies from 1% to 15% in the UK, depending on whether interventions to prevent vertically-acquired HIV infection are taken up by mothers during pregnancy and the perinatal period.

CLINICAL PRESENTATION

In infants receiving no antiretroviral treatment, the majority are asymptomatic for the first few years of life. Generalised lymphadenopathy, hepatosplenomegaly, failure to thrive, parotitis (**Fig. 3.24**) and lymphocytic interstitial pneumonitis are often seen in combination when children become symptomatic. Around 25% of children, however, present in the first year with an AIDS-defining illness (PCP, recurrent bacterial infections, HIV encephalopathy, CMV retinitis, etc.). The situation has changed dramatically in developed countries where HIV infection has moved from being a fatal condition to a chronic one. With widespread antenatal HIV testing of pregnant women, and institution of early antiretroviral therapy for infected infants, infants and children on highly active antiretroviral therapy (HAART) are not developing opportunistic infections or symptomatic disease, as described above, and are surviving well into adulthood.

DIAGNOSIS

A positive HIV antibody test (ELISA) is diagnostic of HIV infection in children over 18 months. In younger infants, because placentally transmitted antibody may persist for up to 18 months, the diagnosis is usually made by a plasma HIV RNA PCR test. By using repeated tests, most children can be diagnosed by the age of 3–4 months. An infant is considered infected if two separate samples are positive, the first taken at 1–2 months and the second taken at 3–4 months. Other laboratory findings may show low CD4 cells (both absolute percentage and total number), lymphopenia, hypergammaglobulinaemia and thrombocytopenia.

AIDS-DEFINING ILLNESS

Pneumocystis pneumonia

This is the most common AIDS-defining illness occurring in up to 30% of children with an AIDS diagnosis. Presentation is usually in the first year of life, often with cough, dyspnoea and tachypnoea. The chest x-ray shows an interstitial pattern of pneumonitis (**Fig. 3.25**); diagnosis is via bronchoalveolar

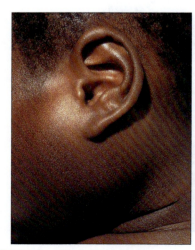

FIGURE 3.24 Parotitis in HIV infection.

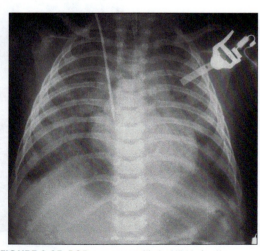

FIGURE 3.25 PCP pneumonitis in HIV infection.

lavage (BAL) with demonstration of typical proto-zoal cysts. Treatment is supportive (infants often require ventilation), along with the administration of high-dose co-trimoxazole and steroids. HIV-infected infants, in developed countries, are usually treated with prophylactic co-trimaxoazole for the first 12-months of their life. This is highly effective at preventing PCP.

Lymphocytic interstitial pneumonitis

Lymphocytic interstitial pneumonitis (LIP) presents as a slowly progressive pulmonary disorder, often with associated cough and obstructive airway symptoms. Generalised lymphadenopathy and parotitis are often common accompaniments, with the presence of digital clubbing indicating severe disease. The chest x-ray shows a reticulonodular infiltrate bilaterally (**Fig. 3.26**). Definitive diagnosis is via a lung biopsy; however, in practice a presumptive clinical diagnosis is usually made, after other causes have been excluded (especially miliary TB). LIP may be asymptomatic; the more severe forms are considered AIDS-defining. The aetiology is not known, although EBV may play a part in the pathogenesis. Treatment is symptomatic and may include bronchodilators, oxygen therapy, steroids and antiretrovirals. A common complication is superadded viral or bacterial pneumonia.

Recurrent bacterial infections

Children with HIV infection are prone to the development of recurrent bacterial infections, including bacteraemia and meningitis, due to the encapsulated organisms (pneumococcus, *Haemophilus influenzae* type b). The most common infections tend to involve the respiratory tract: pneumonia (**Fig. 3.27**), sinusitis, otitis media. Despite the hypergammaglobulinaemia, there is B-cell dysfunction and in some patients IgG2 subclass deficiency. Broad-spectrum antibiotics (third-generation cephalosporins) are given intravenously for serious disease. PCP prophylaxis with daily co-trimoxazole tends to provide some protection against recurrent bacterial infections.

Failure to thrive

This is highly prevalent in less developed countries where the malnutrition associated with AIDS is known as 'slim disease' in the adult HIV population. Due to the progressive immunodeficiency in HIV infection, gastrointestinal pathogens (e.g. *Cryptosporidium, Campylobacter, Salmonella* spp.) often initiate the damage to the gut epithelium leading to chronic diarrhoea and malnutrition. HIV infection itself is probably responsible for a malabsorptive syndrome (**Fig. 3.28**). Treatment consists of specific therapy for any enteric pathogens isolated and dietary manipulation to decrease the malabsorption and increase calorific intake through the use of an elemental formula. In some cases, continuous overnight nasogastric feeding regimens may be required to provide the necessary calories.

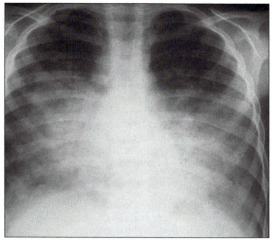

FIGURE 3.26 Reticulonodular infiltrate suggestive of LIP in HIV infection.

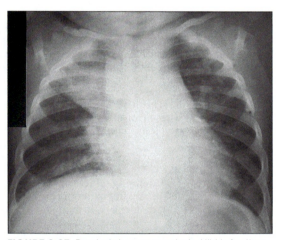

FIGURE 3.27 Bacterial pneumonia in HIV infection.

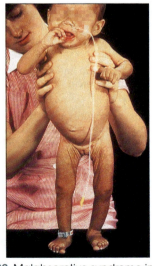

FIGURE 3.28 Malabsorptive syndrome in HIV infection.

HIV encephalopathy

A common early sign is the development of spastic diplegia. There may also be failure to achieve developmental milestones, and in the latter part of the disease, developmental regression and seizures may occur. Opportunistic infections of the CNS, common in adults, need to be excluded. CT scan findings may show cerebral atrophy (**Fig. 3.29**) or basal ganglia enhancement/calcification. Treatment with HAART may lead to some improvement, with reversal of the cognitive and neurological deficits. Without any treatment, the prognosis is bleak (median survival is 11 months).

CMV retinitis

CMV retinitis occurs in around 1–2% of untreated HIV-infected children. It is the most common paediatric ocular infection. White granular lesions with irregular borders and centred around blood vessels (haemorrhagic lesions may be present) are seen on fundoscopy (**Fig. 3.30**). It occurs as a result of systemic infection with CMV that may be otherwise asymptomatic. Young children do not usually complain of visual loss, but tend to present with bilateral ocular involvement, unless adequate screening regimens are in place that will detect early disease. Some centres screen all patients with low CD4 counts (i.e. CD4+ <100), and/or who are viraemic with CMV.

Treatment is with ganciclovir (or foscarnet, if no response). Patients, who have a degree of immune reconstitution as a result of combination antiretroviral therapy can stop long-term suppressive therapy with ganciclovir.

Kaposi's sarcoma

This is a rare AIDS-defining illness in children. It usually presents as a lymphadenopathic variant with massive enlargement of groups of lymph nodes (**Fig. 3.31**). Progressive visceral involvement may occur as well as skin infiltration (**Fig. 3.32**). Recurrent blood-stained pleural effusions, indicating pulmonary/pleural Kaposi's sarcoma, is one manifestation of visceral disease (**Fig. 3.33**). The disease is now thought to be associated with a new herpes virus (HHV-8). Treatment in children has consisted of administration of various chemotherapeutic agents:

- Vincristine, bleomycin and doxorubicin.
- Liposomal daunorubicin.
- Interferon-alpha.

These agents are mainly used for control of disease rather cure. The prognosis is generally poor in those patients with advanced immunodeficiency who have no access to HAART.

TREATMENT

Combination HAART is indicated for patients with an AIDS diagnosis, severe symptomatic disease and in patients with a progressively falling CD4 cell count (CD4 25% of total lymphocytes and/or absolute CD4 counts of fewer than $350/mm^3$). It is also indicated for all infants aged less than 12 months, regardless of clinical, immunological or virological status. HAART has

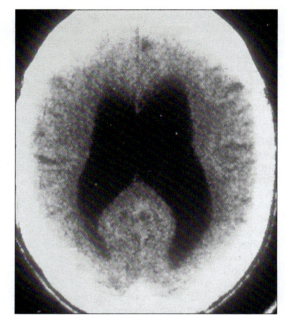

FIGURE 3.29 CT scan showing cerebral atrophy in HIV infection.

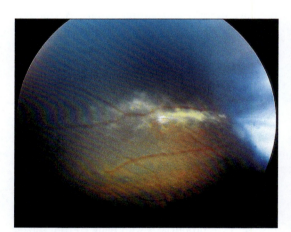

FIGURE 3.30 CMV retinitis in HIV infection.

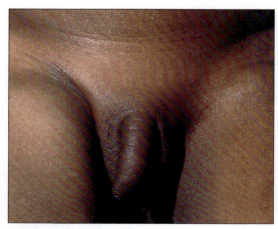

FIGURE 3.31 Kaposi's sarcoma: femoral lymphadenopathy in HIV infection.

increased survival rates, improved immune status and reduced opportunistic infections.

It is usual to start with two nucleoside reverse transcriptase inhibitors (NRTI), such as abacavir and lamivudine, as well as a boosted protease inhibitor (PI), such as lopinavir/ritonavir (kaletra), or a non-nucleoside reverse transcriptase inhibitor (NNRTIs) such as nevirapine or efavirenz. This combination would need to be changed, if or when, there was evidence of therapy failure. Prophylaxis with daily co-trimoxazole is important in the prevention of PCP, if the CD4 count is below 200/mm^3.

All immunisations are indicated in this group of patients, except perhaps BCG, which may be considered for asymptomatic children in those countries with high incidence of TB. Pneumovax, Hib vaccines and meningococcal C conjugate vaccine should also be given.

It is essential that infected children and their families receive comprehensive care that addresses both the medical and psychosocial aspects of this disease. This is best done in a 'family clinic', where both parents and children can be assessed/treated by a multi-disciplinary team that would include an adult physician, a paediatrician, psychologist, social worker, HIV counsellor, physiotherapist and dietician.

PROGNOSIS

As far as the natural history of HIV/AIDS is concerned, two patterns are seen in children with perinatally-acquired disease who have no access to HAART. In around 20–25% of patients, severe immunodeficiency develops in the first year of life with resultant severe opportunistic infections and/or encephalopathy developing. The prognosis in this group of patients is poor, with the majority dying by the age of 2 years. The other 75–80% of infected children have a slower, progressive disease, as is seen in adults. This is also the case in those HIV-infected children who acquired disease via blood products.

Since the introduction of HAART in the mid-1990s, morbidity and mortality have declined dramatically. If HIV-infected patients continue to take their HAART, it is anticipated that survival will be into late adulthood. The problem is adherence to prescribed HAART in the adolescent age group.

PREVENTION

Apart from educating teenagers with regard to the dangers of unprotected sexual intercourse, the main emphasis in preventative strategies has been to try and decrease perinatal transmission rates, through the adminstration of antiretroviral therapy to mothers during the latter part of pregnancy and the intrapartum period, and to the neonate for the first 4 weeks of life. Elective caesarian section has also been shown to exert a protective effect. When these two approaches are combined, with the avoidance of breast-feeding, HIV perinatal transmission rates can be decreased from 15–20% to 1–2%. All of this is obviously dependent on an effective antenatal screening programme being in place.

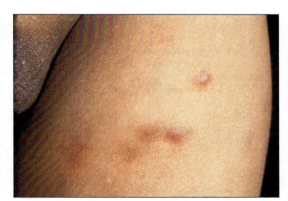

FIGURE 3.32 Kaposi's sarcoma: skin infiltration in HIV infection.

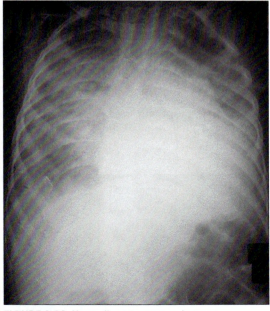

FIGURE 3.33 Kaposi's sarcoma: pulmonary involvement in HIV infection.

CONGENITAL CYTOMEGALOVIRUS

INCIDENCE

CMV is a ubiquitous virus that only infects humans. Transmission occurs horizontally (by direct person-to-person contact through secretions), vertically (from mother to child before, during or after birth) and via blood products from infected donors. Approximately 1% of all live-born infants are infected *in utero* and excrete CMV at birth, making this the most common congenital viral infection.

AETIOLOGY/PATHOGENESIS

CMV is a ubiquitous double-stranded DNA virus that causes primary infection followed by latency established in cells of myeloid lineage. Seropositivity increases with age and in populations from lower socioeconomic status. The majority of children in resource-poor countries are seropositive by 1 year of age compared with a more gradual increase. Congenital infection is thought to be transmitted from maternal blood via the placenta and is 40 times more common following primary infection in the mother during pregnancy than in those who have serological evidence of previous CMV infection.

CLINICAL PRESENTATION

Congenital CMV infection is usually asymptomatic in the majority of babies at birth; however, 10% will have features evident at birth (so-called symptomatic congenital CMV infection) that include intrauterine growth retardation, jaundice, purpura, hepatosplenomaegaly, microcephaly, intracerebral calcification **(Fig. 3.34)** and retinitis. Sensorineural hearing loss is the most common sequelae of congenital infection, occurring more often in those infants with symptomatic infection. Hearing loss may be present at birth or occur later in the first years of life. Developmental delay may also occur in some infants as they grow. In contrast with congenital infection, postnatally-acquired infection (usually acquired though breast milk) is not associated with clinical illness except in preterm infants were systemic infections can occur, including respiratory tract disease.

DIAGNOSIS

CMV infection is usually diagnosed by direct methods or by serology. Direct methods involve either direct viral culture from tissues or through CMV antigen detection either by immunofluorescence or by PCR. Serology is of limited use in those under 1 year of age but may be useful in older children. CMV IgM measurements may indicate primary infection but are only positive in around 70% of congenitally-infected infants. Identification of CMV from samples obtained within the first 3 weeks of life usually indicates congenital infection compared with postnatal infection. Dried blood spots (Guthrie card) taken shortly after birth may be used retrospectively to confirm the presence of congenital CMV using PCR.

TREATMENT

Data in neonates with symptomatic congenital CMV disease involving the central nervous system suggest possible benefit of 6 weeks of IV ganciclovir for protecting against hearing loss and potentially in decreasing developmental impairment at 1–2 years of age. Oral valganciclovir may provide the same benefits although a direct comparative study with IV ganciclovir has so far not been conducted. Antiviral therapy is not recommended routinely in asymptomatic neonates and young infants because of possible drug toxicities, particularly neutropenia. Long-term antiviral use (up to 6 months) is presently being evaluated in an international clinical trial.

PREVENTION

Evaluation of investigational vaccines in healthy volunteers is in progress and recent data from a phase II trial in pregnant women appear promising. CMV-IVIG has been developed for prophylaxis of CMV disease in transplant recipients as well as tested in pregnant women to prevent CMV transmission. However, at present the use of CMV-IVIG cannot be recommended.

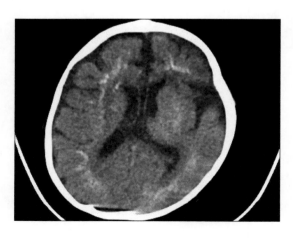

FIGURE 3.34 Congenital CMV with intracellular calcification.

INFECTIOUS MONONUCLEOSIS

INCIDENCE

Although infection usually occurs early in life (more than 90% infected), an acute primary EBV infection is usually subclinical and is not synonymous with infectious mononucleosis (IM), unless typical clinical findings are present. The incidence of IM is highest in the adolescent age group (15–24 years). The virus is excreted in the saliva and spread by direct contact (kissing disease), and typically it spreads through schools and colleges.

AETIOLOGY/PATHOGENESIS

EBV is a herpes virus that has special affinity for B-lymphocytes. Initial infection takes place in pharyngeal epithelial cells followed by spread to B-lymphocytes. In acute stages of IM, the number of infected circulating B-cells may be as high as 20%. Proliferation of EBV is regulated by natural killer cells and T-cytotoxic suppressor cells. Atypical lymphocytes represent T-lymphocytes responding to infected B cells.

CLINICAL PRESENTATION

Typical manifestations of the disease include fever, exudative pharyngitis (**Fig. 3.35**), lymphadenopathy, hepatosplenomegaly and atypical lymphocytosis. Complications include upper-airway obstruction, thrombocytopenia, jaundice, and CNS problems (aseptic meningitis, encephalitis, Guillain–Barré syndrome). EBV is associated with post-transplant lymphoproliferative disease (PTLD). In X-linked lymphoproliferative disease (Duncan disease), patients are unable to control EBV infection and may develop overwhelming infection. Burkitt B-cell lymphoma and nasopharyngeal carcinoma are associated with EBV infection in Africa and Asia, respectively.

DIAGNOSIS

Laboratory diagnosis generally rests on serology: non-specific tests such as mono-spot or the Paul-Bunnell test (heterophile antibody tests), and the more specific tests of identifying antibody against the various viral components of EBV (VCA, EA [D & R], EBNA). Acute infection is characterised by the presence of IgM against VCA. Isolation of virus from oropharyngeal secretions is possible. Quantitative PCR is routinely used in transplant recipients to detect those patients who have EBV reactivation with a view to prevention of PTLD. Non-specific laboratory changes include an absolute lymphocytosis (>10% atypical lymphocytes) often with neutropenia, rarely a haemolytic anaemia with pancytopenia and frequently raised liver enzymes.

TREATMENT

IM is a self-limited disease, hence treatment is supportive. Steroids have been shown to be beneficial in upper-airway obstruction due to tonsillar hypertrophy and adenopathy. Aciclovir has activity against EBV, but clinical trials do not show any clear benefit. Nevertheless, children with EBV-induced lymphoproliferative disease are usually initially treated with aciclovir (or ganciclovir), as well as having their immunosuppressive therapy decreased. Specific monoclonal antibodies (anti-CD20) such as rituximab have been shown to be beneficial in some groups of patients.

PROGNOSIS

Most cases of IM resolve over a period of 2–3 weeks. Death from IM is rare. It is usually the result of overwhelming infection in the immunocompromised host or as a result of complications of the disease.

FIGURE 3.35 Exudative pharyngitis in infectious mononucleosis.

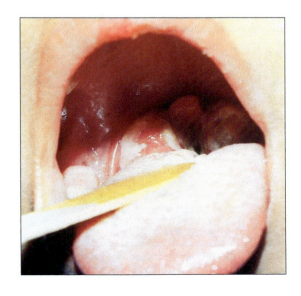

MEASLES

INCIDENCE

Prior to immunisation programmes being instituted, measles was common in childhood, with epidemics occurring every 2–3 years. More than 90% of individuals had symptomatic infection by the age of 10 years. Until the late 1990s, measles was responsible for just under 1 million deaths world-wide, mainly in resource poor countries. Since then, due to increased global immunisation programmes, the death rate from measles has decreased substantially (164,000 in 2008).

AETIOLOGY/PATHOGENESIS

Measles is caused by the measles virus, which is an RNA virus of the genus Morbillivirus, of the Paramyxoviridae family. It is transmitted by droplet infection, with the virus replicating initially in the respiratory tract. During the prodromal period, and for a short time after the rash appears, it is found in nasopharyngeal secretions, blood and urine. Patients are infectious from 4 days before the rash appears, until 4 days after its appearance. The incubation period generally is 8–12 days from exposure to the onset of symptoms.

CLINICAL PRESENTATION

Measles begins with a prodromal period of 3–5 days, which is characterised by a fever, cough, runny nose and conjunctivitis. Koplik's spots (grayish white dots) (**Fig. 3.36**) appear on the buccal mucosa opposite the upper and lower premolar teeth some 24–48 hours before the onset of rash. These are a pathognomonic exanthem of measles and may persist up to 2–3 days after the rash has appeared. The characteristic rash usually appears around the fourth day, as the fever peaks. It is an erythematous, blanching maculopapular eruption (**Fig. 3.37**) that starts at the hairline and spreads down, eventually involving the hands and feet. The rash tends to become confluent and after 2–3 days starts to fade, with clearing over 2–3 days. A brawny desquamation of the skin often follows.

DIAGNOSIS

Clinical diagnosis is based on the presence of a characteristic rash, fever, conjunctivitis, rhinitis, and cough. Salivary tests for detecting the presence of antimeasles IgM antibodies are available for confirming the diagnosis. Serologic tests (ELISA) are also used to detect IgG and IgM antibodies. A nasopharyngeal aspirate can also be used to confirm the diagnosis by performing immunofluorescence testing for the presence of measles antigen. Viral isolation is rarely performed.

COMPLICATIONS

Complications of measles include otitis media, pneumonia, laryngotracheitis and encephalitis. These may occur as a result of the primary viral illness or due to secondary bacterial invasion. Subacute sclerosing panencephalitis (SSPE) is a rare and late complication of measles infection, occurring many years after primary infection. It is characterised by the onset of gradual intellectual deterioration, inco-ordination and seizures.

TREATMENT

No specific treatment is indicated for measles, and treatment is supportive. Patients require appropriate isolation, hydration and administration of antibiotics for any secondary bacterial infections (pneumonia, otitis media). Respiratory support may be required for severe croup or pneumonia. Vitamin A should be given to children who are malnourished, vitamin A deficient or immunodeficient. Antiviral therapy (ribavirin) for giant-cell pneumonia in the immunodeficient host is not established.

PROGNOSIS

Mortality is around 1:1000 and is greatest in infants and adults.

PREVENTION

The priority is routine immunisation with MMR (2 doses, at 15 months and 4 years). In countries where measles is a problem, the first dose of vaccine can be given at 9 months. However, this dose is repeated after 12 months, due to possible lower efficacy in infants <1 year of age, due to the presence of maternal antibodies.

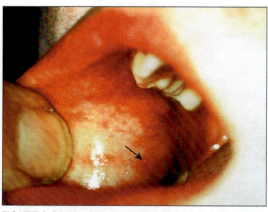

FIGURE 3.36 Koplik's spots present on the buccal mucosa.

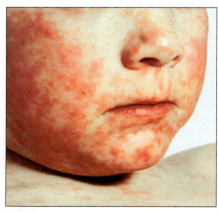

FIGURE 3.37 Measles exanthem – a blanching maculopapular eruption.

NEONATAL HERPES SIMPLEX VIRUS

INCIDENCE

Herpes simplex virus (HSV) infection of the neonate can be acquired during the intrauterine, intrapartum or postnatal period. More than 85% of cases occur following intrapartum transmission. In the UK, the incidence of neonatal HSV infection is much less than in the USA.

AETIOLOGY/PATHOGENESIS

The majority of neonatal HSV infections are due to HSV-2 (75%). Following direct exposure to the virus at delivery, the newborn will develop localised disease on the skin, eye or mouth. In some patients, infection will progress to involve the brain, perhaps by intraneuronal transmission of viral particles, or disseminated disease may occur following the development of viraemia. A higher incidence of neonatal herpes has been documented in babies born to mothers with primary infection (25–50%) as compared to recurrent genital herpes infection (2%).

CLINICAL PRESENTATION

The hallmark of infection is a vesicular eruption (clusters of vesicles on an erythematous base) on the skin (**Fig. 3.38**). Presentation is usually within the first 2–4 weeks of life, and most neonatal infections with HSV can usually be divided into one of the following categories:

- Disease localised to the skin, eyes or mouth (45%).
- Localised CNS disease (usually encephalitis) (30%).
- Disseminated disease with multiple organ involvement, including lungs and liver (25%).

Unfortunately the diagnosis can sometimes be difficult, as skin lesions may not be seen in some patients with disseminated or CNS disease. Disseminated infection may also present with a picture of severe liver dysfunction, mimicking a metabolic disorder, or primarily a sepsis syndrome.

DIAGNOSIS

HSV can be easily cultured from infected tissues. Acute and convalescent sera show rise in antibodies to HSV. Intrathecal synthesis of herpes antibodies can also be detected in HSV encephalitis, as can HSV DNA in the CSF by PCR.

TREATMENT

Aciclovir, 60 mg/kg/d in three divided doses, intravenously for 14 days (21 days for encephalitis or disseminated disease) is recommended. Disease may relapse after discontinuation of therapy. Long-term oral suppressive therapy (Aciclovir) for 6–12 months has recently been shown to be effective. Babies with ocular involvement (keratoconjunctivitis) should also receive a topical antiviral drug (3% vidarabine).

PROGNOSIS

If the diagnosis can be made early when the disease is localised (i.e. skin, eye and/or mouth), antiviral therapy leads to zero mortality and normal development in >90% of infants. Involvement of the brain and disseminated disease leads to mortality rates of 18–50%, with as many as 50% of surviving patients having some form of neurological sequelae.

PREVENTION

Women with active genital lesions at the time of delivery should be delivered by caesarian section. Infants born vaginally to mothers with active genital lesions should be observed closely and have HSV cultures taken at 24–48 hours (eyes, mouth, skin, rectum, CSF). If cultures are positive or should the infant develop symptoms, antiviral therapy should be started. Some authorities recommend starting empiric therapy with aciclovir, at birth, pending results of cultures.

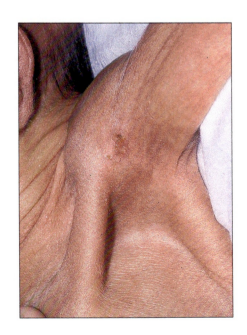

FIGURE 3.38 Neonatal herpes simplex virus infection. Vesicular eruption.

VARICELLA (CHICKEN POX)

INCIDENCE

Chicken pox is a highly contagious disease with an estimated 90% of susceptible household contacts developing the disease after exposure. Varicella tends to occur seasonally (late winter, early spring) and in epidemics. In the UK, virtually the whole of the annual birth cohort (720,000) will develop the infection.

AETIOLOGY/PATHOGENESIS

Varicella zoster virus (VZV) is a herpesvirus and primary infection with this agent results in varicella. The incubation period is usually 14 days (ranging between 10 and 21 days). Transmission occurs from person to person by direct contact or via airborne spread from respiratory secretions. Virus replication occurs in regional cervical lymph nodes following infection of conjunctivae and/or mucosa of the nasopharynx. A primary viraemia ensues in 4–6 days, with viral replication occurring in the liver, spleen and other organs. A secondary viraemia occurs at 10 days, with spread of virus to the skin and subsequent appearance of rash. Children are infectious 1–2 days before the rash appears until crusting of the lesions.

CLINICAL PRESENTATION

Varicella is generally a benign illness characterised by the appearance of a maculopapular vesicular rash, fever, malaise and anorexia. The rash, which may be pruritic, usually crusts over in 5 days and occurs in a centripetal distribution with a characteristic feature of lesions at all stages (macules, papules, vesicles, crusts) being present together (**Fig. 3.39**).

The most common complication is secondary bacterial infection. Other complications include pneumonitis (**Fig. 3.40**), hepatitis, encephalitis and orchitis (**Fig. 3.41**). In the immunocompromised patient, varicella can be life threatening. There is a progressive eruption of numerous, umbilicated and haemorrhagic vesicles, associated with a high-grade fever (**Fig. 3.42**). Pneumonitis is a common manifestation of disseminated disease in this population.

DIAGNOSIS

VZV can be isolated from vesicular fluid early in the illness. Specific diagnosis can also be accomplished by the staining of vesicle scrapings with fluorescein-tagged VZV specific monoclonal antibodies. Electron microscopy of vesicular fluid will identify a 'herpesvirus', while a Tzanck smear will demonstrate multi-nucleated giant cells with intracellular inclusions. The most reliable serological tests to detect specific VZV IgM and IgG are the fluorescent antibody to membrane antigen test (FAMA) and the ELISA assay. PCR tests are also being increasingly used.

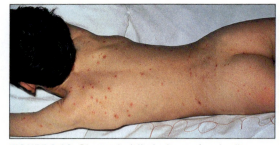

FIGURE 3.39 Characteristic lesions of varicella (chicken pox).

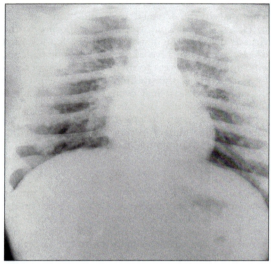

FIGURE 3.40 Pneumonitis in varicella (chicken pox).

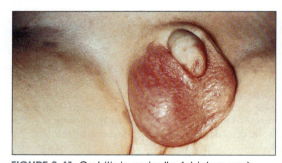

FIGURE 3.41 Orchitis in varicella (chicken pox).

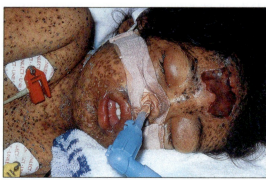

FIGURE 3.42 Varicella (chicken pox) in an immunocompromised patient.

TREATMENT

Simple measures are sufficient for most patients, i.e. fluids, antipyretics and calomine lotion for the spots. Oral aciclovir is not recommended routinely for treatment of uncomplicated chicken pox in otherwise healthy children. It may be considered for the older child (>12 years), or for those patients taking short courses of steroids (or inhaled steroids). Infection in the immunocompromised host should be treated with IV aciclovir 500 mg/m^2 per dose, 3 times daily, for 7–10 days. Children with varicella should not receive salicylates because of the risk of Reye syndrome.

PROGNOSIS

Complications will develop in 5% of normal children, the most common being secondary bacterial infection. Severe complications, requiring hospital admission, are rarer and include secondary bacterial skin infection with sepsis, necrotising fasciitis, encephalitis and pneumonia. In untreated immunocompromised children, one-third of patients will develop disseminated disease, with a mortality of 7%. Varicella is responsible for 20–30 deaths per year in the UK.

PREVENTION

Strict isolation of cases in negative-pressure rooms is necessary if patients are admitted to hospital. Infectivity occurs from 24–48 hours before, until 5 days after the appearance of the rash. Varicella zoster immunoglobulin should be given to susceptible individuals, in contact with chickenpox, if they are at risk of developing severe varicella.

A live-attenuated varicella vaccine is available, but is not part of the UK immunisation schedule. Nevertheless, the two dose vaccination schedule provides about 98% protection in children and about 75% protection in adolescents and adults.

HERPES ZOSTER (SHINGLES)

INCIDENCE

Herpes zoster infection is less common in children than in adults. It is a more common event in the immunosuppressed patient, especially after bone marrow transplantation (BMT). There is an association between the early development of chickenpox and the appearance of zoster in later childhood.

AETIOLOGY/PATHOGENESIS

Shingles occur as a result of reactivation of latent VZV in the dorsal root ganglia after primary infection with chicken pox. When cell-mediated immunity to VZV declines (e.g. onset of immunodeficiency, old age), the virus starts replicating in the ganglia and is transported along the axon to the sensory nerve endings in the skin. Thereafter it replicates locally to produce the characteristic vesicular lesions.

CLINICAL PRESENTATION

The eruptive phase of herpes zoster infection in children starts with the appearance of grouped red papules, which are dermatomal in distribution. These rapidly progress to vesicles, pustules and scab formation in around 5–10 days. The lesions are usually unilateral and may be accompanied by fever and malaise. Pain and tenderness is often felt along the dermatomal distribution a few days before the onset of the rash. The most commonly affected dermatomes tend to be the thoracolumbar (**Fig. 3.43**) and the trigeminal, especially the ophthalmic division (**Fig. 3.44**).

Typically the rash is present for about 7 days. Immunocompromised children may have lesions that are outside the involved dermatomes; prolonged eruption of vesicles may occur as well as disseminated visceral disease.

DIAGNOSIS

The characteristic lesions and their distribution usually make the clinical diagnosis. Viral culture of vesicular fluid and specific serological tests to detect rises in VZV IgG may be helpful. Vesicular scrapings to detect multi-nucleated giant-cells and electron microscopy to detect herpesviruses are less specific tests. PCR tests to detect viral DNA are helpful.

TREATMENT

Immunocompromised children with zoster should receive IV aciclovir 500 mg/m^2/dose, 3 times daily, for 7–10 days. Healthy children with uncomplicated zoster do not require systemic antiviral therapy.

PROGNOSIS

Generally, children are not at risk of postherpetic neuralgia that can cause chronic debilitating pain in adults after resolution of the rash.

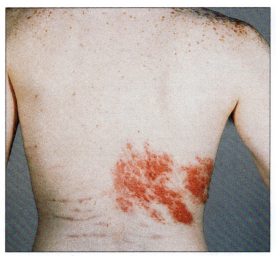

FIGURE 3.43 Thoracolumbar infection in herpes zoster (shingles).

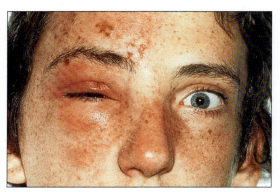

FIGURE 3.44 Ophthalmic infection in herpes zoster (shingles).

Immunocompromised children (e.g. HIV infected children) can have unusual chronic or relapsing cutaneous lesions.

PREVENTION

There is some evidence to suggest that live varicella vaccine may be protective in some groups of immunosuppressed children (haematological malignancies in remission, or on maintenance chemotherapy) against the development of subsequent zoster, compared with a control group who were infected with wild type virus. In the USA, an attenuated live varicella vaccine is available for patients, above 65 years, to prevent shingles.

CONGENITAL TOXOPLASMOSIS

INCIDENCE

The incidence of maternal toxoplasmosis in the UK is thought to be around 1:500 pregnancies. The transmission rate to the fetus is thought be about 40%, with a higher risk of congenital infection being associated with the latter stages of pregnancy. Most infants with congenital toxoplasmosis (CTx) are asymptomatic at birth (90%). The BPSU estimates that about 14 infants per year may be born in the UK with severe symptomatic CTx.

AETIOLOGY/PATHOGENESIS

Toxoplasma gondii is an intracellular coccidian parasite with a world-wide distribution. Members of the cat family are the definitive hosts. Humans acquire the disease by consumption of poorly cooked meat or ingestion of oocysts from soil or contaminated food. When the disease is acquired in pregnancy, transplacental transmission of the parasite may occur with potentially serious sequelae for the fetus and newborn. The severity of CTx is related to the period of gestation when maternal disease was acquired: infection in early pregnancy results in the more severe form of congenital disease.

CLINICAL PRESENTATION

The clinical manifestations include the 'classic triad' of hydrocephalus, intracranial calcification (**Fig. 3.45**) and choroidoretinitis. Other non-specific features that may be seen include jaundice, hepatosplenomegaly, thrombocytopenia, maculopapular rash, dysmaturity, lymphadenopathy, microphthalmia and seizures.

DIAGNOSIS

A diagnosis of CTx can be made by detection of specific *Toxoplasma* IgM or IgA (ELISA/ ISAGA), the persistence of specific IgG antibodies beyond 12 months (passively transmitted antibodies usually disappear by this time in an uninfected child), or the isolation of the parasite by mouse inoculation.

Toxoplasma PCR is available in some centres to detect the presence of parasite DNA in blood, CSF or amniotic fluid. Other investigations that may be helpful include CT of the head, and CSF examination (pleocytosis and high protein).

TREATMENT

All infants with CTx should be treated irrespective of clinical findings. Therapy should be for a total of 12 months and should include the following: pyrimethamine 2 mg/kg/d for the first 2 days, followed by 1 mg/kg/d (maximum of 25 mg/d) for 2 or 6 months, followed by 1 mg/kg once per day every Monday, Wednesday, Friday. Sulfadiazine 100 mg/kg/d, q6h, and folinic acid 10 mg three times weekly. Steroids are given for choroidoretinitis when there is macular involvement.

PROGNOSIS

Most congenital infections are asymptomatic at birth (up to 90%). There is significant mortality among those neonates who are severely symptomatic at birth; most who survive have neurological sequelae. Up to 80% of congenitally infected neonates who are asymptomatic at birth may present later in life with visual impairment, learning disabilities or mental retardation.

PREVENTION

Pregnant women should avoid contact with cats and cat litter and gardening should not be undertaken. Hands should be washed after handling raw meat and vegetables; all meat should be thoroughly cooked before eating.

CRYPTOSPORIDIOSIS

INCIDENCE

Disease prevalence is higher in less developed countries (8.5% compared with 2.1% in industrialised communities). The highest incidence is in young children aged 6–24 months. There are around 4000 reported cases per year in the UK. Symptoms appear after an incubation period of 2–14 days. The main source of transmission is person to person, although animal to human (farm livestock) and waterborne outbreaks have occurred.

AETIOLOGY/PATHOGENESIS

Cryptosporidium species are intracellular coccidian protozoan parasites that invade the epithelial lining of the intestinal and respiratory tracts. Following ingestion of oocysts, excystation occurs with the release of sporozoites that attach to intestinal epithelial cells, forming parasitiphorous vacuoles (**Fig. 3.46**). An asexual intestinal cycle leads to reinfection of enterocytes and a sexual intestinal phase produces oocysts that are excreted in the stools. *C parvum* and *Cryptosporidium h* are the primary parasites that infect humans.

CLINICAL PRESENTATION

Infection in immunocompetent individuals results in a self-limited diarrhoeal illness (average of 10 days), associated with low-grade fever, anorexia, abdominal pain and weight loss. The infection in immunocompromised patients, especially those with defective cellular immunity, is characterised by chronic profuse watery diarrhoea, malabsorption, extreme weight loss and, in some cases, a fatal outcome. Disseminated disease (pulmonary, biliary tract) may also be seen in this population.

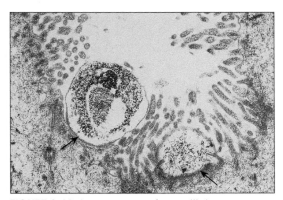

FIGURE 3.46 Appearance of parasitiphorous vacuoles at biopsy in cryptosporidiosis.

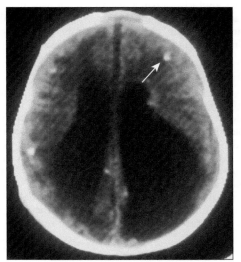

FIGURE 3.45 Intracranial calcification in congenital toxoplasmosis.

DIAGNOSIS

Definitive diagnosis is made by microscopic identification of oocysts in stool specimens stained with a modified acid-fast technique, or by identification of the organism in jejunal tissue obtained at biopsy. At least three separate stool specimens should be examined before considering the test to be negative.

TREATMENT

To date there is no fully effective therapeutic agent against *Cryptosporidium* spp. Paramomycin, azithromycin, nitazoxanide and hyperimmune bovine colostrum have all been used with limited success. The FDA, however, has approved a 3 day course of nitazoxanide for treatment of all people 1 year of age and older with diarrhoea associated with cryptosporidiosis. Supportive therapy, along with adequate fluid replacement (with or without parenteral nutrition) is important.

In HIV patients, antidiarrhoeal agents are also often used as symptomatic treatment.

PROGNOSIS

In infected immunocompetent children, diarrhoeal disease is self-limited usually lasting up to 2 weeks. This is not the case for children who are immunocompromised. The chronic severe diarrhoea may lead to malnutrition and weight loss. Antibiotic therapy is usually prescribed for these children, and recovery is seen when there is immune reconstitution.

PREVENTION

Immunocompromised patients should boil their drinking water and avoid contact with potential sources of infection (such as farm animals and pets). People with diarrhoea should not use public swimming pools.

CYSTICERCOSIS (NEUROCYSTICERCOSIS)

INCIDENCE

The disease is endemic in rural areas of Latin America, South East Asia and Africa. Prevalence is high in areas with poor sanitation and where swine are fed. Autopsy studies in some areas show that up to 3.5% of the population have cysticercosis.

AETIOLOGY/PATHOGENESIS

The disease is caused by infection with the larval stage (cysticerci) of the pork tapeworm, *Taenia solium* (**Fig. 3.47**). It is acquired by ingesting eggs of the pork tapeworm that are shed in the faeces of human carriers of tapeworm (these acquire the adult tapeworm through eating inadequately cooked pork). Autoinfection is also a recognised route of infection. Between 24 and 72 hours after the eggs are ingested, larvae hatch and penetrate the small intestinal wall and then migrate via the circulation, to sites throughout the body. Symptoms appear when a granulomatous reaction eventually ensues around dead or dying cysts.

CLINICAL PRESENTATION

Symptoms depend on the location, size and number of cysticerci. Any tissue can be affected, the most common being brain, subcutaneous tissue, muscle and eye. Painless lumps under the skin are characteristic of subcutaneous cysticerci. Involvement of the CNS (neurocysticercosis) presents mainly as epilepsy in more than half of affected patients, some 4–8 years after infection. Other neurological symptoms that may be seen include transient hemiplegia, obstructive hydrocephalus and meningitis.

DIAGNOSIS

Neurocysticercosis is diagnosed by a CT scan of the head (**Fig. 3.48**) or MRI (**Fig. 3.49**). These show multiple enhancing and non-enhancing cysts that later may become calcified. The enzyme-linked immunotransfer blot detects antibody to *Taenia solium* and is the best serological test available.

TREATMENT

Cysticidal therapy is beneficial in those children with multiple cysts, viable cysts or symptomatic disease. The two drugs used for this indication are albendazole (15 mg/kg/d in 2 divided doses for 4 weeks) and praziquantel (50 mg/kg/d in 3 divided doses for 2–4 weeks). Albendazole is preferred over praziquantel because of fewer drug interactions, e.g. with anticonvulsants. Dexamethazone is usually given during the first week of treatment to reduce the inflammatory reaction induced by the dead larvae. Anticonvulsants may also be required.

PROGNOSIS

80–90% of patients respond to medical therapy with complete disappearance or regression in cyst volume.

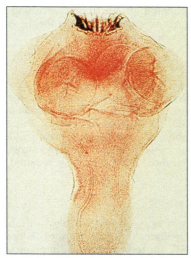

FIGURE 3.47 *Taenia solium* (cysticercosis).

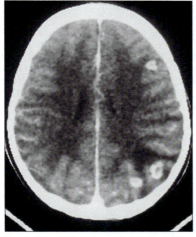

FIGURE 3.48 Appearance of the head (CT scan) in cysticercosis.

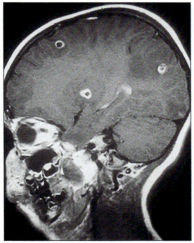

FIGURE 3.49 Appearance of the head (MRI) in cysticercosis.

Around 60% of patients remain seizure-free after cysticidal therapy. Patients who have a single ring-enhancing lesion often have spontaneous resolution of the lesion.

PREVENTION

Eating raw or undercooked pork should be avoided. Stool examination of the patient and close family contacts should be carried out. Those harbouring the adult tapeworm should be treated.

INVASIVE ASPERGILLOSIS

INCIDENCE

Aspergillus species are ubiquitous saprophytic moulds present in the environment. The incidence of disease varies in different groups of immunocompromised patients, from around 4–8% in patients undergoing BMT, 5–25% in patients with acute leukaemia and 25-40% in patients with chronic granulomatous disease (CGD). They are second only to *Candida* species in the frequency of opportunistic mycoses. Outbreaks of disease have been reported on cancer and transplant units that are in close proximity to construction sites.

AETIOLOGY/PATHOGENESIS

Infection with the organism is usually initiated by inhalation of air-borne spores. In the immunocompromised host, *Aspergillus* then tends to invade blood vessels resulting in infarction, necrosis and haematogeneously disseminated disease. *A fumigatus* is the usual cause of invasive disease, although *A flavus* is also important.

CLINICAL PRESENTATION

Occurs almost exclusively in immunocompromised patients, especially those with prolonged and profound neutropenia, or defects in neutrophil function. The most common clinical presentation is pulmonary aspergillosis. These patients present with persisting fever not responding to antibiotics, abnormal chest x-ray (often with new infiltrates appearing) (**Fig. 3.50**), cough, haemoptysis and pleuritic chest pain. Other clinical syndromes indicating disseminated disease include: cutaneous disease (**Fig. 3.51**), spinal osteomyelitis, cerebral abscess (**Fig. 3.52**) and renal involvement.

DIAGNOSIS

Definitive diagnosis requires histopathological evidence of *Aspergillus* hyphae in tissue, as well as isolation of an *Aspergillus* species in culture. Histopathological stains reveal dichotomously branched and septate hypahae. Galactomannan (GM) antigen testing of blood and other biological fluids may be helpful in diagnosing invasive aspergillosis. GM is a polysaccharide released from aspergillus during active growth.

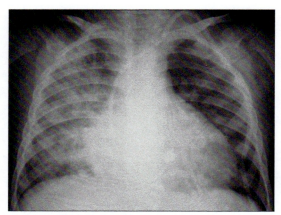

FIGURE 3.50 Invasive aspergillosis, chest x-ray.

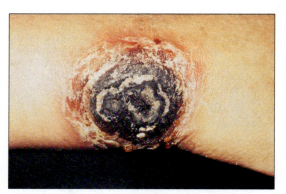

FIGURE 3.51 Invasive aspergillosis, skin lesion.

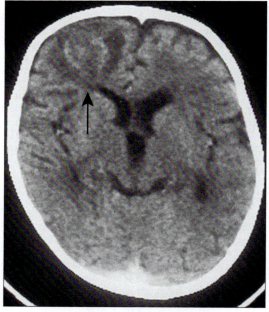

FIGURE 3.52 Invasive aspergillosis, cerebral abscess.

CT scanning of the lungs, revealing multiple nodules, can be a helpful adjunct for the early diagnosis of invasive aspergillosis.

TREATMENT

Ambisome (or voriconazole) is the treatment of choice; length of therapy should be for at least 6–12 weeks, but may be longer especially in patients with CGD. In seriously ill patients, an echinocandin (caspofungin, micafungin) is often added to the ambisome or voriconazole therapy. Surgical resection of localised lesions may be required in some patients.

PROGNOSIS

Mortality rates are around 60–70%, with the highest rate being observed in subgroups of children undergoing BMT for severe combined immunodeficiency (SCID) or haematological malignancies. Earlier diagnosis and therapy as well as the future development of effective prophylactic regimens will lead to lower mortality.

PREVENTION

Some evidence supports the use of oral itraconazole and posaconazole as fungal prophylaxis in high-risk patients. Nursing patients in air-filtered areas (high-efficiency particulate arrestance, HEPA) also decreases exposure of patients to high *Aspergillus* counts.

NEONATAL SYSTEMIC CANDIDIASIS

INCIDENCE

Over the past two decades, there has been a significant increase in the incidence of systemic candidiasis in NICU patients, especially in very low birth weight (VLBW) infants (<1500 g). Although *Candida* infections range from superficial colonisation to widely disseminated, life-threatening disease, the incidence of invasive or systemic candidiasis has had the most dramatic increase. These infections may affect 1.6% to 12.9% of VLBW infants in NICU.

AETIOLOGY/PATHOGENESIS

Members of the genus *Candida* are ubiquitous, and form a heterogenous group of single-cell eukaryotic, dimorphic organisms, which grow as yeast cells **(Fig. 3.53)**. Although *C parapsilosis* and *C glabrata* have increased exponentially over the last 10 years, *C albicans* remains the most frequently isolated yeast species among infected neonates. Up to 63% of *Candida* species isolated from blood cultures of infected neonates are *C. albicans* (*C parapsilosis* 29%, *C glabrata* 6%).

Most *Candida* infections are nosocomially acquired. *Candida* species colonise the human gastrointestinal tract of neonates, and disseminated infection results from translocation across the gastrointestinal epithelium of commensal *Candida* spp. Main risk factors for systemic candidiasis are prematurity and low birth weight, prolonged use of indwelling intravascular catheters, the administration of multiple course of broad-spectrum antibiotics and use of total parenteral nutrition (TPN).

CLINICAL PRESENTATION

Although individual organ system involvement (e.g. UTI, meningitis) can occur, infection occurs much more often as a component of disseminated *Candida* infection from haematogenous spread. Catheter-related infections and disseminated candidiasis, usually involving the kidney, heart, eye and CNS are the clinical syndromes that are most often seen. The incidence of catheter-related infections increases if the catheter has been in place for more than 7 days. Neonates exhibit non-specific signs of sepsis (feeding intolerance, apnoea, hyperglycaemia and temperature instability), but no evidence of multi-organ involvement. Prompt removal of catheter may be indicated. The suspicion or diagnosis of candidal infection should prompt an investigation to see whether organ systems are involved (ultrasound of kidneys, ophthalmic exam, ECHO, and in some instances, a spinal tap). Renal cadidiasis may be manifested by the presence of 'fungal balls' in kidney; candidal endophalmitis **(Fig. 3.54)** is also the result of haematogenous spread of *Candida* spp. to the eye.

DIAGNOSIS

Diagnosis of candidiasis is made by isolation of the fungus from blood.

Blood culture may be positive in 80% of infected neonates. The best sensitivity has been achieved using the lysis-centrifugation method. Other techniques, with at least equal sensivity, include the BACTEC and BacT/Alert. A screening test for identification of *C. albicans* involves the incubation of yeast organisms in serum or plasma for 2–3 hours, at 37°C, and looking for the production of a 'germ tube'. Non-albicans *Candida* sp. do not develop 'germ tube' formation.

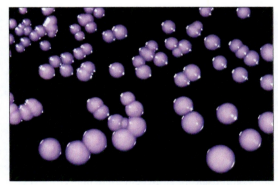

FIGURE 3.53 Neonatal systemic candidiasis showing typical colonies of *Candida* spp.

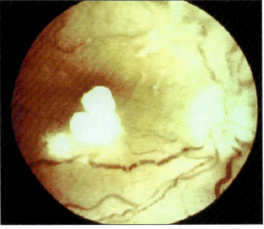

FIGURE 3.54 *Candida* endophthalmitis in neonatal systemic candidiasis.

TREATMENT

Recommendations for treatment of neonatal candidiasis include the conventional amphotericin or ambisome +/− flucytosine. The latter is not used as monotherapy, but recommended by some experts, to be used in combination with amphotericin or ambisome when CNS, renal or cardiac disease is diagnosed. Micafungin (an echinocandin) has also been used for neonatal candidiasis, and has shown the same efficacy as ambisome.

Most disseminated disease requires 4–6 weeks of treatment (6 weeks for endocarditis). The Infectious Diseases Society of America recommends a minimum of 2–3 weeks of systemic therapy after negative blood, urine and CSF culture have been obtained, along with resolution of clinical findings.

PROGNOSIS

The smaller the infant, the greater the likelihood of systemic infections to develop. The overall morbidity and mortality for disseminated candidiasis approaches 30%. In VLBW infants (<1,500 g) mortality rate is 28–32%, while in extremely low birth weight infants (<1000 g) mortality rate is 37–40%. Thus factors determining prognosis, apart from the degree of prematurity, include severity of illness, and rapidity of institution of appropriate antifungal therapy.

PREVENTION

Avoidance where possible of broad-spectrum antibiotics. Prophylactic use of antifungal drugs (e.g. fluconazole) in infants less than 1500 g. Avoid prolonged use of central and peripheral intravascular catheters. Consider removal of intravascular catheters when *Candida* sp. is cultured from a blood specimen taken from a catheter.

MALARIA

INCIDENCE

Each year, world-wide, there are more than 200 million cases of malaria, with around 1 million deaths (mainly African infants). In the UK, around 1600 cases of imported malaria are seen each year, with 10–15% occurring in children. Most cases (80%) are due to *Plasmodium falciparum* acquired in Africa, with between 10 and 20 deaths reported each year.

AETIOLOGY/PATHOGENESIS

Malaria is caused by invasion of erythrocytes by one of the species of intracellular protozoa of the genus *Plasmodium*. Those species infecting humans are: *P falciparum* (**Fig. 3.55**), *P vivax*, *P ovale*, *P malariae* and *P knowlesi*. Transmission of the parasite is usually through the bite of an infected female *Anopheles* mosquito.

The severe complications seen in *P falciparum* malaria are the result of the high parasitaemia, followed by sequestration of parasitised red blood cells in deep vascular beds (including the cerebral vasculature). Vascular occlusion subsequently occurs with resultant tissue anoxia and the development of clinical symptoms, including a diffuse encephalopathy in cerebral malaria.

CLINICAL PRESENTATION

Symptoms tend to be paroxysmal with high fever, chills, sweating and headaches in a cyclical pattern. Jaundice and anaemia, as a result of haemolysis, as well as hepatosplenomegaly, may be found on physical examination. *P falciparum* tends to cause the most severe disease, ranging from cerebral malaria (**Fig. 3.56**), renal failure, shock, pulmonary oedema, hypoglycaemia and haemoglobinuria ('blackwater fever').

DIAGNOSIS

A thick smear, stained by Giemsa, identifies the presence of malarial parasites in the peripheral blood and a thin smear identifies the type of malarial species causing disease, as well as parasite count (reported as percentage of red blood cells parasitised). Rapid diagnostic tests (RDT), which detect parasite antigens in the blood, are often used in non-hospital settings in less developed countries. The presence of thrombocytopenia is also suggestive of malaria.

TREATMENT

All children with malaria due to *P falciparum* require admission to hospital. Recent guidelines from WHO recommend IV artesunate be used preferentially over quinine as the drug of choice for severe falciparum malaria. A dose of 2.4 mg/kg IV of artesunate, at 0, 12 and 24 hours, then once daily until oral therapy is tolerated. Oral therapy consists of 6 doses of artemether + lumefantrine(0, 8, 24, 36, 48 and 60 hours). An alternative orally is 7 days of quinine + (clindamycin or doxycycline).

If artesunate is not available, IV quinine dihydrochloride is given by a loading dose of 20 mg/kg over 4 hours, followed by 10 mg/kg every 8 hours, until the patient can tolerate oral medications. Oral quinine + (clindamycin or doxycycline) is given for 7 days. For other strains of malaria, chloroquine is the drug of choice (25 mg/kg of base, over 48 hours), followed by primaquine for 14 days to prevent relapse in *P. vivax* and *P. ovale* infections.

Atovaquone and proguanil are both used in combination to prevent and treat malaria, especially in countries where malaria is common.

PROGNOSIS

In endemic areas, infants and young children tend to be at highest risk of infection, as are non-immune visitors to these areas. In cerebral malaria, there is a mortality rate of 15–20%, with obvious focal neurological deficits occurring in 10–20%. These deficits tend to get better over 1–6 months, although a 2-year follow-up of Ugandan children with cerebral malaria noted 25% had some cognitive impairment.

PREVENTION

The following general measures should be adopted to prevent mosquito bites: use of bed nets impregnated with permethrin, wearing of appropriate clothing (i.e. long sleeves, trousers), and the use of insect

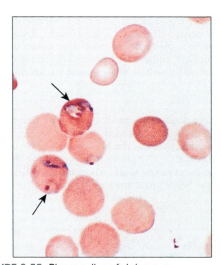

FIGURE 3.55 *Plasmodium falciparum.*

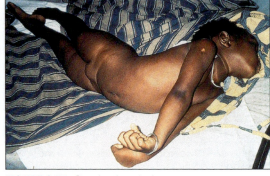

FIGURE 3.56 Cerebral malaria.

repellants. Prophylactic antimalarials should be taken 1–2 weeks before departure to an endemic area and continued for 4 weeks after returning.

SCHISTOSOMIASIS (URINARY)

INCIDENCE

The disease is endemic in Africa, the Middle East, Asia and South America. The presence of the specific snail host and the inappropriate disposal of human excreta in the environment are essential in maintaining endemicity of the disease. World-wide, approximately 200 million people are infected with the 5 major species of schistosomes.

AETIOLOGY/PATHOGENESIS

Schistosoma haematobium is a blood fluke (trematode) that inhabits the venous plexuses of the urinary bladder. Large amount of eggs are laid by the female every day. The eggs retained in the tissues cause a tissue reaction with the formation of multiple granulomas and eventual fibrotic lesions, leading to obstructive uropathy. The expelled eggs hatch in fresh water and the liberated miracidiae penetrate the body of the snail intermediate host. Cercariae are eventually released that penetrate the skin of a human swimmer, and then migrate to the lung and liver and finally to the venous plexus of the bladder.

CLINICAL PRESENTATION

The early manifestations in children infected with *S haematobium* are frequency, dysuria and terminal hematuria. Symptoms of obstructive uropathy (straining, dribbling, incomplete emptying of the bladder and constant urge to urinate) occur in advanced infection. End-stage disease results in hydronephrosis (**Fig. 3.57**) and uraemia. CNS involvement is occasionally seen.

DIAGNOSIS

Microscopic examination of centrifuged urine, collected between 12 and 2 pm, demonstrates the characteristic *S haematobium* eggs with the lateral spine (**Fig. 3.58**). Egg excretion in urine often peaks between noon and 2 pm. Biopsy of the bladder mucosa may be necessary if urine tests are negative. IV pyelogram (IVP) and cystoscopy indicate the extent of the disease. Serological tests (ELISA, RIA) to detect schistosomal antibodies are available.

TREATMENT

Praziquantel: 2 oral doses of 20 mg/kg in 1 day. Some authorities recommend this to be repeated after 2 weeks.

PROGNOSIS

Egg/worm burden has been shown to be related to severity of disease. Urinary tract lesions are reversible

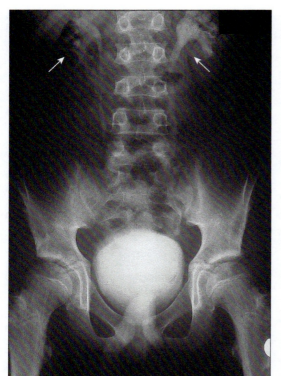

FIGURE 3.57 Hydronephrosis in schistosomiasis (urinary).

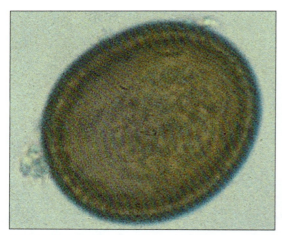

FIGURE 3.58 Characteristic *S haemotobium* egg, with lateral spine.

if treatment is initiated early in the course of the illness. In advanced disease, despite parasitological cure, surgical intervention may be required. An association between chronic schistosomiasis and bladder cancer has been noted.

PREVENTION

Health education along with treatment of infected hosts and proper disposal of human excreta are the mainstays of prevention. Travellers should avoid freshwater streams and lakes.

VISCERAL LEISHMANIASIS (KALA-AZAR)

INCIDENCE

Visceral leishmaniasis (VL) is endemic in many countries worldwide but 90% of VL cases occur in India, Bangladesh, Nepal, Sudan, Ethiopia and Brazil. In Europe, VL may occur along the Mediterranean coast of southern Europe. Cases of VL occurring in non-endemic areas have usually had a travel history to an endemic country.

AETIOLOGY/PATHOGENESIS

VL is a zoonosis caused by *Leishmania* species (*L donovani, L infantum* and *L chagasi*), which are intracellular protozoan parasites. They are transmitted through the bite of the female phlebotomine sand-fly. The incubation period for VL typically ranges from 2 to 6 months.

CLINICAL PRESENTATION

Following inoculation through the bite of an infected phlebotomine sand-fly, parasites spread throughout the mononuclear macrophage system to the spleen, liver and bone marrow. The typical presenting features include fever, anorexia, failure to thrive, hepatosplenomegaly, lymphadenopathy and pancytopenia. Untreated VL is nearly always fatal. Reactivation of latent VL may also occur in those who become immunocompromised, including people with HIV or those undergoing transplantation.

DIAGNOSIS

Definitive diagnosis is made by demonstration of the parasite in the spleen and bone marrow (**Fig. 3.59**). Splenic aspiration has the highest sensitivity but also the highest risk. Lymph node aspiration is also used in some parts of the world for rapid identification of parasites. Serological testing is also used, but false

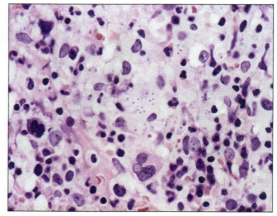

FIGURE 3.59 Visceral leishmaniasis. Bone marrow showing intracellular *Leishmania* organisms (amastigotes).

positives can occur due to other infectious diseases such as trypanosomiasis.

TREATMENT

First-line treatment for VL is liposomal amphotericin B for a total of 10 days duration although shorter courses and lower doses are being studied in high-prevalent, resource-limited settings. Sodium stibolgluconate is an alternative treatment although it carries a high risk of toxicity, particularly cardiac. Recent concerns about antimonial resistance in India and Nepal mean that these drugs will be less effective in South Asia. Recently oral miltefosine for 28 days has been shown to have similar efficacy to liposomal amphotericin and has the advantage of not requiring IV therapy.

PROGNOSIS

Prompt and early diagnosis and treatment results in complete recovery.

PREVENTION

So far vaccines and drugs for preventing infection are not available. The best way of preventing leishmaniasis is by protecting against sand-fly bites.

KAWASAKI DISEASE

See also Chapter 1 Emergency Medicine, page 9 and Chapter 17 Rheumatology, page 518.

INCIDENCE

The disease is most prevalent in Japan, where epidemics occur every 3 years. In the UK there are around 90–120 cases reported each year with an estimated incidence of 15 per million children, which is probably an underestimate of the true incidence of the disease. About 80% of affected patients are under 4 years of age. There is little evidence for person-to-person transmission, although siblings of index cases have been affected as have some contacts of index cases.

AETIOLOGY/PATHOGENESIS

Clinical features suggest an infectious aetiology, however a microbial agent has not been conclusively implicated. Current evidence suggests the disease is the result of superantigen activity (i.e. a toxin with superantigen properties is able to cause widespread activation of the immune system with massive cytokine release and consequent initiation of generalised inflammatory changes and vasculitis). The pathological lesion in Kawasaki disease is thus a vasculitis affecting small to medium-sized musculoelastic arteries throughout the body but with a predilection for the coronary vessels. Medial disruption and formation of coronary artery aneurysms (CAA) may occur.

CLINICAL PRESENTATION

Kawasaki disease is an acute febrile illness of unknown aetiology, affecting predominantly infants and young children. It is a leading cause of acquired heart disease in children. It is characterised by a prolonged remittent fever, mucositis (**Fig. 3.60**), conjunctivitis, polymorphous skin rash (**Fig. 3.61**), cervical adenopathy and oedema of the hands and feet with subsequent skin desquamation (**Fig. 3.62**). Cardiac involvement with coronary arteritis and aneurysm formation (**Fig. 3.63**) may occur, with fatal consequences.

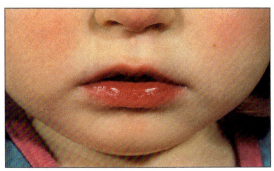

FIGURE 3.60 Mucositis in Kawasaki disease.

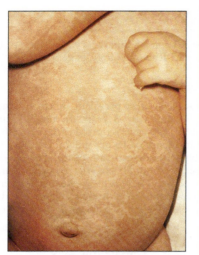

FIGURE 3.61 Polymorphous skin rash in Kawasaki disease.

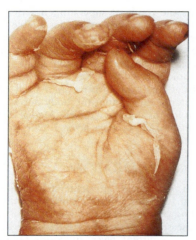

FIGURE 3.62 Desquamation of the hand in Kawasaki disease.

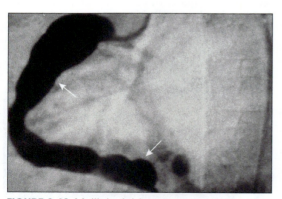

FIGURE 3.63 Multiple right coronary artery aneurysms on angiogram in Kawasaki disease.

DIAGNOSIS

The diagnosis is based on the presence of five of six principal clinical criteria (mentioned above), without other explanation for the illness. Laboratory investigations are non-specific: normochromic normocytic anaemia, leukocytosis, thrombocytosis (in the second week), raised ESR and CRP, along with hypoalbuminaemia may be present.

TREATMENT

A single high dose of IVIG (2 g/kg) given over 10–12 hours, within the first 10 days of the illness, along with the initiation of high-dose aspirin therapy (100 mg/kg/d in 4 divided doses) is the mainstay of treatment. Once the fever has defervesced (or on the 14th day) the aspirin is reduced to 3–5 mg/kg once daily as antiplatelet therapy and continued for 2–3 months. Some patients may require additional doses of immunoglobulin if symptoms persist.

ECHOs are obtained at diagnosis, 1 week into the illness and at 4–6 weeks after the start of the illness. If CAA are detected, dipyridamole may be added to the aspirin therapy and continued indefinitely.

PROGNOSIS

In patients not receiving high-dose immunoglobulin within the first 10 days of the illness, the incidence of CAA is 15–30%. In treated patients the incidence is less than 5%. Regression of CAA may occur in around 50% of patients over a 1–2 year period. Sudden death from coronary thrombosis and myocardial infarction occurs in approximately 1–2% of untreated patients.

FURTHER READING

Diphtheria
Daskalaki I. Corynebacterium diphtheriae. In: Long S, Pickering L, Prober C (eds). *Principles and Practice of Pediatric Infectious Diseases* (4th edn). Philadelphia: Elsevier Saunders, 2012, pp. 754–9.

Tetanus
Arnon S. Tetanus (*Clostridium tetani*). In: Kliegman RM, Stanton BF, St Geme JW, Schor NF, Behrman RE (eds). *Nelson Textbook of Pediatrics* (19th edn). Philadelphia: Elsevier Saunders, 2011, pp. 991–4.

Meningococcal infections
Pollard AJ, Faust SN, Levin M. Meningitis and meningococcal septicaemia. *J Roy Coll Phys* 1998;32:319–28.

Tuberculosis
Shingadia D, Novelli V. Diagnosis and treatment of tuberculosis in children. *Lancet Infect Dis* 2003;3:624–32.

Tuberculous meningitis
Farinha N, Razali B, Holzel H, Morgan G, Novelli VM. Tuberculosis of the central nervous system in children: a 20 year survey. *J Infect* 2000;41:1–8.

Non-tuberculous mycobacterial infections
Sharland M. Non-tuberculous mycobacterial infection. In: Sharland M (ed). *Manual of Childhood Infections*, 3rd edn. Oxford: Oxford University Press, 2011, pp. 649–54.

Cat-scratch disease
Batts S, Demers DM. Spectrum and treatment of cat-scratch disease. *Pediatr Infect Dis J* 2004;23:1161–2.

Lyme disease
Stanek G, Wormser GP, Gray J, Strie F. Lyme borreliosis. *Lancet* 2012;379:461–73.

Pyogenic liver abscess
Kaplan S. Pyogenic liver abscess. In: Feigin RD, Cherry JD, Demmler-Harrison GJ, Kaplan S (eds). *Feigin & Cherry's Textbook of Pediatric Infectious Diseases* (6th edn). Philadelphia: Saunders Elsevier, 2009, pp. 689–93.

Staphylococcal toxic shock syndrome
Lappin E, Ferguson AJ. Gram-positive toxic shock syndromes. *Lancet Infect Dis* 2009;9:281–90.

Tularaemia
Nigrovic LE, Wingerter SL. Tularemia. *Infect Dis Clin North Am* 2008;22:489–504.

HIV infection and AIDS
Seeborg FO, Shearer WT, Hanson CI. Impact of HIV and AIDS. In: Feigin RD, Cherry JD, Demmler-Harrison GJ, Kaplan S (eds). *Feigin & Cherry's Textbook of Pediatric Infectious Diseases* (6th edn). Philadelphia: Saunders Elsevier, 2009, pp. 2618–42.

Congenital cytomegalovirus
Kimberlin DW, Lin CY, Sánchez PJ, *et al.* Effect of ganciclovir therapy on hearing in symptomatic congenital cytomegalovirus disease involving the central nervous system: a randomised, controlled trial. *J Pediatr* 2003;43:16–25.

Infectious mononucleosis
Katz BZ. Epstein-Barr Virus (Mononucleosis and Lymphoproliferative Disorders). In: Long S, Pickering L, Prober C (eds.). *Principles and Practice of Pediatric Infectious Diseases.* New York: Churchill Livingstone, 2003, pp. 1059–68.

Measles
Mason WH. Measles. In Kliegman RM, Standon B, St Geme J, Schor NF, Behrman RE(eds). *Nelson Textbook of Pediatrics* (20th edn). Philadelphia, Elsevier 2011, pp. 1069–75.

Neonatal herpes simplex virus
Whitley RJ. Herpes Simplex Infections. In: Glaser R, Jones JE (eds). *Herpes Virus Infections.* New York: Marcel Decker, 1994, pp. 1–58.

Varicella (chicken-pox)
Grose C. Varicella zoster virus infection: chickenpox, shingles and varicella vaccine. In: Glaser R, Jones JE (eds). *Herpes Virus Infections.* New York: Marcel Decker, 1994, pp. 117–85.

Herpes zoster (shingles)
Grose C. Varicella zoster virus infection: chickenpox, shingles and varicella vaccine. In: Glaser R, Jones JE (eds). *Herpes Virus Infections.* New York: Marcel Decker, 1994, pp. 117–85.

Congenital toxoplasmosis
Montoya JG, Liesenfeld O. Toxoplasmosis. *Lancet* 2004; 363:1965–76.

Cryptosporidiosis
American Academy of Pediatrics. Cryptosporidiosis. In: Pickering LK (ed). *Red Book: 2012 Report of the Committee on Infectious Diseases* (29th edn). Elk Grove Village, Ill: American Academy of Pediatrics, 2012, pp. 296–98.

Cysticercosis (neurocysticercosis)
American Academy of Pediatrics. Tapeworm disease (taeniasis and cysticercosis). In: Pickering LK (ed). *Red Book: 2012 Report of the Committee on Infectious Diseases* (29th edn). Elk Grove Village, Ill: American Academy of Pediatrics, 2012, pp. 703–5.

Invasive aspergillosis
Steinbach WJ. Pediatric aspergillosis: disease and treatment differences in children. *Pediatr Infect Dis J* 2005;24:358–64.

Neonatal systemic candidiasis
Pappas PG, Kauffman CA, Andes D, *et al.* Clinical Practice Guidelines for the Management of Candidiasis: 2009 Update by the Infectious Disease Society of America. *Clin Infect Dis* 2009;48:503–35.

Malaria
Crawley J, Chu C, Mtove G, Nosten F. Malaria in children. *Lancet* 2010;375:1468–81.

Schistosomiasis (urinary)
Maguire JH. Trematodes (schistosomes) and other flukes. In: Mandell GL, Bennett JE, Dolin R (eds). *Principles and Practice of Infectious Diseases*, 7th edn. New York: Elsevier, 2010, pp. 3595–606.

Visceral leishmaniasis
Van Griensven J, Diro E. Visceral leishmaniasis. *Infect Dis Clin North Am* 2012;26:309–22.

Kawasaki disease
Brogan PA, Bose A, Burgner D, *et al.* Kawasaki disease: an evidence based approach to diagnosis, treatment, and proposals for future research. *Arch Dis Child* 2002;86:286–90.

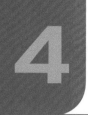

Respiratory Medicine

Colin Wallis, Helen Spencer and Sam Sonnappa

CYSTIC FIBROSIS

INCIDENCE

The incidence of cystic fibrosis (CF) is approximately 1 in 2500 in Caucasians with a wide variation, although usually lower frequency, in other ethnic groups. Carriers are normal healthy individuals with a population frequency of 1 in 20–25 in the UK.

AETIOLOGY/PATHOGENESIS

Cystic fibrosis (CF) is an autosomal recessive disease caused by a gene defect on the long arm of chromosome 7. The most common mutation in Caucasians is ΔF508, accounting for some 70% of the gene mutations seen in Northern Europeans. Over 1,000 other mutations have been described, a number of which are specific to other ethnic groups. Although there is some evidence of a phenotype – genotype correlation especially in relation to pancreatic sufficiency, the phenotype is unpredictable. A number of environmental factors as well as phenotypical impact from modifier genes will all influence the final clinical phenotype.

The gene defect codes for an abnormal protein, the cystic fibrosis transmembrane regulating (CFTR) protein. This principally controls a chloride channel on the cell surface with associated effects on some sodium transport channels which, when abnormal, results in unusually viscid and sticky secretions in tubular structures of the lung, sinuses, liver and the pancreas. It may also have a role in the immune defence of the respiratory epithelium, therefore promoting bacterial infection. There is also an absence of the vas deferens in males leading to infertility in many cases. Diabetes mellitus is also an increasingly common complication in adolescents and adults and the importance of bone health is receiving increasing attention as patients are now surviving into middle age. The liver can also be affected over time leading to hepatic cirrhosis.

CLINICAL PRESENTATION

Neonatal screening for CF is now a routine test on a heel prick sample in neonates in the UK. Whereas previously, the most common presentations of CF were recurrent chest infections, failure to thrive and steatorrhoea, the majority of newborns are now identified with no clinical signs. Other modes of presentation include neonatal bowel obstruction due to meconium ileus in about 10–15% of cases (**Fig. 4.1**).

Delayed diagnoses are still occurring in those who were born prior to the neonatal screening programme. Nasal polyposis, pancreatitis, periportal cirrhosis, bronchiectasis and male infertility are features of a late diagnosis. Other cases may be detected by antenatal detection of bowel echogencity or as part of family screening with a known CF proband.

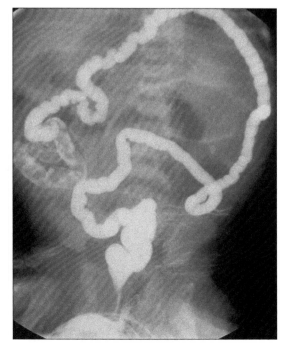

FIGURE 4.1 Meconium ileus in cystic fibrosis. Contrast study showing micro-colon.

DIAGNOSIS

The diagnosis of CF is by identification of two CF disease-causing mutations, which is possible with extended gene testing in over 90% of cases. Elevated levels of sweat chloride remains a major diagnostic criteria in those with typical clinical features in whom two genes cannot be specifically identified. Most children develop respiratory symptoms early in life and may present with signs of pancreatic insufficiency even before the screening results are available. Pancreatic insufficiency is confirmed by low levels of faecal elastase. The chest disease is highly variable in severity. Early changes can be found on specialist lung function testing even by 3 months of age. A pattern of recurrent lower respiratory tract infections, obstruction by viscous mucus and heightened inflammatory response leads to a destructive process to the airways and ultimately bronchiectasis (**Fig. 4.2**) with finger clubbing (**Fig. 4.3**). Common organisms cultured from the secretions include *Staphylococcus aureus*, *Haemophilus influenzae* and *Pseudomonas aeruginosa*, although the spectrum of growth cultures is increasing to include additional pathogens such as *Aspergillus*, non-tuberculous mycobacteria, *Burkholderia* complex and *Stenotrophomonas*.

TREATMENT

Prophylactic flucloxacillin is currently used from diagnosis to delay the onset of chronic staphylococcal infection as long as possible. As age increases there may be persistent symptoms of cough, chronic sputum production and wheeze related to the development of long-term airway damage and bronchiectasis. The major pathogen that increases in prevalence with age is *P aeruginosa*. When initial infection occurs it should be treated with oral ciprofloxacin and inhaled colomycin in an attempt to achieve eradication. Prophylactic inhaled colomycin or tobramycin may be needed long term. Intensive 2 week courses of IV antibiotics are often necessary to control *Pseudomonas*-related lung infection. *Burkholderia cepacia* is another important organism, usually multi-resistant, which can cause severe and even fatal lung disease in a small but important number of cases. The role of non-tuberculous mycobacteria are receiving increasing attention as a disease-causing pathogen in CF.

Cross-infection between patients is best prevented by separation and avoidance of physical contact. Treatment of the chest requires physiotherapy by a number of techniques in many cases on a daily basis (**Fig. 4.4**).

Bronchodilators and inhaled corticosteroids are useful for those with significant wheeze or asthma. Mucolytic agents such as nebulised hypertonic sodium chloride and DNase may also be of significant benefit in children with CF who have reduced lung function and significant cough and sputum production. Bilateral lung transplantation is an option for those with end-stage lung disease. However, the supply of donors is very limited, with survival rates in the order of 60% at 5 years post-transplant (see lung transplant).

Pancreatic insufficiency is seen in over 80% of CF cases and requires supplementation with pancreatic enzymes. Given in sufficient amounts a normal or energy-rich diet is well tolerated. The exact dose of daily enzymes is individualised by the CF dietician. Most children will receive additional vitamin supplementation with careful monitoring of vitamin A and D levels during the annual review.

Other important bowel related problems include distal intestinal obstruction syndrome (DIOS) which requires treatment with lactulose, oral acetylcysteine, gastrografin or 'kleen prep' depending on its severity. Intestinal obstruction can occur due to this problem or secondary to adhesions from previous surgery or stricture formation. CF-related diabetes mellitus is seen in children and increasingly in adults. Assessment of glucose handling should be part of the annual review of all older children with CF. Liver dysfunction leading to hepatic cirrhosis is another problem

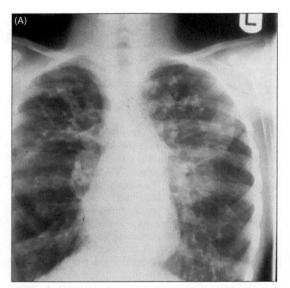

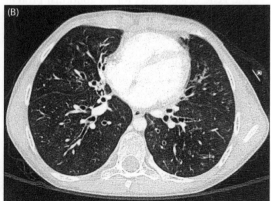

FIGURE 4.2 (A) Chest x-ray and (B) CT scan of advanced cystic fibrosis lung disease. There is severe overinflation, generalised bronchial wall thickening, cystic destruction and bilateral bronchiectasis.

seen in 10–15% of children, especially in adolescence. This can lead to splenomegaly, portal hypertension, oesophageal varices and haematemesis. The use of ursodeoxycholic acid may be helpful in slowing the progress of hepatic disease over time. Liver transplantation is useful in those with end-stage disease.

PROGNOSIS

Long-term survival in cystic fibrosis is increasing steadily with a current expected median life expectancy expected to extend beyond 45 years in a neonate diagnosed with CF today. Current research is targeting the cellular mechanisms of the disorder with the use of novel cell transport enhancing proteins. It is anticipated that therapies aimed at modifying and correcting the cellular behaviour of the CFTR protein will target specific gene mutations in the future. Gene therapy trials using a non-viral vector are currently ongoing.

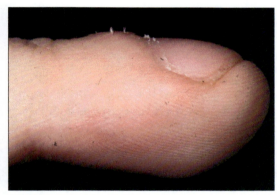

FIGURE 4.3 Finger clubbing.

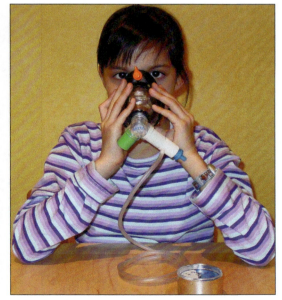

FIGURE 4.4 A child using a PEP mask to assist with sputum clearance.

CHRONIC LUNG DISEASE OF PREMATURITY

Chronic lung disease (CLD) of prematurity also referred to as bronchopulmonary dysplasia (BPD) is the primary respiratory complication that develops as a consequence of mechanical ventilation and oxygen supplementation for acute respiratory distress after premature birth.

INCIDENCE

The overall incidence of CLD of prematurity is estimated at 25% of survivors born before 32 weeks of gestation. However, the true incidence is unknown due to regional differences in the definitions of CLD of prematurity.

AETIOLOGY/PATHOGENESIS

CLD of prematurity represents the response of the lungs to acute injury during a critical period of lung growth. The complex interactions between several adverse stimuli, such as inflammation, hyperoxia, mechanical ventilation and infection on the immature lungs contribute to CLD of prematurity.

BPD was first described about four decades ago in premature neonates with severe respiratory distress syndrome (RDS), who had been exposed to aggressive mechanical ventilation and high concentrations of inspired oxygen. This 'old' form of BPD seen in the presurfactant era was characterised by extensive inflammatory and fibrotic changes in the airways and lung parenchyma, has been largely replaced in more recent years (the postsurfactant era), by a new form of the condition that occurs in much more immature infants (<32 weeks gestation and averaging <1000 g in birth weight), often with less severe RDS and less obvious iatrogenic injury. The 'new' BPD, now referred to as CLD of prematurity, is mainly a developmental disorder in which the immature lung fails to reach its full structural complexity, developing fewer, larger alveoli with a global reduction in the surface available for gas exchange. The airways are somewhat spared, and inflammation is usually less prominent than in the 'old' BPD.

CLINICAL PRESENTATION

Recurrent wheezing and frequent viral respiratory tract infections requiring hospital admission in the early years of life is very common, in infants born before 33 weeks of gestation. In addition, recurrent or persistent respiratory exacerbations may be due to structural lesions such as, tracheobronchomalacia, subglottic stenosis and chronic aspiration from gastro-oesophageal reflux or swallow dysfunction. Chronic cough and wheeze may persist to school age. Symptoms resembling asthma with spirometric evidence of airflow limitation are often wrongly labelled as asthma. Although there is some overlap of symptoms, the causal mechanisms, risk factors, therapeutic response and natural history are different. Clinical improvement is usually seen over time and symptoms progressively subside.

DIAGNOSIS

- The diagnosis of BPD is currently based on the need for supplemental oxygen for at least 28 days after birth, and its severity is graded according to the respiratory support required at near term gestation (36 weeks postmenstrual age) (**Table 4.1**). However, prematurity *per se* may to some extent result in long-term respiratory symptoms and lung function abnormalities irrespective of the duration of oxygen dependence in the neonatal period.
- The investigative work-up in a premature infant who is oxygen or ventilator dependent includes CT chest to evaluate extent of lung disease (**Figs 4.5, 4.6**), gastro-oesophageal reflux work-up, bronchoscopy and bronchogram for tracheobronchomalacia (**Fig. 4.7**) and ECHO for pulmonary hypertension.

TREATMENT

- Oxygen supplementation for hypoxaemia (SpO_2 < 92%).
- Mechanical ventilation: some infants with established severe CLD of prematurity require prolonged ventilator assistance with larger tidal volume breaths and a slower rate to improve ventilation inhomogeneity. Children with chronic hypoventilation and/or severe tracheobronchomalacia and hypercarbia will require tracheostomy with prolonged ventilatory support.
- Pharmacological treatment includes treatment with diuretics, bronchodilators, inhaled or systemic corticosteroids and antireflux medication.

PROGNOSIS

Although most children with CLD of prematurity show gradual symptomatic improvement with growth, they have reduced respiratory reserve with substantive obstructive lung disease that persists into adulthood.

TABLE 4.1 Diagnostic criteria for establishing CLD of prematurity according to gestational age

	Less than 32 weeks	More than 32 weeks
Time of assessment	36 weeks postmenstrual age	>28 days but <56 days postnatal age
Mild CLD of prematurity	Breathing room air at 36 weeks postmenstrual age	Breathing room air by 56 days postnatal age
Moderate CLD of prematurity	Need for <30% O_2 at 36 weeks postmenstrual age	Need for <30% O_2 to 56 days postnatal age
Severe CLD of prematurity	Need for >30% O_2 ± PPV or CPAP at 36 weeks postmenstrual age	Need for >30% O_2 ± PPV or CPAP at 56 days postnatal age

CPAP: continuous positive airway pressure; PPV: positive pressure ventilation

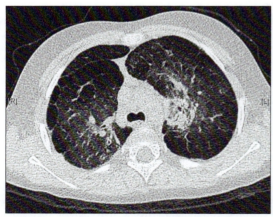

FIGURE 4.5 A CT scan of a child with chronic lung disease of prematurity showing extensive changes with fibrosis, air trapping, areas of collapse and bronchial wall thickening in the perhilar regions.

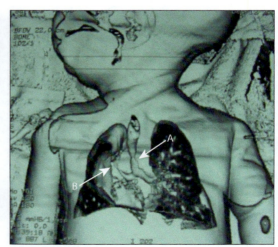

FIGURE 4.6 CT reconstruction showing a fixed narrowing mid trachea following prolonged intubation and suctioning (A) and malacia of the right upper lobe bronchus (B) as a consequence of severe prematurity.

Respiratory medicine

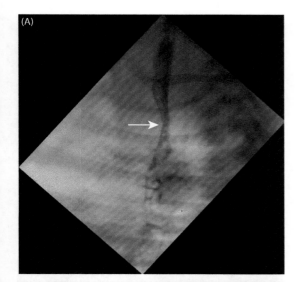

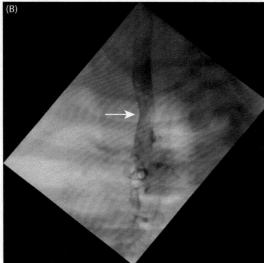

FIGURE 4.7 A contrast tracheogram of a premature infant with recurrent apnoea and cyanosis demonstrating significant tracheal malacia (A), which distends to normal dimensions following a continuous positive pressure of 10 cm during the contrast study (B).

PRESCHOOL WHEEZE

INCIDENCE

Wheezing in the preschool years is extremely common and it is estimated that approximately 1 in 3 children will have at least one episode of wheeze prior to their third birthday, and by 6 years of age this figure increases to 1 in 2 children.

AETIOLOGY/PATHOGENESIS

Wheeze in preschool children is mostly associated with viral upper respiratory tract infections, which can recur frequently, and is usually not associated with any underlying airway inflammation, at least between episodes. Spontaneous resolution of wheezing occurs in some of these children, and in others, wheeze can persist, and these children are at risk of developing asthma as conventionally defined, in mid-childhood. Allergic sensitisation before age 3 years, respiratory syncytial virus (RSV) and rhinovirus associated wheezing illnesses in the early years, genetic predisposition, poor pulmonary function, recurrent wheeze in the first 3 years of life, parental history of asthma, atopy, multiple-trigger wheeze are all described as risk factors for persistence of wheezing from preschool to school age.

CLINICAL PRESENTATION

The natural course of wheezing disorders in childhood is quite heterogeneous and distinguishing between phenotypes is clinically important since aetiology, pathophysiology, potential for therapy and outcome may differ. However, there are a confusing number of terms used to describe preschool wheeze phenotypes, due to poor agreement on definitions, large overlap in phenotypes and because patients can move from one phenotype to the other. Wheeze phenotypes based on age at onset and duration of wheeze and atopic statuses have limited utility in a clinical setting. However, the phenotypes of episodic (viral) wheeze and multiple-trigger wheeze based on symptom-pattern of wheeze, can be applied clinically, allowing prospective rational treatment planning.

Episodic (viral) wheezers

These children wheeze only with viral respiratory tract infections and are symptom free between episodes/infections. The common causative agents include rhinovirus, RSV, corona virus, metapneumovirus, parainfluenza virus and adenovirus. The associated risk factors include atopy, prematurity and exposure to tobacco smoke. Episodic (viral) wheeze may be transient (disappear by the age of 6 years); persistent (continue as episodic [viral] wheeze into school years); change to multiple-trigger wheeze; or disappear at a later age. Recent evidence suggests that preschool episodic (viral) wheezers have normal pulmonary function.

Multiple-trigger wheeze

In these children, although the commonest trigger for the wheeze is a viral respiratory tract infection, wheeze also occurs between episodes/infections, triggered by other causes such as allergen or dust exposure, tobacco smoke, exercise, laughter and ambient air pollution. Children with multiple-trigger wheeze are believed to be at a higher risk of developing asthma, although this is currently speculative. Multiple-trigger wheeze may also be transient, persistent or late onset. Multiple-trigger wheezers have abnormal pulmonary function compared with healthy controls and episodic (viral) wheezers. Furthermore, multiple-trigger wheeze is the most significant feature associated with abnormal pulmonary function independent of atopic and current symptom status.

DIAGNOSIS

Diagnosis is based on clinical history and symptoms. However, if children are asymptomatic when being evaluated, the term wheeze as reported by parents may not be representative of the actual respiratory symptoms and a therapeutic trial may be indicated to confirm the diagnosis.

DIFFERENTIAL DIAGNOSIS

Although most cases of recurrent wheeze in the preschool years are triggered by viral illnesses the differential diagnosis is broad and several conditions as mentioned below have to be considered in children with atypical presentations:

- Laryngotracheomalacia.
- Foreign body in the airway.
- Chronic aspiration from gastro-oesophageal reflux or swallow dysfunction.
- Vascular ring or congenital tracheal stenosis (**Fig. 4.8**).
- Congenital lung lesions.
- Tracheo-oesophageal fistula.
- Cystic fibrosis.

TREATMENT

Limited treatment options are available and a trial of intermittent montelukast is suggested as the safest treatment for episodic (viral) wheeze. However, in some children with recurrent episodic (viral) wheeze and associated risk factors, a therapeutic trial of low-dose inhaled corticosteroids is suggested.

In multiple-trigger wheezers, a therapeutic trial of low-dose inhaled corticosteroids with or without intermittent montelukast is suggested.

PROGNOSIS

Multiple-trigger wheeze, onset and duration of wheeze and presence of atopy potentially influence disease progression along with a host of associated risk factors. Inhaled corticosteroids do not prevent disease progression when used as prophylaxis at an early age, but they do have some effect on symptom control and pulmonary function in preschool children at high risk of developing asthma. Wheeze severity scores and asthma predictive indices may be useful tools, but are not of much value in predicting future asthma in the individual child.

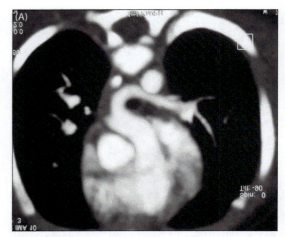

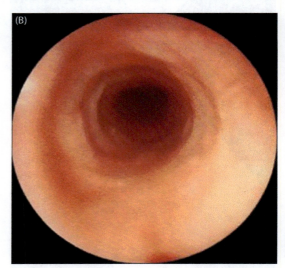

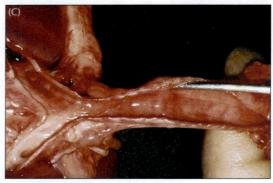

FIGURE 4.8 A contrast CT (A) showing a vascular ring and long segment tracheal stenosis visualised further on the bronchoscopy image (B) and pathological specimen (C).

ASTHMA

Asthma is a diverse respiratory condition related to several biological, immunological and physiological mechanisms that produce multiple phenotypes, which further interact with genetic and environmental factors to produce variability in disease severity and expression.

INCIDENCE

Asthma affects approximately 7 million children worldwide with consistently higher prevalence reported in urban compared with rural children. The potential protective effect of microbial exposure may account for the lower prevalence in rural environments.

AETIOLOGY/PATHOGENESIS

A number of risk factors are recognised for the development of asthma. These include frequent wheezing during the first 3 years of life, parental history of asthma, history of eczema, allergic rhinitis, wheezing with triggers other than colds, peripheral eosinophilia of ≥4%, allergic sensitisation to aeroallergens and foods. Other factors that may contribute to the risk of developing asthma are exposure to tobacco smoke, air pollution, frequent antibiotic use in infancy, obesity and genetic susceptibility.

Asthma is characterised by airway inflammation with resultant symptoms and altered airway function. Most patients have airway remodelling, which includes reticular basement membrane thickening, epithelial fragility, airway smooth muscle hypertrophy and hyperplasia, extracellular matrix deposition and mucous-secreting gland hypertrophy. The onset and course of airway inflammatory changes and remodelling in children of all ages is not fully characterised, but several studies show that by 6 years of age, children with persistent asthma symptoms demonstrate poor lung function, airway inflammation and remodelling, which is typical of adult asthma.

CLINICAL PRESENTATION

The probability of asthma is high in a child who presents with frequent or recurrent wheeze, cough, difficulty breathing and chest tightness. Symptoms can occur in response to, or are worse after, exercise or other triggers such as exposure to pets, cold or damp air, or with emotions or laughter. Symptoms can be worse at night and early mornings in some children. When symptomatic, widespread wheeze is heard on auscultation and there is improvement in symptoms and lung function in response to bronchodilator administration.

DIAGNOSIS

- Airflow obstruction with air trapping (**Fig. 4.9**) and bronchodilator reversibility assessed by spirometry (**Fig. 4.10**) and raised fractional exhaled NO (a marker of eosinophilic airway inflammation) may provide support for a diagnosis of asthma.
- In children with a high probability of asthma, it is reasonable to proceed to a trial of treatment and reserve further investigations to those with poor/ no response.

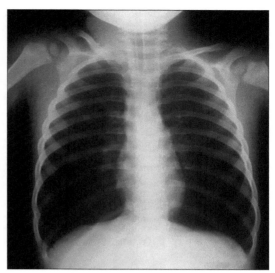

FIGURE 4.9 Severe overinflation with air trapping in asthma.

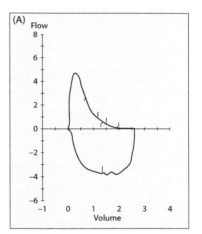

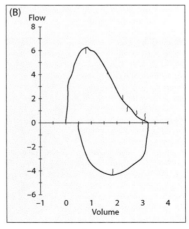

FIGURE 4.10 Flow volume loops of a child before bronchodilator showing a classical 'scooped out' appearance of the expiratory loop (A) and after bronchodilator (B). There is improvement in the peak expiratory flow and FEV_1.

85

- In children with a low probability of asthma, other conditions should be considered and further investigations planned accordingly (**Table 4.2**).

TREATMENT

The aim of asthma management is to control symptoms and improve quality of life. Control of asthma according to the British Thoracic Society (BTS) guidelines for the management of asthma is defined as:

- No daytime symptoms or night time awakening due to asthma.
- No need for rescue medication.
- No exacerbations.
- No limitations on activity including exercise.
- Normal spirometric lung function.

Step 1: for those with mild and intermittent symptoms, short acting β_2 agonists work effectively as short-term relievers.

Step 2: inhaled corticosteroids (ICS) given twice daily as preventive medication are the mainstay of asthma treatment, administered via a spacer device. The dose of ICS should be titrated to the lowest dose at which effective asthma control is achieved, as

administration of ICS ≥400 µg/d of beclometasone (BDP) or equivalent may be associated with systemic side-effects, such as growth failure and adrenal suppression.

Step 3: long-acting β_2 agonist (LABA) should be considered as first add-on therapy, if symptom control is suboptimal at a dose of 400 µg/day of BDP or equivalent.

Step 4: if there is a response to LABA, but optimal symptom control is not achieved then increasing ICS to a maximum of 800 µg/day of BDP and/or leukotriene receptor antagonists should be considered with a specialist referral.

Step 5: in the small minority of children not responding to step 4, daily oral corticosteroids in the lowest dose that can achieve symptom control should be considered.

PROGNOSIS

Several studies show that ICS control symptoms and maintain lung function in the majority of children with asthma, but are not disease modifying.

TABLE 4.2 Differential diagnosis of asthma in children

Vascular rings
Gastro-oesophageal reflux
Swallow dysfunction and aspiration
Congenital heart disease with congestive cardiac failure
Vocal cord dysfunction
Cystic fibrosis
Non-CF bronchiectasis
Inhaled foreign body (**Fig. 4.11**)
Tracheobronchomalacia
Hypersensitivity pneumonitis
Airway compression by mediastinal lymph nodes

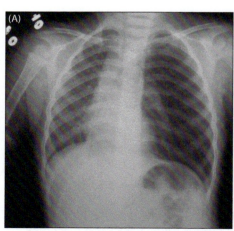 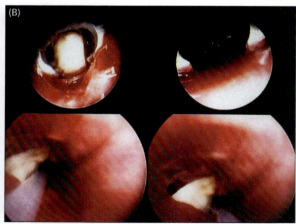

FIGURE 4.11 A child presenting with acute wheezing and unilateral overinflation on chest x-ray (A) shows on rigid bronchoscopy (B) to have inhaled a peanut into the left main bronchus leading to a ball valve overinflation.

BRONCHIOLITIS

The term "bronchiolitis" refers to inflammation of the bronchioles, but is a clinically diagnosed acute respiratory disorder.

INCIDENCE

Bronchiolitis mainly affects children under 2 years of age and incidence peaks at age 3–6 months. It is seasonal occurring between late autumn and early spring, when viruses are widespread in the community. It is estimated that around 33% of all infants will develop bronchiolitis (from all viruses) in their first year of life. Of these children 70% are infected with RSV and 22% develop symptomatic disease.

AETIOLOGY/PATHOGENESIS

Bronchiolitis is primarily caused by viral infections, particularly RSV, which accounts for around 75% of cases. Other viruses, such as rhinovirus, influenza, parainfluenza, adenovirus and human metapneumovirus have also been implicated.

The viral infection starts in the upper respiratory tract and spreads to the lower airways in a few days resulting in inflammation of the bronchiolar epithelium, with peribronchial infiltration of white blood cells and oedema of the submucosa and adventitia. Plugs of sloughed, necrotic epithelium and fibrin in the airways cause significant small airway obstruction resulting in hyperinflation, air trapping, atelectasis and ventilation/perfusion mismatch leading to hypoxemia.

CLINICAL PRESENTATION

Infants characteristically present with rhinorrhoea that is followed within 1–2 days by onset of a dry wheezy cough, tachypnoea and chest wall recessions. The infant may be irritable and refusing feeds. On auscultation prolonged expiratory phase, high-pitched expiratory wheeze and fine inspiratory crackles may be heard. Apnoea can be the presenting feature, especially in the very young and in premature infants.

Most infants tend to deteriorate clinically in the first 72 hours of the illness, before symptom improvement. Children with other comorbidities such as, prematurity, CLD of prematurity and congenital heart disease are at increased risk of severe RSV disease.

DIAGNOSIS

- There is no role for any diagnostic tests in the routine management of bronchiolitis in the community.
- In the hospital setting, detection of the causative virus is helpful in reducing nosocomial spread. The diagnosis of RSV and other viruses causing bronchiolitis has improved with newer techniques such as real-time PCR.
- Chest radiograph, although non-specific, typically shows bilateral hyperinflation with patchy areas of peribronchial infiltrates, collapse or consolidation (**Fig. 4.12**).

DIFFERENTIAL DIAGNOSIS

- Pulmonary causes:
  - Preschool wheezing disorders.
  - Pneumonia.
  - Congenital lung disease.
  - CF.
  - Inhaled foreign body.
- Non-pulmonary causes:
  - Congenital heart disease.
  - Sepsis.
  - Severe metabolic acidosis.

TREATMENT

Most children with bronchiolitis are managed at home, with careful observation and adequate fluid administration. Children with moderate to severe respiratory distress should be hospitalised, with a low threshold for hospitalisation in those with other comorbidities.

Antivirals such as nebulised ribavirin are not recommended in the treatment of acute bronchiolitis. There is no role for systemic or inhaled corticosteroids and leukotriene receptor antagonists in the treatment of acute bronchiolitis. The mainstay of treatment is supportive therapy:

- Oxygen supplementation for hypoxaemia (SpO_2 <92%).
- Maintain fluid balance: consider nasogastric feeding in infants who cannot maintain oral intake.
- While inhaled bronchodilators and nebulised ipratropium or epinephrine are not routinely recommended, a careful therapeutic trial of inhaled bronchodilators is an option which can be continued if there is a positive clinical response.
- The use of nasal CPAP can be helpful in those who have significant respiratory failure.
- Prophylactic therapy: palivizumab is a humanised monoclonal RSV antibody that does not prevent infection but is used for prophylaxis against severe RSV bronchiolitis. It is given intramuscularly in five, monthly doses in winter (in the UK usually beginning in November). It is recommended in high-risk groups, such as children with chronic lung disease, who are on supplemental O_2, infants under 6 months of age with significant congenital heart disease and children under 2 years of age with severe congenital immune deficiency.

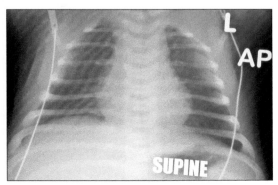

FIGURE 4.12 A child with severe bronchiolitis showing areas of hyperinflation and peribronchial thickening.

PROGNOSIS

Acute bronchiolitis is associated with later respiratory morbidity, the mechanisms of which are poorly understood. It is controversial whether there is prior genetic or environmental susceptibility to respiratory morbidity, or whether the bronchiolitis illness is the primary insult to the growing lung.

PNEUMONIA

INCIDENCE

Pneumonia is responsible for a significant morbidity worldwide and is a leading killer of children in developing countries causing an estimated 1.9 million deaths globally in children under the age of 5 years. The European incidence of community-acquired pneumonia is approximately 33/10,000 in children aged 0–5 years and 14.5/10,000 in children aged 0–16 years.

AETIOLOGY

Pneumonia usually begins as nasopharyngeal colonisation followed by spread into the lower respiratory tract. The source of the infection can be community acquired or nosocomial. Bacteria, viruses, atypical organisms and fungi are all known to cause pneumonia. Respiratory viruses appear to be responsible for approximately 40% of cases of community-acquired pneumonia in children who are hospitalised, particularly in those under 2 years of age, whereas *Streptococcus pneumoniae* is responsible for 27–44% of community-acquired pneumonia. **Table 4.3** lists causative organisms according to age.

CLINICAL PRESENTATION

Typical presenting features include fever, cough, tachypnoea, breathlessness or difficulty in breathing, chest wall recessions and hypoxia in severe infections. Crackles heard on auscultation increases the likelihood of a diagnosis of pneumonia. Wheeze in young children suggests a viral aetiology and in older subjects the possibility of *Mycoplasma pneumoniae* infection. Mycoplasma infections in older children are associated with headache and myalgia and *Chlamydia trachomatis* infections in neonates are associated with sticky eyes.

In terms of severity, the WHO recommends hospital admission in children with chest wall recessions. In a developed world setting, the BTS guidelines regarding admission to hospital are shown in **Table 4.4**.

DIAGNOSIS

Radiological findings are accepted as the gold standard for defining pneumonia, but chest radiographs are not routinely indicated in children suspected of having pneumonia. The BTS guidelines suggest that a chest radiograph be considered in a child <5 years old, with a fever >39°C of unknown origin and without features typical of bronchiolitis (**Figs 4.13–4.16**). Microbiological investigations are not generally recommended for those being managed in the community, but blood cultures should be performed in all hospitalised children.

TABLE 4.4 British Thoracic Society guidelines – factors indicating need for admission of a child with pneumonia

Temperature >38.5°C
Oxygen saturations ≤92%
Respiratory rate >70/min in infants or >50/min in older children
Nasal flaring, intermittent apnoea, grunting
Moderate to severe chest wall recessions
Infant not feeding or signs of dehydration in older children
Tachycardia
Capillary refill time ≥2 sec

TABLE 4.3 Organisms causing pneumonia according to age

- Neonates
Common organism: Group B streptococci, gram-negative enteric bacteria, CMV, *Ureaplasma urealyticum, Listeria monocytogenes, Chlamydia trachomatis*
Less common: *Streptococcus pneumoniae*, Group D *Streptococcus*, anaerobes

- Infants
Common organisms: RSV, parainfluenza viruses, influenza viruses, adenovirus, metapneumovirus, *Streptococcus pneumoniae, Hemophilus influenzae, Mycoplasma pneumoniae, Mycobacterium tuberculosis*
Less common: *Bordetella pertussis, Pneumocystis jirovecii*

- Preschool children
Common organisms: RSV, parainfluenza viruses, influenza viruses, adenovirus, metapneumovirus, *Streptococcus pneumoniae, Hemophilus influenzae, Mycoplasma pneumoniae, Mycobacterium tuberculosis*
Less common: *Chlamydia pneumoniae*

- School age
Common organisms: *Mycoplasma pneumoniae, Chlamydia pneumoniae, Streptococcus pneumonia, Mycobacterium tuberculosis*, respiratory viruses

When pulmonary tuberculosis is suspected, consecutive early morning, preprandial, preambulatory gastric washings are indicated and are more sensitive than bronchoalveolar lavage (BAL). Measuring acute phase reactants are not of any clinical utility.

TREATMENT

Treatment can be divided according to whether the child is treated in the community or admitted to hospital.

In the community:
- In the developing world oral co-trimoxazole and amoxicillin are found to be effective.
- In the developed world children are usually treated with amoxicillin with or without clavulanic acid or with a macrolide when mycoplasma infection is suspected.

In the hospital:
- Supportive:
  - Oxygen supplementation for hypoxaemia (SpO$_2$ <92%).
  - IV fluids if the child is dehydrated.
  - Antipyretics and analgesics.
- Specific:
  - Oral amoxicillin with or without clavulanic acid are the antibiotics of choice, and a macrolide may be added when mycoplasma infection is suspected. IV antibiotics are indicated only if the child is unable to tolerate oral antibiotics. Optimal duration of treatment is unknown but most recommend 5–7 days.

PROGNOSIS

The outcome is usually complete recovery. Some children go on to develop acute complications such as pleural empyema. Long-term complications

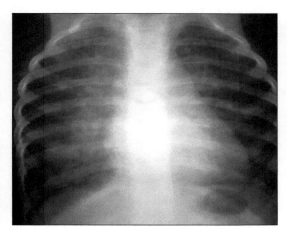

FIGURE 4.13 A plain chest x-ray revealing diffuse reticulonodular shadowing and blurring of the right cardiac margins in a child with an adenoviral pneumonia.

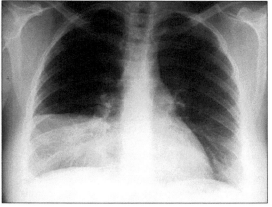

FIGURE 4.14 X-ray of a patient with a dense right middle lobe pneumonia showing obliteration of the right cardiac border but preservation of the right diaphragmatic shadow secondary to a pneumococcal pneumonia.

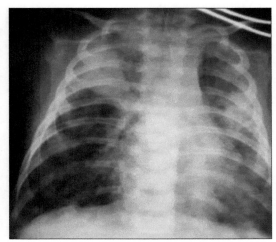

FIGURE 4.15 A child with bordetella pertussis showing diffuse patchy changes in both lung fields and segmental atelectasis of the right upper lobe.

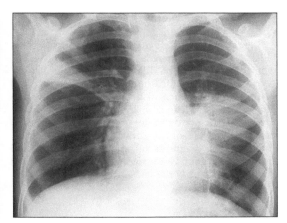

FIGURE 4.16 A child with a *Mycoplasma pneumoniae* showing diffuse changes predominantly affecting the lingula with segmental collapse of the right upper lobe.

Pneumonia

such as bronchiectasis are more likely to occur where there is an underlying abnormality including recurrent aspiration, immune deficiency or malnutrition.

EMPYEMA

Empyema is a fibropurulent collection in the pleural space, which in children usually occurs as a complication of bacterial pneumonia caused most commonly by *Streptococcus pneumoniae* and *Staphylococcus aureus*.

AETIOLOGY/PATHOGENESIS

The incidence of childhood empyema is increasing worldwide affecting about 3.3 per 100,000 children and nearly 1 in 150 children hospitalised with pneumonia progress to empyema. The pleural space normally contains about 0.3 ml/kg body weight of pleural fluid. Pneumonia can cause pleural inflammation and the resulting increased vascular permeability allows migration of inflammatory cells into the pleural space. This consequently leads to an exudative pleural effusion which progresses to an empyema due to bacterial invasion across the damaged epithelium.

CLINICAL PRESENTATION

Children commonly present with typical pneumonia symptoms, such as fever, cough, breathlessness, exercise intolerance, poor appetite, abdominal pain and malaise. They may have pleuritic chest pain and lie on the affected side to splint the involved side. On examination, a pleural collection is suggested by decreased chest expansion, dull note on percussion and reduced or absent breath sounds on the affected side. Some children may be hypoxic due to ventilation–perfusion mismatch.

DIAGNOSIS

Blood tests include haemoglobin, acute phase reactants such as total white cell and neutrophil counts, CRP.

Pleural collection is evident on a chest radiograph (**Fig. 4.17**) unless there is a 'white out' (**Fig. 4.18**) when it is difficult to differentiate from collapse/consolidation. An ultrasound scan of the chest will confirm the presence of a pleural fluid collection (**Fig. 4.19**) and can also guide chest drain insertion with the sonographer marking the optimum drainage site. CT of the chest is not routinely indicated for the diagnosis of empyema. Pleural fluid should be sent for Gram stain, bacterial culture and 16sPCR to identify the causative organism.

TREATMENT

- Supportive:
  - Oxygen supplementation for hypoxaemia (SpO_2 <92%).
  - IV fluids if the child is dehydrated.
  - Antipyretics and analgesics.

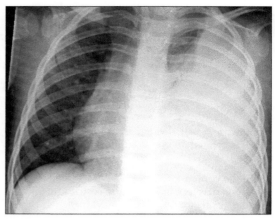

FIGURE 4.17 Chest radiograph showing a large left-sided pleural effusion with obliteration of the costophrenic angle.

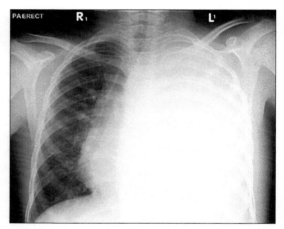

FIGURE 4.18 Chest radiograph in a child with pleural effusion showing a 'white out' of the left hemithorax and mediastinal shift.

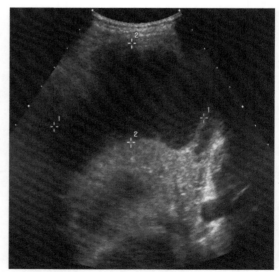

FIGURE 4.19 Chest ultrasound on patient in **4.17** showing the presence of pleural fluid (between markers).

- IV antibiotics (start with a broad-spectrum empirical cover against *S pneumonia, S pyogenes and S aureus*). Further antibiotic management should be rationalised according to microbiological results.
- Specific treatment:
  - The primary treatment of choice is chest drain insertion with instillation of intrapleural urokinase twice a day for 3 days (40,000 units in 40 ml of 0.9% sodium chloride for children ≥1 year, and 10,000 units in 10 ml of 0.9% sodium chloride for children <1 year). Chest drain is removed when there is minimal discharge (40–60 ml/24 h).
  - Surgical opinion for video-assisted thoracoscopic debridement is indicated as rescue therapy if there is poor or no clinical and radiological response to the primary approach.

Therapeutic response is monitored by blood tests measuring acute phase reactants and a chest radiograph performed after completion of the urokinase course. Patients can be discharged from hospital if they remain afebrile for 24 hours after chest drain removal. Oral antibiotics are continued for 1–2 weeks.

PROGNOSIS

The majority of affected children are previously healthy and make a complete recovery. Most chest radiographs are abnormal at discharge but return to normal between 3 and 6 months.

NON-CF BRONCHIECTASIS

Bronchiectasis is a descriptive term for a pathological state characterised by chronic dilatation and suppuration of the bronchi and bronchioles.

INCIDENCE

The incidence of non-CF bronchiectasis has decreased markedly in the developed countries with improved immunisation programmes, better hygiene and nutrition, reduced crowding and early access to medical care. However, non-CF bronchiectasis remains common among the disadvantaged groups in affluent countries, with a reported incidence of 15–20 per 1,000 children among the Alaskan Upiks and Australian aborigines. While non-CF bronchiectasis remains common in the developing world, it is difficult to estimate the prevalence.

AETIOLOGY/PATHOGENESIS

Non-CF bronchiectasis results from a variety of airway injury and predisposing conditions that lead to recurrent or persistent airway infection and injury (Table 4.5). Studies report an unidentified cause in 25–48% of all children with non-CF bronchiectasis. The severity and distribution of bronchiectasis is heterogeneous and varies according to aetiology and host response.

TABLE 4.5 Causes of non-CF bronchiectasis in children

1. Impaired immunity
   - Primary immunodeficiency disorders
   - Ectodermal dysplasia
   - Ataxia telangiectasia
   - Bloom syndrome
   - DNA ligase I defect
   - Secondary immunodeficiency (HIV infection, immunosuppressive treatment)
2. Altered pulmonary host defence
   - Primary ciliary dyskinesia (**Figs 4.20, 4.21**)
   - Impaired mucociliary clearance
3. Airway injury caused by infections
   - Pulmonary tuberculosis
   - Severe measles bronchopneumonia
   - Pertussis
4. Airway injury caused by recurrent aspiration pneumonia
   - Gastro-oesophageal reflux disease
   - Swallow dysfunction with aspiration (as seen in neurodevelopmental disorders)
   - Tracheo-oesophageal fistula
5. Syndromes associated with bronchiectasis
   - Young syndrome
   - Yellow nail lymphoedema syndrome
   - Marfan syndrome
   - Usher syndrome
   - Mounier-Kuhn syndrome
   - Williams–Campbell syndrome
   - Ehlers–Danlos syndrome
6. Others
   - Retained foreign body in the airways
   - Autoimmune diseases
   - Allergic bronchopulmonary aspergillosis

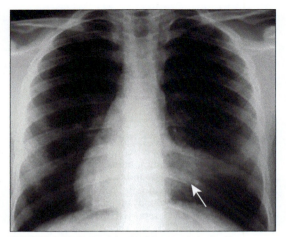

FIGURE 4.20 Bronchiectasis associated with primary ciliary dyskinesia showing a chest x-ray with situs inversus and consolidation in the left hemithorax (anatomical right lung).

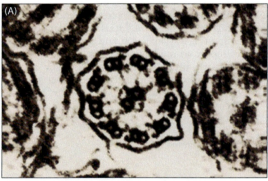

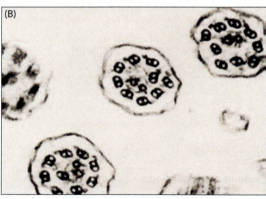

FIGURE 4.21 Electromagnetic cross-sectional studies of a normal cilium (A) and abnormal cilia (B) showing radial spoke defect.

The initial trigger for the bronchiectatic process is unknown, but persistent infection with inadequate mucous clearance appears to be a primary offending factor. Mucous clearance in bronchiectasis is affected by a combination of factors, such as airflow limitation, abnormal quality and quantity of mucous production and bacterial elements that cause ciliary slowing, dyskinesia and mucous stasis. This leads to a vicious cycle of decreased mucociliary clearance, increased bacterial colonisation and persistent infection.

CLINICAL PRESENTATION

Children usually present with chronic or recurrent cough with sputum production.

Some children may present with wheeze, shortness of breath and failure to thrive. On clinical examination digital clubbing may be present and persistent crackles with or without wheeze may be heard on auscultation.

DIAGNOSIS

- A baseline chest X-ray should be performed in all patients but mild cases of bronchiectasis may not be evident.
- High resolution CT (HRCT) scan of the lungs is generally accepted as the gold standard to establish the diagnosis of bronchiectasis (**Figs 4.22, 4.23**) and should be performed in all patients when there is a clinical suspicion.

Once the diagnosis of bronchiectasis is confirmed on HRCT, further investigations should be performed to establish cause and severity of disease. These tests are not indicated in all patients and a step-wise prioritisation of investigations is suggested depending on the clinical features of the individual patient.

- Lung function (spirometry) should be assessed in all children old enough (usually age 5 years and above) to perform the tests.
- Sputum or cough swabs for microbiology.
- Serum immunoglobulins to screen for immunodeficiency.
- Sweat test for CF.
- Gastrointestinal investigations such as 24-hour pH study, impedance study and upper gastro-intestinal barium studies to rule out gastro-oesophageal reflux, and video fluoroscopy to rule out swallow dysfunction and aspiration.
- Nasal NO as a screening test and ciliary investigations to rule out primary ciliary dyskinesia, particularly in those patients who present with associated symptoms of rhinitis and sinusitis.
- Flexible bronchoscopy when a single lobe is affected, and in some patients with frequent infections where a pathogen is not identified.

TREATMENT

Early diagnosis and treatment reduces the morbidity associated with non-CF bronchiectasis. However, therapy has been largely empirical based on therapeutic strategies in CF bronchiectasis. The goal of treatment is to prevent disease progression, reduce infective exacerbations and maintain or improve pulmonary function. This is achieved by:

- Identification and treatment of underlying conditions, such as, primary immunodeficiency, gastro-oesophageal reflux disease.
- Early treatment of acute infective exacerbations with antibiotics.

- Prophylactic antibiotics to suppress microbial load.
- Airway clearance techniques.
- Immunisation: pneumococcal vaccine and annual influenza vaccine is recommended.
- Some children with airflow limitation and bronchodilator response on spirometry may benefit from a trial of inhaled corticosteroids.
- In localised bronchiectasis not responding to medical treatment, surgical removal of damaged segments or lobes may be considered to avoid 'spill-over' infection of other lobes of the lung.

PROGNOSIS

Non-CF bronchiectasis in children is potentially reversible and disease progression is preventable with early diagnosis and appropriate treatment.

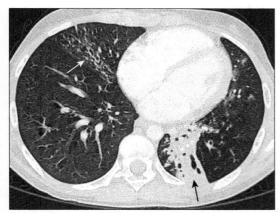

FIGURE 4.22 High resolution CT chest scan in 13-year-old female with common variable immunodeficiency. There is bronchiectasis with mucus plugging in the right middle lobe (white arrow). There is (chronic) collapse with bronchial dilatation of the left lower lobe, clearly seen on CT scan (black arrow).

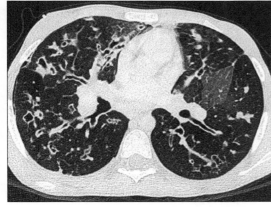

FIGURE 4.23 CT scan showing severe established bronchiectasis of unknown cause.

INTERSTITIAL LUNG DISEASE

Childhood interstitial lung disease (ILD) is a spectrum of a heterogeneous group of rare lung diseases resulting from varied pathogenic processes that include genetic factors, associated systemic diseases and pathological inflammatory responses to stimuli.

INCIDENCE

ILD is extremely rare with an estimated prevalence of 3.6 cases/million children.

AETIOLOGY/PATHOGENESIS

Within the spectrum of childhood ILD, conditions of known aetiology (such as hypersensitivity pneumonitis, storage disorders, connective tissue disorders [**Fig. 4.24**], pulmonary vasculitides, surfactant dysfunction mutations [**Figs 4.25, 4.26**]), and conditions of unknown aetiology (such as desquamative interstitial pneumonia, lymphoid interstitial pneumonia, non-specific interstitial pneumonia and pulmonary alveolar proteinosis, among several others) have been described. Some ILDs are unique to infants, such as diffuse developmental disorders (acinar dysplasia, congenital alveolar dysplasia, alveolar capillary dysplasia) and specific conditions of undefined aetiology, such as neuroendocrine cell hyperplasia of infancy and pulmonary interstitial glycogenosis.

CLINICAL PRESENTATION

There is a high incidence of prematurity (28%) and neonatal onset of symptoms and a family history of lung disease (34%). Common presenting features are dyspnoea, cough and wheeze, exercise intolerance, failure to thrive and frequent respiratory infections. On physical examination, tachypnoea, chest wall retractions are often observed and fine crackles are commonly heard. In severe cases hypoxemia, clubbing and signs of pulmonary hypertension may be present. A five point severity of illness score based on symptoms, presence or absence of hypoxaemia and pulmonary hypertension has been shown to be prognostic. (**Table 4.6**)

DIAGNOSIS

Diagnosis is made by a combination of clinical, functional, radiological and pathological findings. An individualised systematic approach is essential in the evaluation of childhood ILD due to the extensive differential diagnosis. Investigations are performed to assess severity of the disease and to try to identify the aetiology or predisposing condition (**Table 4.7**).

TREATMENT

- Supportive:
  - Oxygen supplementation for hypoxaemia (SpO_2 <92%).
  - Adequate nutrition.
  - Annual influenza vaccination.

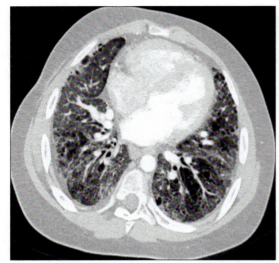

FIGURE 4.24 CT chest in an 11-year-old boy with systemic lupus erythematosus, showing extensive interstitial lung disease. Diffuse ground glass attenuation, cystic changes and diffuse fibrosis with some honeycombing is seen.

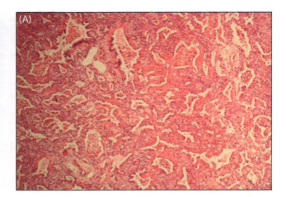

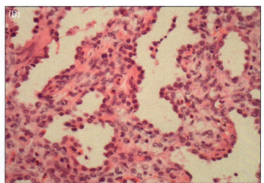

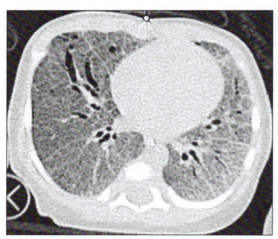

FIGURE 4.25 CT chest in a neonate with ABCA3 deficiency showing widespread interlobular septal thickening and diffuse hazy ground glass opacification. There are proximally dilated bronchi in both lungs, particularly prominent in the right middle lobe with scattered small subpleural lucencies in the right lung, suggesting subpleural cystic change, probably due to barotrauma.

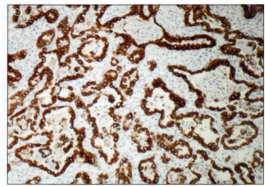

FIGURE 4.26 Lung histopathology of patient from Figure 4.25. There is marked thickening of the interstitium, type 2 pneumocyte hyperplasia and accumulation of macrophages without evidence of inflammatory infiltrates (A and B – H&E stains). The lung structure is simplified and immunostaining for cytokeratin (C) confirms type 2 pneumocyte hyperplasia. Surfactant protein gene analysis confirmed ABCA3 deficiency.

TABLE 4.6 Childhood ILD illness severity score

Score	Symptoms	O$_2$ <90% during sleep/exercise	O$_2$ <90% at rest	Pulmonary hypertension
1	No	No	No	No
2	Yes	No	No	No
3	Yes	Yes	No	No
4	Yes	Yes	Yes	No
5	Yes	Yes	Yes	Yes

TABLE 4.7 Step-wise diagnostic evaluation of childhood ILD

1. To assess illness severity
   - Chest X-ray
   - HRCT of chest
   - Pulmonary function tests
   - Pulse oximetry and arterial blood gases (resting, sleeping and during exercise)
   - Echocardiogram
2. To identify predisposing disorders
   - Gastro-oesophageal reflux work-up
   - Swallow assessment
   - Blood tests for primary and acquired immunodeficiencies
3. To determine aetiology
   - Blood tests for surfactant defects, connective tissue disorders and others as indicated by clinical evaluation
   - BAL
   - Lung biopsy

- Treatment when specific condition is not identified:
  - Systemic corticosteroids are the treatment of choice in most children with ILD. While there is a lack of randomised, controlled trials, a trial of oral prednisolone at 2 mg/kg/d is usually indicated.
  - IV-pulsed methylprednisolone at 30 mg/kg administered over 1 hour daily, for 3 consecutive days and repeated monthly is a common alternative to regular prednisolone as it is equally effective with fewer side-effects.
  - Other cytotoxic agents that can be tried when corticosteroids have failed or as steroid sparing treatment include hydroxychloroquine, azathioprine, cyclophosphamide, methotrexate and ciclosporin.
- Specific therapy when predisposing/underlying condition is identified:
  - Patients with underlying systemic disorders need primary treatment for that disorder, such as anti-TNF and monoclonal antibody therapy for pulmonary vasulitides and connective tissue disorders.
  - Large volume BAL and granulocyte-macrophage colony stimulating factor therapy for pulmonary alveolar proteinosis.
  - Oral prednisolone and removal of causative allergen in hypersensitivity pneumonitis.
- Lung transplantation: for some lethal disorders, such as surfactant protein B deficiency and alveolar capillary dysplasia, lung transplantation is the only choice of treatment. This is currently only available in a few centres internationally and the long term outcomes of infant lung transplant is unknown.

PROGNOSIS

The clinical course is extremely variable from complete resolution without treatment in conditions such as neuroendocrine hyperplasia of infancy, to resolution or remission on treatment for some forms of desquamative interstitial pneumonitis, to progression and early death in some forms of surfactant protein deficiency. A high ILD illness severity score (**Table 4.6**) at the time of initial assessment has been shown to be associated with decreased survival.

CHRONIC ASPIRATION

AETIOLOGY

Chronic aspiration principally of liquid or semi-solid foodstuffs is a major cause of respiratory pathology in children. It is often associated with gastro-oesophageal reflux but is also strongly associated with swallowing incoordination. Principal presenting features include recurrent episodes of wheezing and lower respiratory tract infection with overinflation of the lungs seen on x-ray. When major aspiration occurs the episodes may be life threatening.

The condition is exacerbated by oesophageal motility disorders such as those occurring in tracheo-oesophageal fistula or hiatus hernia. In children with underlying neurological abnormalities that cause incoordination of sucking or swallowing, the risk of aspiration 'over the top' is greatly increased. Rarely there may be a more direct connection between the oesophagus and the airway such as occurs in cleft larynx or in H-type tracheo-oesophageal fistula. A number of children who recurrently aspirate have no cough reflex so that inhaled material is not expelled from the lungs as it should be under these conditions.

DIAGNOSIS

This should include an upper gastrointestinal contrast study to evaluate oesophageal motility and to rule out underlying anatomical defects such as hiatus hernia, pyloric narrowing resulting in hold up to gastric emptying or malrotation of the upper small bowel. A video fluoroscopy study examines the swallowing reflex in specific detail especially with different consistencies of food including liquids, semi-solids and solids. This will demonstrate spill-over or recurrent aspiration into the trachea and also the efficiency of the cough reflex in the face of such stimulation. A particularly severe example is illustrated in Fig. **4.27**. A tracheo-oesophageal fistula requires specific investigation with a tube oesophagram carried out by an experienced radiologist. Gastro-oesophageal reflux also requires investigation with a pH study, sometimes in combination with impedance measurements or a radio isotope milk scan. There is no gold standard test to prove that aspiration has occurred. There is interest in the value of alveolar lavage sampling for chemicals such as pepsin or cytological evaluation of lipid laden macrophages.

TREATMENT

This depends on the nature of the underlying lesion and varies from feeding of specific consistencies of food to complete abstinence of oral feeding in those

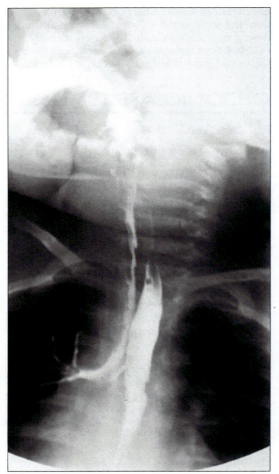

FIGURE 4.27 A contrast swallow showing acute aspiration 'over the top' into the tracheobronchial tree.

with the worst problems. Gastro-oesophageal reflux can be treated with thickening of the feeds and pro-kinetic agents such as domperidone and H2 antagonists or proton pump inhibitors. Physically propping up the infant to no greater than 30 degrees may help to control reflux.

If medical measures fail then a Nissen's fundoplication with or without gastrostomy is the treatment of choice.

PROGNOSIS

Some children with swallowing difficulties in infancy who are otherwise neurologically normal outgrow these problems with time. Children with cerebral palsy and associated swallowing incoordination may require long term gastrostomy feeds. Manipulation of feeding position and feed consistency can benefit the less severely affected but requires regular monitoring.

PNEUMOTHORAX

AETIOLOGY

Pneumothorax occurs when there is presence of air in the pleural space outside the lung. This can occur either due to rupture of the lung surface itself or by external puncture of the thoracic wall. Pneumothorax occurs for a variety of reasons, shown in **Table 4.8**. Spontaneous pneumothorax is not uncommon in adolescent males even in the absence of other underlying lung pathology. In other cases, there may be intrinsic pulmonary anomalies such as congenital cysts or connective tissues disorders (e.g. Ehlers–Danlos syndrome). Some cases are familial. External trauma to the chest including direct injury can allow puncture of the pleural surface to occur with air escape.

CLINICAL PRESENTATION

This includes the sudden onset of chest pain in association with breathlessness and cyanosis. Physical examination may reveal mediastinal shift and hyper-resonance to percussion on the affected side. If the air is under tension this is a dangerous situation and there will be tracheal shift to the opposite side. The condition may be associated with air leak elsewhere such as surgical emphysema onto the chest wall, abdomen, into the neck or down the arm.

DIAGNOSIS

Chest x-ray will show the pneumothorax (**Figs 4.28, 4.29**) and any associated air leaking elsewhere such as into the mediastinum or subcutaneous tissue.

TABLE 4.8 Causes of pneumothorax

• Spontaneous	Idiopathic Familial e.g. Ehlers–Danlos syndrome Congenital subpleural blebs/cysts
• Trauma	Penetrating or blunt chest injury
• Foreign body aspiration	
• Asthma	
• Cystic fibrosis	
• Iatrogenic	Intubation Positive pressure ventilation Venous cannulation Bronchoscopic biopsy
• Pneumonia	Bacterial Viral
• Rare diseases	Histiocytosis Congenital lobar emphysema Congenial cystic malformation
• Toxic inhalation	

TREATMENT

This consists of direct evacuation of air from the pleural cavity by chest tube drainage. In those with minor symptoms spontaneous recovery can occur and is assisted by the administration of oxygen, which increases its content in the pneumothorax space and therefore hastens absorption. Otherwise a chest tube should be inserted into the appropriate area under local or general anaesthesia and placed on direct suction. The drain should be placed under a water seal so that air does not leak back into the pleural cavity. If the chest drain shows continuous bubbling this is an indication that there is a broncho-pleural fistula and that other interventions such as surgical correction or pleurodesis may be required. Nowadays, thoracoscopic intervention can be particularly helpful in this situation.

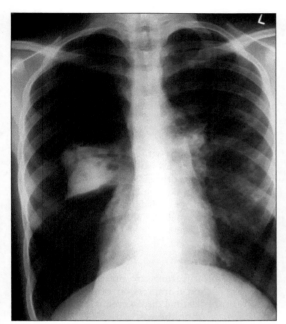

FIGURE 4.28 The x-ray of a child with a large right-sided pneumothorax resulting in complete collapse of the right lung.

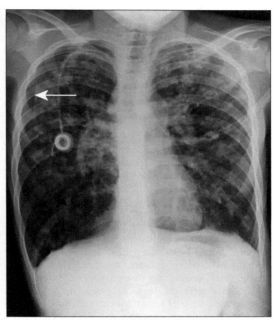

FIGURE 4.29 A plain film of a child with severe CF lung disease shows an incidental finding of a pneumothorax at the right apex (arrowed).

PIERRE ROBIN SEQUENCE

INCIDENCE

The incidence of Pierre Robin sequence (anomalad) is probably about 1 in 30,000 live births. The micrognathia is usually obvious at birth and results in significant airway obstruction. This varies greatly in severity, causing minimal problems in some and major airway obstruction in others. These infants often have significant feeding problems.

AETIOLOGY/PATHOGENESIS

There is a combination of upper airway anomalies including micrognathia, glossoptosis and cleft palate. It is usually sporadic but must be differentiated from other conditions such as Stickler syndrome where there is an associated myopia and hypotonia and which has an autosomal dominant inheritance.

TREATMENT

In the mildest cases prone positioning may be sufficient to overcome airway obstruction. However, in those with significant problems, the best approach is the use of a nasopharyngeal tube. This is inserted through the nose to lie just above the epiglottis but over the back of the tongue, so relieving the airway obstruction. Positioning of the airway is critical and should be confirmed by a lateral neck x-ray (**Fig. 4.30**). Many infants will need supplemental nasogastric feeding for satisfactory calorie intake and normal growth. In most cases the airway can be removed by 6–9 months of age. Severe cases of upper airway obstruction may not be relieved by the use of the nasal prong and a tracheostomy may be required. Some centres will consider the role of mandibular jaw distraction in refractory cases.

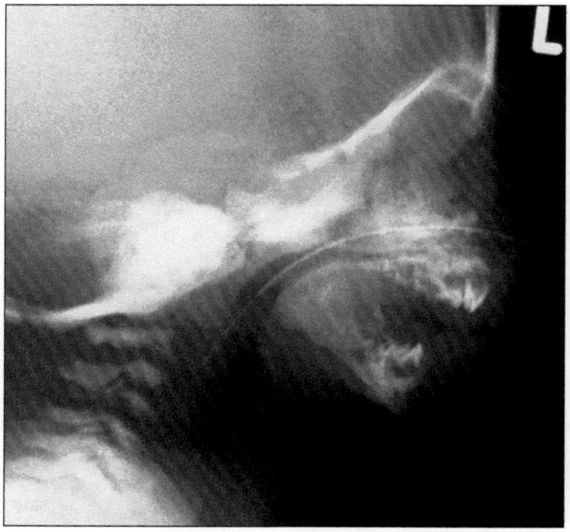

PULMONARY AGENESIS, APLASIA AND HYPOPLASIA

In pulmonary agenesis, there is no development of the lung beyond the carina. Bilateral pulmonary agenesis occurs at the single respiratory bud stage and is incompatible with life. Unilateral pulmonary agenesis may be associated with complete tracheal rings.

In unilateral pulmonary aplasia, it is common to find either a rudimentary bronchus that ends blindly (**Fig. 4.31**) or enters a very underdeveloped and non-functioning lung. If some functioning lung is present the term hypoplasia is used. Anomolous venous drainage can be associated with left-sided congenital hypoplasia (see scimitar syndrome below). The unaffected lung or lobes can function normally apart from the compensatory overinflation to fill the empty hemithorax.

CLINICAL PRESENTATION

Children may present with single lung agenesis, aplasia or hypoplasia as an isolated finding. Frequently, however, there are other associated anomalies (often on the ipsilateral side) such as renal agenesis, ear, tracheal, cardiac or radial limb defects. Curiously, congenital abnormalities are more associated with right-sided agenesis.

DIAGNOSIS

The anatomical features are present on chest x-ray following a clinical impression of decreased breath sounds or mediastinal displacement. A CT scan with contrast to outline the vasculature (CT angiogram) is usually warranted to identify the underlying anatomy more accurately and can be useful in revealing lung remnants not readily visible on the plain film.

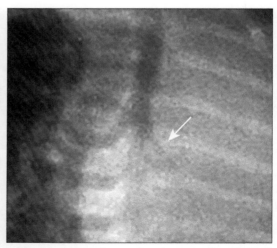

FIGURE 4.30 A nasopharyngeal prong of correct length inserted into the nose of a child with Pierre Robin sequence, allowing the prong tip to lie beyond the tongue but just above the epiglottis.

FIGURE 4.31 Chest x-ray showing opacity of the left hemithorax; a penetrated view of the large airways reveals the presence of a carina with a left-sided complete aplasia confirmed on subsequent CT scan.

PROGNOSIS

Many children suffer no ill-effects and can lead healthy lives although they may experience a reduction in respiratory reserve for exercise or chest infections. Treatment is supportive. With growth there may be a distortion of the chest wall on the lung deficient side. Pulmonary hypertension is rare. Scoliosis may need monitoring during puberty.

SCIMITAR SYNDROME

Scimitar syndrome applies to a dysmorphic condition of the right lung classically represented by hypoplasia of the right lung with a corresponding mediastinal shift where the entire right lung drains into the right atrium or inferior vena cava and systemic collaterals are present. There are many variations on both arterial supply and venous drainage but the syndrome pertains particularly to abnormalities of the whole lung. Although the term 'scimitar syndrome' is in common use, we would suggest that all complex abnormalities of lung structure and blood supply are described anatomically, clearly defining the structure of the airways and pulmonary lobes, detailing the arterial supply to each area, and documenting the venous drainage of the lungs.

CLINICAL PRESENTATION

Children can present with recurrent respiratory tract infection or the abnormality may be an incidental finding on plain chest films (**Fig. 4.32**). In the scimitar syndrome, x-rays show right-sided pulmonary hypoplasia and often, but not always, demonstrate the scimitar sign of a shadow produced by the draining vein. A case of left-sided scimitar syndrome has been reported but almost always it occurs as a dysplastic right lung.

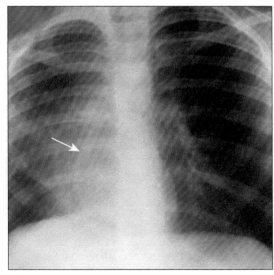

FIGURE 4.32 A classical scimitar syndrome showing a small left lung with a clearly visible 'scimitar' vein running along the right heart border.

DIAGNOSIS

Pulmonary function is rarely compromised. The lesion may present as an incidental finding.

TREATMENT

Occasionally excess blood flow to the lung can result in shunting with breathlessness or exercise limitation. In this situation it is possible to embolise the abnormal systemic arterial supply. Surgical correction of other vascular anomalies may also be indicated. If the area has become infected and there is significant lung damage, then removal of the affected area is recommended as it may become bronchiectatic.

CONGENITAL PULMONARY AIRWAY MALFORMATIONS

There are a collection of congenital abnormalities of lung growth that occur in the first trimester during the early developmental stages of lung formation. Traditionally they were considered as separate entities but it is becoming clear that there is a spectrum of abnormalities and that hybrid forms occur. For this reason the umbrella term 'congenital pulmonary airway malformations' or 'congenital pulmonary foregut malformations' has been suggested. Although individually rare, the incidence has increased over the last decade following the advent of high resolution antenatal ultrasound examination of the fetal lung. This has resulted in some difficult clinical decisions especially related to the entirely asymptomatic small lesion.

Although it is recognised that there is considerable overlap in all these entities, it is helpful to consider them in the following broad groups as frequently the radiological or histological features of one lesion may predominate:

- Bronchogenic cysts.
- Congenital overinflation lesions.
- Congenital cystic lung lesions.
- Sequestrated lung segments.

BRONCHOGENIC CYST

Abnormal budding of the bronchial tree can occur either in early gestation, producing a mediastinal or central cyst or later during lung development, producing peripheral lesions. These bronchogenic cysts are thin-walled with ciliated columnar lining that may contain cartilage, smooth muscle, glands or even gastro-oesophageal mucosa. They can be fluid or air-filled.

Clinical presentation

Functionally most bronchogenic cysts are asymptomatic at birth although the central lesions may compress the airway and impact on ventilation. Peripheral lesions may have a space occupying effect that may not be present immediately after birth.

Diagnosis

The plain chest x-ray may be sufficient to diagnose the cyst although a CT scan is often useful to delineate the structure in the mediastinal forms (**Fig. 4.33**). A ventilation perfusion scan will demonstrate the functional effects and is a useful investigation following removal of the lesion to document postsurgical recovery of the affected lung.

Treatment

Surgical resection of these lesions is recommended even if asymptomatic due to the high incidence of infection. Reports suggest that 75–95% of these cysts become infected although the number of asymptomatic lesions in the general population is unknown.

CONGENITAL LOBAR OVERINFLATION

Over-distension of a lobe or lobule following partial bronchial obstruction and a ball-valve effect can result in emphysematous-like changes to the lobe. Purists will point out that the term emphysema in this situation is incorrect and alveolar overdistension with normal parenchymal architecture is more accurate. For these reasons the term congenital lobar overinflation is preferred to congenital lobar emphysema. In congenital lobar overinflation, a bronchial obstruction is only clearly identified in fewer than a quarter of the cases and in many lesions, no cause is found. There is considerable overlap with the radiological picture of bronchial atresia where a cystic lesion, often fluid filled, and thought to represent the atretic bronchus, can be seen on HRCT. The distal lung remains hyperinflated and can have compressive effects.

Clinical presentation

Usually the abnormality is confined to a lobe and the left upper lobe is the most common. Most present in the neonatal period, with respiratory distress due to compression by the overdistended lobe.

Diagnosis

Diagnosis is usually evident on plain x-ray (**Fig. 4.34**) although CT scans demonstrate the changes well and may image the offending bronchial lesion (**Figs 4.35, 4.36**). A ventilation–perfusion (VQ) scan (**Fig. 4.37**) will confirm the matched perfusion/ventilation defect that is represented by the hyperinflated lobe.

Treatment

Severe respiratory distress requires urgent surgical intervention. Selective intubation of the unaffected lung can significantly improve the cardiorespiratory status during preparation for surgery. For milder cases, a period of observation can prove very useful. Some children will have respiratory distress during viral infections, especially during the first 2 years of life, requiring surgical removal of the lobe.

Congenital lobar overinflation (especially associated with bronchial atresia) can be an asymptomatic finding and produce no long-term effects or vulnerabilities. For these lesions, a conservative approach is appropriate with good long-term outcome.

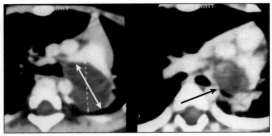

FIGURE 4.33 CT images of a bronchogenic cyst lying to the left of the carina (left image, white arrow) and closer related and impacting on the lumen of the left main bronchus (right image black arrow).

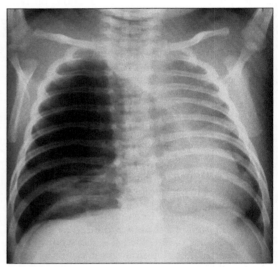

FIGURE 4.34 A plain x-ray of a child with a large right upper lobe congenital overinflation with compression of the lower lobe and herniation of the upper lobe across the midline.

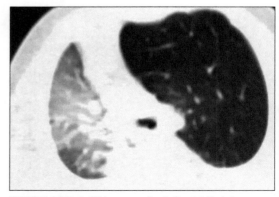

FIGURE 4.35 A CT image of a left middle lobe hyperinflation showing the distended lobar volume with deviation of the mediastinum and a paucity of blood vasculature to that lobe.

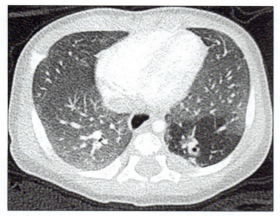

FIGURE 4.36 A characteristic image of bronchial atresia is present with left lower lobe overinflation and the centrally place atretic bronchus.

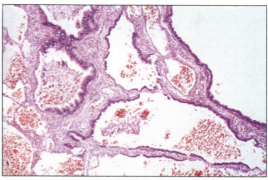

FIGURE 4.38 A histological section of a type 2 CCAM showing thickened alveolar walls, microcystic changes and abnormal proliferating epithelium.

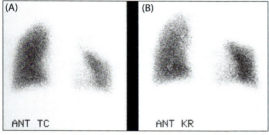

FIGURE 4.37 The VQ scan of a patient with a left upper lobe congenital hyperinflation showing absent matched ventilation (A) and perfusion (B) on these anterior views.

CONGENITAL CYSTIC ADENOMATOID MALFORMATION

Congenital cystic adenomatoid malformations (CCAMs) occur as a result of an antenatal abnormality of lung development. Adenomatous overgrowth of tissue is lined by proliferating bronchial or cuboidal epithelium with intervening normal portions of lung. Traditionally they are divided into types depending on their histological appearance, for example: type 1 with multiple large thin-walled cysts; type 2 with multiple even spaced cysts smaller in size (**Fig. 4.38**); type 3 that is a bulky firm mass with small regular spaced cysts.

Clinical presentation and treatment
The lesion is frequently detected antenatally and if very large and associated with other congenital abnormalities may lead to discussions regarding the long-term future of the pregnancy. During the second and third trimester there can be significant intrauterine shrinkage of these lesions. Postnatally, a CCAM can present in different ways:

- A large mass may present as a space occupying lesion. Clinically there is evidence of respiratory distress with mediastinal shift and a plain chest x-ray reveals a large cystic lesion (**Fig. 4.39**) with the anatomy further defined on CT imaging (**Fig. 4.40**). Surgical removal is indicated and

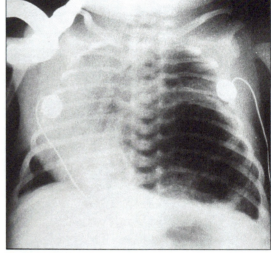

FIGURE 4.39 A plain x-ray of a CCAM showing a multi-cystic expansile lesion in the left middle lobe. This lesion required early surgical resection due to its space occupying effect and impact on surrounding lobes.

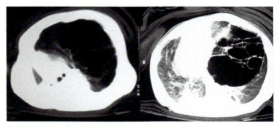

FIGURE 4.40 CT images of the patient in 4.39 demonstrating the large multi-cystic lesion with impact on surrounding lobes and mediastinal shift.

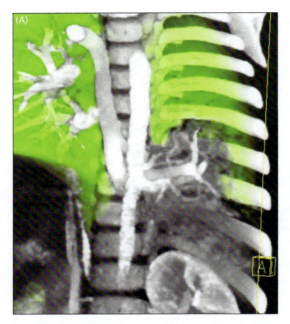

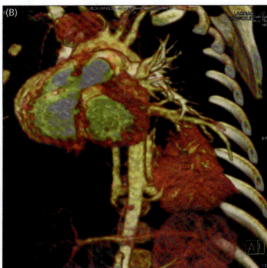

FIGURE 4.41 CT images of the same sequestrated segment showing abnormal blood supply to a sequestered lung segment (grey lesion) lying above the diaphragm on the left (A). The arterial supply is from the aorta and drainage is via the azygous system (B).

outcome depends on the degree of hypoplasia of the remaining lobes following the intrauterine compression. With improved surgical outcome there are now reports of good long-term results even with large lesions.

- Occasionally a CCAM can become infected and require treatment with antibiotics prior to surgical removal. A child who has a severe pneumonia (especially repeated involvement of the same area) or fails to achieve radiological clearance of the infection needs detailed imaging to exclude a congenital cystic lesion.
- A CCAM can be an incidental finding or asymptomatic lesion. Antenatal scanning may document a CCAM that is either completely asymptomatic at birth or very small such that it is not clearly seen on plain chest x-ray. Although some practitioners advocate removal of the lesion thereby preventing any risk of infection or malignant change, the natural history of an asymptomatic CCAM is not well described and many centres would now consider a conservative non-surgical approach to the small lesion.
- There are very rare reports of malignant change occurring within a CCAM. It is unclear whether these lesions are true CCAMS or congenital lung malignancies *de novo*.

PULMONARY SEQUESTRATION

There are two forms of sequestrated lung conditions – an intrapulmonary form that lies with the lobe (most commonly the lower lobes), and an extra lobar form that is enveloped in its own pleural covering, also commonly lying medially below the lower lobes.

A pure sequestration has no bronchial supply and exists from an arterial feeding vessel arising from the systemic system – most commonly the aorta but occasionally from the celiac axis. Venous drainage is either via the pulmonary veins or via an anomalous route to the right atrium.

It is very common to find a hybrid lesion combining elements of both a CCAM and sequestration. For this reason a HRCT scan with contrast is recommended to identify abnormal feeding vessels and venous drainage (**Fig. 4.41**)

Treatment

The management of sequestrated lung segments is controversial. There is a small but unquantifiable risk of infection. Occasionally, if the feeding vessel is particularly large, there can be an arterial steal of blood through the lesion although cardiac failure is very rare. At present the decision between surgical removal and conservative monitoring is individual.

LUNG TRANSPLANTATION

INTRODUCTION

Lung transplantation is a treatment option for those with end-stage parenchymal or vascular lung disease. Bilateral sequential lung transplantation is now the commonest procedure undertaken. Heart–lung transplants are becoming increasingly rare, not only because of the shortage of donors available but also because of increased recognition that right heart recovery is possible in patients with severe idiopathic pulmonary arterial hypertension. Heart–lung transplant is required if there is significant left ventricular dysfunction or an uncorrectable heart defect with pulmonary hypertension. Single lung transplantation is usually only considered in adult patients with non-suppurative lung disease. Living lobar donation (receiving two lower lobes from two living donors) is considered in a few centres in the world.

Although survival has improved over the years lung transplant does not offer a cure and has been described as a trade of one disease for another chronic 'lung transplant' condition. However, most patients will have rapid and sustained improvement in quality of life after transplantation.

INDICATIONS

Paediatric lung transplantation remains a relatively rare procedure with approximately 100 patients receiving a transplant worldwide each year (International Society Heart and Lung Transplant registry data). Lung transplantation is considered when the child is either failing maximal medical therapy or has no medical treatments available, has a poor quality of life and a predicted survival without transplant of less than 2 years (**Table 4.9**). Early referral to the transplant centre is advisable to allow careful assessment and education of the child and family. The commonest indications for transplant are age dependent, but CF and pulmonary hypertension (idiopathic or secondary to congenital heart disease) are the commonest indications in the older age group. One of the greatest challenges for the lung transplant team is to try to decide the right time to list a patient for transplant, with the aim being to confer a survival benefit but not list the patient so late that they are unlikely to receive an organ in time. This decision is based on an individual patient basis involving many different clinical, physiological and quality of life factors and is not based on a single physiological measurement such as FEV_1. Other factors such as height and blood group are also taken into

TABLE 4.9 Indication for lung transplantation assessment

Cystic fibrosis	$FEV_1 < 30\%$ or
	Rapidly declining FEV_1
	Young, female
	Acute exacerbation requiring ICU
	Recurrent pneumothorax
	Recurrent haemoptysis not controlled with embolisation
	Oxygen dependent
	Hypercapnea
	Desaturation <90% with exercise
	Poor quality of life
Pulmonary arterial hypertension	NYHA Functional class III or IV
	Commencement of IV vasodilator therapy
	Declining haemodynamics/ECHO
	6 min walk test <350 metres
	Syncope
	Haemoptysis
Surfactant protein deficiencies	Surfactant protein B deficiency – at diagnosis
	Surfactant protein C, ABCA3 deficiency have a more variable course – refer when evidence of interstitial lung disease and clinical deterioration
Pulmonary veno-occlusive disease and pulmonary capillary haemangiomatosis	At diagnosis
Other interstitial lung disease	Progressive clinical decline and decrease in lung function despite medical therapy
Obliterative bronchiolitis	Progressive clinical decline and decrease in lung function despite medical therapy

TABLE 4.10 Contraindications to lung transplantation (may be centre specific)

Absolute
- Malignancy in the last 2 years, with the exception of cutaneous squamous and basal cell tumours
- Untreatable advanced dysfunction of another system (although combined lung/other organ transplants can be considered in some centres)
- Active infection – pulmonary TB, chronic active hepatitis B, chronic active hepatitis C (biopsy proven)
- Congenital or acquired immunodeficiency
- Chronic infection with *Burkholderia cenocepacia* (previous genomovar III)
- Severe chest wall/spinal deformity
- Refractory non-adherence

Relative
- Critical clinical condition, e.g. acute sepsis, invasive ventilation, extracorporeal membrane oxygenation
- Colonised with highly resistant bacteria, fungi or mycobacterium
- Severely abnormal body mass index (high or low)
- Absent or unreliable social support system
- Severe or symptomatic osteoporosis
- Neuromuscular weakness
- Pleurodesis
- Active vasculitis/collagen disorders

TABLE 4.11 Common complications seen after lung transplant

Complication	
Infection	Infections are common during the first 6 months post transplant when immunosuppression level is highest
	Patients are at increased risk of bacterial, viral, fungal and pneumocystis infection
Acute rejection	Rejection is most common in the first year after transplant
	Can present with non-specific symptoms of malaise, low-grade fever and cough or breathlessness
Hypertension	Affects 69% patients within 5 years
Renal impairment	Usually secondary to tacrolimus and is progressive
	Abnormal creatinine in 25–30% patients after 5 years
	1–2% patients will need dialysis or renal transplant
Diabetes	Commonly seen in children with cystic fibrosis, who may be in a prediabetic state before transplant
	Corticosteroids and tacrolimus can potentiate
	Affects 36% patients within 5 years
Bronchiolitis obliterans syndrome	Affects 35% patients within 5 years
Hyperlipidaemia	Affects 15% patients within 5 years
Post-transplant lymphoproliferative disease (PTLD)	Usually EBV driven
	Affects 11% patients within 5 years
	Treated with reduced immunosuppression, rituximab and occasionally chemotherapy
Gastro-oesophageal reflux disease	Moderate to severe reflux is common after transplant and may have an impact on graft function
Other malignancy	<1% patients at 5 years
Growth	May be decreased because of long-term corticosteroid use

account when assessing possible waiting time. It is important in view of the limited organs available to ensure that patients have a reasonable chance of a successful outcome following transplantation and so part of the assessment process involves screening for any absolute or relative contraindications (**Table 4.10**). Although there are a number of generally agreed complete contraindications there may be some centre specific relative contraindications that will differ between lung transplant centres. A number of countries, including the USA and Europe, now use a lung allocation scoring system incorporating different factors such as diagnosis and a number of physiological measurements to prioritise patients waiting for transplant. The aims of such systems are to decrease the numbers of deaths on the waiting list and make the best use of limited organs available.

OPERATION

A clamshell incision or transverse thoracosternotomy (**Fig. 4.42**) is most commonly performed with the paediatric patient on cardiopulmonary by-pass. The size of most paediatric patients precludes the alternative method of ventilating via double lumen endotracheal tubes and bilateral thoracotomy, commonly used in the adult population. The lungs are explanted and the donor lungs are implanted with anastamosis of the bronchus, pulmonary artery and pulmonary vein. The bronchial circulation is not re-anastamosed. The lungs are then gradually inflated and the child weaned from by-pass. Postoperatively patients are extubated as rapidly as possible, usually within 24–48 hours unless there is evidence of allograft dysfunction and rehabilitation is commenced.

TREATMENT

Depending on centre preference, approximately 50% patients will receive an induction agent such as basiliximab an interleukin 2-receptor antagonist or a cytolytic at the time of transplant. After transplant, patients are usually maintained on three immunosuppressive medications life-long, which include prednisolone, a calcineurin inhibitor such as

tacrolimus or ciclosporin and a cell cycle inhibitor such as mycophenolate mofetil (MMF) or azathioprine. Prophylaxis to protect against *Pneumocystis jirovecii* pneumonia, CMV and fungal infection are required by many patients but there is little evidence to decide optimal length of prophylaxis therapy and management is centre specified.

COMPLICATIONS

Complications following lung transplantation are common. A delicate balance is required avoiding under-immunosuppression risking rejection and over-immunosuppression, which may increase the risks of infection, post-transplant lymphoproliferative disease (PTLD) and the various side-effects of drugs that have a narrow therapeutic window. Patients undergo intense surveillance following transplant to monitor allograft function and to check for complications. It can be difficult to distinguish between infection and rejection both clinically and radiologically, and so patients are sent home with a hand held spirometer and asked to measure their lung function on a daily basis, reporting back to the transplant centre if there is a 10% drop in their baseline spirometry. Flexible bronchoscopy and transbronchial biopsy and lavage are required to rule out acute cellular rejection and infection (see **Figs 4.43, 4.44**). Commonly encountered complications following transplant are shown in **Table 4.11**.

PROGNOSIS

Current international 5-year survival figures following paediatric lung transplant is 54% in the current era 2002–2010. (ISHLT registry data) The major impediment to long-term survival is bronchiolitis obliterans syndrome (BOS), a likely state of chronic rejection that can present with indolent cough and shortness of breath, initially with exercise. The clinical term BOS was developed to describe patients who have an irreversible drop in their baseline lung function of at least 20% (graded 1–3, drop of

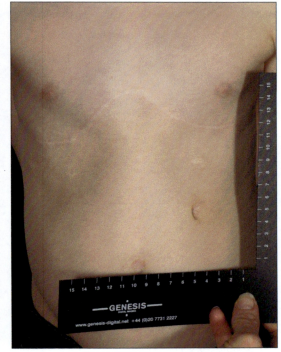

FIGURE 4.42 Clam shell incision; note also the midline laparotomy scar from Nissen fundoplication and gastrostomy scar.

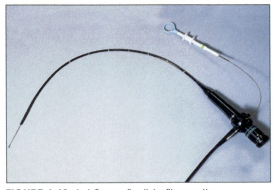

FIGURE 4.43 A 4.9 mm flexible fibreoptic bronchoscope (Olympus, Japan) with alligatorhead transbronchial biopsy forceps inserted through the suction channel. Used for monitoring of pulmonary allografts.

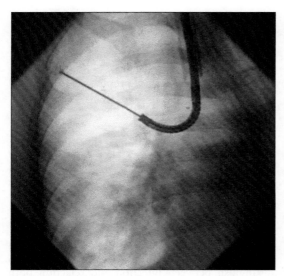

FIGURE 4.44 Fluoroscopic appearance of position of transbronchial biopsy forceps through the flexible fibreoptic bronchoscope.

20–50%). The pathophysiology of the development of BOS is complex and our understanding of the various immune and non-immune factors associated with the development of BOS is emerging. It is now recognised that the single group currently described as having BOS have a much more heterogeneous physiological and histological phenotype and may be better described as having chronic lung allograft dysfunction. Patients may have a typical BOS obstructive lung function defect or a restrictive lung function defect (restrictive allograft syndrome). Some patients with apparent BOS have a neutrophilic component and can be treated successfully with azithromycin with reversal of lung function abnormalities. Our understanding of the implications of the development of donor specific antibodies and antibody-mediated rejection are also emerging and may be much more important than previously suspected.

CONCLUSION

Lung transplantation can offer a select group of patients with end-stage lung disease a survival benefit and an excellent quality of life.

FURTHER READING

General
Chernick V, Boat TF, Wilmott RW, Bush A (eds). *Kendig's Disorders of the Respiratory Tract in Children*. Philadelphia: Saunders, 2006.

Cystic fibrosis
Hodson ME, Geddes DM (eds). *Cystic Fibrosis*, 2nd edn. London: Arnold, 2000.

Chronic lung disease of prematurity
Baraldi E, Filippone M. Chronic lung disease after premature birth. *N Engl J Med* 2007;357:1946–55.

Preschool wheeze
Brand PL, Baraldi E, Bisgaard H, *et al*. Definition, assessment and treatment of wheezing disorders in preschool children: an evidence-based approach. *Eur Respir J* 2008;32(4):1096–110.
Guilbert TW, Morgan WJ, Zeiger RS, *et al*. Long-term inhaled corticosteroids in preschool children at high risk for asthma. *N Engl J Med* 2006;354(19):1985–97.
Morgan WJ, Stern DA, Sherrill DL, *et al*. Outcome of asthma and wheezing in the first 6 years of life: follow-up through adolescence. *Am J Respir Crit Care Med* 2005;172(10):1253–8.
Robertson CF, Price D, Henry R, *et al*. Short-course montelukast for intermittent asthma in children: a randomized controlled trial. *Am J Respir Crit Care Med* 2007;175(4):323–9.

Asthma
British Guideline on the Management of Asthma. *Thorax* 2008;63(Suppl 4):iv1–121.
Guilbert TW, Morgan WJ, Zeiger RS, *et al*. 2006, see above.
Castro-Rodriguez JA, Holberg CJ, Wright AL, Martinez FD. A clinical index to define risk of asthma in young children with recurrent wheezing. *Am J Respir Crit Care Med* 2000;162:1403–6.

Bronchiolitis
AAP Guideline. Diagnosis and management of bronchiolitis. *Pediatrics* 2006;118:1774–93.
Zorc JJ, Hall CB. Bronchiolitis: recent evidence on diagnosis and management. *Pediatrics* 2010;125:342–9.

Pneumonia
Harris M, Clark J, Coote N, *et al*. British Thoracic Society guidelines for the management of community acquired pneumonia in children: update 2011. *Thorax* 2011;66(Suppl 2):ii1–23.
Ranganathan SC, Sonnappa S. Pneumonia and other respiratory infections. *Pediatr Clin North Am* 2009;56:135–6.

Empyema
Balfour-Lynn IM, Abrahamson E, Cohen G, *et al*. BTS guidelines for the management of pleural infection in children. *Thorax* 2005;60(Suppl 1):i1–21.
Sonnappa S, Cohen G, Owens CM, *et al*. Comparison of urokinase and video-assisted thoracoscopic surgery for treatment of childhood empyema. *Am J Respir Crit Care Med* 2006;174:221–7.

Bronchiectasis
Barbato A, Frischer T, Kuehni CE, *et al*. Primary ciliary dyskinesia: a consensus statement on diagnostic and treatment approaches in children. *Eur Respir J* 2009;34:1264–76.
Haidopoulou K, Calder A, Jones A, Jaffe A, Sonnappa S. Bronchiectasis secondary to primary immunodeficiency in children: longitudinal changes in structure and function. *Pediatr Pulmonol* 2009;44:669–75.
Li AM, Sonnappa S, Lex C, *et al*. Non-CF bronchiectasis: does knowing the aetiology lead to changes in management? *Eur Respir J* 2005;26:8–14.
Redding GJ. Bronchiectasis in children. *Pediatr Clin North Am* 2009;56:157–71.

Respiratory medicine

Interstitial lung disease

Das S, Langston C, Fan LL. Interstitial lung disease in children. *Curr Opin Pediatr* 2011;23:325–31.

Deutsch GH, Young LR, Deterding RR, *et al.* Diffuse lung disease in young children: application of a novel classification scheme. *Am J Respir Crit Care Med* 2007;176:1120–8.

Aspiration

Wallis C, Urquhart D. Aspiration and the lung. In: *Pediatric Aerodigestive Disorders*. Brigger M, Hardy S, Hartnick CJ (eds). San Diego; Plural Publishing, 2009.

Pneumothorax

Choudhary AK, Sellars ME, Wallis C, Cohen G, McHugh K. Primary spontaneous pneumothorax in children: the role of CT in guiding management. *Clin Radiol* 2005;60(4):508–11.

Pierre Robin sequence

Abel F, Bajaj Y, Wyatt M, Wallis C. The successful use of the nasopharyngeal airway in Pierre Robin sequence: an 11-year experience. *Arch Dis Child* 2012;97(4):331–4.

Congenital lung lesions

Bush A. Prenatal presentation and postnatal management of congenital thoracic malformations. *Early Hum Dev* 2009;85(11):679–84.

Lung transplantation

Adler FR, Aurora P, Barker DH, *et al.* Lung transplantation for cystic fibrosis. *Proc Am Thorac Soc* 2009;6(8):619–33.

Faro A, Mallory GB, Visner GA, *et al;* American Society of Transplantation executive summary on pediatric lung transplantation. *Am J Transplant* 2007;7:285–92.

International Society of Heart and Lung Transplantation https://www.ishlt.org/

Lammers AE, Burch M, Benden C, *et al.* Lung transplantation in children with idiopathic pulmonary arterial hypertension. *Pediatr Pulmonol* 2010;45(3):263–9.

Further reading

5 Cardiology

Michael Burch and Sian Pincott

DEVELOPMENTAL CARDIOLOGY

The first major organ to function in the developing embryo is the heart. The early heart needs to accommodate and circulate blood to provide nutrition and oxygen to the developing embryo. The heart develops in the cardiogenic region at the caudal end of the embryonic germ disc. On day 19 a pair of lateral endocardial tubes begin to develop in response to chemical triggers. At the same time the major vessels of the body develop and connect with these lateral symmetrical tubes. Folding of the early embryo brings these two endocardial tubes together in the midline, where they fuse by a process of apoptosis (programmed cell death) at their contact surfaces. This fusion results in a single straight cardiac tube comprising an outer myocardium of inherently contractile cardiac myocytes and inner endocardium with cardiac jelly extracellular matrix between the two layers. This single cardiac tube continues to develop in the region that will become the thorax.

By day 21 the simple single cardiac tube has started to undergo a sequence of foldings, constrictions and expansions creating primitive cardiac chambers. Folding of the simple cardiac tube is enforced by the relative restriction of the thorax surrounding it as it grows. Septation then occurs creating the two atria, two ventricles and their corresponding systemic and pulmonary connections. Over the following 5 weeks the organ evolves into the more mature and recognisable cardiac structure (**Fig. 5.1**). By day 22 cardiac activity is observed, initially irregular contractions which soon become more co-ordinated peristaltic motion passing craniocaudally along the heart structure.

In utero the fetus exchanges its waste products for oxygen and nutrition via the placenta. Oxygenated blood leaves the placenta via the umbilical vein and enters the inferior vena cava either directly through the ductus venosus or indirectly through the liver. This oxygenated umbilical vein blood also mixes with deoxygenated blood from the lower half of the fetus in the inferior vena cava before passing into the right atrium. Approximately 25% of this oxygenated blood bypasses the pulmonary vasculature by flowing through the foramen ovale directly from the right atrium into the left. From here it is conducted through the left ventricle and supplies the coronary arteries, brain and upper body; only a small proportion is delivered via the descending aorta to supply the lower part of the body.

The superior vena cava drains the upper body circulation into the right atrium where the flow dynamics direct it through the tricuspid valve into the right ventricle and into the pulmonary trunk. A small

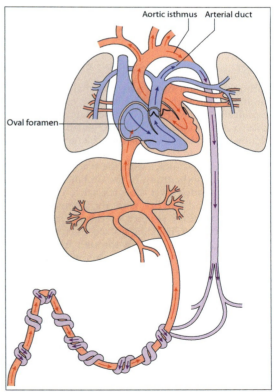

FIGURE 5.1 Illustration of fetal circulation, red indicating oxygenated blood originating from the placenta, and blue indicating deoxygenated blood.

proportion of this blood continues through the pulmonary vascular tree, necessary for the continued development of the peripheral pulmonary vasculature, but the majority is diverted through the ductus arteriosus into the descending aorta to mix with the small amount of oxygenated blood that supplies the lower parts of the body. Deoxygenated blood is then transferred back to the placenta via two umbilical arteries. These umbilical arteries originate from the paired dorsal aortae in early fetal life, and later form new connections with the internal iliac arteries bilaterally. Pulmonary vascular resistance is high and systemic vascular resistance low in fetal life, permitting this circulation which evolves further after birth.

TIME LINE OF CARDIAC DEVELOPMENT

Understanding normal cardiac development helps us comprehend how and why things may go wrong; disruption of the complicated processes involved in cardiac development can lead to congenital heart defects. In addition to developmental aberrations *in situ* in the growing cardiac structure, different cell types migrate to the primitive heart during its development and are important in the correct anatomical progression of the organ. For example, neural crest cells that are associated with craniofacial and peripheral nervous system development travel to the heart where they are important in septation of the cardiac outflow tract. Aberrations in the migration and development of these cells present as cardiac defects and also explain the association often observed between malformations in two body systems concurrently, in this example cardiac and craniofacial malformations.

CARDIAC CHANGES AFTER BIRTH

Although certain cardiac defects may be tolerated *in utero*, after birth they can become more clinically significant. After delivery the neonate needs to be able to survive independently, oxygenating itself efficiently. A number of circulatory changes occur after birth to facilitate this.

On delivery contact with the placenta is broken by clamping and cutting of the umbilical cord. The placenta provided a very low resistance vascular bed antenatally and on breaking this connection the systemic vascular resistance of the neonate consequently increases. The ductus venosus closes as there is no longer blood flowing through it to support its patency, reducing the venous return to the right atrium and lowering the right atrial pressure. The neonate takes its first breath, displacing fluid from the lungs and replacing it with air. This lung expansion results in a reduction in pulmonary vascular resistance, an increase in blood flow to the lungs and a resultant reduction in pressure in the pulmonary artery. As blood flow though the pulmonary vasculature increases, left atrial pressure rises above that of the right atrium causing the foramen ovale to close. As arterial oxygen concentration increases, placental prostaglandin levels fall and blood flow through it diminishes, the ductus arteriosus begins to close. The duct usually completely closes over the first 2–3 weeks of postnatal life.

CARDIAC ASSESSMENT

History and examination form the crucial foundation for assessment of a patient with a cardiac disorder. The information that is determined at this stage allows selection of the most appropriate investigations followed by focused and timely management of the condition encountered.

HISTORY

The patient history details should include antenatal and gestation information covering factors such as maternal disease, medications and environmental exposures, to drugs and alcohol for example. Birth history, gestation and birth weight provide important indicators for both cardiac and non cardiac disorders. Prematurity is associated with persistent patent ductus arteriosus, birth asphyxia with pulmonary hypertension and myocardial dysfunction, for example. Family history of cardiac disorders, miscarriage, early or sudden unexplained death of family members or atypical seizure should be sought.

Cardiac symptoms should also be detailed: cyanosis, breathlessness, poor feeding, growth issues, reduced exercise tolerance, stridor, wheeze, grunting, orthopnoea, chest pain, palpitations, fits, faints and 'funny turns' can all have cardiac significance and should be explored in detail. A full systems enquiry may also reveal associated symptoms of cardiac disease. Current and previous medication details can provide insight into management of related symptoms and disorders as will current therapeutic strategies.

The social history should explore the impact of the cardiac illness on the child in terms of growth, schooling and social isolation or stigmatisation. The illness of a child will additionally have emotional and financial impact on the parents and potentially affect siblings and future children. Coping strategies and contingency plans can be discussed and support, medical, social and educational, offered when necessary.

EXAMINATION

Initial inspection gives a good indication as to the severity of the presenting illness and the need for resuscitation or rapid early management (**Table 5.1**). Dysmorphic features and general growth are also easily observed. The remainder of the full examination follows the standard protocol of inspection, palpation, percussion and auscultation. All children should have their height and weight plotted on an appropriate growth chart.

INVESTIGATIONS

History and examination of the patient will determine which investigations, if any, should most appropriately be performed. Traditionally ECG and chest x-ray (CXR) are the initial investigations performed in most circumstances but with the growing availability of echocardiograms (ECHO) these are increasingly utilised. The CXR can be used to establish the position, basic anatomy and abnormalities of the heart, major vessels, lungs, thoracic and upper abdominal structures (**Table 5.2**).

TABLE 5.1 The cardiovascular examination

	Assessment
Inspection	Well/unwell Growth Dysmorphic features Scars Chest/spinal deformity or asymmetry Cyanosis – central/peripheral Pallor Icterus Clubbing Jugular venous pressure – height and waveform Dentition Respiratory rate/distress
Palpation	Pulses (rate/rhythm, volume/character/delay, presence/absence in upper/lower limbs) Tracheal position Precordium Apex position (displacement/dextrocardia) Heaves (parasternal/substernal/apical) Thrills (suprasternal/supraclavicular) Chest wall movement Liver (enlarged/pulsatile) Spleen (enlarged/displaced) Oedema (dependent)
Percussion	Respiratory assessment Ascites Liver margin
Auscultation	Cardiac (diaphragm and bell of stethoscope) Areas (apex, parasternal border, aortic, pulmonary, back) Heart sounds (intensity/splitting) Added sounds Murmurs (timing/site/radiation/grade/variation) Manoeuvres (valsalva/rolling onto side) Respiratory (air entry/added sounds) Bruits (cranial/renal) Blood pressure

TABLE 5.2 The chest x-ray

Structure	Observation
Heart	Position: left, right, central Apex: left or right Size: cardiothoracic ratio usually <50% (55–60% in neonates); large heart seen in large shunt lesions, dilated cardiomyopathy, pericardial, effusion Shape: 'boot' tetralogy of Fallot, triscuspid atresia; 'egg' transposition of the great arteries; 'snowman' supracardiac anomalous pulmonary venous drainage Contour: size of pulmonary artery, position of aortic arch
Lungs	Lung fields: collapse, consolidation Pulmonary vascularity: Increased: truncus arteriosus, transposition of the great arteries, total anomalous pulmonary venous drainage Decreased: pulmonary atresia, Ebstein anomaly, tetralogy of Fallot, tricuspid atresia, critical pulmonary stenosis Bronchial branching pattern can indicate atrial morphology with isomerism (e.g. bilateral left bronchial branching = two left atria)
Skeleton	Spine: kyphosis, scoliosis Ribs: notching may be seen in coarctation
Thymus	Not obvious after neonatal period
Abdominal viscera	Abdominal situs: usual, inverted or ambiguous
Diaphragm	Abnormal elevation may be due to phrenic nerve palsy, loss of lung volume, hepatomegaly

ELECTROCARDIOGRAM

The ECG is useful for assessing the cardiac rate, rhythm, conduction abnormalities, chamber enlargement, muscular hypertrophy and strain. The ECG should always be evaluated within the clinical context also taking into consideration the age of the patient, as certain parameters assessed by the ECG change as the child grows. ECGs are readily available and do not require expensive or complicated equipment.

ECHOCARDIOGRAM

ECHO is a non-invasive technique that can be used at the bedside to investigate cardiac conditions; it is particularly suited to assessing structural congenital lesions. ECHO has replaced assessment by cardiac catheterisation and angiography in most situations. As well as examining cardiac structure, it can be used to assess cardiac function, monitor haemodynamics within the chambers and great vessels and diagnose conditions such as effusion or tamponade.

CARDIAC CATHETERISATION

ECHO and MRI have replaced cardiac catheterisation and angiography for anatomical assessment, and MRI is beginning to replace it for haemodynamic assessment. However, it remains an essential tool for the cardiologist, particularly as it can be combined with therapeutic interventional procedures. Angiography is particularly useful in assessing highly complex anatomy, for example in pulmonary atresia with major aortopulmonary collaterals where individual vessel injections are required.

Interventional cardiac catheterisation

Percutaneous or minimally invasive approaches are steadily replacing open cardiac surgery procedures. Vascular access is usually secured percutaneously via the femoral artery or vein, though in neonates the umbilical vessels may be accessed instead. For nearly 50 years balloon septostomy has been performed to improve oxygenation in transposition of the great arteries, and balloon dilatation of valves and recoarctation became widespread in the 1980s. In the 1990s atrial septal defect (ASD) occlusion devices were widely adopted. The relatively new specialty of paediatric interventional cardiology has developed as many other lesions have continued to be added to the list of percutaneous procedures, including patent ductus occlusion, shunt occlusion, stent insertion in narrowed arteries and ductal stenting replacing shunt insertion in some cases. It has even become possible to insert valves percutaneously and perform complex palliation of single ventricle anatomy in conjunction with surgeons as a 'hybrid' operation (**Fig. 5.2**).

CARDIAC MAGNETIC RESONANCE IMAGING

MRI is being increasingly utilised for detailed cardiac assessment. MRI is non-invasive and uses no radiation. This modality can create detailed three

dimensional imaging allowing accurate visualisation of the cardiac and vascular structures as well as facilitating calculation of blood flow and muscle mass. For accurate imaging, the child needs to remain still for the duration of the scan and patients also need to be able to follow commands to perform breath-holds for optimum data collection. Smaller children may, therefore, require a general anaesthetic or sedation for this procedure. As MRI scanners use powerful magnets to form the images, precautions must be taken with metal items near the scanner. Unfixed metal objects are not permitted in the vicinity of an MRI scanner and fixed metal items need to be checked. Patients with cardiac pacemakers should not be allowed near the scanner as their internal metal pacemaking wires may become dislodged due to the magnetic force, although some new pacemakers are MRI compatible. Surgical clips or fixed internal prostheses may, however, be permitted but can interfere with the quality of images obtained.

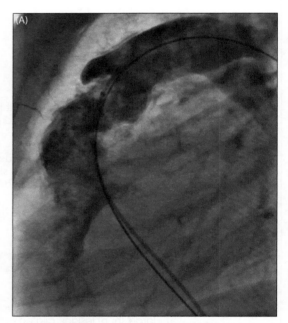

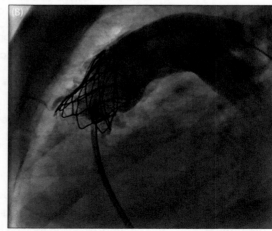

FIGURE 5.2 Images before (A) and after (B) percutaneous pulmonary valve insertion.

Increasingly MRI is combined with cardiac catheterisation in hybrid laboratories, with the facility to perform an intervention in one room and slide the patient through to the MRI scanner. This facility is also useful for combined assessment of pressure and flow to calculate pulmonary vascular resistance in children with suspected pulmonary hypertension.

CONGENITAL HEART DISEASE

Significant congenital heart defects have a collective incidence of approximately 1 in 125 live births. This statistic does not include the incidence of those less severe lesions that are not identified until childhood or adulthood. The fetal incidence of congenital heart defects is also significantly higher than the incidence at birth, owing to the risk of spontaneous abortion and still-birth associated with severe cardiac lesions; in addition to this some parents decide to terminate a pregnancy where a life-limiting cardiac lesion has been identified. Congenital heart defects may be diagnosed *in utero* by ECHO: gross lesions may be identified at the routine 20 week antenatal scan, and the field of fetal ECHO is evolving to permit earlier detection and diagnosis of congenital heart defects. Many units now offer first trimester scanning.

The heart is functionally developed in the first 8 weeks of fetal life, a period during which many women are unaware they are pregnant. The developing fetus may be exposed to teratogens during this period such as alcohol and drugs, which may result in cardiac malformations. Even when pregnancy is anticipated and planned the cause of the majority of congenital cardiac lesions is not identified. Published data on antenatal diagnosis in the UK showed less than 25% of cases were diagnosed; however, in many units this is now over 30%. Data from the Czech Republic showed that detection rates were lesion specific and in the recent era 95.8% of hypoplastic left heart disease cases were detected but only 25.6% of cases of transposition were diagnosed. This is because of the difficulty in obtaining outflow tract views compared to the more easily obtained 4 chamber view of the heart, where it is relatively straightforward to see a hypoplastic left ventricle. When an abnormality is detected on a screening scan at the local unit the patient is referred to a fetal cardiology unit for detailed scanning and counselling.

Certain factors are associated with an increased risk of a congenital heart defect (**Table 5.3**).

TABLE 5.3 Risk factors and associated cardiovascular defects

Risk factor	Association
Drugs	
Warfarin	Ventricular septal defect
Lithium	Ebstein anomaly
Phenytoin	Pulmonary stenosis, aortic stenosis, coarctation of the aorta, patent ductus arteriosus
Carbamazepine	Atrial septal defect, patent ductus arteriosus
Sodium valproate	Tetralogy of Fallot, ventricular septal defect
Oestrogen and progesterone	Ventricular septal defect, tetralogy of Fallot, transposition of the great arteries
Amphetamines and cocaine	Septal defects
Alcohol	Septal defects, tetralogy of Fallot, transposition of the great arteries
Infection	
Rubella	Patent ductus arteriosus, pulmonary stenosis, septal defect
Maternal disease	
Diabetes mellitus	All congenital heart lesions, most commonly transposition of the great arteries, ventricular septal defects and cardiomyopathy
Systemic lupus erythematosus	Congenital complete heart block
Phenylketonuria	Tetralogy of Fallot
Genetic/inherited	
Chromosomal defects:	Approximately 30% of live births with a chromosomal defect will have an associated cardiac lesion
Trisomy 13 (Patau syndrome)	Ventricular septal defect, patent ductus arteriosus
Trisomy 18 (Edwards syndrome)	Ventricular septal defect, patent ductus arteriosus, pulmonary stenosis

(Continued)

TABLE 5.3 *(Continued)* Risk factors and associated cardiovascular defects

Risk factor	Association
Trisomy 21	5% of all congenital heart disease is associated with trisomy 21; atrioventricular septal defects
Turner syndrome	Coarctation of the aorta, aortic stenosis
Klinefelter syndrome	Atrial septal defect, patent ductus arteriosus
Contiguous gene defects	
Beckwith–Wiedemann syndrome	Cardiac hypertrophy
Di George syndrome	Conotruncal lesions (i.e. involving conus/outflow tracts): truncus arteriosus, interrupted aortic arch, Fallot tetralogy
Williams syndrome	Supravalvular aortic stenosis, peripheral pulmonary artery stenosis
Single gene defects	
Noonan syndrome	Hypertrophic cardiomyopathy, pulmonary stenosis
Marfan syndrome	Aortic root dilatation progressing to dissection, mitral valve prolapsed, mitral and aortic regurgitation
Holt–Oram syndrome	Atrial septal defect (secundum)
Apert syndrome	Pulmonary stenosis, ventricular septal defect
Ehlers–Danlos syndrome	Aortic dissection, atrial septal defects, mitral valve prolapse
Carpenter syndrome	Septal defects, patent ductus arteriosus, pulmonary stenosis
X-linked inheritance	
Duchenne muscular dystrophy	Cardiomyopathy
Other associations	
Imperforate anus	Ventricular septal defect, tetralogy of Fallot
Trachea-oesophageal fistula	Septal defects, tetralogy of Fallot
Diaphragmatic hernia	Various lesions
VACTERL	Ventricular septal defects, tetralogy of Fallot
CHARGE syndrome	Septal defects, tetralogy of Fallot, double-outlet right ventricle
Goldenhar syndrome	Ventricular septal defects, tetralogy of Fallot
Alagille syndrome	Peripheral pulmonary stenosis, tetralogy of Fallot

Family history is important in the context of congenital lesions, not only because of the risk of recurrence in offspring (risk doubles from approximately 5% to 10% of a congenital lesion being present in offspring if the mother is affected) but also because of inheritable conditions that are associated with cardiac complications. Family history in a first-degree relative is therefore an indication for referral to a fetal cardiology unit for detailed scanning.

Both functional and structural cardiac disorders may be genetically determined. Some maternal diseases such as diabetes mellitus are similarly associated with congenital cardiac disorders and are also indications for fetal cardiac scanning. Exposure to certain drugs during the first trimester is an indication of detailed fetal cardiac scanning.

There are many congenital heart lesions, below are the 10 that are most commonly encountered.

VENTRICULAR SEPTAL DEFECT

INCIDENCE

Ventricular septal defects (VSDs) are the most common type of congenital cardiac malformations accounting for approximately 30% of cardiac lesions at birth.

AETIOLOGY

The cause of VSDs is not known, but they may occur in isolation or be associated with several congenital syndromes. VSDs can occur at any site in the ventricular septum but most commonly they are located in the perimembranous region (**Fig. 5.3**). Approximately two-thirds of VSDs close spontaneously and others may reduce in size but remain patent. A left to right shunt of blood across the defect increases pulmonary blood flow, which may progress to pulmonary vascular disease, especially if the defect is large.

CLINICAL PRESENTATION

The signs and symptoms of a VSD depend on the size of the defect (**Fig. 5.4**). Small lesions may be asymptomatic but may be associated with a loud pansystolic murmur caused by the high pressure blood flow from the left to the right ventricle. They may also be

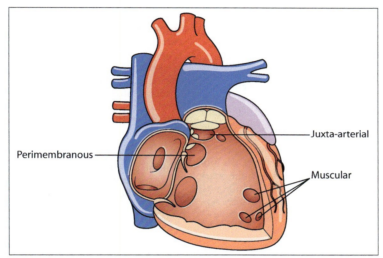

FIGURE 5.3 Illustration of the ventricular septum demonstrating the location of the different types of defects.

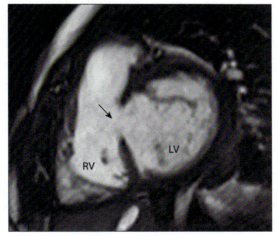

FIGURE 5.4 Single diastolic frame from a cardiac MRI balanced SSFP cine-loop, showing a basal short-axis view of the ventricles and demonstrating a large inlet-muscular VSD (arrow). This patient had a pulmonary artery band put into place during infancy, thus there is no significant left ventricle dilatation from volume loading.

associated with a palpable thrill. Larger lesions may present with recurrent chest infections, failure to thrive or poor feeding secondary to heart failure. Across larger defects ventricular pressures tend to equalise and turbulence is less than that encountered across small defects; as a result the systolic murmur is likely to be soft and occasionally absent. A mid-diastolic murmur may be audible at the apex due to high flow across the mitral valve when pulmonary blood flow is more than double the systemic blood flow.

DIAGNOSIS

Most VSDs are suspected clinically and confirmed by ECHO. ECHO is used to diagnose and locate the defect and Doppler ultrasound techniques can be used to assess pulmonary pressures (derived from the velocity across the defect) and also measure the degree of shunting across the lesion.

There may be no ECG or CXR abnormalities with small VSDs. Moderate lesions may show left ventricular hypertrophy on ECG, cardiomegaly and plethoric lung fields on CXR. Large VSDs show left ventricular hypertrophy on ECG, sometimes right ventricular hypertrophy and eventually abnormal pulmonary vascular changes on x-ray. The degree of left ventricular hypertrophy correlates with the degree of interventricular shunting, right ventricular hypertrophy indicating the degree of elevation of pulmonary vascular pressure. In developing countries, delayed diagnosis of large lesions is more common and pulmonary vascular disease can develop, eventually leading to right to left shunting and cyanosis (Eisenmenger syndrome) when surgical closure is no longer possible.

TREATMENT

If a child presents in heart failure this can be medically managed initially, although there is a tendency to earlier intervention, rather than let a child struggle on medical therapy. Surgical VSD closure may be required if the child is not thriving or has chronic cardiac failure, or if there is pulmonary hypertension (without pulmonary vascular disease, which is a contraindication). Large defects must be closed before pulmonary vascular disease develops as this will reduce life expectancy.

Closure of large VSDs is generally surgical although transcatheter techniques may be used, particularly if the lesion is within the muscular part of the ventricular septum. Transcatheter closure of perimembranous defects with the earlier generation of devices carried a higher risk of heart block compared with open surgery, although newer devices are being developed.

PROGNOSIS

The majority of VSDs close spontaneously in the first 5 years of life. Small defects do not usually require intervention whereas larger lesions are closed by catheter methods or surgery. The mortality from surgical repair of VSDs is low.

PATENT DUCTUS ARTERIOSUS

INCIDENCE

Patent ductus arteriosus (PDA) is the second most common structural cardiac lesion and is more common in premature than term babies and also in neonates with respiratory distress syndrome. PDA is more common in females than males at term.

AETIOLOGY

The ductus arteriosus is a normal fetal structure that provides the communication between the pulmonary artery and the aorta *in utero*, and as such is not a defect. The failure of it to close within the neonatal period is not normal; the duct usually closes in the first few hours after delivery. PDA is most commonly associated with prematurity but can also accompany almost any other cardiac structural abnormality. In some so-called 'duct-dependent congenital cardiac defects', ductal patency is essential for the baby to survive after birth. Pulmonary vascular disease can develop in large PDAs if the lesion permits significant left to right shunting.

CLINICAL PRESENTATION

Clinical findings depend on the size of the PDA. In the preterm infant an increasing oxygen demand can alert the clinician to the possibility of a patent ductus.

Small lesions are often detected incidentally on examination when a continuous (machinery) murmur through both systole and diastole is heard, loudest at the upper left sternal edge. Larger lesions are associated with full pulses and an active precordium but are not always associated with a murmur, the child may present with symptoms of heart failure. In developing countries late presentation is more common and if pulmonary vascular disease develops, the direction of blood flow in the shunt may reverse (Eisenmenger syndrome) to a right to left directional flow, resulting in cyanosis and clubbed toes (not fingers).

DIAGNOSIS

Small PDAs may result in no abnormality on CXR or ECG. Large PDAs cause left atrial and left ventricular enlargement initially, with later right ventricular hypertrophy; ECG shows an increase in left-sided voltages and CXR demonstrates cardiomegaly and pulmonary plethora changes. ECHO confirms the lesion and Doppler studies assist in evaluation of pulmonary artery pressure.

TREATMENT

Treatment of the presenting condition such as heart failure should be instituted where appropriate. A small duct with no murmur so called 'silent ductus' seen on ECHO is usually left alone in the UK. However, some argue that as an endocarditis risk exists all PDAs should be closed. Evidence of left heart enlargement on echocardiography is usually an indication for closure. Larger defects require intervention and in both small and large lesions closure of the duct is either performed using catheter techniques or surgery. Surgical closure is preferred when the duct lesion is large or when the patient is small, although increasing skill in interventional techniques and newer devices allows transcatheter closure of large defects in infants (**Fig. 5.5**). If irreversible pulmonary vascular disease has already developed closure of the duct is contraindicated.

In premature babies first-line treatment of PDA is medical with a prostaglandin synthesis inhibitor such as indomethacin (conversely prostaglandin is used to maintain patency of the ductus in duct-dependent lesions). If medical management fails then surgical intervention is usually preferred to transcatheter procedures.

PROGNOSIS

Spontaneous closure of the PDA is rare outside the neonatal period. Cardiac failure can develop in infants with a significant PDA and Eisenmenger syndrome can result during early adult life. Following successful duct closure however, there is no restriction on physical activity or life expectancy.

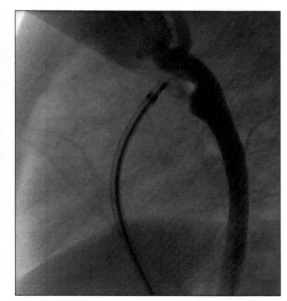

FIGURE 5.5 Lateral view of transcatheter insertion of an Amplatzer PDA closure device.

PULMONARY STENOSIS

INCIDENCE

Pulmonary stenosis accounts for just under 10% of congenital cardiac lesions. It is most commonly valvar, but it may also be subvalvar or supravalvar (in the main pulmonary artery, at the bifurcation or more distally involving peripheral pulmonary arteries).

AETIOLOGY

PS may form part of a more complex lesion and is also associated with various syndromes (e.g. Noonan syndrome). Pulmonary arterial stenosis is associated with Williams syndrome and congenital rubella. Peripheral pulmonary artery stenosis is also seen as an iatrogenic consequence of cardiac surgery to the pulmonary arteries (e.g. arterial switch for transposition).

CLINICAL PRESENTATION

The intensity of the systolic murmur heard in PS depends on the size and site of the obstruction. Valvar PS causes a midsystolic murmur on the pulmonary area associated with an ejection click and the second heart sound may be delayed with the pulmonary component being quiet. Pulmonary arterial stenosis is often associated with a widely transmitted murmur over the front and the back, on the side of the lesion. In the neonate, critical pulmonary stenosis can result in right to left shunting through the patent foramen ovale, resulting in cyanosis in this duct-dependent lesion. The majority of cases of PS are however, asymptomatic in childhood. Severe lesions present similarly with signs of heart failure such as fatigue and cyanosis if there is a patent foramen ovale and a right to left shunt develops. Patients with significant lesions may also present acutely with effort-related dizziness or syncope.

DIAGNOSIS

In mild PS, ECG and CXR are normal; as the stenosis becomes more marked evidence of right ventricular hypertrophy is observed. ECHO is diagnostic and permits measurement of the transpulmonary gradient using Doppler ultrasound.

TREATMENT

Mild PS should be monitored with measurement of the transpulmonary gradient on ECHO. The lesion at which intervention is considered varies with age and the individual unit. However, most units would intervene when the gradient was over 64 mmHg (~4 m/s Doppler) even if asymptomatic. Treatment should be instituted early in symptomatic patients. Transcatheter balloon valvuloplasty is the treatment of choice (**Figs 5.6, 5.7**). If the valve is severely dysplastic, as is sometimes encountered in Noonan syndrome, valvuloplasty is not always possible or successful.

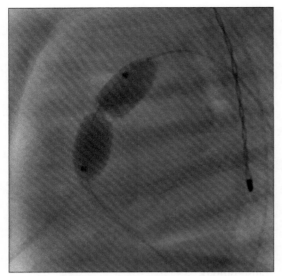

FIGURE 5.6 Transcatheter balloon valvuloplasty of critical pulmonary stenosis. The balloon is sited across the pulmonary valve and on inflation demonstrates 'waisting' at the stenosis.

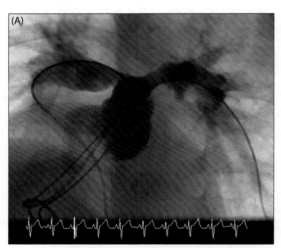

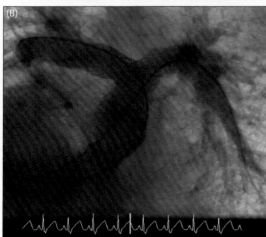

FIGURE 5.7 Pulmonary artery stenosis at the bifurcation before (A) and after (B) stenting.

PROGNOSIS

Peripheral pulmonary artery stenosis can resolve or improve with growth in Williams syndrome but can progress in iatrogenic postoperative stenosis; mild or moderate valvar PS is often stable and does not progress. The risk of intervention in PS is low, although not zero.

COARCTATION OF THE AORTA

INCIDENCE

Coarctation of the aorta (CoA) accounts for approximately 10% of congenital cardiac lesions; it is more common in males than females and is associated with another cardiac defect in approximately 50% of cases. Females with CoA should have the possible diagnosis of Turner syndrome considered and investigated.

AETIOLOGY

This congenital narrowing of the aorta usually occurs distal to the left subclavian artery in the thoracic aorta, and occasionally the abdominal aorta may be involved. Coarctation may occur proximal or distal to the ductus arteriosus.

CLINICAL PRESENTATION

Severe coarctation is another duct-dependent lesion and can present with neonatal collapse as the ductus arteriosus closes; in less severe cases, cardiac failure will develop during infancy or early childhood. Less severe cases are not duct dependent and may not present until later in life with complications of hypertension. The association of coarctation with other cardiac lesions also influences the clinical presentation of the patient.

Depending on the severity of the narrowing, patients may present with general systemic signs such as tachypnoea, dyspnoea and hepatomegaly. A systolic bruit may be heard posteriorly between the scapulae indicating turbulence at the site of coarctation; additional murmurs may be audible if collateral vessels develop. Femoral pulses are weak or impalpable in CoA, this being a diagnostic clinical finding. Other examination findings depend on the site of the coarctation. If the lesion is before the left subclavian artery, right upper limb pulses will be full, left upper limb pulse poor and blood pressure in the left arm and lower limbs will be the same. Narrowing of the aorta after the left subclavian artery results in both upper limb pulses and pressures being equal with low perfusion pressure of the lower limbs.

DIAGNOSIS

Weak or absent femoral pulses in a newborn is diagnostic for CoA. The ECG may be normal or show changes indicating right ventricular hypertrophy in the neonate and left ventricular hypertrophy on the older child. Cardiomegaly may be seen on CXR, and rib notching may be identified in the older child due to formation of collateral vessels.

ECHO and MRI are diagnostic (**Fig. 5.8**). ECHO diagnosis is more difficult in the older child.

TREATMENT

Neonatal CoA is managed surgically but if a child presents with acute collapse prostaglandin E1 or E2 is used in resuscitation in an attempt to prevent the ductus arteriosus closing. Surgical repair is usually by end-to-end anastomosis after resection of the narrowed region, although in the past the left subclavian was used as a flap repair (and if treated in this way the

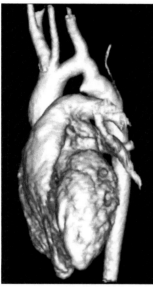

FIGURE 5.8 A 3D volume-rendered image created from a cardiac MRI gadolinium-contrast angiogram, acquired in the first pass of contrast through the aortic arch. The image demonstrates a classic, juxtaductal coarctation of the aorta, in a left-sided arch, with a small collateral artery arising distal to the coarctation.

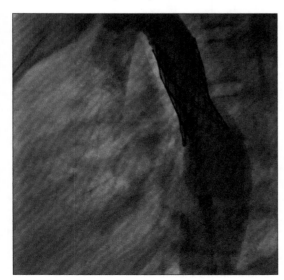

FIGURE 5.9 Covered stenting of coarcted region of the aorta.

left arm pulse is absent at follow-up checks). In older patients balloon dilatation and stenting may be performed by interventional catheterisation (**Fig. 5.9**). Recoarctation is also treated by balloon dilatation.

PROGNOSIS

Untreated CoA invariably results in hypertension and heart failure at some stage. Hypertension can result in intracranial aneurysm formation and cerebrovascular accidents that may have severe sequelae. Recoarctation may occur after treatment and patients should be monitored long-term.

ATRIAL SEPTAL DEFECT

INCIDENCE

ASDs account for approximately 7% of congenital cardiac disorders. They may occur in isolation or in association with other structural lesions or syndromes. ASDs occur more commonly in females than males.

AETIOLOGY

The aetiology of ASDs is not known, but they are associated with several syndromes such as Holt–Oram; dominant inheritance of ASDs in some families is well recognised. ASD is an acyanotic defect of abnormal communication across the atrial septum with left to right shunting. The defect may occur at different positions in the atrial septum, most commonly in the ostium secundum (70%) at the position of the fossa ovalis after incomplete development of the septum secundum (**Figs 5.10, 5.11**). Ostium primum defects (~25% of ASDs) occur at the lower part of the atrial septum when the septum primum fails to extend to the endocardial cushions. Sinus venosus defects (5% of ASDs) are located at the top of the atrial septum after failure of absorption of the sinus venosus into the right atrium, the right upper lobe pulmonary vein then often draining into the lower part of the superior vena cava (partial anomalous pulmonary venous drainage).

The patent foramen ovale is not generally considered to be an abnormal lesion even if its patency continues throughout life. PFOs usually close spontaneously but their presence is associated with the risk of the 'bends' in divers and are a contraindication to SCUBA diving. There is still debate over whether PFOs increase the risk of stroke, and some believe migraine is worse in patients with PFO.

CLINICAL PRESENTATION

ASDs rarely present symptomatically in childhood. Larger defects if not diagnosed and managed may result in an older child presenting with fatigue or recurrent chest infections. Symptoms often do not occur until adult life.

DIAGNOSIS

Typical clinical findings include fixed splitting of the second heart sound, an ejection systolic murmur is loudest in the pulmonary region due to increased blood flow across the pulmonary valve and sometimes a diastolic flow murmur from tricuspid flow. ECG may show mild right ventricular hypertrophy, incomplete right bundle branch block is often present. CXR may show enlargement of the heart particularly the right atrium and pulmonary arteries. ECHO confirms the diagnosis and locates the lesion, Doppler flow studies can measure the size of the shunt. Transoesophageal ECHO can detect small defects more accurately.

TREATMENT

Closure of those lesions that do not spontaneously resolve is mainly by interventional catheterisation although some larger or more complicated defects may require surgical repair. Corrective procedures are usually performed in the preschool age group.

PROGNOSIS

Small ASDs often close spontaneously in infancy; some medium sized defects closing by preschool age but larger lesions rarely do. Prognosis after corrective surgery or intervention is good and life expectancy is normal if performed before adult life.

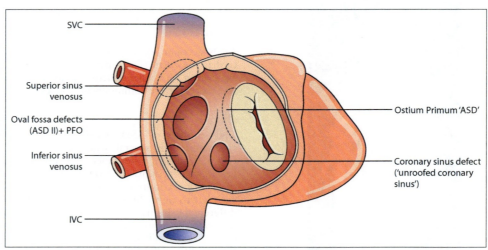

FIGURE 5.10 Illustration of atrial defects demonstrating the position of atrial wall defects and patent foramen ovale (PFO). ASD: atrial septal defects; IVC: inferior vena cava; SVC: superior vena cava.

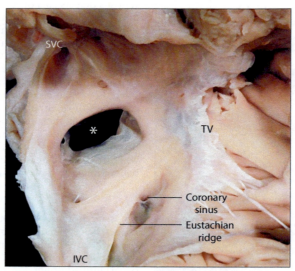

FIGURE 5.11 Postmortem specimen highlighting a septum secundum defect (*) where insufficient septal tissue has grown to cover the ostium secundum and foramen ovale or oval fossa. The defect here appears oval although may be circular or fenestrated if tissue strands bridge the defect. IVC: inferior vena cava; SVC: superior vena cava; TV: tricuspid valve.

FALLOT TETRALOGY

INCIDENCE

Fallot tetralogy is the most common cyanotic cardiac lesion and represents approximately 10% of all congenital heart defects. The 22q11 deletion lesion (Di George syndrome) is associated with this lesion and some units will screen all cases for this deletion; others will only perform the genetic tests if there are other markers such as right aortic arch, aberrant subclavian, absent thymus or dysmorphic features.

AETIOLOGY

The four anomalies associated with Fallot tetralogy are subvalvar pulmonary stenosis, an outlet VSD, overriding aorta and right ventricular hypertrophy (**Fig. 5.12**). The morphology of tetralogy of Fallot results from the VSD being malaligned and consequently there are varying degrees of abnormal anterior displacement of the remaining infundibular septum, allowing the aorta to override, the right ventricular outflow to be obstructed and right ventricular hypertrophy to develop.

CLINICAL PRESENTATION

Severity of the symptoms depends on the degree of right ventricular outflow tract obstruction/pulmonary stenosis from the deviated infundibulum. If pulmonary stenosis is severe, there will be neonatal cyanosis; however, generally subvalvar stenosis progresses in infancy resulting in cyanosis developing over the first year of life. As there is a trend to correction in early infancy, it is rare to see clubbing and even the hypercyanotic spells are now uncommon. The latter can present as cyanosis or pallor, frequently on crying. In developing countries where infant correction is not performed, it is not uncommon to see the child assume a squatting position during these spells to alleviate symptoms. This position increases the systemic vascular resistance,

reducing the right to left shunting and improving pulmonary perfusion and oxygenation. On examination, infants have an ejection systolic murmur loudest at the upper left sternal edge, this murmur diminishes as right ventricular outflow obstruction increases. There is no murmur associated with the VSD as it is large with equal ventricular pressures on either side. The child may have a parasternal heave and a thrill in the pulmonary area, and the pulmonary component of the second heart sound is quiet.

DIAGNOSIS

Right ventricular hypertrophy is seen on ECG and CXR. Pulmonary oligaemia, small central pulmonary arteries and the enlarged right ventricle often give the appearance of a boot-shaped heart on x-ray. In approximately 30% a right sided aortic arch is seen. ECHO is diagnostic, and usually further investigation such as cardiac catheterisation is not usually needed to determine the anatomy prior to surgery (**Fig. 5.13**).

TREATMENT

If the child is symptomatic early in neonatal life a systemic–pulmonary shunt is created, such as the modified Blalock–Taussig shunt with an interposition graft between subclavian and pulmonary arteries, with a view to corrective surgery when the child grows. Elective surgical correction is usually performed in infancy with a surgical mortality risk of less than 5%.

PROGNOSIS

If left untreated survival to adult life is unusual although does occur. In adult life, further surgery may be required, typically for pulmonary regurgitation and or recurrent right ventricular outflow obstruction. Ventricular arrhythmias and progressive heart block are also recognised as complications, although may be less common with modern surgical techniques.

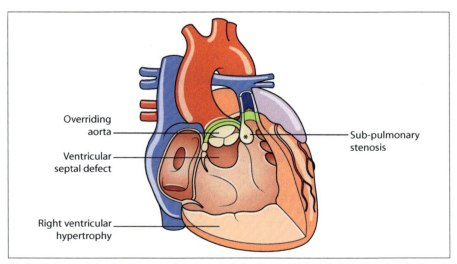

Overriding aorta

Ventricular septal defect

Right ventricular hypertrophy

Sub-pulmonary stenosis

FIGURE 5.12 Illustration of the four anomalies seen in tetralogy of Fallot. *: Abnormal outlet septum (antero-cephalad deviation).

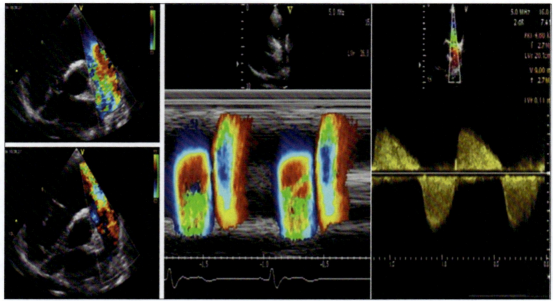

FIGURE 5.13 Postoperative images of Fallot tetralogy seen in 2D colour M-mode and colour wave Doppler. Pulmonary stenosis and pulmonary regurgitation measured by bidirectional flow in Doppler mode.

AORTIC STENOSIS

INCIDENCE

Aortic stenosis (AS) accounts for approximately 5% of congenital cardiac lesions and occurs more commonly in males than females.

AETIOLOGY

Stenosis of the left ventricular outflow tract may be valvar, subvalvar or supravalvar. Valvar and subvalvar lesions can develop in association with other left-sided obstructive lesions. Subvalvar stenosis may be a discrete membrane or a diffuse tunnel-like obstruction. Most AS is mild and obstruction at any level may be progressive.

CLINICAL PRESENTATION

Severe AS can present in the neonatal period with signs of cardiac failure, critical aortic stenosis and aortic atresia being significant duct-dependent lesions. Older children with severe lesions may present with syncope or chest pain on exertion.

Pulses are weak in severe valvar AS. A thrill may be palpable suprasternally and the apex beat may be hyperdynamic. An ejection systolic click indicates a stenotic aortic valve. The aortic component of the second heart sound may be reduced and can be delayed until after the pulmonary component (reversed splitting).

DIAGNOSIS

Left ventricular hypertrophy may be identified by high left-sided voltages on ECG. If stenosis is severe, evidence of myocardial ischaemia or strain may be evident (ST depression and T wave inversion). CXR may be normal in mild stenosis with evidence of left ventricular dilatation in more significant lesions. ECHO is used to identify the site and extent of the stenosis.

TREATMENT

Intervention to reduce the stenosis is indicated if the patient has ECG changes or is symptomatic. As with pulmonary stenosis, the exact gradient at which these changes become apparent and intervention is required varies between individual patients. In general if the pressure gradient between the left ventricle and ascending aorta exceeds 64 mmHg (non-invasively measured by Doppler ultrasonography using the modified Bernoulli equation) treatment is required.

Transcatheter balloon valvuloplasty is preferred to open surgery in most units. This is not curative treatment and later in life aortic valve replacement may be required, often because of aortic regurgitation from the balloon procedure. The usual operation involves the Ross procedure rather than using a prosthetic valve. This involves replacement of the damaged aortic valve with the patient's own pulmonary valve, and replacing the pulmonary valve with a homograft. This process allows growth of the valves and eliminates the need for anticoagulation.

PROGNOSIS

Operative mortality during surgery or interventional catheterisation is generally low except in neonates with critical AS. Those patients with mild lesions or who have responded well to intervention have a near normal life expectancy. Severe stenosis can result in cardiac failure and even moderate lesions can become symptomatic on exertion causing angina, syncope and sudden death; competitive sports should therefore be discouraged in severe stenosis.

TRANSPOSITION OF THE GREAT ARTERIES

INCIDENCE

Transposition of the great arteries (TGA) is the second most common cyanotic cardiac lesion accounting for approximately 5% of all congenital heart disease. It is more common in males than females.

AETIOLOGY

Transposition of the great arteries exists when the pulmonary artery originates from the left ventricle and the aorta from the right ventricle (**Figs 5.14, 5.15**). It is linked with maternal diabetes mellitus and is also found in association many other cardiac lesions. Somewhat confusingly the term transposition is used for two very different conditions: simple transposition and the less common congenitally corrected transposition; the latter is dealt with below in the 'other lesions' section.

CLINICAL PRESENTATION

In simple transposition, two parallel circulations exist with deoxygenated blood circulating from the right atrium to the right ventricle into the aorta and around the body returning via the vena cava to the right sided system; oxygenated blood returns from the lungs into the left atrium, left ventricle and exits via the transposed pulmonary artery back to the lungs. The vascular arrangement of TGA is not compatible with life *ex utero* and survival depends on the presence of other lesions and the patency of fetal structure that permits mixing of oxygenated and deoxygenated blood. Mixing of blood from these two parallel circulations is usually via the foramen ovale and little mixing occurs at ductal level; however, maintaining ductal patency may increase left atrial pressure and therefore shunting across the foramen. A secundum ASD may allow oxygen saturation to be reasonable after delivery and a significant VSD may mean that the baby is only mildly cyanosed. However, for most babies, there is only a foramen ovale and they are very cyanosed at birth. An emergency balloon septostomy is required with a balloon catheter from the femoral vein or umbilicus tearing the atrial septum.

TREATMENT

If transposition is diagnosed on fetal scanning it is wise to deliver the infant in a maternity unit where paediatric cardiology cover can be obtained soon after delivery.

Corrective surgery for simple transposition is the arterial switch repair with anatomical correction for the transposed arteries. The complicating factor for this operation is the transfer of the coronary arteries and if any tension is created on these small arteries after their transfer, there is myocardial ischaemia, which can be fatal.

PROGNOSIS

If the neonatal course is not complicated the long-term outlook is generally very good after surgery, although sometimes pulmonary arterial stenosis can subsequently develop, which may need balloon dilatation or stent placement.

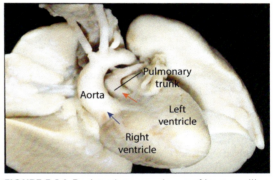

FIGURE 5.14 Postmortem specimen of transposition of the great arteries, the aorta arising from the right atrium and the pulmonary trunk from the left ventricle.

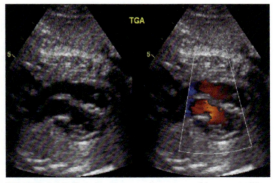

FIGURE 5.15 Fetal echocardiogram of transposition of the great arteries demonstrating the classic double barrel shotgun appearance, highlighted here in Doppler mode.

HYPOPLASTIC LEFT HEART

INCIDENCE

Hypoplastic left heart (HLH) occurs in approximately 2–3 per 10,000 live births, accounting for 2–3% of all congenital heart disease (**Fig. 5.16**). This is likely to be an underestimate as many pregnancies affected by HLH will end in a spontaneous abortion, and if diagnosed antenatally many parents decide to undergo a termination of pregnancy. It is 50% more common in males than females. Left untreated HLH is likely to account for 25–40% of neonatal cardiac deaths. HLH is associated with other birth defects in approximately 10% of cases.

AETIOLOGY

In this lesion the left side of the heart fails to develop. The left ventricle is small and it can be associated with aortic and mitral atresia.

CLINICAL PRESENTATION

HLH is a duct-dependent lesion, which is frequently detected antenatally on ultrasound scan. Early management to maintain ductal patency is required, if undiagnosed ductal closure presents with collapse in the neonatal period.

TREATMENT

Early management involves maintaining patency of the arterial duct with intravenous prostaglandin therapy. As this can occasionally cause respiratory compromise it is essential that ventilatory support be available, if required. Surgical management involves reconstructing the circulation to work effectively with the right ventricle as the single systemic ventricle. To achieve this, the small aorta must be connected to the large pulmonary artery and the aortic arch reconstructed using homograft material. The atrial septum is opened up and a conduit or a shunt inserted onto the pulmonary arteries (as they have been disconnected from the proximal pulmonary artery). This is termed the Norwood operation (**Fig. 5.17**). Later in infancy, a second stage is performed which comprises a Glenn shunt. The total cavopulmonary connection is completed in the pre-school years.

PROGNOSIS

Although results are improving, many children still do not survive the three surgical stages and there is concern that the single (morphologically right) systemic ventricle circulation may fail later in life and transplantation will be needed. However, many children have managed normal schooling and although somewhat limited can enjoy reasonable quality of life.

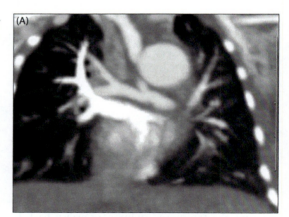

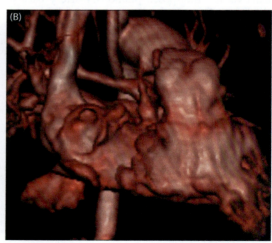

FIGURE 5.16 Single diastolic frame from a cardiac MRI balanced SSFP cine-loop, showing a 4-chamber view of a patient with hypoplastic left heart syndrome.

FIGURE 5.17 Stage 1 Norwood procedure imaged by CT angiography (A) and by 3D reconstruction (B) showing the pulmonary artery shunt.

ATRIOVENTRICULAR SEPTAL DEFECT

INCIDENCE

Atrioventricular septal defects (AVSD) account for approximately 5% of all congenital heart disease, affecting 2–3 live births per 10,000. AVSD is commonly associated with Trisomy 21.

AETIOLOGY

This is the typical cardiac lesion seen in trisomy 21, although it can occur in any child. In the past it has been called an endocardial cushion defect or an AV canal. It is essentially a large hole in the middle of the heart that involves the atria and ventricles. There is also a deformity of the inlet valves, which are no longer mitral and tricuspid, but become a common inlet valve with leaflets bridging across linking the two sides of the valve (**Figs 5.18, 5.19**).

TREATMENT

The repair typically involves two patches and a reconstruction of the single valve into two inlet valves. As the hole is typically very large, surgery must be performed early to prevent pulmonary vascular disease developing and is rarely left more than 6 months.

PROGNOSIS

A good surgical outcome is achieved in most cases but the reconstructed inlet valves sometimes have residual incompetence which occasionally needs further surgery.

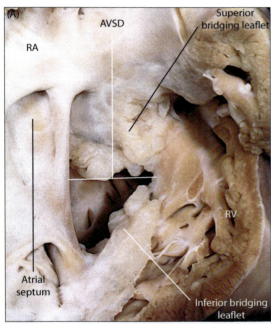

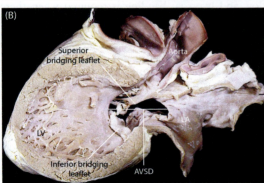

FIGURE 5.18 Atrioventricular septal defect (AVSD) viewed from the right (A) and left (B) side of the heart at postmortem. LA: left atrium; LV: left ventricle; RA: right atrium; RV: right ventricle.

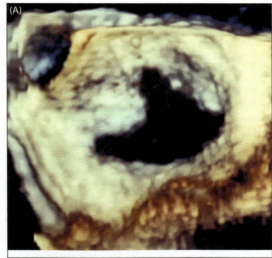

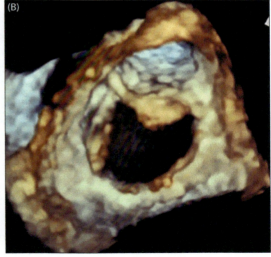

FIGURE 5.19 3D ECHO reconstruction image of an atrioventricular septal defect showing the common AV valve.

OTHER CARDIAC LESIONS

TOTAL ANOMALOUS PULMONARY VENOUS DRAINAGE

AETIOLOGY

In total anomalous pulmonary venous drainage (TAPVD) the pulmonary veins do not connect to the left atrium. Communication may be supracardiac (into the superior vena cava), cardiac (into the right atrium), infracardiac (below the level of the diaphragm into the IVC, ductus venosus or portal vein) or a combination of connections.

Approximately one-third of lesions have a degree of pulmonary venous obstruction; obstruction may occur at several sites and is typically associated with infracardiac TAPVD. As there is common mixing of the blue and red blood in the right atrium before crossing the foramen ovale there is a variable degree of cyanosis, which is worse when there is obstruction and pulmonary oedema. The neonate with obstructed TAPVD may present with a respiratory distress picture and may show a 'ground glass' appearance on CXR, which causes confusion. The neonate will deteriorate with fluid boluses as the lung congestion increases. Unobstructed TAPVD often presents in the first few months with failure to thrive and recurrent chest symptoms. The CXR may show an unusual cardiac outline with a 'cottage loaf' appearance, the enlarged ascending channel giving the silhouette shape. ECG shows right atrial and right ventricular hypertrophy in both obstructed and unobstructed types. ECHO is diagnostic and demonstrates any coexistent lesions. The results of cardiac surgery are generally good although dependent on clinical condition and unless pulmonary vein stenosis occurs the long-term outcomes are excellent.

TRICUSPID ATRESIA

AETIOLOGY

When the tricuspid valve fails to form, or is atretic, blood entering the right atrium is forced to leave via a patent foramen ovale or ASD. The right ventricle is hypoplastic. Other cardiac lesions are also associated with tricuspid atresia, VSDs are usually present and their size determines the amount of pulmonary blood flow.

CLINICAL PRESENTATION

Cyanosis is always present and may be severe from birth if there is little VSD flow, or present as hypoxic spells in older infants as the VSD limits flow. Other presenting signs and symptoms may be attributable to the associated cardiac lesions. Sometimes the great arteries may be transposed, in which case the pulmonary artery arises from the left ventricle and there is high pulmonary flow and mild cyanosis. Flow may need to be limited by pulmonary artery banding and sometimes the limited VSD flow to the right ventricle and aorta results in coarctation. More usually the pulmonary artery arises from the small right ventricle and there may be pulmonary stenosis. These children are often very cyanosed at birth and reliant on a PDA to maintain the circulation to their lungs.

ECG may show right atrial enlargement, left ventricular hypertrophy and left axis deviation. Left ventricular hypertrophy may be visualised on CXR and pulmonary markings depend on the haemodynamics caused by the associated lesions.

ECHO is used to determine the anatomical structures.

TREATMENT

The surgical strategy used in treatment of tricuspid atresia is similar to that for double inlet left ventricle below.

DOUBLE INLET LEFT VENTRICLE

This lesion is also called univentricular heart and typically both inlet valves open into a 'single' ventricle, although it is rarely single and a posterior hypoplastic ventricle is usually identifiable on detailed scanning. The management is rather like tricuspid atresia and depends on the arterial connections (i.e. which are from the hypoplastic ventricle), the size of the VSD and any associated lesions, which, just like tricuspid atresia, may limit pulmonary or systemic flow. There may be associated pulmonary stenosis and systemic outflow obstruction or coarctation.

Initial surgery depends on the associated lesions. In the cyanosed infant, a palliative systemic to pulmonary anastomosis (e.g. Blalock shunt) may be required initially to improve pulmonary blood flow and hypoxia; banding is required when there is excessive pulmonary flow. Ultimately treatment for double inlet left ventricle, like all single ventricle circulations such as tricuspid atresia, pulmonary atresia with intact septum and hypoplastic left heart, aims for a total cavopulmonary circulation (Fontan) where the single ventricle pumps blood around the body and the pulmonary circulation drains by passive flow. Usually this is staged with a Glenn shunt preceding the total cavopulmonary connection. A Glenn shunt is typically superior vena cava to both pulmonary arteries (bidirectional) (**Fig. 5.20**). When the inferior vena cava is connected to the pulmonary arteries this is called a total cavopulmonary connection or Fontan operation.

Cardiology

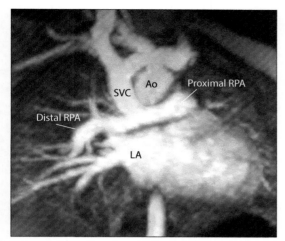

FIGURE 5.20 Cardiac MRI gadolinium-contrast angiogram, acquired in the second pass of contrast. This near-coronal view demonstrates a surgical bidirectional cavopulmonary connection in a patient whose underlying cardiac defect is pulmonary atresia, with intact ventricular septum. Ao: aorta; LA: left atrium; RPA: right pulmonary artery; SVC: superior vena cava.

PULMONARY ATRESIA WITH AN INTACT SEPTUM

Like tricuspid atresia this lesion is associated with a hypoplastic right heart with an obligatory atrial shunt (**Fig. 5.20**). It is always a duct-dependent cyanotic lesion. Staged palliation (Blalock followed by Glenn then total cavopulmonary connection) is the aim although the prognosis is less good than with tricuspid atresia. There may be complicated coronary artery anatomy via sinusoidal connections to the right ventricle, which worsen the prognosis.

PULMONARY ATRESIA WITH A VSD

When there is a VSD associated with pulmonary atresia the lesion is completely different and can be like an extreme tetralogy with a fairly straightforward two ventricle repair, or there can be no associated pulmonary arteries and only major aortopulmonary collateral arteries (MAPCAs). In this situation repair is tremendously challenging.

EBSTEIN ANOMALY

Ebstein anomaly describes a malformed tricuspid valve where the posterior and septal leaflets are displaced inferiorly, effectively atrialising part of the right ventricle. The remaining right ventricle is small and unable to function efficiently, reducing pulmonary blood flow and resulting in varying degrees of cyanosis. Development of this lesion is associated with maternal lithium use during pregnancy.

Presentation varies with the severity of the lesion; severe symptoms in the neonatal period generally have a bad prognosis (cardiomegaly can be extreme) but mild lesions may not even present until adult life. Atrial arrhythmias can result from the raised right atrial pressure and supraventricular tachycardias may occur. Surgical repair with the Cone operation has improved outcomes.

INTERRUPTED AORTIC ARCH AND TRUNCUS ARTERIOSUS

These lesions are associated with Di George syndrome. Rarely, some children have both interruption and truncus. Interruption is a duct-dependent lesion and can present with neonatal collapse and poor perfusion as the duct closes. A common arterial trunk usually presents later with heart failure and mild cyanosis. Surgical results have improved and most children will now survive.

CONGENITALLY CORRECTED TRANSPOSITION

This is rare problem that can cause confusion because of the term transposition. In this condition (if there are no associated lesions) the blood circulates normally and there is no cyanosis. The transposition term is used because the characteristic morphology of the ventricles is reversed. There is a typical left ventricle shape on the venous circulation side pumping blood to the lungs and a morphological right ventricle pumping blood to the aorta. Therefore the arteries are transposed onto the wrong ventricles. While this may seem simply of academic interest, the right ventricle is not best suited to left ventricular function. Of clinical importance, there are often other associated lesions such as VSD, pulmonary outflow obstruction, dextrocardia and heart block.

Isolatated congenitally corrected transposition may often go undetected and life expectancy is good with patients reaching middle age or older. Life expectancy is slightly reduced as the right ventricle functions as the systemic ventricle and may fail in late adult life. Coexistent lesions invariably result in earlier diagnosis and management of these defines the outcome and survival for the patient.

VASCULAR RING AND SLING

The most common vascular ring is caused by a double aortic arch encircling the trachea and oesophagus causing compression of these structures (**Fig. 5.21**). A right aortic arch combined with an aberrant subclavian artery passing behind the oesophagus with a duct or ligament can also complete a ring. Vascular rings can be associated with other cardiac lesions, typically VSD or conotruncal abnormalities. Vascular slings occur when the aberrant vasculature partially surrounds the trachea and oesophagus. The left pulmonary artery may arise from the right pulmonary artery and compress the trachea (**Fig. 5.22**). Sometimes there may be severe tracheal abnormalities including complete tracheal rings, which may need extensive tracheal reconstruction. An isolated aberrant subclavian artery is very common in normal children and is very rarely responsible for feeding problems.

If the obstruction is significant symptoms can present in infancy. The respiratory signs associated with vascular rings are usually present from birth and are typically stridor and wheeze. Recurrent chest infections may occur as a result of feed aspiration. As solids are introduced oesophageal compression can result in dysphagia and failure to thrive. Severe obstruction may cause bronchomalacia, tracheomalacia, cyanosis and respiratory arrest.

ECHO can usually diagnose the problem but cardiac MRI can define the anatomy of the lesion more precisely. Bronchoscopy can help explore the tracheal disease and a barium swallow may suggest vascular compression; however, neither investigation is diagnostic.

Surgical management is indicated if the child is symptomatic. The vascular ring can be divided by a left thoracotomy approach and aortopexy may be considered to reduce tracheal compression. If a slide tracheoplasty is needed this is highly specialised surgery available at very few centres.

Prognosis is good if the vascular ring is divided successfully; however' the extent of tracheal obstruction determines the final outcome. A ring or sling that previously caused significant obstruction may cause long-term feeding or airway compromise despite vascular correction.

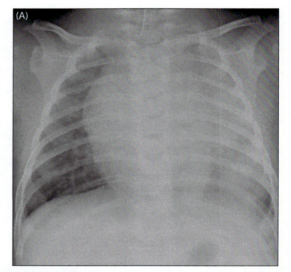
(A)

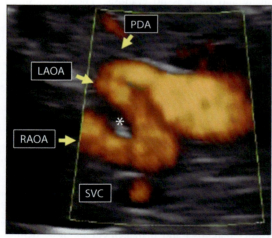

FIGURE 5.21 Fetal power Doppler angiography showing a double aortic arch. LAOA: left aortic arch; PDA: patent ductus arteriosus; RAOA: right aortic arch; SVC: superior vena cava.

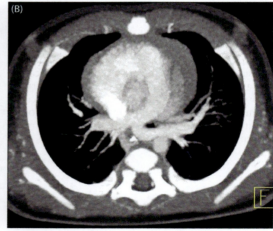
(B)

FIGURE 5.22 Imaging of a patient with a pulmonary sling, the chest x-ray (A) showing mediastinal shift to the right, the compressed small trachea demonstrated on CT (B).

Cardiology

128

HEART MUSCLE DISEASE

Heart muscle disease is less common than congenital heart disease with an incidence of around 1 in 2,500 for the most common lesion, dilated cardiomyopathy (DCM).

DILATED CARDIOMYOPATHY

In DCM, the heart is dilated and as a result contracts inefficiently. DCM can be the end stage of metabolic disease, be caused by toxins such as anthracyclines, develop as a consequence of chronic tachycardias or as a result of nutritional deficiency such as vitamin D deficiency and hypocalcaemia. The majority of cases are probably sporadic or caused by inherited mutations of cardiac structural proteins. Genetic causes are varied with many cases considered isolated lesions, but all modes of inheritance are described. Detailed screening for cardiomyopathies using panels of genes or whole exome screening is undertaken in some centres. If clinically suspected, some more common genetic lesions can be screened for; these include Barth syndrome (X-linked with cyclical neutropenia) and lamin A/C mutations (often associated with skeletal myopathy and abnormal rhythms). The cardiomyopathy associated with Duchenne and Becker muscular dystrophy rarely causes symptoms before later teenage years.

In most cases of DCM, symptoms can be controlled with medical therapy for many years, but a few cases do deteriorate more rapidly, resulting in cardiomyopathy being the most common indication for paediatric heart transplantation in Europe.

The cornerstone of long-term treatment for cardiac failure is currently with angiotensin converting enzyme inhibitors, beta-blocker (particularly carvedilol) and spironolactone. Other treatments are more geared to symptom control such as diuretics and perhaps digoxin (if the latter is used in low dose with low levels to reduce the risk of sudden death).

MYOCARDITIS

Myocarditis can cause confusion with DCM as the ECHO appearances are similar. Typical acute myocarditis however tends to demonstrate less dilatation and lacks the thin walls of DCM. Many aetiologies for myocarditis have been described; viruses are the most common cause particularly enteroviruses (these can be particularly destructive to the myocardium) but parvovirus is also common, adenovirus, influenza, chickenpox and EBV are all know to cause myocardial inflammation. Other causes need to be considered in endemic areas such as Chagas disease, HIV, hepatitis C, Dengue fever and diphtheria. Treatment for myocarditis is largely symptomatic as little evidence for immunosuppression exists.

Severe cases may need mechanical circulatory support to allow a period of myocardial rest and hopefully recovery.

PERICARDITIS

The causes of myocarditis are also implicated in pericarditis, although an isolated pericardial effusion may also be bacterial and purulent, or related to autoimmune diseases such as systemic lupus erythematosus and juvenile idiopathic arthritis. Pericardial effusion is a well recognised complication of cardiac surgery in children and can be very severe causing cardiac tamponade, particularly after ASD surgery.

HYPERTROPHIC CARDIOMYOPATHY

In contrast to DCM, the heart in hypertrophic cardiomyopathy (HCM) is very thickened; the heart contracts strongly and often the outflow is obstructed. Most commonly it is associated with sarcomeric protein mutations and is a dominantly inherited condition. Sudden death is well recognised and high risk cases are candidates for implantable cardioverter defibrillators. In children, dysmorphic syndromes that affect components of RAS-mitogen activated protein kinase, such as Noonan, Leopard, Costello and neurofibromatosis type 1 are associated with HCM. Metabolic diseases associated with HCM include Pompe syndrome, which exhibits severe hypertrophy in the neonatal period and mitochondrial disease that often demonstrates impaired systolic function and hypertrophy.

RESTRICTIVE CARDIOMYOPATHY

This uncommon cardiomyopathy is a physiological diagnosis with impaired filling. Usually the prognosis is poor with complications including arrhythmias, thromboembolic disease, pulmonary hypertension and heart failure. Treatment is very difficult. It can be associated with some neuromuscular diseases such as BAG -3 abnormalities and myofibrillary problems.

ARRHYTHMOGENIC RIGHT VENTRICULAR CARDIOMYOPATHY

Arrhythmogenic right ventricular cardiomyopathy (ARVC) is very rare in the first decade of life and tends to be a problem of teenagers and young adults, with a high risk of sudden death. Although predominantly a disease of the right ventricle, the left can also be involved. It is autosomal dominantly inherited but genetically heterogeneous.

ENDOCARDITIS

Endocarditis is uncommon but remains a very serious disease that can cause severe destruction of the valves. Gram-positive organisms (e.g. alpha haemolytic streptococcus, particularly *Streptococcus viridans*) and *Staphylococcus aureus* are the most common causes, although many other pathogens are implicated and pneumococcal disease can be very destructive. The pathogens are more complex in the neonate and immunosuppressed. Rheumatic heart disease is the major cause of endocarditis in developing countries, whereas in the developed world it is more associated with congenital heart lesions or indwelling central lines. In most nations, the advice on antibiotic cover for dental or surgical procedures has been relaxed because the perceived risk of endocarditis is so low; however, good dental hygiene and the avoidance of high risk procedures, such as body piercing and tattoos is advised.

KAWASAKI DISEASE

In Kawasaki disease, an inflammatory myocarditis or pericarditis may occur at presentation. However, the major cardiac manifestation is the development of coronary artery aneurysms. Early treatment with immunoglobulin reduces the incidence of aneurysm formation; however, aneurysms are still seen, often in atypical cases or those that occur in infancy when it can be more difficult to recognise and give immunoglobulin early enough. Very large aneurysms are more liable to complications that include rupture (rarely) and stenosis with myocardial infarction. Stenosis can be treated by coronary stenting or bypass grafting. The long-term prognosis is still not defined but there is concern that even those without aneurysms may be at risk of accelerated atheromatous disease.

ARRHYTHMIAS

The most common paediatric arrhythmia is supraventricular tachycardia from an accessory pathway. Most acute paediatricians are now familiar with using adenosine intravenously and this is usually effective. Atrial flutter and ectopic atrial tachycardias are much less common in children. Although they may not be abolished by adenosine, the increase in block at the atrioventricular node will often reveal the blocked atrial activation or flutter waves more clearly.

Ventricular tachycardias are uncommon in children. Narrow complex ventricular tachycardias originating from the His bundle are seen postoperatively related to oedema and swelling. Broad complex tachycardias can be related to heart muscle disease (see HCM and ARVC above). There are also genetically inherited 'ion channelopathies' such as long QT syndrome (**Fig. 5.23**) and Brugada syndrome, that can result in ventricular arrhythmias. Brugada syndrome may have a characteristic ECG with right bundle branch block with ST segment elevation, which may be provoked with specific drug testing, e.g. ajmaline (**Fig. 5.24**). Catecholaminergic ventricular tachycardia is a genetic arrhythmia recognised in paediatrics and can often present in the first decade. There can be a characteristic bidirectional ventricular tachycardia with alternating changes in the axis. A history of syncope induced by exercise, anxiety, startle response, fever or a family history of sudden death or death during sleep would suggest a channelopathy.

Drug treatment can be successful for ventricular tachycardias, but cardioverter-defibrillators are increasingly used. There is increasing use of transcatheter ablation of arrhythmias particularly for Wolff–Parkinson–White where there may be a risk of sudden death (not from the re-entrant pathway

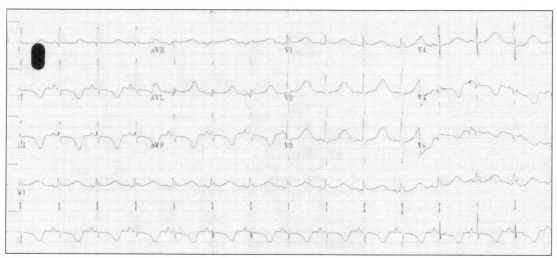

FIGURE 5.23 ECG showing long QT syndrome.

but where there is the possibility of rapid conduction of atrial flutter in the accessory pathway). Ablation is not always successful and recurrence of arrhythmias is seen. The risk of ablation is low but not zero, heart block being one of the more serious complications. Heart block itself can be congenital and associated with maternal lupus, anti-Ro antibody or congenital heart disease, such as congenitally corrected transposition. Cardiac surgery can result in heart block if sutures are near the conduction tissue. Pacemaker leads can be placed on the epicardium by an open surgical procedure or the endocardium; the latter is usually performed by cardiologists using a transvenous route although some units prefer to preserve veins for later in life as pacing is a lifelong therapy. The box is placed in the pectoral or abdominal position. There is increased use of biventricular pacing to improve cardiac synchrony and preserve cardiac function (**Fig. 5.25**).

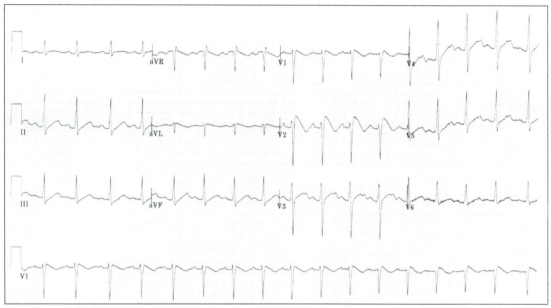

FIGURE 5.24 ECG of Brugada syndrome.

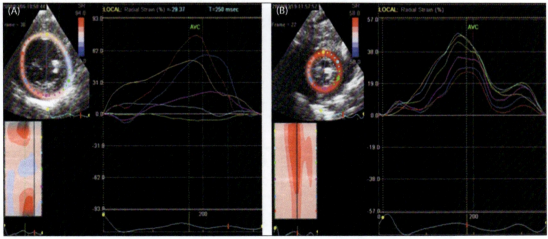

FIGURE 5.25 Speckle tracking echocardiography showing cardiac muscle motion before (A) and after (B) resynchronisation pacing therapy. In the first image muscle wall motion is dys-synchronous and ineffective; following pacing the heart muscle motion is more co-ordinated resulting in functional improvement of cardiac output.

HEART TRANSPLANTATION

The most common cardiothoracic transplantation is heart transplantation. In Europe the main indication is DCM, although congenital heart disease is an increasingly common indication. Children with severe cardiac failure may require mechanical support before transplantation is possible. Extra corporeal membrane oxygenation is used in some instances but is only a short-term support. For small children an external pneumatic device is used called the Berlin heart. There is a high incidence of major thromboembolic complications but children have been supported for many months with these devices. More advanced devices using continuous flow technology are implanted in adults and are suitable for adolescents. These devices have much lower risk of thrombosis. They are fully implantable although an external drive-line is still needed. The patients can go home and are fully mobile unlike those using the Berlin heart. Efforts are being made to transfer the technology to smaller children in the coming decades.

Most children survive heart transplantation and in the current era approximately 60% will survive 10 years after transplantation. However, very long-term survival is uncertain as accelerated coronary artery disease limits the allograft survival. Although cellular rejection is now very rare with modern immunosuppression, the drugs themselves may have side-effects that include increased risk of infections, chronic kidney disease and malignancy, particularly EBV driven lymphoma. Antibody-mediated rejection is more widely recognised as cellular rejection becomes less common, and is difficult to treat effectively.

Heart–lung transplantation is rarely performed due to donor organ shortage. There is instead a tendency to use the lungs and heart separately to benefit two recipients (**Fig. 5.26**). Indications for heart–lung transplantation are also limited and generally the procedure is reserved for treatment of adults with congenital heart conditions with associated Eisenmenger syndrome. For both heart and lung transplantation, a regimen of tacrolimus and mycophenolate mofetil (and prednisolone for lung transplant) is becoming the most common immunosuppression regime.

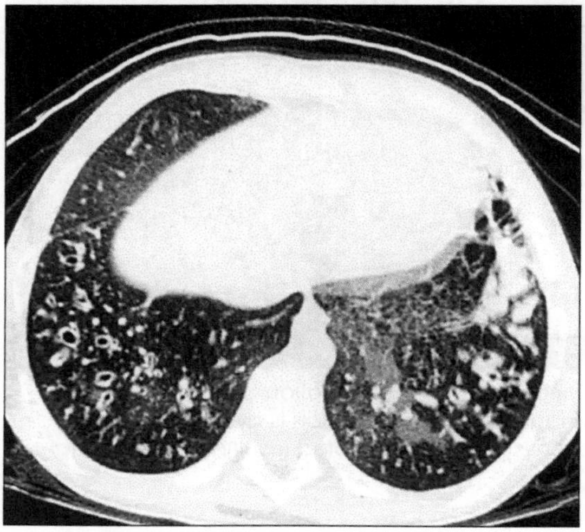

Tracheal transplantation is beginning to be introduced to treat conditions such as tracheal agenesis or stenosis. The procedure is different to heart and lung transplantation in that a decellularised graft is prepared *ex vivo* with the recipient patient's own stem cells and growth factors to produce a new trachea. As a result immunsuppression is not required as the tissue transplanted is recipient compatible.

Acknowledgements: we would like to thank Ms Gemma Price, Gemma Price Designs and the following staff at Great Ormond Street Hospital for Children NHS Foundation Trust for the provision of images for this chapter: Dr Marina Hughes, Consultant Paediatric Cardiologist, Clinical Lead for Cardiac MRI; Dr Juan Kaski, Consultant Paediatric Cardiologist; Dr Sachin Khambadkone, Consultant in Paediatric and Adolescent Cardiology; Dr Jan Marek, Consultant Cardiologist and Director of Echocardiography; Dr Catherine Owens, Consultant Paediatric Radiologist.

FURTHER READING

Apitz C, Webb GD, Redington AN. Tetralogy of Fallot. *Lancet* 2009;374(9699):1462–71.

Feinstein JA, Benson DW, Dubin AM, *et al.* Hypoplastic left heart syndrome: current considerations and expectations. *J Am Coll Cardiol* 2012;59(1 Suppl):S1–42.

Hijazi ZM, Awad SM. Pediatric cardiac interventions. *J Am Coll Cardiol Cardiovasc Interv* 2008;1(6):603–11.

Kantor PF, Lougheed J, Dancea A, *et al*; Children's Heart Failure Study Group. Presentation, diagnosis, and medical management of heart failure in children: Canadian Cardiovascular Society guidelines. *Can J Cardiol* 2013;29(12):1535–52.

Lewin MB, Stout K. *Echocardiography in Congenital Heart Disease.* Elsevier, 2011 ISBN: 978-1-4377-2696-1.

Marek J, Tomek V, Skovránek J, Povysilová V, Samánek M. Prenatal ultrasound screening of congenital heart disease in an unselected national population: a 21-year experience. *Heart* 2011;97(2):124–30.

Nies M, Sekar P. Advances in noninvasive imaging in pediatric cardiology. *Adv Pediatr* 2013;60(1):167–85.

Park MK. *Park's Pediatric Cardiology for Practitioners.* Philadelphia: Mosby, 2008. ISBN: 978-0-323-16951-6.

Park MK. *The Pediatric Cardiology Handbook*, 4th edn. Philadelphia: Mosby, 2010. ISBN: 978-1-4160-6443-5.

Wilson W, Osten M, Benson L, Horlick E. Evolving trends in interventional cardiology: endovascular options for congenital disease in adults. *Can J Cardiol* 2014;30(1):75–86.

FIGURE 5.26 End-stage cystic fibrosis on CT imaging.

Cardiology

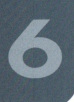

6 Dermatology

Veronica Kinsler and John Harper

VASCULAR LESIONS – TUMOURS

INFANTILE HAEMANGIOMA

Infantile haemangioma is a common endothelial cell tumour of infancy. It resolves spontaneously over time but may require treatment depending on site, size and associated complications (**Figs 6.1–6.4**).

HISTORY

Lesions are not usually present at birth, but appear within the first weeks of life. They grow for around 6 months, stabilise and involute spontaneously over 2–10 years.

CLINICAL PRESENTATION

- Superficial, deep, or mixed.
- Superficial component is bright red, deep component is blue-ish
- Palpable as a soft lump.
- Single or multiple.

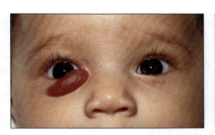 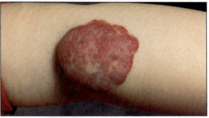

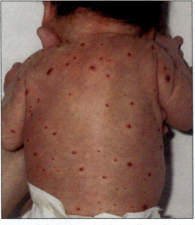

FIGURES 6.1–6.3 Infantile haemangioma. **6.1**: below right eye threatening vision, requires treatment; **6.2**: right arm, showing signs of spontaneous resolution; **6.3**: multiple or miliary, requires screening for internal lesions.

Infantile haemangioma

133

TREATMENT

Treatment is conservative for the majority, but patients should be referred to a paediatric dermatologist if the lesion is:

- Near important structures, e.g. eye, nose, mouth, subglottic.
- Ulcerated.
- Bleeding significantly.
- Multiple (5 or more) – requires screening for internal haemangiomata.
- Very large, where there is possibility of consumptive coagulopathy and/or cardiac failure.
- Plaque-like – head and neck lesions may be associated with intra-cerebral anomalies and/or cardiac or large vessel anomalies (PHACES syndrome).

Systemic treatment of choice is currently oral propranolol. For ulceration +/– bleeding, treatment is wound care, +/– pulsed-dye laser therapy. For consumptive coagulopathy, treatment is supportive, +/– surgery/embolisation. In cardiac failure, treatment is supportive and surgery/embolisation may need to be considered.

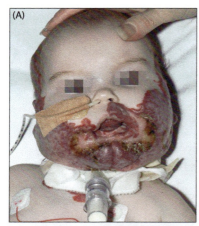

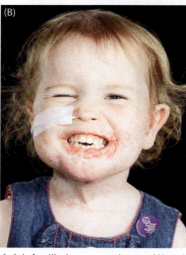

FIGURE 6.4 Infantile haemangioma: (A) extensive plaque-like haemangioma associated with subglottic lesion requiring tracheostomy, showing resolution with propranolol treatment (B).

RARE VASCULAR TUMOURS

Patients should be referred if the history is not typical, or examination reveals a hard lump on palpation. Possible diagnoses include rapidly-involuting congenital haemangioma (RICH), non-involuting congenital haemangioma (NICH), Kaposiform endothelioma, tufted angioma, haemangiopericytoma and others. Diagnosis usually requires biopsy.

VASCULAR LESIONS – MALFORMATIONS

CAPILLARY MALFORMATIONS

STORK MARK

This is a very common flat pink lesion, present at birth. It is usually located on the forehead, eyelids, occiput, neck or midline of the back. It may be V-shaped on the forehead/occiput. Facial lesions fade, occipital tend not to. The lesions are not pathological so there is no active management needed.

PORT WINE STAIN

This is a relatively common congenital and permanent malformation of capillaries (**Fig. 6.5**). It may

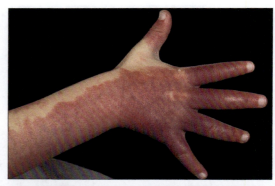

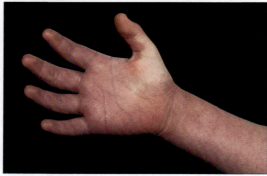

FIGURE 6.5 Port wine stain of the right hand and forearm.

Dermatology

be associated with ocular and/or neurological abnormalities (Sturge–Weber syndrome) when affecting the forehead/upper eyelid, or with other genetic conditions (for example the PIK3CA-related overgrowth syndromes, and others).

History

The lesion is present from birth; it will not grow independently but is permanent. The lesion changes colour intensity with heat/emotion.

Clinical presentation

- Red/purple lesion.
- Well-defined edges.
- Not palpable in childhood, may become lumpy over time.
- Blanches on pressure.
- Neurology, head circumference, full systems examination should be checked.

Treatment

- Refer to paediatric dermatology for assessment of response to pulsed-dye laser therapy and camouflage make-up.
- If any lesion affects the forehead or the upper eyelid, refer to the ophthalmologist for urgent assessment to include intraocular pressure on day 1 of life, as glaucoma can be present from birth.
- Refer for neurological assessment +/– MRI/MRA of brain if affecting the forehead or the upper eyelid.
- May be associated with over-growth of underlying tissue.
- Skin biopsy (if capillary malformation not on the face) for genotyping, if associated with other abnormalities.

VENOUS MALFORMATIONS

Congenital slow-flow malformations of the veins is a relatively rare condition. Rarely, they can be inherited as part of familial venous malformations syndromes.

HISTORY

Malformations are present from birth but may not be noticed initially (**Fig. 6.6**). They occur as bluish discolouration, lumps, pain or swelling and change in size with activities and posture.

CLINICAL PRESENTATION

- Variable, but palpable lumps, visible bluish discolouration is common.
- May be able to reduce lumps with change of posture.
- Variably growth dysregulation of underlying tissue, often seen in association with a smaller affected limb.
- Measurement of limbs for discrepancy if appropriate (**Fig. 6.7**).

TREATMENT

- Patients should be referred for investigation.
- Ultrasound Doppler/MRI to assess flow and extent of malformation.
- Assessment of possible associated abnormalities.
- Sclerotherapy or surgery if required.
- Skin biopsy for histopathology and genotyping can be helpful. Blood for genotyping if familial presentation.

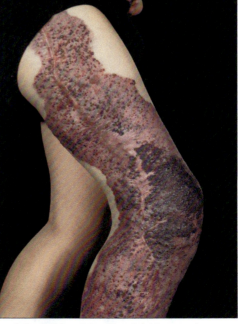

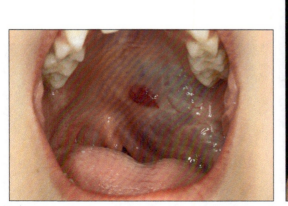

FIGURES 6.6, 6.7 Venous malformation. **6.6**: Involving the palate; **6.7**: involving the right leg, and associated with growth dysregulation and lymphatic component.

ARTERIOVENOUS MALFORMATIONS

These involve rare congenital high-flow malformations of arteries and veins. They are often difficult to manage and are associated with significant morbidity.

HISTORY

Lesions may be visible at birth and present with red/blue/skin-coloured area, swelling, ulceration or bleeding. They may enlarge at puberty.

EXAMINATION

- Often in the head/neck area.
- Varies from flat red area to swollen blue mass; vessels can be palpable.
- Warm to the touch, often pulsatile on palpation or auscultation.
- Check cardiovascular system – rarely there is also high-output cardiac failure.

Management

- Refer to paediatric dermatologist.
- Ultrasound Doppler/MRI/angiography to assess flow, extent of lesion and feeding vessels.
- Embolisation/surgery if possible.

POSTINFLAMMATORY PIGMENTARY CHANGES

Normal skin pigmentation can be increased or decreased during and following inflammation.

VITILIGO

Vitiligo is an acquired macular depigmentation associated with autoimmune conditions. Childhood onset may have a better prognosis.

HISTORY

Lesions are not present at birth, often gradually worsening, starting in new sites. There is a predilection for perioroficial and extensor surface skin. Patients may have a family history of autoimmune conditions.

EXAMINATION

- Complete skin depigmentation – milky white lesions (**Fig. 6.8**).
- Not palpable.
- Clear-cut edges.
- Usually symmetrical, occasionally segmental.

MANAGEMENT

- Refer to paediatric dermatologist for therapy – topical steroids and/or calcineurin inhibitors, light therapy.
- Consider single measurement of thyroid function and autoantibodies.

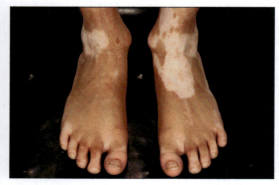

FIGURE 6.8 Vitiligo affecting knees and feet.

Dermatology

HYPOMELANOTIC MACULES

HISTORY

Lesions can be present at birth; patients may develop new lesions but existing lesions are usually static in childhood. They can occur at any site and may be associated with tuberous sclerosis.

EXAMINATION

- Hypopigmented lesions.
- Classic oval shape (**Figs 6.9, 6.10**).
- Not palpable.
- Any site but the trunk is common.
- Check for other cutaneous signs of tuberous sclerosis: facial angiofibromas, shagreen patches, periungual fibromas.
- Check neurology, abdomen, heart, blood pressure.

MANAGEMENT

- Refer for full assessment of tuberous sclerosis:
  - MRI brain.
  - Abdominal ultrasound.
  - Ophthalmological assessment.
  - Cardiac ECHO and ECG.
- Investigation of family members if diagnosis of TS is confirmed.

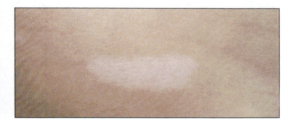

FIGURE 6.9 Isolated hypomelanotic macule.

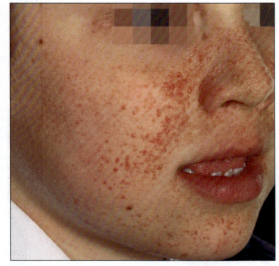

FIGURE 6.10 Facial angiofibromas (adenoma sebaceum) seen in tuberous sclerosis. These can be treated with topical rapamycin.

PIGMENTARY MOSAICISM

HISTORY

Lesions are usually present from birth and may extend later.

EXAMINATION

- Hypo- or hyperpigmented lesions.
- Lesions may follow lines of Blaschko – linear on limbs, whorled on trunk.
- Not palpable.
- Check neurology, teeth, eyes.

MANAGEMENT

- Refer to paediatric dermatologist.
- Ophthalmology and neurology assessment.
- Consider skin biopsy and bloods for genetic analysis.

CAFÉ-AU-LAIT MACULES

HISTORY

Café-au-lait macules (CALMs) can be present at birth; patients may be developing new lesions but existing lesions are static. Lesions are at any site and size (**Fig. 6.11**). Patients may have family history of neurofibromatosis or other genetic condition.

EXAMINATION

- Hyperpigmented lesions.
- Variable shape, size and site.
- Flat, not palpable.

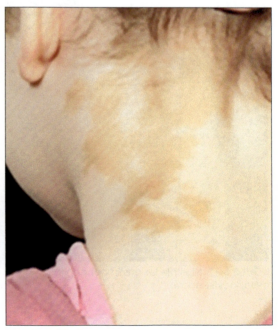

FIGURE 6.11 Café-au-lait macule on the neck.

- Check for other signs of neurofibromatosis types 1 (NF1) and 2: axillary/inguinal freckling, cutaneous neurofibromas, plexiform neuroma, peripheral schwannomas, raised BP, scoliosis, pseudoarthroses, full neurological examination.
- Check for signs of early puberty and bony abnormalities seen in McCune–Albright syndrome.

MANAGEMENT

- Refer to paediatric dermatologist for monitoring of CALMs.
- Yearly ophthalmological assessment for signs of neurofibromatosis 1, plus yearly BP measurement.
- MRI brain not done routinely.
- If NF1 usually would have 6 CALMs of the appropriate size (>0.5 mm prepubertal) by the age of 6 years.

CONGENITAL MELANOCYTIC NAEVI

HISTORY

Lesions are present at birth, at any site, size and number, but often fade at least to some degree, occasionally dramatically (**Figs 6.12–6.14**). Patients may develop new lesions after birth.

EXAMINATION

- Congenital moles, increased skin markings.
- Variable shape, size, site and number.
- Usually palpable, but sometimes not if <0.5 cm.
- Check neurology.

MANAGEMENT

- Conservative if one lesion, refer to paediatric dermatologist for assessment and follow-up for melanoma if:
  - more than one lesion at birth.
  - cosmetic implications.
  - neurodevelopmental abnormalities.
- MRI brain and whole spine if more than one lesion, to look for associated neurological melanosis/structural abnormalities/tumours.

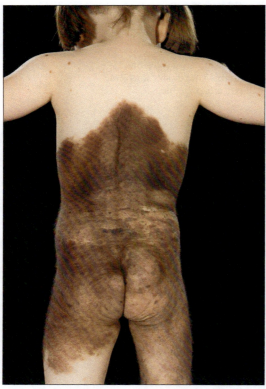

FIGURE 6.12 Multiple lesions in congenital melanocytic naevi.

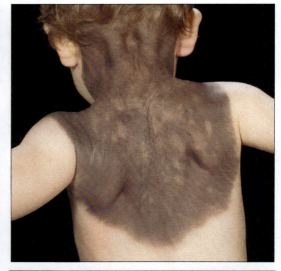

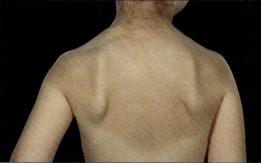

FIGURES 6.13, 6.14 Spontaneous lightening in congenital melanocytic naevi.

BLISTERING CONDITIONS

EPIDERMOLYSIS BULLOSA

Epidermolysis bullosa is a group of rare genetic conditions of mucocutaneous skin fragility. Presentation and clinical course is highly variable dependent on the type (simplex, junctional or dystrophic) and the underlying genetic mutation.

HISTORY

The condition is present from birth, with skin +/– mucosal fragility and blistering in response to minor skin trauma. There may be family history of epidermolysis bullosa may be associated problems such as pain, hoarse cry, failure to thrive, difficulty feeding or secondary infection.

EXAMINATION

- Blistering/skin denudement in sites of handling/ trauma (**Figs 6.15, 6.16**), with scarring in some subtypes.
- Small white papules (milia) in areas of healing.
- Signs of bacterial superinfection.
- Full systems examination with minimal handling.

MANAGEMENT

- Immediate referral to specialist centre for optimisation of skin care, exact diagnosis and management.
- Minimise handling/procedures/observations.
- Pain control, optimisation of nutrition.
- Skin biopsy and gene testing for diagnosis, genetic counselling.

IMMUNOBULLOUS DISORDERS

These are rare acquired blistering conditions, secondary to immunological attack of skin integrity and are often difficult to manage. Conditions include linear IgA disease, pemphigus, pemphigoid and epidermolysis bullosa acquisita. Skin biopsy with immunostaining is diagnostic and informs further management.

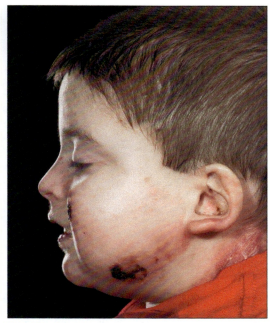

FIGURE 6.15 Blistering and erosions on the face in epidermolysis bullosa.

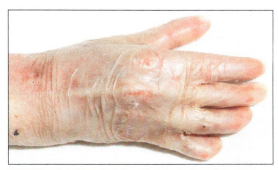

FIGURE 6.16 Scarring leading to 'mitten-hand' deformity in dystrophic epidermolysis bullosa.

INFLAMMATORY CONDITIONS

ECZEMA

Eczema is common in childhood and mainly affects atopic individuals.

HISTORY

Eczema is not present at birth, but there may be family history of atopy, +/− ichthyosis vulgaris. The severity should be assessed – sleep disrupted, failing to thrive, missing school, scratching from itchy skin, steroid requirement.

EXAMINATION

- Red, dry rash (**Figs 6.17, 6.18**).
- Often flexural, but may be widespread (**Fig. 6.19**).
- Often superficially infected – bright red, shiny, may have yellow crusting (**Fig. 6.20**).
- Look for vesicles, roofless or crusted ulcers as signs of eczema herpeticum.

MANAGEMENT

- Daily baths with oily bath additive and soap substitute.
- Regular emollients.
- Appropriate potency topical steroid.
- Refer to paediatric dermatologist for further management if unresponsive, for:
  - for more potent topical steroids +/ topical calcineurin inhibitors.
  - admission and wet dressings.
  - systemic treatment – azathioprine, methotrexate, rarely oral prednisolone or ciclosporin.

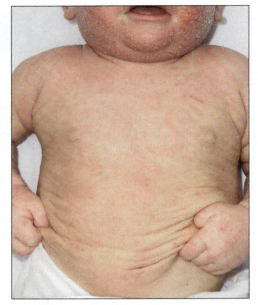

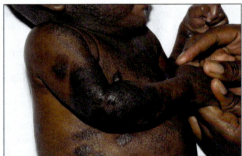

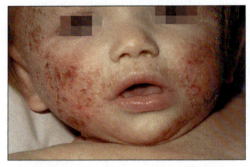

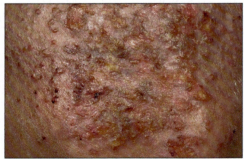

FIGURES 6.17–6.20 Eczema. **6.17**: Eczema is intensely pruritic; **6.18**: it may not appear erythematous on darker skin; **6.19**: facial eczema; **6.20**: close-up of infected eczema.

MORPHOEA (LOCALISED SCLERODERMA)

This is a rare, chronic scarring inflammatory disease of the skin that can affect underlying tissues.

HISTORY

Morphoea is not normally present at birth. Lesions are initially red/pink/purple, particularly at the edges and subsequently pale with scarring. The linear form is most common in childhood. The condition is slowly progressive. Lesions are usually asymptomatic, but long-standing lesions can lead to disability with contractures and wasting. The most severe type is 'en coup de sabre' affecting the scalp and can be associated with neurological problems (**Fig. 6.21**).

EXAMINATION

- Red/pink/purple/pale areas.
- Poorly-defined borders.
- Older lesions atrophic, scarred.
- May be plaque-like or linear.
- Growth of underlying tissues restricted, particularly in the linear form, leading to deformity or asymmetry.

MANAGEMENT

- Refer to paediatric dermatologist.
- Usually requires systemic anti-inflammatory treatment: steroids (short term) and methotrexate.
- Ultrasound/MRI to assess any effect on underlying tissues.

PSORIASIS

Psoriasis is a chronic inflammatory disease of the skin. It is less common in childhood, but may be under-diagnosed as eczema.

HISTORY

The child may have family history of psoriasis. The guttate type may be triggered by bacterial infection, classically streptococcal.

EXAMINATION

- Well-defined red patches with silvery overlying scale (**Fig. 6.22**).
- May be in plaques, classically extensor joint surfaces/scalp, also nappy area (**Fig. 6.23**).
- May be guttate (raindrop-like).
- Check nails for pitting, onycholysis.
- Joints may be affected (psoriatic arthropathy).

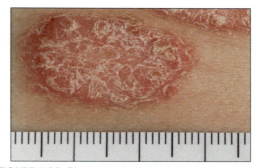

FIGURE 6.22 Close-up of abdominal plaque psoriasis.

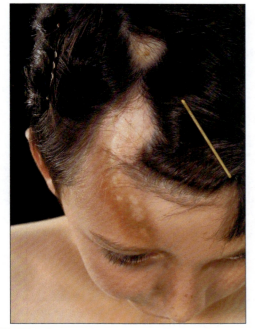

FIGURE 6.21 Morphea en coup de sabre.

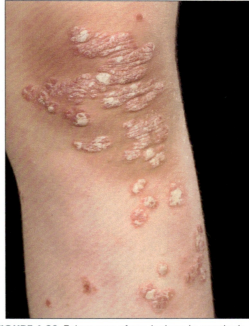

FIGURE 6.23 Extensor surface lesions in psoriasis.

MANAGEMENT

- Screen for streptococcal infection if guttate.
- Topical treatment of skin lesions with moisturisers, vitamin D analogues, steroids, coal-tar derivatives, dithranol.
- Topical treatment of scalp lesions with oil-based moisturisers, tar-based shampoo, topical steroids or vitamin D analogues.
- Refer to paediatric dermatologist if failing to respond to conventional topical treatment or if there is a sudden deterioration and the child is systemically unwell (erythroderma or generalised pustular psoriasis). Options for systemic treatment include methotrexate and the newer biological anti-tumour necrosis factor (TNF) agents.

LUMPS AND BUMPS

ANOGENITAL WARTS

HISTORY

Warts are not normally present at birth. They comprise persistant asymptomatic warts in the perineal region, often slowly progressive. Any history of maternal anogenital warts or of family members' warts of any sort and maternal history of vaccination against HPV should be ascertained. There should be direct questioning of social circumstances and for child abuse.

EXAMINATION

- Whole perineal area, for warts, other infections, anatomy.
- Whole child for any signs of child abuse.

MANAGEMENT

- Warts:
  - conservative in most cases, with monitoring.
  - can type warts if necessary to match with maternal type.
  - ablative therapies are painful in this area.
  - topical treatment with podophyllin or imiquimod.
- Suspected child abuse:
  - refer immediately to duty child protection officer.

MOLLUSCUM CONTAGIOSUM

HISTORY

Lesions are not normally present at birth and are progressive, with the appearance of papular lesions. They are itchy and occasionally secondarily infected. There is often contact history. Lesions can be severe in the immunocompromised child.

EXAMINATION

- Groups of flesh-coloured umbilicated papules (**Fig. 6.24**).

MANAGEMENT

- Conservative for the majority, may take 2 years to resolve.
- Ablative treatment with cryotherapy is of limited value.
- Imiquimod application may be appropriate for the immunocompromised child.

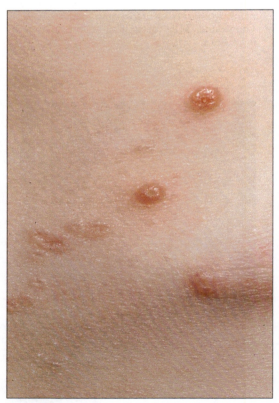

FIGURE 6.24 Molluscum contagiosum – papular lesions showing umbilication.

SEBACEOUS NAEVUS

HISTORY

Naevus is present from birth, often on the scalp but can be elsewhere. It usually flattens after 6 months and then remains static in childhood until puberty.

EXAMINATION

- Yellowish/skin-coloured raised naevus (**Fig. 6.25**).
- Well-defined edges.
- Slightly shiny/oily.
- No overlying hair.

MANAGEMENT

It is usual to refer for removal before the age of puberty as rarely can become malignant thereafter; whether this is absolutely necessary is questionable.

APLASIA CUTIS

HISTORY

This is present from birth, usually on the scalp. There is absent skin, usually healed with scarring at birth but occasionally open at birth.

EXAMINATION

- Defect of scalp skin, atrophic/sunken once healed (**Fig. 6.26**).
- No overlying hair.
- Well-defined edges.
- Can be single or multiple, any size.
- Check neurology and general examination for other defects if linear sebaceous naevus.

MANAGEMENT

- Consider skull x-rays, +/– MRI to look for under-lying bony defect and intracerebral abnormalities if the lesions are large or multiple, or there is the clinical impression of a bony defect.
- If only a skin defect, management is conservative, but if large may require plastic surgery.
- Skin biopsy for genotyping if associated with extracutaneous abnormalities.

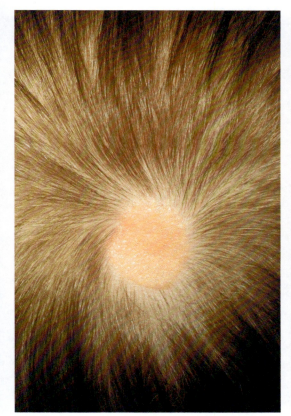

FIGURE 6.25 Sebaceous naevus in scalp.

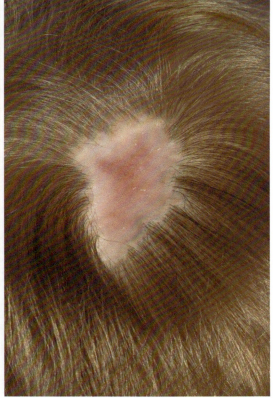

FIGURE 6.26 Aplasia cutis of scalp.

OTHER IMPORTANT CONDITIONS

ACRODERMATITIS ENTEROPATHICA

This is a rare skin condition of infancy caused by failure of zinc absorption (genetic – true acrodermatitis enteropathica) or as a result of acquired dietary zinc insufficiency, and is reversed by zinc supplementation.

HISTORY

Progressive skin lesions affecting the nappy area, face, hands/feet are not present at birth but often begin after the child is weaned onto solid food. Lesions are unresponsive to any topical therapies.

EXAMINATION

- Well-defined erythematous encrusted skin lesions (**Figs 6.27, 6.28**).
- Child may be failing to thrive with diarrhoea.
- Alopecia common.

MANAGEMENT

- Confirm diagnosis by measuring serum zinc level.
- Oral zinc supplementation reverses skin findings within days/weeks.
- Monitor zinc levels – may require supplementation for life.
- Blood DNA for genotyping if genetic cause suspected.

INCONTINENTIA PIGMENTI

This is an X-linked dominant genetic condition lethal to males. It is mosaic in females and caused by mutations in the *NEMO* gene.

HISTORY

There are four stages of skin lesions, which can overlap:

- Blistering and erythematous lesions in the first few weeks of life.
- Verrucous lesions in the first few months.
- Hyperpigmented flat lesions in the first few years.
- Hypopigmented atrophic lesions in later childhood/adult.

Patients may have problems with teeth, eyes, hair growth and neurology and there may be family history on the mother's side.

EXAMINATION

- First two stages of skin lesions follow lines of Blashko – linear on the limbs, whorled on the trunk (**Figs 6.29, 6.30**).
- May be alopecia.
- Check teeth, eyes, neurology.

MANAGEMENT

- Conservative for skin lesions.
- Refer for genetic testing and counselling.
- Refer to ophthalmology, dentistry, neurology for appropriate imaging and follow-up.

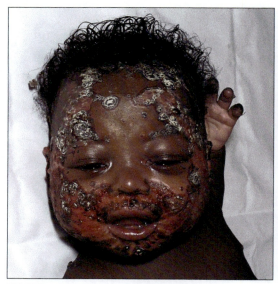

FIGURE 6.27 Facial lesions in acrodermatitis enteropathica.

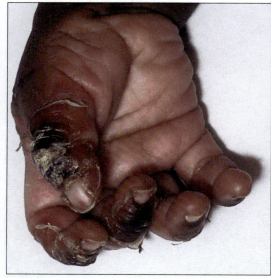

FIGURE 6.28 Acral lesions in acrodermatitis enteropathica.

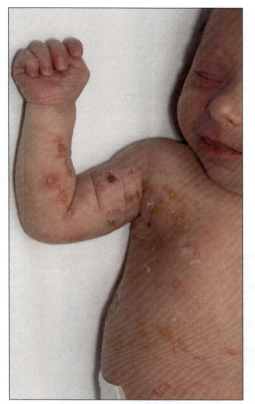

FIGURE 6.29 Vesiculoverrucous lesions following Blashko's lines in incontinentia pigmenti.

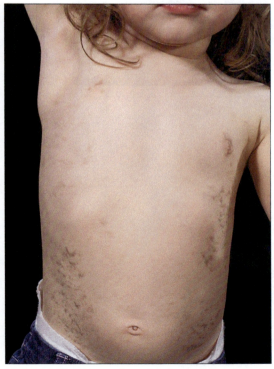

FIGURE 6.30 Chinese-figurate pigmentation phase in incontinentia pigmenti.

CUTANEOUS MAST CELL DISEASE

This is a rare skin condition of mast cell overproliferation, either local (solitary mastocytoma) or widespread (urticaria pigmentosa, diffuse cutaneous mastocytosis), which very rarely affects other organ systems. It is generally less severe than adult disease and usually improves with age.

HISTORY

The disease may be present at birth, with single (solitary mastocytoma [SM]) or multiple (urticarial pigmentosa [UP]) itchy lesions anywhere on the skin and diffuse erythema, blistering, thickening of skin and itch (diffuse cutaneous mastocytosis [DCM]). Lesions are persistent over years. If severe, the patient may have flushing, diarrhoea, abdominal pain and wheezing, which do not necessarily indicate systemic mastocytosis, rather systemic effects of cutaneous mast cell release.

EXAMINATION

- SM or UP lesions are red/brown and thickened, urticate on stroking (Darier sign).
- DCM is Darier positive over whole skin and the child may be generally unwell.

MANAGEMENT

- Oral antihistamines and mast cell stabilisers.
- Avoid known precipitants of mast cell degranulation, including codeine, certain anaesthetic drugs and radiological contrast. Refer to a textbook for a full list of drugs and other agents.
- May cause anaphylaxis: consider epipen prescription if appropriate.

ICHTHYOSIS

Ichthyosis is a group of genetic skin conditions caused by abnormalities of epidermal structure, resulting in dry scaly skin. Ichythosis vulgaris is common, associated with atopic eczema and alterations in the filaggrin gene. The other ichthyoses are rare.

HISTORY

The more severe forms can be associated with collodion baby (collodion membrane at birth, shed after few weeks). Dry scaly skin, often from birth, is present in rarer forms. Patients have difficulty regulating body temperature and there may be a build up of skin scales in the ears. There may be family history of ichthyosis.

EXAMINATION

- Dry scaly skin, may be worse in certain areas dependent on type (**Figs 6.31– 6.33**).
- Skin may be normal colour or red or blistered, dependent on type.
- Scalp may be involved with hair growth reduced.
- Palms may be hyperlinear.
- Check neurology as rare types are associated with neurological abnormality.

MANAGEMENT

- For ichthyosis vulgaris moisturisers only.
- For the more severe forms refer to paediatric dermatologist.
- Intensive moisturising regime, oral retinoid therapy for severe ichthyosis if indicated.
- Genetic testing and counselling.

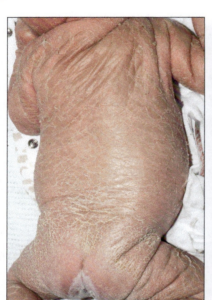
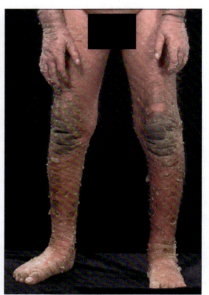
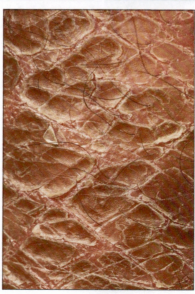

FIGURES 6.31–6.33 Hyperkeratosis and scaling in different autosomal recessive ichthyosis.

LINEAR EPIDERMAL NAEVI

This is a heterogeneous group of congenital lesions assumed to be caused by genetic mosaicism, which can be associated with other abnormalities. Different types are related to the cell of origin, e.g. keratinocytic or adnexal.

HISTORY

Epidermal naevi are usually present from birth and can extend after birth. They can be associated with other congenital abnormalities.

EXAMINATION

- Follow Blashko's lines (**Fig. 6.34**).
- Palpable epidermal lesions.
- Variable colour and texture dependent on type (**Fig. 6.35**).
- Check for other abnormalities.

MANAGEMENT

- Laser therapy can be useful in certain types.
- Surgical excision is possible for small lesions.
- Refer for genetics opinion as there is a possibility of gonadal mosaicism with certain types.

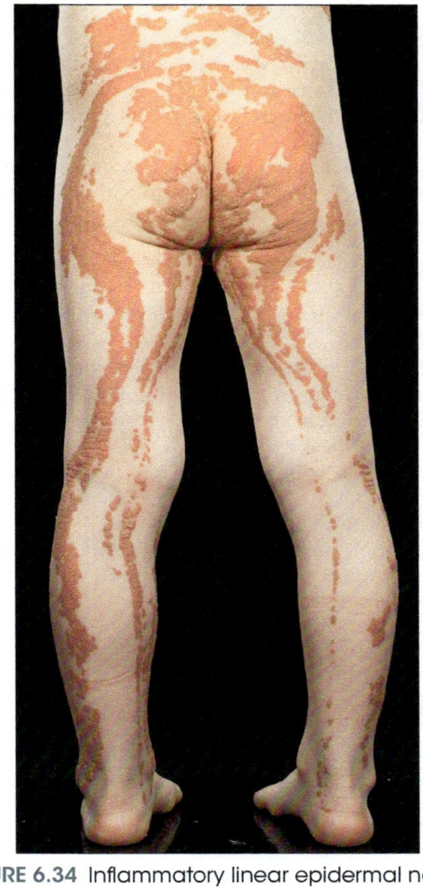

ECTODERMAL DYSPLASIA

Ectodermal dysplasia is a heterogeneous group of genetic conditions defined clinically as abnormalities of two of the following ectodermal structures: skin, hair, nails and teeth. It is very variable in severity and can be part of a broader syndrome.

HISTORY

There may be family history with variable inheritance patterns. Abnormalities may be obvious from birth or not until early childhood. Hair may have no or reduced rate of growth or increased breakage. Sweating may be reduced, leading to over-heating or febrile convulsions. The child may have reduced vision or hearing and may have reduced tear production and recurrent conjunctivitis.

EXAMINATION

- Child and other family members if appropriate.
- Dystrophic nails.
- Sparse or brittle hair, absent eyebrows/lashes/ body hair.
- Skin may be dry or eczematous.

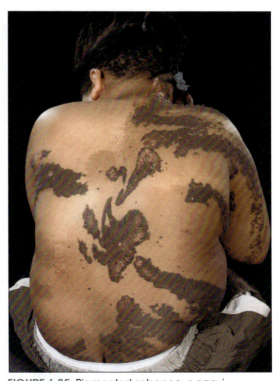

FIGURE 6.35 Pigmented sebaceous naevi.

FIGURE 6.34 Inflammatory linear epidermal naevi.

- Teeth may be reduced in number and/or abnormal in shape (**Fig. 6.36**).
- Characteristic facial features in X-linked hypohydrotic type (**Fig. 6.37**).
- Check for other congenital abnormalities, e.g. clefting.
- Growth may be reduced.

MANAGEMENT

- Ophthalmology and hearing check.
- Moisturisers for skin.
- Dental assessment and long-term management.
- Refer family to genetics for counselling.

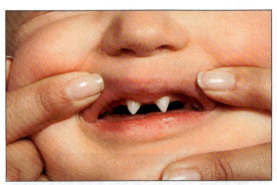

FIGURE 6.36 Reduced and abnormal teeth in ectodermal dysplasia.

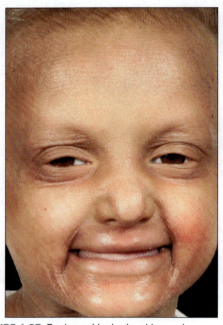

FIGURE 6.37 Reduced hair, dry skin and characteristic facial features in X-linked hypohydrotic ectodermal dysplasia.

PAEDIATRIC DERMATOLOGICAL EMERGENCIES

STEVENS–JOHNSON SYNDROME AND TOXIC EPIDERMAL NECROLYSIS

These conditions comprise a rare but severe mucocutaneous reaction to infectious agents or drugs (most commonly NSAIDs, antibiotics and anticonvulsants). Toxic epidermal necrolysis (TEN) is usually more rapid in onset than Stevens–Johnson syndrome (SJS), more severe, affects more of the skin surface and has a poorer outcome.

HISTORY

There is a preceding infection or history of medication. SJS is often caused by *Mycloplasma pneumoniae* in children; TEN is usually caused by a drug (as listed above). The child systemically unwell before onset of mucocutaneous signs. There is a sudden onset of rash and mucous membrane involvement with worsening of the clinical picture (**Figs 6.38–6.40**).

EXAMINATION

- Child is unwell – can be severely toxic.
- <10% skin involved in SJS, >30% in TEN.
- Skin lesions are initially red, may be target-like, subsequently large areas of blistering and skin necrosis.
- At least two mucous surfaces are involved in SJS, always including the mouth with characteristic crusting of lips.

MANAGEMENT

- Urgent admission; TEN requires intensive care or burns unit.
- Stop potentially causative medication.
- Treat with appropriate antibiotic(s) if infection considered a likely cause.
- Fluid and heat management.
- Refer to an ophthalmologist.
- Scrupulous eye and oral care.
- Skin and blood cultures for sepsis.
- For TEN, treatment options include intravenous immunoglobulin, methylprednisolone and anti-TNF biological agent.

Dermatology

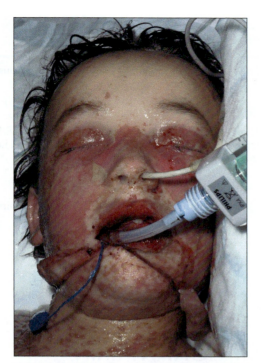

STAPHYLOCOCCAL SCALDED SKIN SYNDROME

HISTORY

There may be a history of preceding skin lesion/infection. The patient has sudden onset fever and systemic illness with diffuse redness of the skin and development of blistering/desquamation.

EXAMINATION

- Toxic unwell child.
- Diffuse erythema, +/− superficial skin peeling.
- Nikolsky's sign is positive (minimal shearing pressure causes skin separation).
- May be the focus for staphyloccal entry.

MANAGEMENT

- Urgent admission.
- Specialist dermatology nursing.
- Skin swab and blood cultures.
- IV antibiotics to cover *Staphylococcus* sp.

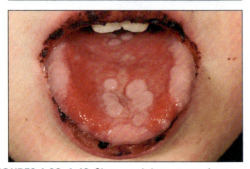

FIGURES 6.38–6.40 Stevens–Johnson syndrome and toxic epidermal necrolysis. **6.38**: Acute phase followed by gradual resolution; **6.39, 6.40**: typical oral lesions.

COLLODION BABY AND HARLEQUIN ICHTHYOSIS

These are two distinct clinical entities; however they have in common a similar approach to basic management soon after birth. A collodion baby is encased in a so-called collodion membrane at birth. It is usually associated with underlying genetic ichthyosis (of variable severity). The most severe is harlequin ichthyosis (HI). HI is potentially fatal, but good early management optimises the chance of survival.

HISTORY

A thickened membrane is present around the skin at birth, which eventually sheds. There may be family history of ichthyosis.

EXAMINATION

- Child's temperature may be unstable.
- Membrane may be red, cracking, forming plates (HI).
- Edges of facial orifices may be retracted (ectropion, eclabion).
- Chest/limbs digits may be constricted (HI).

MANAGEMENT

- Refer to paediatric dermatologist.
- Specialist dermatology nursing in regulated temperature and humidity.
- Scrupulous eye care – ophthalmology opinion.
- Occasionally skin is near normal after the collodion membrane is shed, but if not refer family to geneticist for gene testing and counselling.
- For HI consider early oral retinoid therapy.
- Optimise fluid balance; nutritional support if feeding difficult.

ECZEMA HERPETICUM

There is herpes simplex viral infection on a background of eczema. It carries significant mortality.

HISTORY

There is history of preceding eczema and of familial herpes simplex infection.

EXAMINATION

- Vesicles or roofless blisters.
- Child may be systemically unwell.

MANAGEMENT

- Admission for IV aciclovir and treatment of underlying eczema.

GENERALISED PUSTULAR PSORIASIS

This is rare in childhood but potentially very serious. It may be the presenting episode of psoriasis.

HISTORY

There may be history of preceding psoriasis, with acute exacerbation/onset of the skin condition. The child is systemically unwell.

EXAMINATION

- Erythroderma (redness all over) and scaling, with overlying multiple sterile superficial pustules.
- Child toxic and unwell.

MANAGEMENT

- Urgent admission.
- Systemic ciclosporin/methotrexate/biologicals.
- Specialist dermatology nursing.
- Genetic testing for interferonopathies.

MALIGNANT SKIN CONDITIONS

LANGHERHANS CELL HISTIOCYTOSIS

- Proliferation of Langerhans cells in the skin and/or other organs.
- Skin lesions tend to be truncal +/– in scalp, similar in appearance to seborrhoeic dermatitis.
- Skin biopsy is diagnostic.
- Clinical presentation and course are highly variable.
- Management varies between topical treatments and systemic chemotherapy.

MALIGNANT MELANOMA

Malignant melanoma is very rare in childhood. Known predisposing factors are very large or multiple congenital melanocytic naevi, familial melanoma syndromes, and DNA repair defects.

OTHERS

Other malignant conditions include cutaneous leukaemic deposits, rare vascular tumours (see above), squamous cell carcinomas, basal cell carcinomas and cutaneous T-cell lymphoma.

FURTHER READING

Ezzedine K. Lim HW, Suzuki T, *et al.* Revised classification/ nomenclature of vitiligo and related issues: the Vitiligo Global Issues Consensus Conference. *Pigment Cell Melanoma Res* 2012;25:E1–13.

Ferrandiz-Pulido C, Garcia-Patos V. A review of causes of Stevens-Johnson syndrome and toxic epidermal necrolysis in children. *Arch Dis Child* 2013;98:998–1003.

Halvorson CR. An approach to urticaria. *Cutis* 2012;90:E1–7.

Happle R. The group of epidermal nevus syndromes. Part I. Well defined phenotypes. *J Am Acad Dermatol* 2010;63:1–22; quiz 23-24.

Harper JI, Oranje AP, Prose NS. *Textbook of Paediatric Dermatology*, 2nd edn. Oxford: Blackwell Science, 2006.

Hernandez-Martin A, Aranegui B, Martin-Santiago A, Garcia-Doval I. A systematic review of clinical trials of treatments for the congenital ichthyoses, excluding ichthyosis vulgaris. *J Am Acad Dermatol* 2013;69:544–9.

Itin PH, Fistarol SK. Ectodermal dysplasias. *Am J Med Gen* Part C, Seminars in medical genetics 2004;131C:45–51.

Khorsand K, Sidbury R. Recent advances in pediatric dermatology. *Arch Dis Child* 2014;99:944–8.

Kinsler V, Bulstrode N. The role of surgery in the management of congenital melanocytic naevi in children: a perspective from Great Ormond Street Hospital. *J Plastic Reconstruct Aesthetic Surg* 2009;62:595–601.

Luu M, Frieden IJ. Haemangioma: clinical course, complications and management. *Br J Dermatol* 2013;169:20–30.

Mann JA, Siegel DH. Common genodermatoses: what the pediatrician needs to know. *Pediatr Ann* 2009;38:91–8.

McAleer MA, Flohr C, Irvine AD. Management of difficult and severe eczema in childhood. *Br Med J* 2012;345:e4770.

Mellerio JE. Epidermolysis bullosa care in the United Kingdom. *Dermatol Clin* 2010;28:395–6.

Noguera-Morel L, Hernandez-Martin A, Torrelo A. Cutaneous drug reactions in the pediatric population. *Pediatr Clin North Am* 2014;61:403–26.

Posso-De Los Rios CJ, Pope E. New insights into pustular dermatoses in pediatric patients. *J Am Acad Dermatol* 2014;70:767–73.

Tollefson MM. Diagnosis and management of psoriasis in children. *Pediatr Clin North Am* 2014;61:261–77.

Torrelo A, Alvarez-Twose I, Escribano L. Childhood mastocytosis. *Curr Opin Pediatr* 2012;24:480–6.

Waelchli RAS, Robinson K, Chong KW, Martinez AE, Kinsler VA. New vascular classification of port wine stains: improving prediction of Sturge-Weber risk. *Br J Dermatol* 2014;171:861–7.

Weibel L, *Sampaio MC, Visentin MT, Howell KJ, Woo P, Harper JI.* Evaluation of methotrexate and corticosteroids for the treatment of localized scleroderma (morphoea) in children. *Br J Dermatol* 2006;155:1013–20.

7 Ophthalmology

Ken K. Nischal

Ophthalmology obviously is important for the surveillance and assessment of vision and visual development in the child, but in a childrens hospital it often plays a key role in diagnosis, disease surveillance and timing of therapeutic intervention. This chapter should allow the paediatrician to understand these many roles.

ANATOMY OF THE EYE

See **Figs 7.1–7.3** for terminology of eye anatomy. See **Fig. 7.4** for description of eye movements.

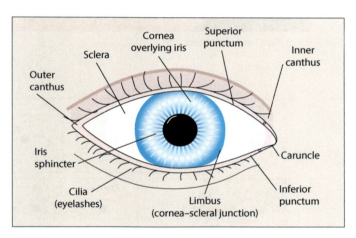

FIGURE 7.1 External landmarks of the eye and periocular region.

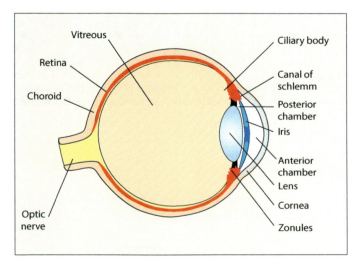

FIGURE 7.2 Cross-section of the globe.

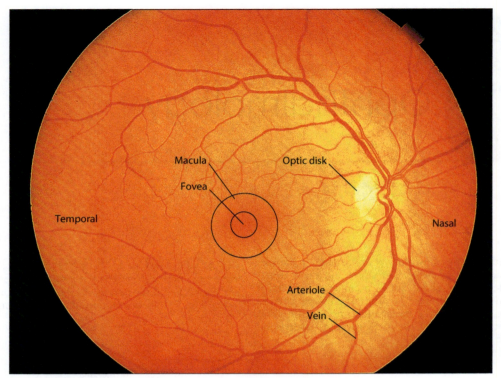

FIGURE 7.3 Fundus landmarks.

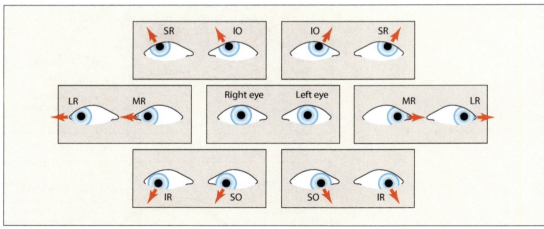

FIGURE 7.4 Schematic showing the field of action of the extraocular muscles. IO: inferior oblique; IR: inferior rectus; LR: lateral rectus; MR: medial rectus; SO: superior oblique; SR: superior rectus.

VISUAL DEVELOPMENT

VISUAL MILESTONES

It is essential to understand normal visual milestones: The chart (**Fig. 7.5**) provides an easy guide to these. Delayed visual maturation (DVM) may be seen in otherwise healthy children, which resolves by 6 months of age. Complex DVM is when there is a pathology explaining a degree of visual impairment but the child is exhibiting a more profound visual impairment. Under these circumstances the child may still have DVM that is preventing him/her from reaching their visual potential (which may not be normal due to the underlying pathology).

AMBLYOPIA

This is the commonest cause of decreased vision in childhood, affecting 2–3 in every 100 children. It occurs when the neural pathways between the affected eye and the brain fail to develop, usually due to lack of stimulation. The earlier the onset of amblyopia, the greater the depth of the deficit. The critical period for visual development is probably between the first and eighth weeks of life; visual disruption during this period can cause dense amblyopia.

Amblyopia has numerous causes; the commonest are strabismus, visual deprivation (e.g. due to congenital cataract), significant difference between refractive error in the two eyes (anisometropic), significant bilateral refractive errors (ametropic) and significant astigmatism (meridional). Amblyopia is reversible by occlusion therapy of the better or good eye, with early detection and treatment offering the best outcome.

Behaviours	Neo	6wks	3m	4m	5m	6m	9m	12m
Blinks to flash	+	+	+	+	+	+	+	+
Turns to diffuse light	+	+	+	+	+	+	+	+
Fixes and follows near face	+ −	+ −	+	+	+	+	+	+
Watches an adult at 0.75m	+ −	+	+	+	+	+	+	+
F & F dangling ball at 6.5cm		+ −	+	+	+	+	+	+
Watches adult at 1.5m		+ −	+ −	+	+	+	+	+
Converges to 6.5cm			+ −	+	+	+	+	+
Fixates 2.5cm brick at 3.3m				+ −	+	+	+	+
Blinks to threat				+ −	+	+	+	+
Watches adult at 3m					+ −	+	+	+
Fixates 1.25cm sweet					+ −	+	+	+
Fixates 1.25mm sweet						+ −	+	+

☐ = upper limit of normal behaviour

FIGURE 7.5 Observable visual behaviour (after Blanche Stiff and Patricia Sonksen). F&F: fixates and follows.

LIDS

ABLEPHARON

- Incidence – very rare.
- Aetiology – absent or hypoplastic lids that occur as a developmental anomaly.
- Clinical presentation: exposed globe with lids that cannot close and may appear everted but cannot be inverted back to normal shape/position. It is often seen with macrostomia.
- Diagnosis: clinical.
- Differential diagnosis: congenital everted lid (seen with chlamydia infection) and lid easily everted back to normal shape/position.
- Treatment: protect exposed cornea with lubrication/contact lenses, until lids are reconstructed.
- Prognosis: poor if cornea exposure is not tackled early.

CRYPTOPHTHALMOS

- Incidence: rare.
- Aetiology: developmental anomaly.
- Clinical presentation: the upper and lower eyelids are fused together so that the skin of the forehead passes onto the skin of the cheeks. Most often associate with Fraser syndrome (*Fryn 1* gene).
- Diagnosis: clinical, with only differential being anopthalmos but here lids are separated but there is a very small palpebral fissure.
- Treatment: reconstruction of eyelids but the visual function is often limited.
- Prognosis: poor for vision.

COLOBOMA

- Incidence: rare.
- Aetiology: developmental anomaly.
- Clinical presentation: incomplete formation of upper/lower lid(s) (**Fig. 7.6**).
- There is association with Goldenhar syndrome (upper lid), amniotic band syndrome and other clefting syndromes (usually lower lid).
- Treatment: lubrication in the first instance to prevent exposure keratopathy. Early referral to oculoplastic surgeon to allow reconstruction of lid(s).
- Prognosis: good once repair is achieved.

EPICANTHUS

- Incidence: common.
- Aetiology: developmental anomaly.
- Clinical presentation: a vertical fold of skin on either side of the nose, sometimes covering the inner canthus (but may be a normal ethnic variant). It can give the impression of pseudostrabismus.
- Diagnosis: clinical.
- Prognosis: usually resolves with age.

ENTROPION

- Incidence: uncommon.
- Aetiology: may be congenital or acquired (usually due to cicatrising conjunctivitis but very rare in children).
- Clinical presentation: inturing of lower eyelid(s), which can cause corneal problems.
- Dignosis: clinical; differential includes epiblepharon, which is due to an excess skin fold causing the lashes only to turn in.
- Treatment: surgical correction is straightforward.
- Prognosis: good.

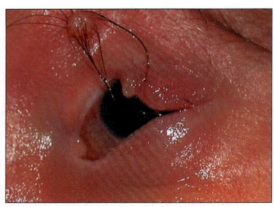

FIGURE 7.6 Upper lid coloboma.

ECTROPION

- Incidence: uncommon.
- Aetiology: usually acquired due to shortening/cicatrisation of the lid skin. It is often seen in icthyosis (harlequin baby).
- Diagnosis: clinical by exposure of tarsal conjunctiva.
- Treatment: depends on aetiology but emollient use in cases of icthyosis often causes resolution. Rarely surgical correction is needed.

SYMBLEPHARON

- Incidence: rare.
- Aetiology: usually acquired but may be congenital. Acquired types are seen in Stevens–Johnson syndrome, toxic epidermal necrolysis, alkali injuries to the eyes, ocular cicatricial pemphigoid and rarely, epidermolysis bullosa (recessive types usually).
- Clinical presentation: connection between the lid and conjunctiva (**Fig. 7.7**).
- Treatment: prevention is the best approach in conditions where symblepharon may be acquired; topical lubrication and steroids may be needed but ophthalmic opinion must be sought early. Once formed amniotic membrane may be used to treat after resection of the symblepharon.
- Prognosis: prevention is the best treatment but after amniotic membrane graft the results are usually good.

BLEPHARITIS

- Incidence: much more common than originally thought.
- Aetiology: inflammation of the eyelid margins (**Fig. 7.8**), with or without chalazion (blocked meibomian gland). The anterior type usually affects the lashes while the posterior type is caused by meibomian gland dysfunction.
- Clinical presentation: recurrent chalazia, chronic red eyes or chronically crusted lids.
- Differential diagnosis: conjunctivitis; exclude molluscum contagiosum or chlamydia infection if a chronic unilateral red eye.
- Association: usually isolated but may be associated with acne rosacea. Absent meibomian glands may be seen in ectodermal dysplasia.
- Treatment: lid hygiene. Topical antibiotics and mild steroids may be needed and occasionally systemic antibiotics may be needed. Treatment is necessary to prevent corneal complications (vascularisation/keratitis).
- Prognosis: moderate since the condition may never totally resolve but the signs and symptoms can be controlled to prevent ocular damage

STYE

- Incidence: very common.
- Aetiology: this is an infected eyelash follicle (**Fig. 7.9**).
- Treatment: removal of the eyelash accelerates resolution. Occasionally topical antibiotics may be needed.

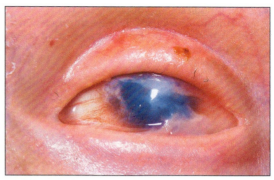

FIGURE 7.7 Neglected epidermolysis bullosa resulting in symblepharon of the lower lid and bulbar conjunctiva (see Chapter 6 Dermatology, page 139). Also shown is keratinisation and scarring of the cornea due to exposure keratopathy.

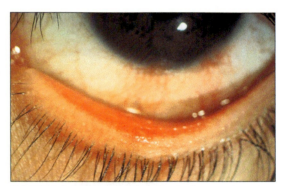

FIGURE 7.8 Blepharitis of the lower lid margin with phlycten of the lower limbus.

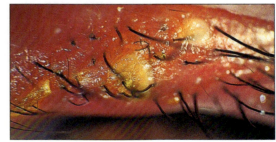

FIGURE 7.9 Stye.

MOLLUSCUM CONTAGIOSUM

- Aetiology: common eyelid tumour (see also Chapter 6 Dermatology, page 142) caused by a poxvirus.
- Clinical presentation: it is often situated on the lid margin and should be looked for in cases of follicular or chronic conjunctivitis. The lesions are small umbilicated nodules (**Fig. 7.10**).
- Treatment: usually self-limiting but if conjunctivitis is troublesome then curettage of lid lesions may be needed.
- Prognosis: good.

CAPILLARY HAEMANGIOMA

These are a vascular anomaly (see Chapter 6 Dermatology, page 133) that histologically displays abundant endothelial cells with narrow vascular channels. They are the commonest tumours of eyelids or orbits in childhood.

Systemic associations include Kasabach-Merritt syndrome (thrombocytopenia due to platelet pooling within one or more large haemangiomas) and Maffucci syndrome (haemangiomas and enchondromas). If the haemangioma is flat and plaque-like, PHACES syndrome should be considered (**Fig. 7.11**).

TREATMENT

The natural history of capillary haemangiomas is that they appear 2–3 weeks after birth, grow rapidly until 4 months of age and then stop growing by 6 months, regressing thereafter. The position of the haemangioma may result in visual deprivation by causing a ptosis, amblyopia from astigmatism or rarely compress the optic nerve if the haemangioma is intraconal in position. Treatment now involves use of systemic beta-blockers, which has superseded intralesional and/or systemic steroids. Some cases still demand surgical excision. Occlusion of the unaffected eye may be needed to prevent amblyopia developing in the affected eye. The complication of hypoglycaemia should be considered when treating with systemic beta-blockers.

PROGNOSIS

Excellent with the advent of systemic beta-blockers.

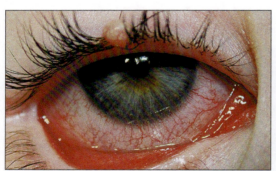

FIGURE 7.10 Molluscum contagiosum – raised papillomatous lesion with a central core containing virus particles.

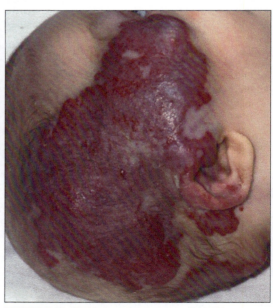

FIGURE 7.11 Flat haemangioma in PHACE.

PORT WINE STAIN

The aetiology is unclear.

CLINICAL PRESENTATION

The lesion is a dermal capillary vascular anomaly that may occur in the periocular region (**Fig. 7.12**); see also Chapter 6 Dermatology, page 134. Ocular associations include episcleral haemangioma, iris heterochromia (affected iris darker than unaffected one), choroidal haemangioma and glaucoma. Systemic associations include Sturge–Weber syndrome and cutis marmorata telangectasia congenita.

TREATMENT/PROGNOSIS

If periocular, there is increased risk of developing glaucoma and the child should be seen regularly to exclude this. The patients at highest risk of developing glaucoma are those with Sturge–Weber syndrome, or those in whom an isolated port wine stain affects both lids, episclera, choroid and causes iris heterochromia. Glaucoma can be difficult to manage because of the risk of choroidal haemorrhage/detachment if filtration surgery is performed. Topical prostaglandin analogues such as latanoprost and bimatoprost have been reported as causing serous retinal detachment in the presence of choroidal hemangioma.

Prognosis is guarded if glaucoma is severe and patient has neurological deficit with Sturge–Weber syndrome.

PTOSIS

Ptosis may be myogenic, neurogenic or mechanical.

CLINICAL PRESENTATION

There is lowered upper lid margin position. It may be measured in terms of palpebral aperture or marginal reflex distance. The latter is the distance of the upper lid margin to the central corneal reflection when using a torch as a target for the patient to look at. This should be 3.5–4.5 mm.

Systemic associations include syndromes such as blepharophimosis, Noonan, Saethre–Chotzen, Freeman–Sheldon and Kabuki and in mitochondrial cytopathies (such as Kearnes–Sayre syndrome). Ptosis may be a presenting feature of myasthenia gravis or myotonic dystrophy.

TREATMENT/PROGNOSIS

Ptosis may be due to dysfunction or absence of the levator palpebrae superioris muscle. Dysfunction may allow strengthening of the muscle while absence needs a frontalis sling (i.e. attaching the lid to the frontalis muscle). Ptosis can cause amblyopia either because of stimulus deprivation (if severe ptosis) or astigmatism (mild to moderate ptosis). In any case, prompt ophthalmic referral is required. Care should be taken so as not to cause exposure keratopathy if ptosis repair is undertaken. If it is mechanical then the cause needs to be removed, e.g. a large haemangioma.

Prognosis is good.

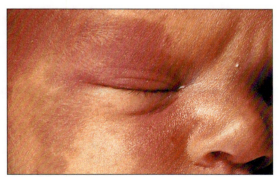

FIGURE 7.12 Port wine stain affecting the periocular region.

LID RETRACTION

AETIOLOGY/CLINICAL PRESENTATION

This includes thyroid eye disease (lid signs such as retraction [**Fig. 7.13**] and lid lag seen in 25–60% of paediatric cases), Parinaud syndrome, Marcus–Gunn jaw winking and primary congenital idiopathic lid retraction. Lower lid retraction is seen in cherubism (a rare, inherited condition characterised by fibro-osseous lesions of the maxilla and mandible recently localised to chromosome 4p16.3).

TREATMENT/PROGNOSIS

No treatment is required except lubricating drops or ointment, used at night if there is evidence of lid lag and incomplete closure of the lids when asleep. Treat the underlying cause.

Prognosis is good.

PRESEPTAL CELLULITIS

AETIOLOGY/CLINICAL PRESENTATION

In children, this is most commonly due to contiguous ethmoid sinusitis. Patients present with infection of the lid without orbital involvement (**Fig. 7.14**). There may be erythematous swollen eyelids that may be tense.

TREATMENT/PROGNOSIS

Full ocular examination without dilation of pupils including visual acuity, eye movements, colour vision, pupil reactions and fundoscopy. Systemic antibiotics and referral to ENT team, who usually decide on the type of imaging. Review to ensure no progression to orbital cellulitis (see later).

Prognosis is good.

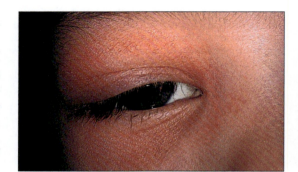

FIGURE 7.14 Preseptal cellulitis.

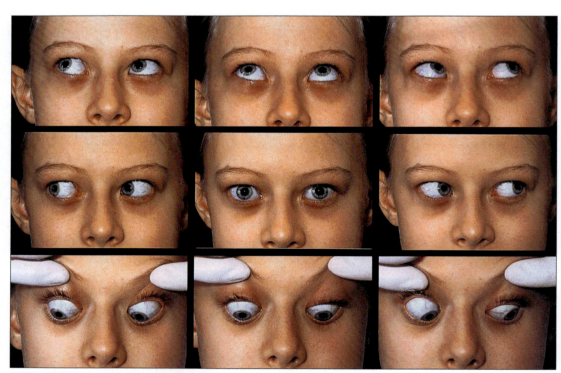

FIGURE 7.13 Lid retraction in thyroid eye disease. Eye movements are normal.

Ophthalmology

LID LAG

- Aetiology: most commonly seen in congenital ptosis (usually unilateral) but also seen in thyroid eye disease and, rarely, polyneuritis.
- Clinical presentation: delay or absence of normal downward excursion of upper lid on downgaze.
- Treatment: may need lubrication if incomplete eyelid closure at night.
- Prognosis: good.

THE WATERING EYE

- Incidence: not uncommon.
- Aetiology: epiphora (watering of the eye) is due to a congenital blockage of the nasolacrimal duct.
- Clinical presentation: lacrimal massage usually improves the situation but occasionally probing under general anaesthetic is needed. Very rarely, the lacrimal sac becomes expanded due to the distal blockage and the child presents with a dacryocoele (**Fig. 7.15**). If this becomes infected it is termed a dacryocystitis.
- Treatment: if probing of the nasolacrimal duct fails then the child may need primary intubation with silicone tubes or a dacrocystorhinostomy.

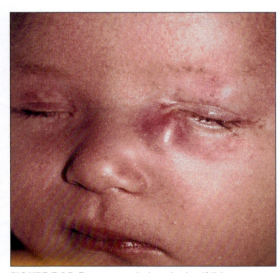

FIGURE 7.15 Dacryocoele in a baby. If this becomes infected it is termed dacryocystitis.

MICROCORNEA

- Incidence: an uncommon condition, defined as any cornea less than 10 mm in horizontal diameter.
- It is often associated with hypermetropia, colobomas of the iris, cataracts, persistent hyperplastic primary vitreous, retinopathy of prematurity, angle closure glaucoma, infantile glaucoma and chronic open angle glaucoma. Systemic associations include Ehlers–Danlos syndrome, Marfan syndrome, Rieger syndrome, Norrie syndrome, Trisomy 21 (Down syndrome), progeria, rubella, Turner syndrome, Waardenburg syndrome, Weil–Marchesani syndrome, Warburg micro syndrome, cataract microcornea syndrome and acroreno-ocular syndrome.

No active treatment is needed other than surveillance for complications. Prognosis is dependent on any complications such as glaucoma.

CORNEA PLANA

- Incidence: rare.
- Aetiology: cornea plana is a flat cornea with a curvature of less than 43 diopters. There are two types CNA1 (dominant) and CNA2 (recessive).
- Ocular associations include sclerocornea, infantile glaucoma, angle closure glaucoma, chronic open angle glaucoma, retinal aplasia, anterior synechiae, aniridia, congenital cataracts, ectopia lentis, choroidal coloboma, blue sclera, iris coloboma, pseudoptosis and microphthalmos. Systemic associations include osteogenesis imperfecta and epidermolysis bullosa (see Chapter 6 Dermatology, page 139).
- Treatment: review to exclude glaucoma and correct any refractive error.
- Prognosis: dependent on any complications that may arise.

MEGALOCORNEA

- Incidence: rare.
- Aetiology: megalocornea is a cornea with a horizontal diameter of more than 13 mm that is not progressive. If the cornea is enlarged in the presence of congenital glaucoma (**Fig. 7.16**), it is not defined as megalocornea. It is usually inherited as an X-linked recessive trait in most instances, but maybe dominantly inherited.
- Megalocornea most often occurs by itself, but other associated ocular conditions include anterior embryotoxon, mosaic corneal dystrophy, glaucoma. Systemic associations include Alport syndrome, craniosynostosis, dwarfism, Down syndrome, facial hemiatrophy, Marfan syndrome, mucolipidosis type II and megalocornea–mental retardation syndrome.

Treatment: children often need lubrication especially at night. Sometimes the lower lid lashes will rub on the cornea and this must be watched for to prevent corneal infections.

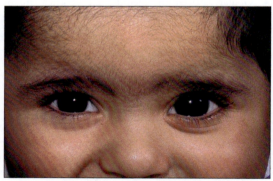

FIGURE 7.16 Bilateral congenital glaucoma with the left eye bigger than the right eye. Large corneas associated with congenital glaucoma are not termed megalocornea.

KERATOCONUS

INCIDENCE/AETIOLOGY

Keratoconus is a common condition affecting the cornea. Why it occurs is unclear but may be hereditary and may be induced by chronic rubbing.

CLINICAL PRESENTATION

This disorder results in a central or paracentral thinning of the cornea, leading to poor visual acuity due to irregular and/or high astigmatism as the cornea bulges outward in a cone shape. Using direct ophthalmoscopy and a dilated pupil an oil droplet sign is seen. Other signs include scissoring of the light reflex on retinoscopy, slit lamp signs (Fleischer's ring, which is a brown deposition of iron in the epithelium at the base of the cone; Vogt's striae, which are small, thin, parallel striations in Descemet's membrane in the area of the cone, which with gentle pressure on the globe will momentarily disappear; prominent corneal nerves; endothelial guttata; and posterior shagreen). Rizutti's sign is that of a conical reflection nasally as a penlight is shone across the cornea from the temporal side. This tends to be a late sign of keratoconus, as is Munson's sign – a bulging of the lower eyelid anteriorly in downgaze, as a result of the cone pushing on the eyelid.

It is associated with atopy, aniridia, blue sclera, congenital cataracts, ectopia lentis, microcornea, Leber's congenital amaurosis, retinitis pigmentosa, retinopathy of prematurity, and vernal conjunctivitis. Associated systemic conditions include Apert syndrome, atopy, brachydactyly, Crouzon syndrome, Down syndrome, Ehlers–Danlos syndrome type IV and VI, Raynaud syndrome, syndactyly, xeroderma pigmentosa and other connective tissue disorders.

TREATMENT

In mild to moderate cases contact lenses will correct the visual loss. In cases of acute hydrops, topical dehydrating, lubricating and steroid agents are needed. In severe cases, penetrating or deep lamellar corneal transplant is required. Collagen cross-linking is becoming more accepted as a treatment in adults and a few centres in Europe are also offering this for progressive keratoconus in children. Essentially UV light is applied to a cornea soaked with riboflavin. This causes collagen cross-linking and stabilises the keratoconic progression.

Ophthalmology

CONGENITAL CORNEAL OPACIFICATION

SCLEROCORNEA

- Incidence: rare.
- Aetiology: usually developmental.
- Clinical presentation: this is a congenital, non-inflammatory extension of opaque scleral tissue and fine vascular conjunctival and episcleral tissue into the peripheral cornea obscuring the limbus (**Fig. 7.17**). It is best considered as peripheral sclerocornea where it is associated with cornea plana. It is usually bilateral in 90% of cases. Its use when describing total congenital corneal opacification is incorrect and misleading.
- Associations are common and include glaucoma, cataract, colobomas of the iris and choroid, cornea plana, aniridia, angle abnormalities, and microphthalmos. Associated systemic abnormalities include spina bifida occulta, cerebellar abnormalities, cranial abnormalities, Hallermann–Streiff syndrome, Smith–Lemli–Opitz syndrome, osteogenesis imperfecta and hereditary osteonychodyplasias.
- Treatment: review to exclude glaucoma and cataract development. Appropriate treatment with spectacles and contact lenses to treat the hypermetropia that often accompanies these cases. Cases of total corneal opacification should not be labelled sclerocornea.

PETERS' ANOMALY

- Incidence: rare.
- Aetiology: usually developmental.
- Clinical presentation: usually bilateral congenital central corneal opacity with defects in the posterior corneal stroma, Descemet's membrane and endothelium, with or without iridolenticular and/or keratolenticular adhesions. Its use as a 'waste paper basket' diagnosis has led to much confusion in genotype/phenotype correlation studies. It is better considered an anterior segment developmental anomaly due to iridocorneal adhesions or keratolenticular adhesion or both.
- Ocular associations include glaucoma, cataract, Axenfeld–Rieger syndrome, aniridia, microphthalmia, persistent hyperplastic primary vitreous (PHPV) and retinal dysplasia. Systemic abnormalities include craniofacial anomalies, central nervous system abnormalities, fetal alcohol syndrome, chromosomal abnormalities and **Peters plus syndrome** (a rare autosomal recessive disorder comprising short-limbed dwarfism, cleft lip and/or palate, brachydactyly and learning difficulties).
- Treatment: review to exclude glaucoma and cataract. Treatment of glaucoma if present. If bilateral, corneal transplant should be considered. Unilateral cases should be treated with transplant if the better eye is not normal.

Prognosis: varies with degree of anterior chamber disorganisation. The less the disorganisation, the better the prognosis.

TOTAL CONGENITAL CORNEAL OPACIFICATION

- Incidence: rare – this condition has previously been called sclerocornea incorrectly.
- Aetiology: it is almost always developmental and due to lens-related issues, e.g. failure of lens to separate from the cornea or a dysgenetic or absent lens.
- Clinical presentation: presents as totally opaque cornea most commonly with corneal vascularisation and glaucoma.
- Treatment: control of glaucoma is essential and while corneal transplant can be done prognosis is poor due to the abnormal/absent lens.

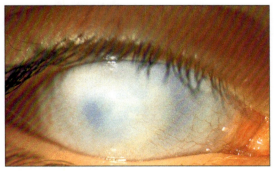

FIGURE 7.17 Sclerocornea.

CORNEAL DYSTROPHIES

See **Table 7.1**. Only those dystrophies that commonly affect children are described.

TABLE 7.1 Differential diagnosis of neonatal corneal opacity

Aetiology	Age of onset	Corneal signs	Other
INFECTIOUS DISEASE			
Herpes simplex (Type II)	4–10 days	Unilateral corneal ulcer, positive fluorescein staining, often in a geographic configuration	Viral culture for herpes
Rubella	Birth	Diffuse corneal oedema, often associated with cataracts	Serology including IgM
Neisseria gonorrhoeae	2–3 days	Diffuse punctate staining with possible corneal ulceration	Gram stain and culture
TRAUMA			
Tears in Descemet's membrane	Birth	Vertical corneal striae with oedema in the area of breaks in Descemet's membrane	History of forceps delivery often associated with soft tissue injury of the face
Corneal perforations with amniocentesis	Birth	Local corneal opacity with possible iris adhesions	Amniocentesis; traumatic cataract
DYSGENESIS SYNDROMES			
Peters' anomaly	Birth	Central corneal opacity may extend to the limbus; iridocorneal strands	60% with glaucoma
Sclerocornea	Birth	Peripheral corneal opacity associated with flattening of the cornea	May be associated with other anterior segment anomalies
Limbal dermoid	Birth	Limbal mass; yellow-white in appearance; may also have hair follicles	May be isolated or associated with Goldenhar syndrome
DYSTROPHIES			
Congenital hereditary endothelial dystrophy (CHED)	Birth to several months	Bilateral diffuse corneal oedema; corneal thickening; corneal diameter normal	Attenuated or absent endothelium; autosomal dominant or recessive
Posterior polymorphous dystrophy (PPD)	Infrequently at birth to first few years of birth	Deep linear opacities and thickening of Descemet's membrane (snail tracks); deep posterior vesicles; corneal oedema	Usually autosomal dominant
Congenital hereditary stromal	Birth	Diffuse, flaky stromal central anterior stromal haze with deeper involvement	
METABOLIC			
Mucopolysaccharidoses (Hurlers-MPS-IH most severe form)	Unusual at birth	Diffuse ground glass appearance through all layers; bilateral and symmetrical	Urinary glycosaminoglycans; autosomal recessive
Mucolipidoses (Type IV)		Anterior and epithelial clouding	Autosomal recessive
Cystinosis (rare)	Rarely at birth, usually first year	White needle-like crystals within corneal stroma; ground-glass appearance	Renal impairment; crystals also in conjunctiva; glaucoma; autosomal recessive
Tyrosinaemia	Neonate	Corneal epithelial deposits	Tyrosine in blood and urine; hyperkeratosis of skin
CONGENITAL			
Congenital glaucoma	Birth to first 6 months of life	Buphthalmos corneal oedema; Haab's striae (horizontal curvilinear breaks in Descemet's membrane due to stretch injury)	Increased ocular pressure; myopic shift; increased cupping

POSTERIOR EMBRYOTOXON

- Aetiology: a prominent, anteriorly displaced Schwalbe's ring seen only on slit lamp examination. Seen in up to 20% of the normal population.
- Associations include Axenfeld–Rieger anomaly and Alagille syndrome (seen in 95% of cases).
- Treatment: none but if associated with Axendfeld–Rieger anomaly the child may need follow-up to exclude glaucoma development.

CORNEAL DEPOSITS

Corneal deposition in the paediatric age group can vary from the simple deposition of iron in the epithelium, with no visual complications, to a full-thickness corneal opacification that can lead to profound amblyopia or even blindness. Proper diagnosis and management of these conditions is important in order to minimise or prevent profound complications.

Corneal deposition may be metabolic in origin or non-metabolic. The **metabolic** causes include the mucopolysaccharidoses (not MPS III – Sanfillippo), the mucolipidoses, glycogen storage disorders (namely Von Gierke disease), sphingolipidoses (namely Fabry disease), Gaucher disease, gangliosidoses, cystinosis, Wilson disease, tyrosinaemia type II, alkaptonuria, Niemann–Pick disease, LCAT deficiency and metachromatic leukodystrophy. **Non-metabolic** causes include corneal blood staining (seen after blunt trauma with blood in the anterior chamber), band-shaped keratopathy (**Fig. 7.18**) (from calcium deposition in the cornea), amyloid deposition and neoplastic causes (i.e. monoclonal gammopathy).

KERATITIS

Keratitis is an inflammation of the cornea. It may affect the epithelium, subepithelium or stroma. Most causes of keratitis are due to infection such herpes simplex keratitis or bacterial keratitis, but there are non-infection-related causes such as neurotrophic ulcer or dry eye.

INSUFFICIENT TEAR PRODUCTION (DRY EYE)

This is insufficient production of aqueous tears leading to epithelial erosions, filamentary keratitis and secondary corneal vascularisation. It is rare in children.

It may be associated with Riley–Day syndrome (familial dysautonomia), ectodermal dysplasia, keratoconjunctivitis sicca (KCS) usually due to primary or secondary Sjögren syndrome and radiation therapy.

Treatment is with adequate lubricating drops and in some cases temporary lacrimal punctal occlusion with silicone punctal plugs to decrease tear drainage. Tarsorraphy should also be considered. Prognosis is reasonable if treated early.

NON-INFECTION-RELATED KERATITIS

The hereditary type is very rare. Aetiology includes autosomal dominant keratitis (*PAX 6*, homeobox gene mutation), ectrodactyly, ectodermal dysplasia and cleft lip and palate syndrome (EEC), ectodermal dysplasia, keratitis–ichthyosis–deafness syndrome (KID), Riley–Day syndrome (familial dysautonomia), epidermolysis bullosa, keratopathy (corneal erosions, epithelial defects) and corneal vascularisation. The child is usually photophobic and has reduced visual acuity (**Fig. 7.19**).

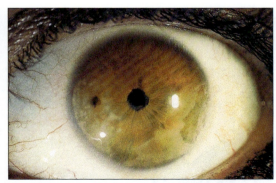

FIGURE 7.18 Band-shaped keratopathy, secondary to uveitis, in a patient with juvenile chronic arthritis. Note also a small, irregular pupil due to posterior synechiae (adhesions of the iris to the anterior capsule of the lens).

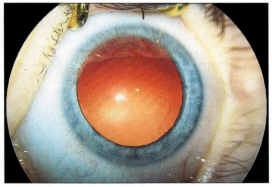

FIGURE 7.19 Keratitis affecting the superior half of the cornea. This was present from birth and progressive.

Treatment depends on the cause, but lubrication is the mainstay together with punctual plugs and/or tarsorraphy.

Inadequate spreading of tears
- Incidence: rare.
- Aetiology: inadequate spreading of tears leads to epithelial erosions or dellen (an area of corneal dessication) and is most commonly seen in lid colobomas, corneal limbal dermoids (**Figs 7.20, 7.21**) most commonly seen in Goldenhar syndrome, facial palsy, Moebius syndrome.
- Treatment: adequate ocular surface lubrication and removal of the cause if possible (e.g. limbal dermoid removal or lid coloboma repair).

Increased evaporation of tears
- Incidence: not uncommon.
- Aetiology: this is usually seen when there is proptosis or when the lids do not close adequately when the child is asleep. Seen in shallow orbits (craniosynostoses), lid colobomas, lagophthalmos, comatosed patients and lid ectropion(e.g. in cases of lamellar icthyosis).
- Treatment: eye ointment to exposed eyes when the child is asleep and regular daily lubrication. Tarsorraphy may be needed and a moist chamber may be needed.

Trauma (including corneal anaesthesia)
The aetiology may be congenital (familial dysautonomia, Goldenhar syndrome, oculofacial syndromes and leprosy) or acquired (damage to the trigeminal nerve due to herpes zoster, herpes simplex, intracranial tumours both pre- and/or postsurgery especially cerebellopontine angle tumours).

Repetitive trauma is the main cause of chronic keratitis and the presence of corneal hypo- or anaesthesia allows repetitive trauma. The accompanying reduced blink reflex reduces corneal wetting and exacerbates such a keratitis.

Treatment is with lubricating agents. Tarsorraphy or botulinum toxin-induced ptosis may be needed.

Avitaminosis A
This is common in some underdeveloped countries and is due to a deficiency of dietary vitamin A intake. It is characterised by a thickening of the corneal epithelium, keratinisation of the epithelium and a diffuse corneal opacity. Secondary pannus and corneal vascularisation can occur. In addition to corneal pathology, white foamy lesions (Bitit's spots) of the temporal conjunctiva occur.

The treatment is protein, calorie, and vitamin A replacement. Prognosis depends on how soon replacement is initiated, as corneal changes can be permanent.

Vernal keratoconjunctivitis
Although seasonal allergic conjunctivitis is extremely common, vernal keratoconjunctivitis with corneal involvement is much less common. It is a severe allergic form of eye disease. It presents with mucoid discharge and lumps on the superior tarsal conjunctiva (papillae) (**Fig. 7.22**), which cause trauma to the superior half of the cornea leading to corneal epithelial erosions, shield ulcers (5% of patients) and corneal vascularisation (micropannus).

There may be limbal infiltration with the presence of Tranta's dots, which are aggregates of eosinophils. Repeated such infiltration may leave a scar in the adjacent cornea in the form of a 'Cupid's bow', called a pseudogerontoxon. This is usually found superiorly and resembles an arcus senilis.

Treatment is with topical antiallergic medication, usually with topical steroid therapy and lubricating agents. Supratarsal steroid injection or topical cyclosporin drops may also be needed in severe cases.

Prognosis is good if treated aggressively.

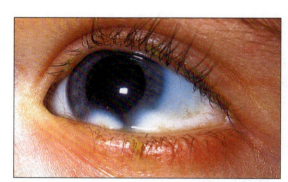

FIGURE 7.20 Limbal dermoids seen in a child with Goldenhar syndrome.

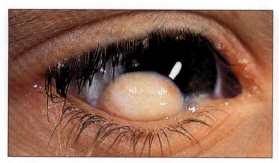

FIGURE 7.21 Very large limbal dermoid, causing difficulty in closure of the eyelids.

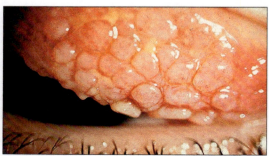

FIGURE 7.22 Giant papillae in vernal keratoconjunctivitis.

INFECTION-RELATED KERATITIS

Herpes simplex

Eye involvement occurs in 13% of newborns with systemic herpes simplex virus (HSV) infection. Herpes keratitis can occur at almost any age in children, as even neonates can become infected as they pass through the birth canal. Infections acquired at birth are usually of herpes simplex virus type 2, while herpes contracted later in life is most often HSV type 1. Primary herpes is the first exposure of the herpes virus to the patient. The hallmark sign of primary herpetic infection is conjunctivitis, which is accompanied by vesicles on the eyelids. Recurrent disease (secondary) can result in dendritic, disciform or interstitial keratitis.

Neonatal herpes simplex keratitis may be the only sign of systemic herpes simplex.

Treatment

Any child who will not open an eye should be considered to have either a foreign body or herpes simplex keratitis until proven otherwise. Examination under anaesthetic should be done in such cases.

Viral cultures from scrapings taken from the edge of any ulcer are necessary. However, PCR for HSV may be performed even on tears or conjunctival swabs from the affected eye.

Herpes simplex keratitis (epithelial) is treated with topical aciclovir while stromal and/or endothelial disease with intact epithelium is treated with topical aciclovir and topical steroids. Systemic aciclovir should be considered if systemic herpes simplex is a possibility.

Varicella-zoster

Corneal involvement is extremely rare, but ocular findings include swollen lids, vesicular lesions of the lids, and varying degrees of keratoconjunctivitis. Infrequently superficial punctate keratitis of the cornea occurs.

Treatment is with oral aciclovir, and topical cycloplegic drops for eye comfort.

Prognosis is usually good.

Chlamydia trachomatis

Trachoma is a cause of blindness world-wide. The causative organism is *Chlamydia trachomatis*, an intracellular parasite. A chronic follicular conjunctivitis results from infection with secondary corneal scarring.

Treatment is with single oral dose of azithromycin and topical erythromycin eye ointment.

Bacterial

Bacterial keratitis is rare and usually seen in children with some type of predisposing factor such as: neurotrophic cornea, contact lenses, trauma, dry eyes, HSV, immunosuppression, immunodeficiency or vitamin deficiency. Keratitis is usually stromal with or without accompanying hypopyon (pus in the anterior chamber).

Culture and Gram stain are required, followed by appropriate intensive topical and oral antibiotics.

Prognosis is variable as residual scarring can affect vision severely.

Fungal

Fungal keratitis is very rare The infection may be due to filamentous fungi such as *Aspergillus* or *Fusarium* spp. or to yeast-like fungi such as *Candida* spp. Most traumatic fungal ulcers are the result of filamentous organisms, while infection by yeasts are most common in patients with immunosuppression or dry eyes.

Clinical suspicion should be raised if there are fuzzy borders of the infiltrate, an elevated infiltrate with initially intact epithelium, satellite lesions and pyramidal or convex hypopyon. Sometimes the infiltrate may be seen to develop pigmentation and this is suggestive of filamentous infection.

Culture and Gram stain are required. Treat with systemic and topical antifungal agents.

Visual prognosis is often guarded and corneal graft may be needed.

CONJUNCTIVA

INFECTION-RELATED CONJUNCTIVITIS

NEONATAL CONJUNCTIVITIS

- Incidence: varies from 1 to 21% depending on the region of the world.
- Aetiology: includes chemical (relatively mild diffuse injection without discharge), gonococcal (copious purulent discharge that may be associated with membrane formations), HSV type II, chlamydia and bacterial.
- Clinical presentation: conjunctival inflammation occurs during the first month of life (ophthalmia neonatorum – **Fig. 7.23**). This is a notifiable condition.
- Treatment: swabs and appropriate topical and (if gonococcal or chlamydial) systemic antibiotics are needed.
- Prognosis: good if treatment is prompt.

BACTERIAL CONJUNCTIVITIS

This is very common, with the commonest causes being *Staphylococcus aureus*, *Streptococcus pneumoniae* and *Haemophilus influenzae*. Membranes and

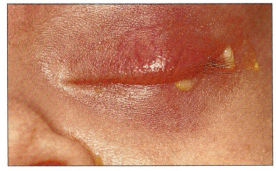

FIGURE 7.23 Ophthalmia neonatorum caused by *Chlamydia* spp.

pseudomembranes may be caused by haemolytic streptococci, gonococcus and *Corynebacterium diphtheriae*.

The conjunctivitis is usually bilateral with mucopurulent discharge, conjunctival hyperaemia and, occasionally, membranes or pseudomembranes.

Treatment is with broad-spectrum topical antibiotics. If membranes or pseudomembranes are present these should be physically removed and an anti-inflammatory topical drop added to the antibiotic.

Swabs should be taken if the discharge is copious or persistent despite topical antibiotics.

VIRAL CONJUNCTIVITIS

Viral conjunctivitis is a common, contagious, usually bilateral condition with the commonest causes being adenovirus, HSV, enterovirus, and EBV. Adenoviral conjunctivitis presents with watery discharge, conjunctival hyperaemia, follicular conjunctivitis, preauricular lymphadenopathy and pseudomembranes in severe cases.

Treatment is with topical antibiotics to prevent secondary bacterial infections.

CHRONIC CONJUNCTIVITIS

This is uncommon. It is usually unilateral but may be bilateral chronic red eye. It may be caused by *Molluscum contagiosum* (molluscum eyelid lesions associated with ipsilateral follicular conjunctivitis), toxic conjunctivitis (aminoglycoside antibiotics, antivirals, glaucoma medication, eye makeup and preservatives), Parinaud's oculoglandular syndrome (follicular conjunctivitis and severe preauricular lymphadenopathy – most commonly caused by cat-scratch fever, tularaemia, sporotrichosis, tuberculosis, and coccidiodomycosis) and blepahrokeratoconjunctivitis.

Molluscum contagiosum causes a self-limiting condition but if the conjunctivitis is too uncomfortable, the child should have an examination under anaesthetic and the eyelid lesion curettaged. For toxic conjunctivitis the offending topical medication should be discontinued if possible. Blepharokeratoconjunctivitis needs to be treated as described above (see Blepharitis).

CHLAMYDIA CONJUNCTIVITIS

This usually unilateral condition causes a follicular conjunctivitis with preauricular lymphadenopathy.

This condition may be sexually transmitted. Therefore, in teenagers a history of sexual activity needs to be sought while in younger children the possibility of sexual abuse must be considered.

Treatment includes taking appropriate swabs and treating with topical and systemic erythromycin, exclusion of pneumonitis and referral to genitourinary medicine to exclude other sexually transmitted diseases. Single dose azithromycin may also be used with topical erythromycin ointment.

NON INFECTION-RELATED CONJUNCTIVITIS

ALLERGIC CONJUNCTIVITIS

Allergic conjunctivitis is a very common, bilateral seasonal or perennial condition.

There is often chemosis (swelling of the conjunctiva), watery discharge and conjunctival hyperaemia with a history of hayfever.

Topical antiallergic medication includes mast cell stabilisers or antihistamines or dual action eyedrops. Systemic antihistamines may also be needed.

ATOPIC KERATOCONJUNCTIVITIS

A not uncommon condition associated with lid eczema, inflammation of the lid margins (blepharitis) and mucoid discharge. Cataracts, keratoconus and retinal detachments may occur. Secondary glaucoma may occur if periocular steroids are used to treat the skin.

Lubricating agents and, if necessary, antiallergy topical and systemic medication may be needed.

Prognosis depends on complications that may occur.

CONJUNCTIVAL PIGMENTATION

BENIGN MELANOSIS

Brown-black patches are seen near the limbus and sometimes in the interpalpebral bulbar conjunctiva. The patches move very easily over the globe and are most commonly seen in pigmented races.

No treatment needed as there is no risk of malignant change.

FLAT DEEP PIGMENTATION

A not uncommon condition in pigmented races. It is due to unilateral subepithelial melanocytosis and as such the pigmentation cannot be moved over the globe. There is a slate-grey appearance, which may be isolated to the eye (melanosis oculi), isolated to the periocular skin (dermal melanocytosis) or involve both eye and skin (oculodermal melanocytosis or naevus of Ota). Naevus of Ota is associated with increased risk of glaucoma and increased risk of uveal melanoma. Oculo- (dermal) melanocytosis is nine times more common in young patients with uveal melanoma than in the general population with uveal melanoma.

Regular observation is needed.

Ophthalmology

ELEVATED CONJUNCTIVAL LESIONS

PIGMENTED NODULES

Naevus

Naevus is a common solitary, well-defined, slightly elevated lesion, which moves freely over globe. Most (75%) are pigmented. Naevi usually are present at the limbus, plica, caruncle and lid margin.

There is rare malignant transformation to melanoma. Rapid growth may be seen around puberty; excisional biopsy may be needed to confirm the diagnosis.

NON-PIGMENTED SMALL NODULES

Phlycten

Phlycten is an uncommon, straw-yellow, slightly elevated lesion usually at or near the limbus, surrounded by hyperaemia (**Fig. 7.8**).

The commonest cause is *Staphylococcus aureus* hypersensitivity seen in blepharitis. It may also be caused by tuberculosis, HSV and *Candida* infection.

If associated with blepharitis then topical antibiotic and topical steroid therapy is used.

NON-PIGMENTED LARGE NODULES

Epibulbar dermoid

An uncommon solid, elevated, congenital lesion, usually located at the limbus. It may have hairs on the surface (**Fig. 7.21**).

Ocular associations include lid coloboma, ocular coloboma, microphthalmos and aniridia, Goldenhar, Treacher–Collins and Franchescetti syndromes.

If the lesion is very large or causing ocular surface wetting problems, it must be removed.

PLAQUE-LIKE CONJUNCTIVAL LESIONS

Pterygium

A wing-shaped, very common fleshy lesion usually at the nasal limbus seen in equatorial regions. It occurs mainly in adults but may be seen in teenagers.

Treatment is rarely needed in teenagers but, in adults, if it encroaches on the corneal central axis it should be removed.

Bitot spot

These are rare foamy plaques temporal to the limbus, seen in avitaminosis A. Vitamin A replacement is needed.

DIFFUSELY ELEVATED CONJUNCTIVAL LESIONS

LYMPHOMA

A very rare diffuse subconjunctival fleshy lesion, which may be bilateral. Smaller patches have been termed 'salmon patches'. It is most commonly associated with non-Hodgkin's or Burkitt's lymphoma.

Excision biopsy followed by systemic therapy from the oncology team is needed.

PLEXIFORM NEUROFIBROMA

An uncommon diffuse, very smooth, elevated lesion extending from the lid to the superior bulbar conjunctiva. It is almost always associated with NF1.

Usually no treatment is needed but occasionally debulking has been considered.

CONJUNCTIVAL TELANGIECTASIA

This is very uncommon. Causes include metabolic (Fabry disease, fucosidosis, galactosialidosis, GM1 gangliosidosis, multiple endocrine neoplasia IIa); haematological (dysproteinaemias, sickle cell anaemia); Louis–Bar (ataxia telangiectasia) syndrome (**Fig. 7.24**); Sturge–Weber syndrome; Rendu–Osler–Weber disease; capillary haemangioma, lymphangioma – conjunctival lesions are more saccular than true telangiectasia. (See also Chapter 8 Neurology, page 213 and Chapter 16 Immunology, page 494.)

Dilated and tortuous bulbar conjunctival vessels are **not** normal. Treatment depends on the aetiology.

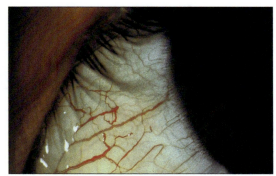

FIGURE 7.24 Telangiectasia of the bulbar conjunctiva in a child with ataxia telangiectasia.

SCLERA

PIGMENTATION OF THE SCLERA

This is uncommon and can be due to metabolic and non-metabolic causes. Metabolic causes include alkaptonuria, haemochromatosis and jaundice, while non-metabolic causes include osteogenesis imperfecta I, Marshall–Smith, Russell–Silver, Roberts, and Ehlers–Danlos VI syndromes, all of which may be associated with blue sclera. It may occasionally also be seen in Marfan, Hallermann–Streiff, Bloch–Sulzberger, Turner and Kabuki syndromes and in high myopia of any cause.

SCLERAL INFLAMMATION

EPISCLERITIS

An uncommon inflammation of the episclera differentiated from scleritis because, unlike scleritis, it is not tender to the touch.

Simple episcleritis often follows a viral illness and is self-limiting. Nodular and diffuse disease may be associated with systemic lupus erythematosus (SLE), juvenile idiopathic arthritis, spondyloarthropathy, inflammatory bowel disease, rheumatic fever, relapsing polychondritis, polyarteritis nodosa and inflammatory bowel disease.

Topical mild steroid is used to treat episcleritis and while this can be recurrent, prognosis is usually good.

SCLERITIS

Scleritis is an uncommon inflammation of the sclera that is tender to touch. It may be diffuse, nodular or necrotising.

Causes include idiopathic, infections, surgically induced (necrotising or diffuse), rheumatic diseases, connective tissue disorders, enteropathies, vasculitides, granulomatous diseases and certain skin disorders.

Treatment includes treating underlying condition and using anti-inflammatory drugs systemically (ono-steroidal or steroidal) to treat the eye initially. Prognosis can be guarded if necrotising, but this is extremely rare in children.

DEVELOPMENTAL ANOMALIES OF THE GLOBE

NANOPHTHALMOS

Nanophthalmos is an uncommon developmental anomaly. The eye is small in its overall dimensions but is not affected by other gross developmental defects nor accompanied by other systemic congenital anomalies. There is high hypermetropia, with short axial length (16–18.5 mm) and a crowded anterior chamber predisposing to glaucoma.

Glaucoma occurs later in life, as do choroidal effusions because of the thickened inelastic sclera. Systemic associations include Kenny Caffey syndrome.

Treatment includes correction of refractive error and review for glaucoma and choroidal effusions.

SIMPLE MICROPHTHALMOS

An uncommon developmental anomaly that may be seen in fetal alcohol syndrome, diabetic embryopathy, myotonic dystrophy, achondroplasia, pseudotrisomy 18, neurodevelopmental delay, isolated growth hormone deficiency, mucopolysaccharidosis VI and mucolipidosis III.

The eye is small but otherwise essentially normal. It may be associated with systemic developmental anomalies in about 50% of cases. Since these eyes have a short axial length they are usually moderately hypermetropic. The corneal diameter can be normal, but cases associated with a systemic disorder can have microcornea. Most patients have a normal best-corrected vision for their age. The late ocular complications seen in nanophthalmos do not occur in simple microphthalmos.

COMPLEX MICROPHTHALMOS

A rare developmental anomaly that may be associated with various syndromes: CHARGE syndrome (coloboma; heart defects; atresia choanae; retarded growth and development or central nervous system anomalies, or both; genital anomalies or hypogonadism, or both; and ear anomalies or deafness, or both); micro syndrome (microphakia, microphthalmos, characteristic lens opacity, atonic pupils, cortical visual impairment, microcephaly, and developmental delay); MIDAS (microphthalmia, dermal aplasia, and sclerocornea – also known as MLS) syndrome; oculodentodigital dysplasia. Multiple chromosomal abnormalities may be present.

Cases tend to be bilateral, and the vision ranges from normal to no light perception, depending on the ocular malformation. Microphthalmos with coloboma is caused by incomplete closure of the embryonic fissure by the seventh week (**Fig. 7.25**). Microphthalmos with cyst is a colobomatous malformation that results from a defective closure of the embryonic fissure. There is typically a protruding mass in the inferior orbit or lid associated with a severely malformed microphthalmic eye (**Fig. 7.26**).

Treatment depends on maximising any vision including cataract surgery if needed. In the presence of a cyst the cyst often needs removing.

ANOPHTHALMIA

A very rare developmental anomaly where the eye appears to be absent. Primary anophthalmos due to failure of the outgrowth of the optic vesicle, unassociated with an abnormality of the neural tube, is the most common type. This must occur during the first 2 weeks of development and is usually bilateral (but asymmetric), sporadic, and, in most cases, the child is otherwise well-formed.

Patients with clinical anophthalmos have been shown to have a high incidence of developmental anomalies involving both eyes (88%), the brain (71%) and the body (58%) (**Fig. 7.27**).

The absence of a normal eye affects normal orbital growth and for this reason orbital expanders may be needed and referral to an oculoplastic surgeon is needed.

Anophthalmia/microphthalmia may be seen in anophthalmia-oesophageal-genital syndrome (SOX2), pituitary abnormalities (OTX2), Matthew–Wood syndrome or PDAC syndrome (STRA6), oculofaciocardiodental syndrome (BCOR), Lenz microphthalmia syndrome (BCOR), MIDAS or MLS syndrome (HCCS), Waardengurg anophthalmia syndrome (SMOC1) and pituitary defects with brain and digital anomalies (BMP4).

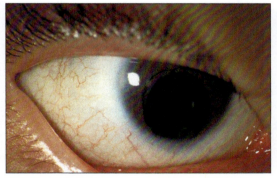

FIGURE 7.25 Microphthalmos with iris coloboma.

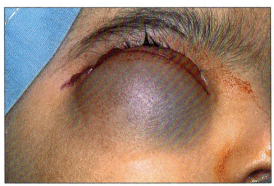

FIGURE 7.26 Microphthalmos with cyst. The cyst is bluish in colour and occupies the major part of the orbit.

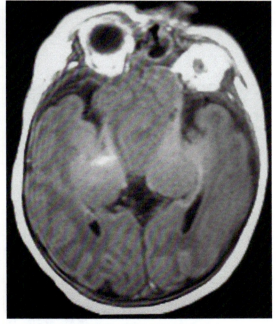

FIGURE 7.27 MRI of a child with clinical anophthalmos. Note the abnormal intracranial findings.

IRIS

CONGENITAL IRIS DEFECTS

IRIS COLOBOMA

An uncommon developmental anomaly due to non-closure of the embryonic fissure in the fifth week of gestation. Typical iris colobomas occur in the infero-nasal quadrant and may involve the ciliary body, choroid, retina and optic nerve.

Iris colobomas may be isolated or associated with ocular features such as retinochoroidal/optic nerve coloboma, microcornea, microphthalmos (**Fig. 7.25**) or both, or microphthalmos with cyst (**Fig. 7.26**). Nystagmus may be seen, as may cataracts. Although iris colobomas can be associated with almost any chromosomal abnormality they are frequently seen in branchio-oculo-facial, cat-eye, CHARGE, 13q deletion, Goltz, triploidy, Patau (trisomy 13), Wolf–Hirschhorn (4p-) and Walker–Warburg syndromes.

Patients should be reviewed for correction of refractive error and cataract progression if lens opacity is present.

ANIRIDIA

The prevalence of aniridia is 1:72000 in two scandinavian countries, with most causes due to mutations in PAX6.

Aniridia (autosomal dominant) is a panocular, bilateral disorder. The most obvious presenting sign is absence of much or most of the iris tissue. In addition to iris involvement, foveal and optic nerve hypoplasia may be present, resulting in a congenital sensory nystagmus and leading to reduced visual acuity to 6/30 or worse. Anterior polar cataracts, glaucoma, and corneal opacification often develop later in childhood and may lead to progressive deterioration of visual acuity. Glaucoma occurs in up to half of all cases.

Associations include Wilm's tumour, genitourinary abnormalities and retarded growth or development (AGR triad) or both (WAGR), or associated with ataxia and neurodevelopmental delay (Gillespie syndrome).

All children with sporadic aniridia should have repeated abdominal ultrasonographic and clinical examinations; molecular genetic evaluation reveals intragenuc mutation only. One protocol advised that the child be seen every 3 months until the age of 5 years, every 6 months until the age of 10, and once a year until the age of 16. If chromosomal deletion is found, 3-monthly scans should be performed and the child transferred to the care of a nephrologist. 50% of patients with aniridia may develop glaucoma and nearly all will develop a keratopathy in adulthood due to limbal stem cell deficiency.

IRIS TRANSILLUMINATION

The congenital causes of iris transillumination include albinism (both ocular and oculocutaneous) when it occurs because of absence of pigmentation in the posterior pigment epithelial layer (**Fig. 7.28**). It may also be seen in the mid peripheral iris in female carriers of X-linked ocular albinism. Other causes include iris hypoplasia; X-linked megalocornea; Marfan syndrome; ectopia lentis et pupillae; microcoria. Small transillumination defects just visible near the iris root in blue-eyed children may be idiopathic with no clinical significance. Rarely, it occurs in association with congenital ocular fibrosis syndrome.

ACQUIRED IRIS DEFECTS

IRIS TRANSILLUMINATION

Aquired causes include: iatrogenic from surgical or laser iridectomy or iridotomy, respectively; pigment dispersion syndrome may be seen in teenagers; it is thought to occur as a result of posterior bowing of the iris resulting in pigment dispersion from lens/iris pigment epithelium friction; herpes zoster ophthalmicus often results in sector iris atrophy; trauma – blunt injury may result in detachment of the iris root (iridodialysis) that results in pseudopolycoria.

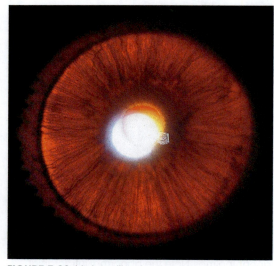

FIGURE 7.28 Iris transillumination seen in a child with ocular albinism.

CHANGES IN IRIS COLOUR

BENIGN PRIMARY IRIS TUMOURS

Brushfield spots
These occur in 38–90% of patients with Down syndrome. Very similar iris findings may occur in normal individuals (Wolfflin nodules).

SECONDARY TUMOURS

Juvenile xanthogranuloma
Juvenile xanthogranuloma (JXG) is a rare condition and iris involvement occurs almost exclusively in infants. Usually unilateral yellow nodules or diffuse infiltration may be seen. It may present with spontaneous hyphaema (blood in the anterior chamber) and/or unilateral glaucoma may occur.

All children with JXG should have ocular screening because even asymptomatic ocular lesions may be associated with glaucoma. Most ocular lesions will regress with topical steroids. Some cases may need systemic steroids and others a small dose of radiotherapy treatment. Prognosis is usually good.

Langerhans cell histiocytosis
See also Chapter 6 Dermatology, page 150, Chapter 12 Oncology, page 353.

Although similar to JXG, which is systemically benign, Langerhans cell histiocytoses (eosinophilic granuloma, Letterer–Siwe and Hand–Schuller–Christian disease) are systemic malignancies and need appropriate chemotherapy. They are rare and usually limited to orbital involvement but iris nodules or choroidal involvement may rarely occur in Letterer–Siwe disease.

Patients should have routine ophthalmic examination and treatment of underlying disease (see treatment details for JXG).

LEUKAEMIA/LYMPHOMA

See also Chapter 11 Haematology.

Leukaemia iris infiltrates, although rare, have been reported with most types of childhood leukaemia and lymphoma. Acute lymphoblastic leukaemia (ALL) is both the most common form of childhood leukaemia and the most likely to be associated with iris infiltration.

Iris infiltration (nodules, spontaneous hyphema, heterochromia, pseudohypopyon with iritis, and/or acute glaucoma) is an ominous finding since the median time of survival after discovery of leukemic iris involvement is 3 months.

Since these are immunocompromised patients anterior chamber aspiration or iris biopsy may be needed to exclude an infectious etiology. Chemotherapy may not be effective and low-dose external radiation has been used successfully despite potential for cataract development.

HETEROCHROMIA IRIDES

The differential diagnosis of paediatric heterochromia irides (**Fig. 7.29**) is extensive but may be classified on the basis of whether the condition is congenital or acquired and whether the affected eye is hypopigmented or hyperpigmented.

HYPOCHROMIC HETEROCHROMIA

- Congenital causes: Horner syndrome; Waardenburg syndrome; piebaldism trait.
- Acquired causes: Fuch's heterochromic cyclitis – rare type of unilateral iritis; nonpigmented iris tumours.

HYPERCHROMIC HETEROCHROMIA

- Congenital causes: iris mammillations – unilateral villiform protuberances that may cover the iris usually in association with oculodermal melanosis or neurofibromatosis (NF); congenital iris ectropion (see page 174); unilateral iris coloboma (affected iris is darker); port wine stain.
- Acquired causes: cataract surgery in children – operated eye is darker in eyes operated early in life; topical medication (e.g. latanoprost, which is a prostaglandin analogue and causes darkening of the iris of the eye being treated); pigmented iris tumours; rubeosis iridis, iris neovascularisation – causes include retinopathy of prematurity, retinoblastoma, Coats' disease, and iris tumours; siderosis – due to intraocular metallic foreign body.

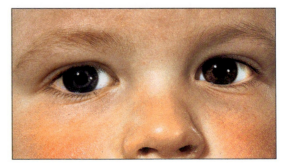

FIGURE 7.29 Heterochromia irides. This child had Waardenburg syndrome.

LEUKOCORIA

A white pupil reflex. It may be caused by:

- Congenital cataract (may be unilateral or bilateral) (**Fig. 7.30**).
- Persistent hyperplastic primary vitreous (a rare congenital, usually unilateral, condition).
- Inflammatory cyclitic membrane.
- Retinal dysplasia (very rare) may be associated with Norrie disease, Bloch–Sulzberger syndrome (incontinentia pigmenti), Warburg syndrome, Patau syndrome (trisomy 13) or Edward syndrome (trisomy 18).
- Tumours and granulomas – retinoblastoma, retinal astrocytoma and toxocaral granuloma.
- Retinal detachment – Retinopathy of prematurity, retinoblastoma, Coats' disease, toxocaral granuloma, and Stickler syndrome.
- Miscellaneous – extensive retinal nerve fibre myelination and large chorioretinal coloboma.

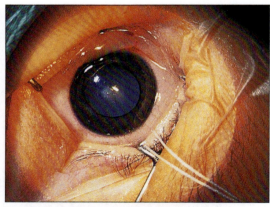

FIGURE 7.30 Leukocoria due to a congenital cataract, at operation.

DYSCORIA

A rare abnormality of the shape of the pupil. Congenital causes include persistent pupillary membranes, iris coloboma, iris hypoplasia and ectopia lentis et pupillae (see below). Acquired causes include posterior synechiae seen in iritis or trauma.

MIOSIS

Uncommonly a pupil or pupils may be less than 2 mm, and may react poorly to dilating drops. This may be due to congenital miosis (microcoria) when there is an absence of the dilator pupillae muscle or fibrous contraction secondary to persistent pupillary membrane. It can be seen in congenital rubella syndrome, Marfan syndrome, in 20% of Lowe (oculocerebrorenal) syndrome and in ectopia lentis et pupillae.

If visual development is thought to be hindered, surgical enlargement of the pupil can be performed. Appropriate management of visual development usually results in good vision.

MYDRIASIS

Rarely a large pupil, usually greater than 4 mm may be seen, and may be true mydriasis or pseudomydriasis.

TRUE MYDRIASIS

This may be congenital but blunt trauma causing iris sphincter rupture, ciliary ganglionitis (unilateral most commonly after chicken pox – also known as Adie's pupil) or acquired neurological disease must be excluded, especially third nerve palsy.

If there is ciliary ganglionitis, accommodation can be affected and the child will need a reading prescription.

PSEUDOMYDRIASIS

Many cases of congenital mydriasis are actually part of the aniridia spectrum. Iris ectropion is eversion of the posterior pigment epithelium onto the anterior surface of the iris.

Congenital iris ectropion is often mistaken as an enlarged pupil. Associated conditions include NF1, Prader–Willi syndrome and facial hemihypertrophy.

Iris ectropion can occur as an acquired tractional abnormality, often in association with rubeosis iridus or as a congenital non-progressive abnormality. Congenital iris ectropion may be associated with congenital and/or developmental glaucoma.

Patients should be reviewed to exclude glaucoma or association. If glaucoma is excluded or treated then the prognosis is good.

CORECTOPIA

An uncommon displacement of the pupil. Normally, the pupil is displaced inferonasally about 0.5 mm from the centre of the iris.

Causes include sector iris hypoplasia, colobomas, ectopia lentis et pupillae and Axenfeld–Rieger anomaly. Intermittent corectopia, with pupils shifting from central to eccentric positions, have been reported during coma and may represent a sign of rostral midbrain dysfunction.

Very rarely if the pupil is very eccentrically displaced then pupilloplasty may be needed to improve the visual axis.

ANISOCORIA

In this not uncommon condition there is a difference in size between the two pupils. The three main causes in childhood that need to be considered are physiological, Horner syndrome and Adie pupil (ciliary ganglionitis).

The child should be examined in bright light and then in the dark. If the anisocoria is physiological then the difference will remain constant and will be no more than 2 mm. If the anisocoria is accentuated in bright surroundings this suggests that the larger pupil is at fault and cannot constrict. The commonest cause for this is ciliary ganglionitis (Adie's pupil).

Examination by slit lamp is performed to detect vermiform iris movements. If the anisocoria is accentuated in the dark, this suggests that the smaller pupil is at fault. The commonest cause for this is Horner syndrome.

HORNER SYNDROME

Horner syndrome comprises miosis, with ipsilateral ptosis and sometimes anhidrosis (**Fig. 7.31**). Congenital Horner syndrome is associated with hypopigmentation of the affected side. Acquired Horner syndrome may be due to: central (first order neurone) lesions; preganglionic (second order) lesions; postganglionic (third order) lesions; metastatic neuroblastoma perhaps causing a congenital Horner syndrome.

Investigation is with pharmacological testing, using 4% cocaine – one drop in each eye. The Horner pupil will NOT dilate. This confirms the presence of Horner syndrome. 24 hours later hydroxyamphetamine 1% can be used in each eye. If the lesion is preganglionic then BOTH pupils will dilate, but in a postganglionic lesion the Horner pupil will not. Alternatively, use 1:1,000 adrenaline into both eyes. In a preganglionic lesion NEITHER pupil will dilate but in a postganglionic one the Horner pupil will dilate.

Even if there is heterochromia irides, metastatic neuroblastoma should be excluded. In an otherwise healthy child, at least a chest x-ray and spot urine vanylymandelic acid.

ADIE SYNDROME

This presents with mydriasis with vermiform iris movements on slit-lamp examination.

The commonest association is chicken pox infection but other viral infections may also cause ciliary ganglionitis.

Accommodation is usually affected and the child may need reading spectacles.

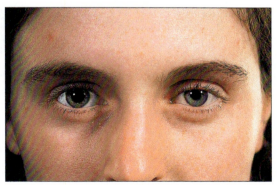

FIGURE 7.31 Left Horner syndrome with the left pupil slightly smaller and the left lid slightly ptotic (droopy).

LENS ANOMALIES

APHAKIA

Aphakia is absence of the lens, most commonly iatrogenic after congenital cataract extraction. Rare causes are spontaneous resorption of a cataract (may be seen in Lowe syndrome and Hallerman–Streiff syndrome), congenital primary aphakia that is extremely rare (usually accompanied by other anterior segment anomalies) and spontaneous complete dislocation of the lens (either traumatic or related to already subluxed lens – see later).

Refractive correction of aphakia is needed and surveillance to exclude glaucoma, which can develop anytime in the patient's life.

ABNORMAL SHAPE

COLOBOMA

Coloboma is rare, but may be associated with other colobomatous ocular defects.

Aetiology is often unclear but refractive treatment is necessary as astigmatism is common.

LENTIGLOBUS

A rare unilateral condition, which usually causes myopia. This may be associated with posterior polar cataract.

ANTERIOR LENTICONUS

A rare bilateral condition with a conoid projection of the anterior surface of the lens centrally; it may be associated with Alport syndrome.

If visual development is hindered, lens extraction is warranted, especially so if a cataract forms.

POSTERIOR LENTICONUS

An uncommon posterior conoid projection of the lens. It is usually isolated but may be seen in Lowe syndrome.

Lens extraction with or without implantation of an intraocular lens is often indicated.

DISLOCATED LENS

This is uncommon but may be seen with ocular associations such as: megalocornea (primary enlarged cornea); severe buphthalmos; very high myopia and aniridia; familial ectopia lentis; ectopia lentis et pupillae; isolated familial microspherophakia. Ectopia lentis et pupillae is an autosomal recessive condition in which there is displacement of the pupil and lens in opposite directions.

Dislocated lens may be seen in systemic associations such as Marfan (**Fig. 7.32**) (fibrillin gene mutation spectrum), Weil–Marchesani, Ehlers–Danlos, Stickler, Kniest syndromes, mandibulofacial dysostosis and osteogenesis imperfecta. Metabolic disorders include homocystinuria, hyperlysinemia and molybdenum cofactor deficiency (including sulfite oxidase deficiency).

Treatment includes exclusion of systemic association. Careful observation with refractive correction to ensure adequate visual development is needed. The child may need lensectomy to improve visual function.

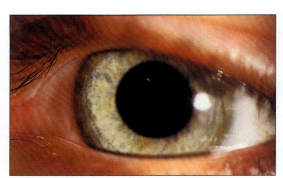

FIGURE 7.32 Dislocated lens in a child with Marfan syndrome.

LENS OPACITY

Lens opacities may be classified in terms of the age at which it occurs or in terms of characteristic lens opacities for certain systemic associations.

CONGENITAL OR INFANTILE CATARACT

(See Figs 7.30, 7.33)

In the UK two-thirds of congenital cataracts are bilateral and one-third unilateral. 31% are associated with systemic disease (6% unilateral and 25% bilateral). 61% are associated with ocular disease (47% unilateral and 14% bilateral). No underlying cause or risk factor can be found in 92% of unilateral and 38% of bilateral cases. Hereditary disease is associated with 56% of bilateral and 6% of unilateral cases.

Therefore, in all bilateral cases unless there is a hereditary risk or associated ocular disease the following investigations should be considered depending on the child's systemic condition:

- Urine: reducing substances (galatosaemia), dipstick for proteinuria (Alport), amino acids (Lowe).
- Serology: TORCH, RBC galactokinase activity, RBC galactose-1-phosphate uridyltransferase activity, serum ferritin, karyotype, calcium, glucose, VDRL phosphorus, alkaline phosphatase.

Possible associations include:

- Hereditary.
- Ocular: persistent hyperplastic primary vitreous, aniridia, iris coloboma, microphthalmos.
- Systemic:
  - Infection: intrauterine infection.
  - Metabolic disease: galactosaemia, neonatal hypoglycaemia, hypocalcaemia.
  - Renal disease: Lowe syndrome, congenital haemolytic syndrome.
  - Chromosomal disorders: trisomy 13 (Patau syndrome) and 18 (Edward syndrome).

  - Neurological disease: Marinesco–Sjögren syndrome (ataxia), Smith–Lemli–Opitz, Zellweger and Sjogren–Larsson syndromes.
  - Skeletal disorders: Conradi syndrome.
  - Skin disorders: ectodermal dysplasia, Rothmund–Thomson, incontinentia pigmenti and Cockayne syndromes.
  - Miscellaneous: Norrie, Rubinstein–Taybi, Turner and Hallermann–Streiff syndromes.

Lensectomy with sparing of the capsule for possible secondary implantation is one treatment option, but lens removal with intraocular implantation has become more common. Amblyopia therapy with correction of the refractive state is essential.

Prognosis is better for bilateral cases than unilateral cases.

JUVENILE CATARACT

These may be:

- Hereditary.
- Ocular: coloboma, ectopia lentis, aniridia, retinitis pigmentosa, and posterior lenticonus.
- Systemic:
  - Renal disease: Alport syndrome.
  - Skeletal disease: Marfan syndrome.
  - Skin disease: atopic dermatitis, Marshall syndrome, lamellar icthyosis.
  - Chromosomal disorders: trisomy 21.
  - Metabolic disease: galactokinase deficiency, Fabry disease, Refsum disease, mannosidosis, diabetes mellitus, hypocalcaemia.
  - Neurological disorders: myotonic dystrophy, Wilson disease.
  - Miscellaneous: chronic uveitis, drug induced (steroids), NF2, Stickler syndrome.

Lens aspiration with implantation is the usual method of treatment. Prognosis is good as long as the visual pathway is otherwise unaffected.

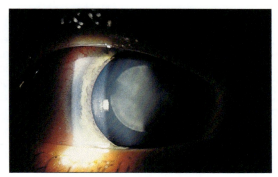

FIGURE 7.33 Congenital lamellar cataract.

BOX 1   RETINOPATHY OF PREMATURITY

The international classification of retinopathy of prematurity (ROP) is used to describe location, extent and stage of the disease. The location of ROP refers to the location relative to the optic nerve. This has been standardised by dividing the retina into three zones. Zone I is an area centred on the optic disc and extending from the disc to twice the distance between the disc and the macula. Zone II is a ring concentric to Zone I that extends to the nasal ora serrata (the edge of the retina on the side of the eye toward the nose). Zone III is the remaining crescent of retina on the temporal (toward the temple) side. The extent of ROP is described by how many clock-hours of the retina are involved. For example, if there is retinopathy extending from 1:00 around to 5:00, the extent of ROP is 4 clock-hours. ROP is a progressive disease. It begins with some mild changes in the vessels, and may progress to more severe changes. The stage of ROP describes how far in this progression the vessels have reached.

- Stage 1 is characterised by a demarcation line between the normal retina nearer the optic nerve and the non-vascularised retina more peripherally.
- Stage 2 ROP has a ridge of scar tissue and new vessels in place of the demarcation line.
- Stage 3 ROP shows an increased size of the vascular ridge, with growth of fibrovascular tissue on the ridge and extending out into the vitreous.
- Stage 4 refers to a partial retinal detachment. The scar tissue associated with the fibrovascular ridge contracts, pulling the retina away from the wall of the eye. Stage 4 is further categorised depending upon the location of the retinal detachment. In Stage 4A, the detachment does not include the macula, and the vision may be good. In Stage 4B, the macula is detached, and the visual potential is markedly decreased.
- Stage 5 ROP implies a complete retinal detachment, usually with the retina pulled into a funnel-shaped configuration by the fibrovascular scar tissue. Eyes with stage 5 ROP usually have no useful vision, even if surgery is performed to repair the detachment.

Plus disease implies dilation and tortuosity of the blood vessels near the optic nerve. It also includes the growth and dilation of abnormal blood vessels on the surface of the iris, rigidity of the pupil and vitreous haze. The presence of plus disease suggests a more fulminant or rapidly progressive course. Rush disease is a term used to describe ROP in zone I with plus disease.

Low birthweight, prolonged supplemental oxygen and respiratory distress syndrome have clearly been shown to be risk factors.

Treatment

If ROP does develop, it usually occurs between 34 and 40 weeks after conception, regardless of gestational age at birth. The laser treatment is applied to the retina anterior to the vascular shunt that does not yet have a blood supply. The purpose of the treatment is to eliminate the abnormal vessels before they lay down enough scar tissue to produce a retinal detachment. Other treatment options include cryopexy, scleral buckle and vitrectomy. Treatment is initiated at threshold disease, which is stage III for 5 contiguous clock hours or 8 non-contiguous clock hours.

HAEMORRHAGES

Haemorrhages may be preretinal, retinal and subretinal.

Preretinal haemorrhages are between the posterior vitreous face and the retina. They may be seen in sickle cell retinopathy, trauma, subarachnoid haemorrhage (Terson syndrome), non-accidental injury (never seen in isolation; widespread retinal and subretinal haemorrhages also seen with or without retinal schisis).

Retinal haemorrhages may be flame shaped, dot and blot or Roth spots (superficial retinal haemorrhage with white centre).

Flame-shaped haemorrhages are seen in retinal vein occlusions, acute papilloedema, optic disc drusen, acute hypertensive retinopathy and retinal perivasculitis (especially early CMV retinitis). Roth spots are seen in severe anaemias, leukaemia, bacterial endocarditis and may also be seen in trauma. Dot and blot haemorrhages may be seen in diabetes mellitus-related retinopathy. The haemorrhage is full thickness in the retina. They may be seen in shaken baby syndrome in association with superficial and subretinal haemorrhages (**Fig. 7.34**) (see Chapter 2 Child Protection, page 35).

Treatment is targeted to the cause. Prognosis depends on severity and depth of haemorrhage.

Subretinal haemorrhages are red, raised areas over which the retinal vessels are clearly visible. They are seen in sickle cell anaemia, Coats' disease (retinal telangiectasia), trauma, shaken baby syndrome and, very rarely, choroidal neovascularisation.

Treatment is targeted to the cause.

HARD EXUDATES

Rare, yellow waxy deposits may occur, which may be retinal (focal, diffuse or macular star) or subretinal. Focal or diffuse hard exudates may be seen in diabetic retinopathy (unusual to see in children), old branch retinal vein occlusion(very rare in children), radiation retinopathy or retinal telangiectasia.

A macular star (stellate pattern of exudates centred on the macula) may be seen in malignant hypertension, papilloedema, neuroretinitis and very rarely retinal angioma (Von Hippel–Lindau syndrome or idiopathic).

Subretinal exudates may be seen in Coats' disease (**Fig. 7.35**) or rarely, with *Toxocara canis* retinochoroiditis.

Treatment for Coat disease has been advocated with removal of subretinal exudates and treatment of vascular anomalies seen in this condition.

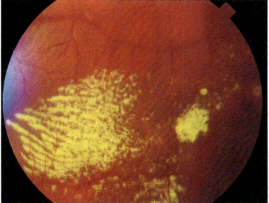

FIGURE 7.35 Hard exudates due to Coats' disease.

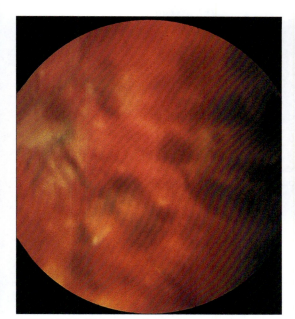

FIGURE 7.34 Widespread retinal haemorrhages in a proven case of shaken baby syndrome.

COTTON WOOL SPOTS

Rarely seen in children, these are small white lesions with fluffy edges that result from localised microvasculature occlusion resulting in ischaemia.

While they may be seen in retinal vein occlusion, acute hypertension, HIV microvasculopathy, ocular ischaemic syndromes, haematological disorders (leukaemia, dysproteinaemias), trauma to chest and long bones (Purtscher retinopathy), systemic vasculitides, especially SLE, should be excluded.

RETINAL NEOVASCULARISATION

Rarely seen in children, retinal ischaemia may result in new vessel formation that can lead to retinal and vitreous haemorrhages as well as tractional retinal detachment. The new vessels may occur within the posterior pole or in the periphery.

The commonest cause in children is peripheral neovascularisation, seen in retinopathy of prematurity, sickle cell disease, familial exudative vitreoretinopathy and incontinentia pigmenti. Posterior pole neovascularisation may be seen in retinal vein occlusion, retinal vasculitis, retinal artery occlusion or radiation retinopathy.

Laser treatment of the ischaemic retina is the principle of therapy. Prognosis depends on the aetiology.

RETINAL VASCULITIS

Extremely rare in children, this present as inflammation around retinal veins (periphlebitis) or retinal arterioles (periarteritis). Periphlebitismay be seen in sarcoidosis, Behçet disease, CMV retinitis, acute retinal necrosis, tuberculosis, frosted branch angitis or idiopathic. Periarteritis may be seen in SLE, dermatomyositis, polyarteritis nodosa or Wegener granulomatosis.

Fundus examination is essential to exclude retinal involvement. If there is involvement systemic immunosuppression is essential.

Prognosis is guarded.

FOVEAL HYPOPLASIA

A rare underdevelopment of the fovea. Nystagmus is usually present and maybe associated with optic nerve hypoplasia. The clue is retinal vessels that go through the fovea and do not arc around it as they should (**Fig. 7.36**).

There is no treatment but PAX6 analysis should be performed.

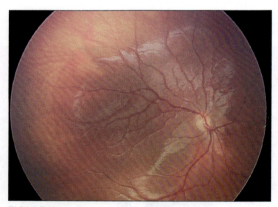

FIGURE 7.36 Foveal hypoplasia.

MACULOPATHY

Very rarely there may be an abnormality of the macula. This may be due to wrinkling, bull's eye appearance or crystalline deposits.

WRINKLED APPEARANCE OF THE MACULA

Striated appearance radiating out from the fovea, which causes a drop in vision. Idiopathic is the commonest cause but may also be seen in juvenile retinoschisis, Bardet–Biedl syndrome and chronic intraocular inflammation.

Vision is often poor and treatment options are limited.

BULL'S EYE MACULOPATHY

Uncommonly there is hyperpigmentation in the centre of the macula, surrounded by a hypopigmented zone, concentric to which is a final hyperpigmented zone.

Causes include long-term chloroquine use, some types of cone dystrophy (**Fig. 7.37**), cone–rod dystrophy, rod–cone dystrophy, juvenile neuronal ceroid lipofuscinosis, benign concentric annular macular dystrophy (usually late onset) and Stargardt disease (macular dystrophy starting in teens).

Prognosis is often guarded. If due to chloroquine the drug should be stopped.

COLOURED MACULAR LESIONS

These are all very rare.

Yellow lesions may be seen in Best's vitelliform macular dystrophy, a dominantly inherited condition that starts in childhood. In the early stages there may be no lesion at the macula but usually there is an egg yolk-like lesion at the macula (**Figs 7.38, 7.39**).

There is no treatment and prognosis is guarded with time.

Cherry-red spots are due to a change in the nerve fibre layer surrounding the fovea, such as ischaemia or deposition of abnormal metabolic by-products, resulting in an accentuation of the normal deep red colour of the fovea, producing the typical cherry-red spot macula.

Causes in children are metabolic disorders such as Tay–Sachs disease, Sandhoff disease, Niemann–Pick disease, generalised gangliosidosis and sialidosis I and II and central retinal artery occlusion.

Prognosis is poor.

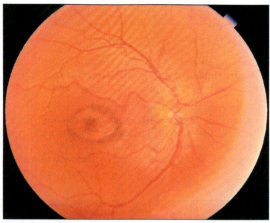

FIGURE 7.37 Bull's eye maculopathy seen in a case of cone retinal dystrophy.

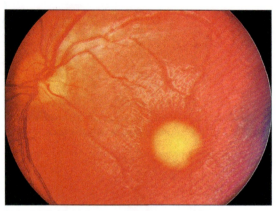

FIGURE 7.38 Yolk-like appearance of Best disease.

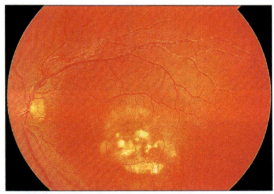

FIGURE 7.39 Scrambled egg appearance of Best disease.

PALE RETINAL LESIONS

INFLAMMATORY LESIONS

These are all rare in children but it is important to consider them in a differential diagnosis of a yellow/white lesion in the retina.

- Single focal lesions: these may be caused by toxoplasmosis (**Fig. 7.40**), toxocariasis (**Fig. 7.41**), candidiasis and cryptococcus. Occasionally pars planitis ('snowbanks' in the inferior peripheral retina) may also be seen. All of these inflammatory conditions are accompanied by vitritis, which makes the view of the fundus hazy.
- Multiple focal lesions: these may be caused by candidiasis, sarcoidosis, Lyme disease, choroidal pneumocystosis, presumed ocular histoplasmosis syndrome, Behçet disease, Vogt–Koyanagi–Harada (VKH) syndrome, sympathetic ophthalmitis and tuberculous choroiditis.
- Diffuse lesions: these may be seen in CMV retinitis (**Fig. 7.42**), acute retinal necrosis, herpes simplex retinitis and measles retinitis.

In all the above cases appropriate serological investigations and radiological examinations need to be undertaken. Joint ophthalmic and rheumatological evaluation improves management of these cases.

Prognosis depends on the diagnosis, with worst prognosis being for retinal necrosis or inflammation affecting the macula.

NON-INFLAMMATORY LESIONS

Most are uncommon with some very rare.

FOCAL PALE LESIONS

These may be due to coloboma of the retina and choroid, 'polar bear tracks', retinal astrocytoma and retinoblastoma.

Coloboma of retina and choroid (**Fig. 7.43**): usually a circular or oval-shaped lesion that may be associated with a coloboma of the optic disc or iris. It is due to incomplete closure of the fetal ocular fissure. Retinochoroidal colobomas may be associated with a serous retinal detachment.

Retinal astrocytoma: a hamartoma seen in 50% of patients with tuberous sclerosis. In children, a pale, almond-shaped lesion lies in the nerve fibre layer. In adults it becomes calcified, showing a mulberry-like lesion. It is usually unilateral.

Early retinoblastoma: small pale lesion, flat, elevated or nodular depending on how early it is detected (see below).

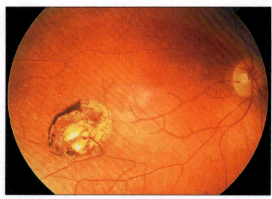

FIGURE 7.40 Extrafoveal toxoplasmosis scar.

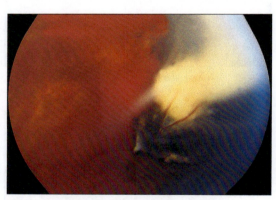

FIGURE 7.41 Peripheral *Toxocara* granuloma.

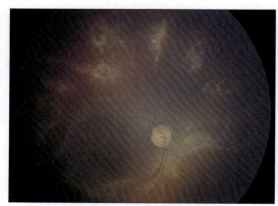

FIGURE 7.42 Cytomegalovirus retinitis.

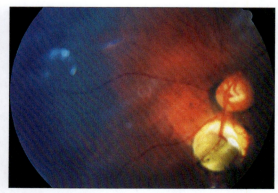

FIGURE 7.43 Retinochoroidal coloboma distinct from the optic disc.

DIFFUSE PALE LESIONS

- Non-hereditary: these include myelinated nerve fibres, high myopia, large coloboma of the optic disc and retina, retinal ischaemia (very are in children) and commotio retinae ('bruising' of the retina after blunt trauma).
- Hereditary: these include albinism, and choroidal dystrophies such as choroideraemia and diffuse choroidal atrophy.

MULTIPLE FOCAL/DISCRETE LESIONS

Hereditary: these includes typical retinitis pigmentosa, atypical retinitis pigmentosa, retinitis pigmentosa-like retinal dystrophy with systemic associations, female carriers of X-linked ocular albinism and female carriers of choroideraemia and angioid streaks. (See **Table 7.2**, for systemic associations of retinitis pigmentosa.)

TABLE 7.2 Systemic disorders associated with retinitis pigmentosa or retinal pigmentary retinopathy

1. Hearing difficulties:
   - Usher syndrome. USH 1: retinitis pigmentosa onset by age 10 years; cataract; profound congenital sensory deafness; labyrinthine defect. USH 2: retinitis pigmentosa onset in late teens; childhood sensory deafness. USH 3: postlingual, progressive hearing loss; variable vestibular dysfunction; onset of retinitis pigmentosa symptoms, usually by the second decade
   - Alstrom syndrome: retinal lesion causes nystagmus and early loss of central vision – in contrast to loss of peripheral vision first, as in other pigmentary retinopathies; dilated cardiomyopathy (infancy)/ congestive heart failure; atherosclerosis; hypertension; renal failure; deafness; obesity; diabetes mellitus
   - Infantile Refsum disease (early onset): mental retardation; minor facial dysmorphism; retinitis pigmentosa; sensorineural hearing deficit; hepatomegaly; osteoporosis; failure to thrive; hypocholesterolemia
   - Classical Refsum disease (late onset): cardinal clinical features of Refsum disease are retinitis pigmentosa, chronic polyneuropathy and cerebellar signs
   - Cockayne dwarfism: precociously senile appearance; pigmentary retinal degeneration; optic atrophy; deafness; marble epiphyses in some digits; photosensitivity; and mental retardation; subclinical myopathy
   - Mucopolysaccharidosis (MPS)
   - Kearns–Sayre ophthalmoplegia: pigmentary degeneration of the retina; deafness and cardiomyopathy are leading features

2. Skin disorders:
   - Refsum disease
   - Cockayne syndrome

3. Renal disorders:
   - Senior–Loken syndrome: renal dysplasia; retinitis pigmentosa; retinal aplasia; cerebellar ataxia; sensorineural hearing loss
   - Rhyns syndrome: retinitis pigmentosa; hypopituitarism; nephronophthisis; mild skeletal dysplasia
   - Bardet–Biedl syndrome: obesity; rod-cone dystrophy; onset by end of 2nd decade hypogonadism; renal anomalies; polydactyly; learning disabilities
   - Cystinosis
   - Alstrom syndrome

4. Skeletal disorders:
   - Bardet–Biedl syndrome
   - Cockayne syndrome
   - Jeune syndrome: chondrodysplasia that often leads to death in infancy because of a severely constricted thoracic cage and respiratory insufficiency; retinal degeneration
   - MPS 1H, 1S, 11,111
   - Infantile Refsum disease

5. Hepatic disorders:
   - Zellweger syndrome: hypotonia; seizures; psychomotor retardation; pigmentary retinopathy and cataracts

6. Neurological/neuromuscular:
   - Kearns–Sayre syndrome
   - Chronic progressive external ophthalmoplegia: retinitis pigmentosa and restricted eye movements
   - Neuronal ceroid lipofuscinosis: characterised by intralysosomal accumulations of lipopigments in either granular, curvilinear, or fingerprint patterns; progressive dementia, seizures and progressive visual failure
   - Hallervorden–Spatz syndrome: retinitis pigmentosa and pallidal degeneration
   - Joubert syndrome: hypoplasia of the cerebellar vermis; saccadic initiation failure; hyperpnea intermixed with central apnea in the neonatal period; retinal dystrophy
   - Infantile Refsum disease
   - Abetalipoproteinemia (Bassen–Kornzweig syndrome): coeliac disease; pigmentary degeneration of the retina; progressive ataxic neuropathy; acanthocytosis

Non-inflammatory lesions

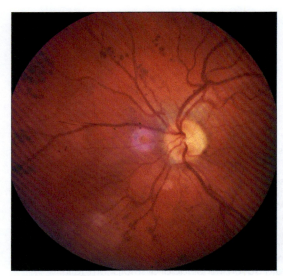

FIGURE 7.44 Bear tracks.

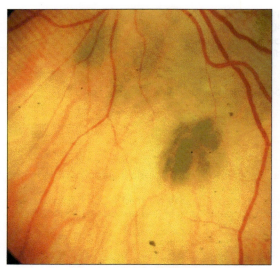

FIGURE 7.45 Single congenital retinal pigment epithelial hypertrophy with halo.

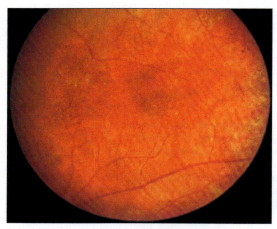

FIGURE 7.46 'Salt and pepper' retinopathy in a case of rubella retinopathy.

OTHER

This includes grouped congenital retinal pigment epithelial (RPE) hypertrophy ('bear tracks') – please note that multiple bear tracks (**Fig. 7.44**) are not associated with familial polyposis coli; it is the single fish-tail type lesion (**Fig. 7.45**), rubella retinopathy and congenital syphilis. Rubella retinopathy is a salt and pepper type pigmentary retinopathy where the vision is usually normal and is caused by congenital rubella (**Fig. 7.46**). Congenital syphilis retinopathy varies from mild ('salt and pepper retinopathy') to severe pigment clumping, similar to retinitis pigmentosa.

All cases need electrodiagnostic and visual field evaluation. Prognosis depends on diagnosis.

RETINAL DETACHMENT

Retinal detachment is very uncommon in children. It is an elevation of the neurosensory retina, which may be **rhegmatogenous** (due to a retinal hole or tear), **exudative** (due to inflammatory exudate), **tractional** (due to traction on the surface of the retina – usually after trauma in children or as a result of untreated retinopathy of prematurity) or **solid** (due to a tumour). A choroidal detachment is most commonly seen in hypotony following intraocular pressure-lowering operations such as trabeculectomy. Here the choroid detaches with the retina still attached.

In a child with high myopia and retinal detachment the possibility of Stickler syndrome must be excluded; vitreous anomalies seen on slit-lamp examination can make the diagnosis.

FOLDS IN THE FUNDUS

These are uncommon and may be fine and multiple or large and single. Fine folds may be due to folds in the retina or the choroid or both. Chorioretinal folds are usually seen in the posterior pole and are usually horizontal. Large single folds are called falciform fold or ligament (**Fig. 7.47**).

Chorioretinal folds may be seen in ocular hypotony, swollen optic discs, choroidal tumours, hypermetropia (long-sightedness, associated with a short ocular axial length), orbital pseudotumour or tumour (haemangioma or neoplasm). Falciform retinal folds are seen in familial exudative vitreoretinopathy, Norrie disease, retinopathy of prematurity and PHPV.

Vitreoretinal evaluation is necessary and prognosis depends on diagnosis.

THE OPTIC DISC

OPTIC DISC SWELLING

Unilateral optic disc swelling is not common but may be due to longstanding ocular hypotony (from any cause), uveitis, posterior scleritis, papillitis/neuritis, neuroretinitis, acute phase of Leber's hereditary optic neuropathy, optic nerve glioma and other compressive lesion.

Bilateral optic disc swelling may be seen more commonly than unilateral and may be due to buried optic disc drusen (**Figs 7.48, 7.49**), papilloedema (**Fig. 7.50**), malignant hypertension, cavernous sinus thrombosis, and bilateral papillitis (**Fig. 7.51**). In papillitis, vision is always affected but not in papilloedema unless it is chronic.

Prognosis is dependent on the cause.

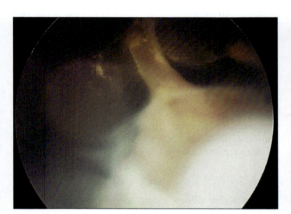

FIGURE 7.47 Thick retinal fold.

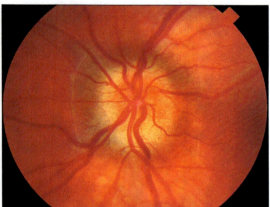

FIGURE 7.48 Swollen optic disc due to optic disc drusen; note the increased retinal vessels crossing the optic disc margins.

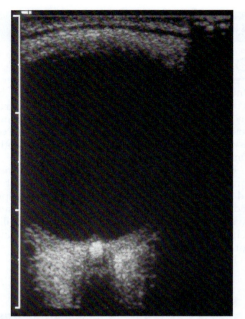

FIGURE 7.49 Ultrasound examination of the case shown in **7.48**. The optic disc drusen are shown as an increased echogenicity at the optic nerve head due to calcification.

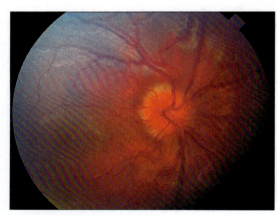

FIGURE 7.50 Papilloedema.

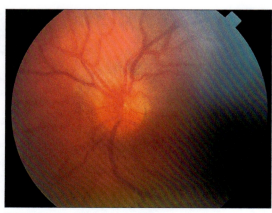

FIGURE 7.51 Bilateral papillitis.

OPTIC ATROPHY

Optic atrophy occurs due to loss of neuronal axons. It may be **primary**, **secondary**, **consecutive**, **primary hereditary**, **secondary hereditary** or associated with contralateral optic disc swelling.

PRIMARY OPTIC ATROPHY

Primary optic atrophy is uncommon but is caused most commonly by gliomas in children but can be due to any space occupying lesion.

Neuroimaging is important. Surveillance with colour vision, visual field analysis and electrodiagnostic testing may be necessary in cases of optic gliomas. Chemotherapy and radiotherapy are treatment modalities. Prognosis may be guarded for vision.

CONSECUTIVE OPTIC ATROPHY

Consecutive optic atrophy is caused by diseases of the inner retina or its blood supply (**Fig. 7.52**), such as retinitis pigmentosa cone dystrophy, diffuse retinal necrosis (e.g. CMV retinitis, acute retinal necrosis and Behçet disease), cherry-red spot at macula syndromes and mucopolysaccharidoses.

Prognosis for vision is usually poor.

SECONDARY OPTIC ATROPHY

Secondary optic atrophy is preceded by swelling of the optic nerve head (**Fig. 7.53**) as a result of swelling, ischaemia, or inflammation – i.e. chronic papilloedema, papillitis. Prognosis depends on the severity of the primary disease.

PRIMARY HEREDITARY OPTIC ATROPHY

This is a rare diffuse optic atrophy with visual loss. It may be simple recessive (onset at 4 years), Kjer juvenile dominant type (onset at about 10 years), recessive diabetes insipidus, diabetes mellitus, optic atrophy and deafness (DIDMOAD) (onset between 5 and 14 years) and Leber's hereditary optic neuropathy (LHON) (onset 16–30 years). Treatment is limited but there is some evidence that progression of LHON can be influenced by smoking and alcohol depending on the mutation found. Prognosis depends on diagnosis.

SECONDARY HEREDITARY OPTIC ATROPHY

These are rare hereditary neurological disorders with optic atrophy that usually present during the first decade of life. They may be Behr (recessive), Friedreich ataxia (recessive), Charcot–Marie–Tooth disease (dominant, X-linked), adrenoleukodystrophies (two types – X-linked recessive and autosomal recessive) or cerebellar ataxia type I (dominant).

Prognosis for vision is guarded.

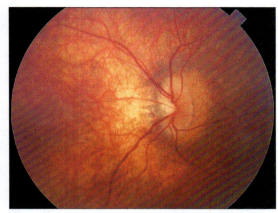

FIGURE 7.52 Retinal arteriolar attenuation in a case of cone dystrophy. The optic disc is tilted, which is a normal variant.

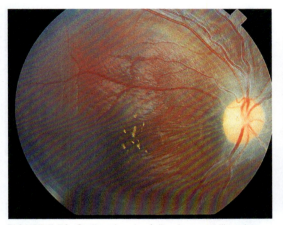

FIGURE 7.53 Optic atrophy following papilloedema.

SMALL OPTIC DISC

The optic nerve may appear small (hypermetropia) or actually be smaller than it should be (tilted disc and optic nerve hypoplasia – **Fig. 7.54**). The latter is uncommon but if seen the possibility of endocrine dysfunction must be excluded in cases of optic disc hypoplasia – classically seen in septo-optic dyplasia. Nystagmus is invariably seen with bilateral optic disc hypoplasia.

Endocrine replacement is important. Visual prognosis depends on degree of hypoplasia.

LARGE OPTIC DISC

This is seen commonly in myopia, congenital optic disc pit, optic disc coloboma (**Fig. 7.55**) and morning glory anomaly.

Bilateral cases of optic coloboma should be investigated with neuroimaging for midline defects. Morning glory anomaly is almost always associated with intracranial abnormalities even if unilateral.

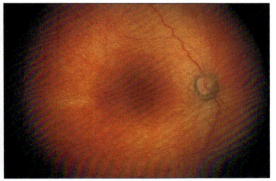

FIGURE 7.54 Optic nerve hypoplasia.

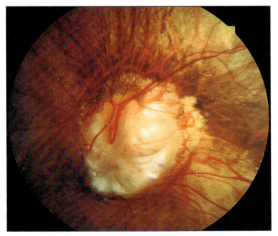

FIGURE 7.55 Marked optic disc coloboma.

LARGE OPTIC DISC CUP

Most normal cups have a cup to disc ratio of 0.3 or less. Physiological cupping (a cup to disc ratio greater than 0.7) is present in about 2% of the normal population, and glaucomatous cupping (**Fig. 7.56**), where there is raised intraocular pressure, with or without increased corneal diameter, increased myopia, Haab's striae and increased axial length.

Treatment depends on severity of the glaucoma but varies from medical topical treatment to laser treatment or surgery. Prognosis for glaucoma depends on how early the glaucoma presents: neonatal and infantile presentation is a worse prognosis than later presenting (juvenile glaucoma).

OPTIC DISC VASCULAR ABNORMALITIES

These may be **congenital** (prepapillary loop, Bergmeister papilla, persistent hyaloid artery, increased disc vessel numbers) or **acquired** (optic disc collaterals, neovascularisation, opticociliary shunts, dragged optic disc vessels). No treatment is needed but in acquired cases the cause must be sought. All causes are rare. Dragged disc vessels may be seen in familial exudative vitreoretinopathy (FEVR) or cicatricial retinopathy of prematurity.

OPTIC DISC HAEMORRHAGES

These are not uncommon and may be due to acute papilloedema, papillitis, infiltrative optic neuropathy, after optic nerve sheath decompression and optic disc drusen. Investigation to exclude early papilloedema are very important as is visual field analysis.

LESIONS OBSCURING THE OPTIC DISC

These are all rare and include primary optic disc tumours, such as capillary angioma (rare, **Fig. 7.57**) and melanocytoma; retinal tumours such as astrocytoma or combined hamartoma of the retina and RPE; infiltrative lesions due to leukaemia (**Fig. 7.58**), tuberculosis granuloma or sarcoid. Treatment is dependent on the diagnosis, as is prognosis.

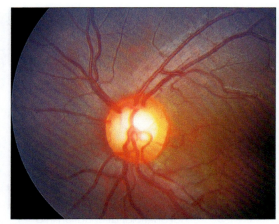

FIGURE 7.56 Optic disc cupping in juvenile glaucoma.

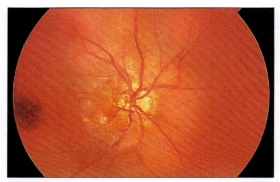

FIGURE 7.57 Retinal capillary angioma on the optic disc in a child with von Hippel–Lindau syndrome.

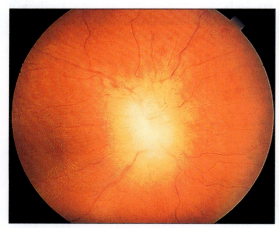

FIGURE 7.58 Leukaemic infiltration of the optic disc.

THE ORBIT

ABNORMALITIES OF GLOBE POSITION

ENOPHTHALMOS

This is when the globe sits further back than normal giving the appearance that the eye on the affected side is smaller.

The commonest cause is trauma resulting in a blow out fracture, but it may be seen in microphthalmos and in self-induced orbital fat atrophy (caused by a child incessantly rubbing his or her eye[s]).

Treatment is repair of orbital wall fracture is essential if it is the cause. In cases of microphthalmos a cosmetic shell can be applied.

EXOPHTHALMOS (PROPTOSIS)

In exophthalmos, the globe sits forward of its normal position. It is better described as proptosis which may be axial (forward without any displacement in any other direction) or non-axial (forward and, for example, down). Axial proptosis is caused by lesions within the cone of extraocular muscles, while non-axial proptosis is caused by lesions outside this cone. Rarely, proptosis may be intermittent (lymphangioma, capillary haemangioma), pulsatile (encephalocoele, orbital roof fracture) or pulsatile with a bruit (congenital arteriovenous communication, which may occur in isolation or as part of Wyburn–Mason syndrome). All causes are rare but proptosis in a child should always raise the differential of rhabdomyosarcoma. This is classically seen around 7 years of age but can be seen earlier or later. Treatment of proptosis depends on the cause but exposure keratopathy can be a complication that can be avoided with copious lunbrication. Prognosis is dependent on cause.

Pseudoproptosis is caused by a large globe (e.g. high myopia, buphthalmos [congenital glaucoma]) lid retraction or contralateral enophthalmos.

PROPTOSIS IN NEONATES AND INFANTS
Tumours
These include capillary haemangioma (see Lids section and **Fig. 7.59**), JXG, teratoma, rhabdomyosarcoma, retinoblastoma (invading the orbit may very rarely present during infancy) and acute leukaemia.

Cystic lesions
These include microphthalmos with cyst, anterior orbital encephalocoele and posterior orbital encephalocoele, which may be associated with NF1.

Shallow orbits
Shallow orbits are seen in patients with craniosynostoses such as Pfeiffer, Crouzon and Apert syndromes.

PROPTOSIS IN CHILDREN
Inflammatory causes

These include:

- Orbital cellulitis: usually secondary to ethmoiditis (**Fig. 7.60**). In severe cases there may be visual compromise and/or development of cavernous sinus thrombosis. Orbital and brain imaging is essential. Treatment includes ENT assessment, intravenous antibiotics and abscess drainage. Prognosis is usually good.
- Pseudotumour: idiopathic orbital inflammation that usually affects children between 6 and 14 years. If it is bilateral, Wegener's granulomatosis must be excluded. Orbital imaging is essential. Treatment is usually with steroids orally.
- Thyroid eye disease: may be seen in children and is associated with lid retraction. Surveillance for optic neuropathy is essential but very rare.

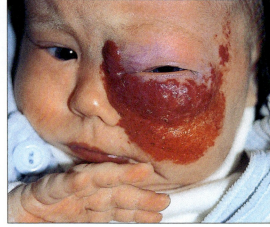

FIGURE 7.59 Left proptosis due to orbital and periorbital capillary haemangioma.

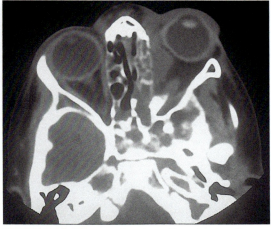

FIGURE 7.60 CT scan showing ethmoid sinusitis and contiguous orbital cellulitis with proptosis.

Benign tumours

- Lymphangioma may present between the ages of 1 and 15 years (**Fig. 7.61**). The lesion may remain stationary for long periods of time or it may suddenly enlarge, either as a result of spontaneous bleeding (chocolate cyst) or in association with an upper respiratory tract infection. Prognosis may be guarded if the tumour keeps growing.
- Plexiform neurofibroma presents in patients with NF1 between the ages of 2 and 5 years with non-axial proptosis.
- Optic nerve glioma may be isolated or associated with NF1 (**Fig. 7.62**). Those associated with NF1 tend to grow much less than those that are not. The eyeball is often turned down slightly as well as being proptosed. Monitoring with colour vision, electrodiagnostics and visual fields is important to evaluate visual function, while neuroimaging is needed to monitor growth of the tumour.

Malignant tumours

See also Chapter 12 Oncology.

- Rhabdomyosarcoma usually presents around the age of 7 years with proptosis, chemosis (swelling of the conjunctiva) and discomfort. Prognosis is good with prompt treatment.
- Metastatic neuroblastoma presents in a similar manner to rhabdomyosarcoma but usually at a younger age (under 5 years) with the primary tumour in the abdomen. Forty percent of metastases affect both orbits. Prognosis may be guarded.

- Langerhans cell histiocytosis. Orbital involvement may be seen and usually affects the superolateral quadrant of the orbit. CT scan shows soft tissue mass with adjacent bony lysis. If isolated the lesion can be curetted out or treated with steroids.
- Acute leukaemia usually presents around 7 years of age with rapid onset proptosis and ecchymosis (bruising in the lids).
- Retinoblastoma may occasionally present with proptosis but only in neglected cases. Retinoblastoma is inherited in an autosomal dominant manner. Genetic analysis is very important to be able to decide if siblings need regular examinations. Treatment depends on the size and location of the tumour. Large tumours with optic nerve involvement are usually treated with enucleation. Small solitary lesions are treated with laser therapy with or without cryotherapy. Chemotherapy is also used to prevent recurrence. While orbital radiation is not used due to the late occurrence of other orbital tumours, local plaque therapy is used. The use of intra-arterial (ophthalmic artery) chemotherapy is controversial. Prognosis is generally good for survival but vision may be lost in the affected eye(s).
- Metastatic Ewing sarcoma is very rare but may present with rapid proptosis, ecchymosis and chemosis.
- Metastatic Wilms tumour may be associated with aniridia.

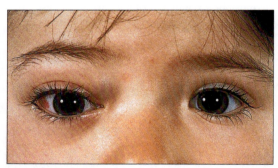

FIGURE 7.61 Proptosis due to orbital lymphangioma.

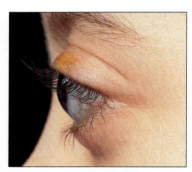

FIGURE 7.62 Proptosis due to optic nerve glioma.

LACRIMAL GLAND ENLARGEMENT

Unilateral enlargement is very uncommon but differential diagnosis includes:

- Dacryoadenitis, usually caused by a viral infection of the lacrimal gland but may be associated with orbital pseudotumour. It is not usually associated with proptosis *per se* but causes the upper lid to develop an 'S' shape and is very tender to touch. Treatment is with pain relief and antibiotics if from an infectious cause, but if pseudotumouor related, steroids are indicated. CT scan is usually needed to make the distinction together with serology.
- Dacryops is due to a dilatation of the major lacrimal ducts secondary to obstruction and again does not usually cause proptosis.
- Pleomorphic adenoma. Very rarely this essentially 'adult' tumour presents in children with a painless, slowly progressive non-axial proptosis. Biopsy may be needed to make the diagnosis. It is very rare.

Bilateral enlargement is also very rare but the differential diagnosis includes:

- Sarcoidosis: may rarely cause bilateral firm enlarged lacrimal glands in children.
- Acute leukaemia. In children a form of acute myeloid leukaemia (chloroma) may cause bilateral lacrimal gland infiltration.

EYE MOVEMENT DISORDERS

See also Chapter 8 Neurology, page 203.

These may be classified as disorders in primary position of gaze, anomalous eye movements and nystagmus. All cases should be referred for ophthalmic opinion.

OCULAR DEVIATION IN PRIMARY GAZE

If a deviation remains stable regardless of the position of gaze of the eyes, it is called comitant. If it does change it is termed non- or in-comitant.

ESODEVIATION

This is a turning in of one or both eyes.

PSEUDODEVIATION

- Epicanthic folds: symmetric corneal reflexes confirm the absence of true esotropia.
- Narrow interpupillary distance seen in hypotelorism.

TRUE ESODEVIATION

Comitant esotropia

Infantile esotropia (**Fig. 7.63**) develops before the age of 6 months with a large and stable angle, cross-fixation (child uses right eye to look to left and *vice versa* as the eyes are so convergent) and normal refraction for age.

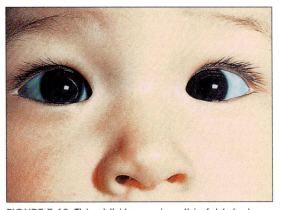

FIGURE 7.63 This child has epicanthic folds but the corneal light reflex on the right cornea is central, while the reflex in the left eye is off the pupil, indicating the presence of a left esodeviation.

- Non-accommodative esotropia: esotropia after 6 months of age with normal refraction.
- Refractive accommodative esotropia: onset is usually between 2 and 3 years, associated with hypermetropia (long-sightedness).
- Non-refractive accommodative esotropia: onset after 6 months but before 3 years. No significant refractive error but excessive convergence for near (called high accommodative convergence: accommodation ratio – AC/A ratio).
- Sensory esotropia: due to reduction in vision, with one eye much worse than the other, which disrupts fusion – e.g. in unilateral cataract.
- Convergent spasm: intermittent esotropia with pseudomyopia and miosis due to accommodative spasm, which may be seen after trauma or due to a posterior fossa tumour but usually has a functional element.

Incomitant esotropia
- VI nerve palsy: may be congenital or acquired (associated with raised intracranial pressure). Esotropia gets worse when looking in the distance.
- Möbius syndrome: bilateral gaze palsies, with esotropia in 50% of cases (due to superimposed VI nerve palsies). There is usually bilateral VII nerve palsies and may be associated V, IX, X nerve palsies.
- Duane syndrome: due to miswiring of the horizontal rectus muscles which leads to cocontraction of the medial and lateral recti. This leads to limited abduction with almost normal adduction (type I), or limited adduction with almost normal abduction (type II) or limited adduction and abduction in equal measures (type III). The eye movements are associated with widening of the palpebral fissure on abduction and narrowing on adduction. Types I and III may present with an esotropia in primary position of gaze. If a child has an abduction deficit but no esotropia in primary gaze, this cannot be a VI nerve palsy and must be Duane syndrome.

EXODEVIATION (THE EYES DIVERGE IN PRIMARY POSITION)
Pseudo-exodeviation
Hypertelorism: look for symmetry of corneal light reflexes.

TRUE EXODEVIATION
Comitant exotropia
- Intermittent exotropia: a common condition with exotropia more commonly present for distance than for near (**Fig. 7.64**). In bright sunlight the child will characteristically close the diverging eye.
- Sensory exotropia: much less common in children than sensory esodeviation.
- Convergence insufficiency: usually seen in older children. Convergence exercises may help but there should be a low threshold to neuroimage if there are any neurological signs or worsening despite convergence exercises.

Incomitant exotropia
- Congenital III nerve palsy: exodeviation and hypodeviation of the affected eye, with ptosis and miosed pupil. There is limitation of upgaze and adduction.
- Acquired III nerve palsy (**Fig. 7.65**): rare. Same signs as in the congenital condition but the pupil is dilated.
- Duane syndrome type II: see above.

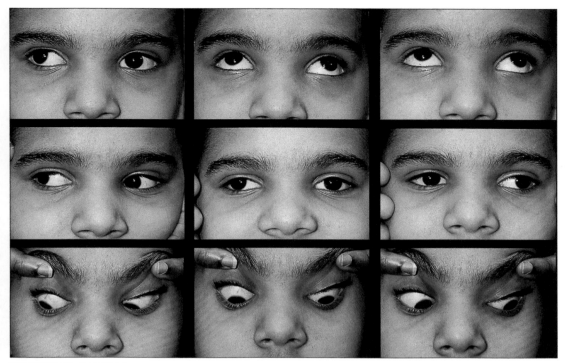

FIGURE 7.64 Exotropia.

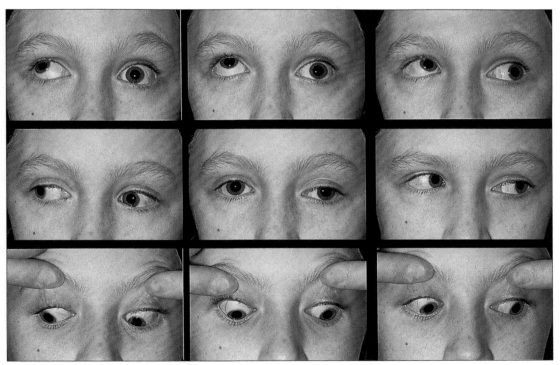

FIGURE 7.65 III nerve palsy (left side).

ANOMALOUS EYE MOVEMENTS

UPSHOOTS IN ADDUCTION (ON VERSION TESTING)

- Inferior oblique overaction: may be primary (usually bilateral and seen with esotropia but also with exotropia occurring in childhood) or secondary (to a superior oblique palsy) (**Fig. 7.66**).
- Duane syndrome I, II, III: see above. Upshoots occur due to a leash effect of a tight lateral rectus muscle secondary to cocontraction of the medial rectus muscle.
- Dissociated vertical deviation: a bilateral condition most commonly seen in association with infantile esotropia. At moments of inattention the eye will move up and then move down to its original position while the fixating eye remains still. It differs from inferior oblique overaction in that the eye may elevate in any position of gaze.
- Craniosynostoses (**Fig. 7.67**): in the syndromic craniosynostoses, e.g. Apert, Pfeiffer, Crouzon, the extraocular muscles are excyclorotated such that the medial rectus now acts as an elevator as well as an adductor.

DOWNSHOOTS IN ADDUCTION (ON VERSION TESTING)

- Duane syndrome I, II or III: see above.
- Brown syndrome: this is not an uncommon condition where the tendon of the superior oblique muscle is unable to pass freely through its pulley (the trochlea, at the superomedial orbital rim). This results in restriction of elevation in upgaze usually just in the adducted position. As a result there may be a coincident downshoot in adduction on version testing. It is usually idiopathic but may be acquired due to inflammation at the trochlea or trauma.
- Superior oblique overaction: may be primary and usually seen with intermittent exotropia in older children (late teens).

LIMITATION OF ABDUCTION

- VI nerve palsy (**Fig. 7.68**): there is always an esotropia in primary position of gaze. In Duane I and II there may not be an esotropia in primary position of gaze.
- Any restrictive myopathy of the medial rectus: myositis, pseudotumour, and very rarely, thyroid eye disease.

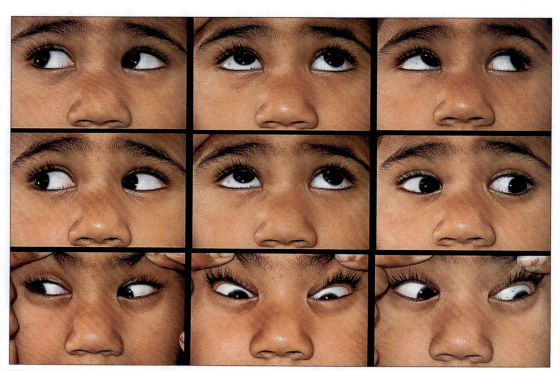

FIGURE 7.66 Right superior oblique palsy. The right eye does not depress in adduction as well as it should do. There is also a mild right inferior oblique overaction (there is a slight upshoot of the right eye in adduction).

LIMITATION OF ADDUCTION

- III nerve palsy **(Fig. 7.65)**: may be congenital or acquired (see above).
- Internuclear ophthalmoplegia (INO): a lesion in the medial longitudinal fasiculus leading to ipsilateral adduction limitation and contralateral eye abducting nystagmus.
- Myasthenia gravis: very rare but may mimic adduction deficit.
- Acute myositis: restriction of movement in the direction of the field of action of the affected muscle.
- Duane syndrome II and III.

LIMITATION OF HORIZONTAL VERSIONS OR GAZE PALSIES

- Any lesion of the paramedian pontine reticular formation (**PPRF**) causes ipsilateral gaze palsy.
- One-and-a-half syndrome: a lesion of the PPRF/abducens nucleus and adjacent medial longitudinal fasiculus causing an ipsilateral gaze palsy and ipsilateral INO. A right-sided neurological lesion would lead to inability for either eye to look to the right, the right eye could not adduct (part of the INO) but the left eye could abduct but only with a nystagmus.

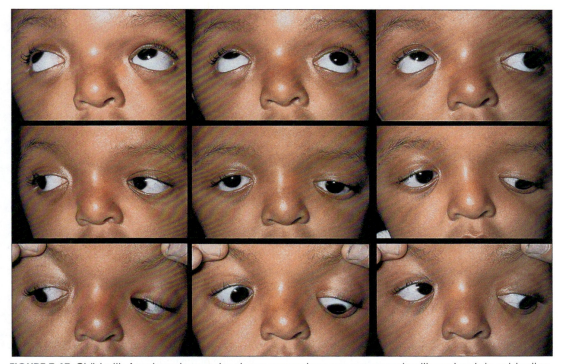

FIGURE 7.67 Child with Apert syndrome who shows anomalous eye movements with upshoots in adduction and coincident downshoots in abduction. This child also demonstrates a V pattern: when the child looks up, the eyes diverge, compared to when the child looks down. There is also a right depression deficit.

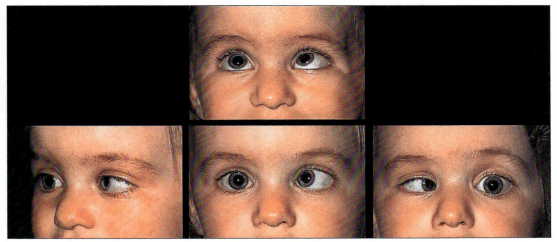

FIGURE 7.68 Left esotropia due to left VI nerve palsy (left abduction deficit).

- Bilateral pontine lesions result in total horizontal gaze palsies.
- Fisher syndrome: a rare variant of Guillain-Barré syndrome, which may present in children with ophthalmoplegia, ataxia and areflexia, though the initial presentation may be one of horizontal gaze palsy or an INO.

LIMITATION OF VERTICAL EYE MOVEMENT (ONE OR BOTH EYES)

- **P**alsy of a muscle: superior rectus, inferior oblique (upgaze affected) and inferior rectus, superior oblique palsy (downgaze affected).
- Orbital floor fracture: causing entrapped inferior rectus muscle and restriction of elevation.
- Orbital space occupying lesion: such as capillary haemangioma, plexiform neurofibroma.
- Symblepharon: attachment of lid to globe will cause restriction of elevation or depression. This may be congenital and seen in clefting syndromes but also may be acquired, seen in epidermolysis bullosa, alkali injuries.
- Brown syndrome: see above. Deficit in elevation.
- Monocular elevation deficit: formerly called double elevator palsy. This may be due to idiopathic tightening of the inferior rectus muscle or idiopathic with no evidence of inferior rectus tightening.

VERTICAL GAZE PALSY

- Parinaud syndrome: decreased upgaze, large pupils, convergence insufficiency and, convergence – retraction nystagmus. In children one of the commonest causes is a pinealoma.
- Hydrocephalus: stretching of the posterior commissure results in loss of upgaze with or without tonic downward deviation of the eyes ('sunset' sign).
- Metabolic causes: may affect vertical eye movements. Tay–Sachs disease may cause impairment of vertical and later horizontal gaze. Niemann–Pick variants may also cause vertical gaze anomalies.

GENERALISED LIMITATION OF OCULAR MOVEMENTS

This may be due to multiple ocular motor palsies or to other causes.

Due to multiple ocular motor palsies
- Cavernous sinus lesions: very rare but may be a complication of orbital cellulitis. Tumours are very rare as are caroticocavernous fistula.
- Superior orbital fissure lesion: rare but tumours of the orbit may cause problems here (e.g. leukaemia) or rarer infections (such as aspergilloma in immunocompromised children). Tolosa–Hunt syndrome (idiopathic granulomatous inflammation that is painful during the acute phase) may affect the superior orbital fissure or cavernous sinus.
- Brainstem lesions: usually encephalitis but tumours of the brainstem (glioma) may also present with ophthalmoplegia.

Due to other causes
- Chronic progressive ophthalmoplegia: may be associated with a mitochondrial cytopathy in which case it may be isolated or part of the Kearns–Sayre syndrome, oculopharyngeal dystrophy.
- Myotonic dystrophy: may be seen in children either as the congenital variant or type I autosomal dominant variant, which has demonstrated anticipation.
- Drug toxicity: most commonly seen with phenytoin.
- Acquired saccadic initiation failure (ocular motor apraxia): may be seen in lesions in the frontoparietal cortex. Both vertical and horizontal saccades are affected. May be seen in Gaucher III. In congenital saccadic initiation failure, vetical saccades are unaffected.
- Metabolic causes: Tay–Sachs disease, and occasionally other lipid-storage diseases.
- Congenital fibrosis syndrome: familial condition that may affect all muscles. Often, however, the eyes are fixed in a downward position with bilateral ptosis and chin up head position.

ABNORMAL HEAD POSITIONS

OCULAR CAUSES

- Nystagmus (**Fig. 7.69**): a null position is a position of the eyes in the orbits where the nystagmus is most dampened; in this position the child sees better. The child adopts an abnormal head position so that the eyes are in the null position but the child is able to look straight ahead.
- Unilateral ametropia (usually astigmatism): results in a head turn but rarely also a head tilt.
- Strabismus: a child will usually develop an abnormal head posture to reduce the amount of diplopia. As a rule the head will turn or be moved in the direction of the underacting muscle(s). In order to see if the head posture is due to strabismic problems one eye should be patched; if it is strabismic in origin then the head posture will improve.

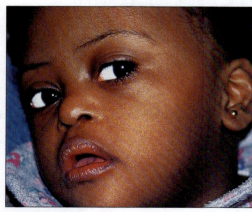

FIGURE 7.69 Child with nystagmus who adopts an abnormal head posture to improve vision by holding the eyes in the null position.

TYPES OF ABNORMAL HEAD POSTURE

- Chin elevation: bilateral ptosis, any cause of elevation deficit (unilateral or bilateral – see above), nystagmus (null position with eyes in downgaze) and in certain types of horizontal strabismus (such as A or V pattern deviations where the eyes are almost straight in downgaze but either develop an esodeviation or exodeviation in upgaze).
- Chin depression: nystagmus with null position of eyes in upgaze, and A or V pattern deviations (with eyes straight in upgaze but not in downgaze).
- Head tilt: may be caused by a superior oblique palsy (commonest cause – see **Fig. 7.66**), Brown syndrome, and rarely posterior fossa tumour.
- Head turn: lateral rectus or medial rectus palsy, Duane syndrome, nystagmus with null position in lateral gaze, manifest latent nystagmus (the nystagmus in the fixating eye dampens if that eye is adducted), homonymous hemianopia, unilateral deafness and ametropia (see above).

NYSTAGMUS

CHARACTER OF NYSTAGMUS

- Horizontal jerk: a combination of slow drift with fast corrective phase. The 'nystagmus' direction is the same as the fast corrective phase.
- Pendular: nystagmus velocity is the same in both directions but on lateral gaze this usually develops a horizontal jerk component.
- Oblique: due to a combination of horizontal and vertical directions of pendular nystagmus.

EARLY ONSET NYSTAGMUS

- Manifest nystagmus: is usually benign but may be acquired. It is uniplanar, dampens on convergence and worsens on eccentric fixation.
- Latent nystagmus: no nystagmus with both eyes open but horizontal jerk nystagmus is seen when one eye is covered. Most commonly seen with infantile esotropia but may be seen with other early onset deviations. The fast phase is towards the uncovered fixating eye.
- Manifest-latent nystagmus: usually seen with infantile esotropia and dissociated vertical deviation. The nystagmus becomes worse when one eye is occluded.
- Spasmus nutans: an early onset (3–18 months) unilateral or bilateral small amplitude high frequency horizontal nystagmus often associated with head nodding. It is most often idiopathic with resolution by 3 years of age but it may be due to an optic pathway glioma.
- Roving nystagmus: severe disruption of visual function may lead to this and the commonest causes are Leber's congenital amaurosis (severe retinal dystrophy) or optic nerve hypoplasia (bilateral).

LATER ONSET NYSTAGMUS

- Coarse horizontal jerk nystagmus: usually seen in cerebellar disease, with fast phase ipsilateral to the lesion.

- Torsional nystagmus: if pure then this is usually only seen in central vestibular disease such as syringomyelia or syringobulbia associated with Arnold–Chiari malformation, demyelination and very rarely, lateral medullary syndrome in children.
- Downbeat nystagmus: usually seen in lesions at the craniocervical junction (e.g. Arnold–Chiari malformation), drug toxicity (phenytoin, carbamazepine), trauma, hydrocephalus and demyelination.
- Upbeat nystagmus: usually seen in cerebellar degenerations (e.g. ataxia telangiectasia) and encephalitis; in babies a retinal dystrophy should be excluded (especially cone dystrophy).
- Gaze-evoked nystagmus: may be seen with lesions of the vestibulocerebellum axis, brainstem or cerebral hemispheres or after a gaze palsy or with drug toxicity (phenytoin and carbemazipine).
- Periodic alternating nystagmus: the direction of the nystagmus reverses. It may be congenital idiopathic but is usually seen with Arnold–Chiari malformation or cerebellar disease, trauma or demyelination.
- Rebound nystagmus: attempt to maintain eccentric gaze results in gaze evoked nystagmus, which dampens and sometimes reverses direction. On returning to primary gaze a transient nystagmus develops. It is usually seen in cerebellar disease.
- See-saw nystagmus: pendular nystagmus in which one eye elevates and intorts while the other eye depresses and extorts and then the eyes reverse. The commonest cause is chiasmal or parasellar tumours but it may also be seen in albinism as a transient finding, head trauma and syringobulbia.
- Internuclear ophthalmoplegia: the abducting eye has nystagmus (see above) and is due to a lesion in the medial longitudinal fasiculus.
- Monocular nystagmus: may be seen in spasmus nutans, unilateral deep amblyopia, superior oblique myokymia and optic nerve glioma.
- Convergence-retraction nystagmus: seen in Parinaud syndrome (see above).

OCULAR CAUSES OF NYSTAGMUS

Disruption of vision will lead to nystagmus. There may be obvious (usually bilateral) ocular disease such as corneal opacities, congenital cataract, microphthalmos, aniridia and oculocutaneous nystagmus or less obvious ocular disease such as retinal dystrophy (usually cone dystrophy or Leber's congenital amaurosis), ocular albinism, X-linked congenital stationary night blindness, optic nerve hypoplasia and early onset optic atrophy.

Depending on the cause nystagmus may be improved with drugs or surgery. Anomalous head posture may be treated by recessions of the extraocular muscles. Recently, for certain types of nystagmus, tenotomy and reattachment surgery has been advocated but this is still in its infancy.

FURTHER READING

Basic and Clinical Science Course (BCSC) - Section 6: Pediatric Ophthalmology and Strabismus. 2014–2015. American Academy of Ophthalmology. http://store.aao.org/clinical-education/product-line/basic-and-clinical-science-course-bcsc/2014-2015-basic-and-clinical-science-course-section-06-pediatric-ophthalmology-and-strabismus.html

Fleck BW. Management of retinopathy of prematurity. *Arch Dis Child Fetal Neonatal Ed* 2013;98(5):F454–6.

Nentwich MM, Rudolph G. Hereditary retinal eye diseases in childhood and youth affecting the central retina. *Oman J Ophthalmol* 2013;6(Suppl 1):S18–25.

Papageorgiou E, McLean RJ, Gottlob I. Nystagmus in childhood. *Pediatr Neonatol* 2014;55(5):341–51.

Petrs-Silva H, Linden R. Advances in gene therapy technologies to treat retinitis pigmentosa. *Clin Ophthalmol* 2014;8:127–36.

Salt A, Sargent J. Common visual problems in children with disability. *Arch Dis Child* 2014;99:1163–8.

Scanga HL, Nischal KK. Genetics and ocular disorders: a focused review. *Pediatr Clin North Am* 2014;61(3):555–65.

Taylor D, Hoyt C (eds). *Pediatric Ophthalmology and Strabismus*, 4th edn. Oxford: Elsevier. 2011.

Wright KW, Spiegel PJ (eds). *Pediatric Ophthalmology and Strabismus*, 2nd edn. New York: Springer Verlag, 2002.

Ophthalmology

8 Neurology

Fenella Kirkham, Adnan Manzur and Stephanie Robb

NEUROLOGICAL EXAMINATION: CRANIAL NERVES

Although neurological examination cannot always be performed in the correct order in young children, it is important to aim to perform the core components. Careful observation of the child's natural behaviour often gives diagnostic clues, but some areas (such as visual fields and acuity) must be formally tested.

THE EYE

See also Chapter 7 Ophthalmology.

It is essential to examine visual fields and visual acuity in every patient.

In schoolchildren, **visual fields** can be compared by confrontation with the examiner's own, ideally with each eye separately with a finger (**Fig. 8.1**) or a white pin to assess the peripheral visual field and then with a red pin (**Fig. 8.2**) to assess the central visual field, but it is better to examine both fields together with wiggling fingers than to omit testing, as most abnormalities, e.g. homonymous hemianopia after stroke or bitemporal quadrantanopia in craniopharyngioma, are detected. If this is not possible, a toy on a string is brought in from behind the child's head and a second examiner distracts, e.g. with a puppet and observes visual behaviour.

Pendular nystagmus, or loss of the direct and consensual pupillary response to light, implies poor visual acuity. Under the age of 2 years, a rapid screen of visual acuity can be conducted using small sweets and then the smaller 'hundreds and thousands' cake decorations. In formal testing, the infant's visual behaviour when shown two black and white grids of different spacing and width is observed; if he only looks at the larger it is assumed that he cannot see the smaller. Being able to recognise buttons is a rapid test of gross vision in a verbal child. Formally, from around the age of 27 months, acuity can be

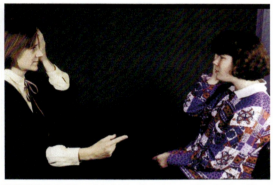

FIGURE 8.1 Visual field testing to confrontation. The patient is about 1 metre away and is looking at the examiner's eye. The test object (finger or white pin) is halfway between the patient and the examiner.

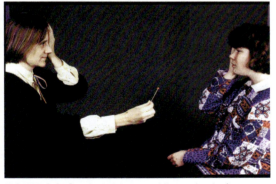

FIGURE 8.2 Central vision and the extent of any blind spot is tested with a red pin.

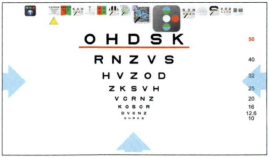

FIGURE 8.3 Visual acuity testing: tablet computer apps may replace the Snellen chart for formal testing of visual acuity in older children who can read.

tested with five or seven letters by asking the child to match the letters they see at 6 metres and show them to a carer using a second chart. Visual acuity can be tested with a Snellen chart at 6 metres (20 feet) in children who can read letters. Visual acuity testing apps are now available for tablet computers (**Fig. 8.3**). Adequate fundoscopy often requires the pupils to be pharmacologically dilated (see Chapter 7 Ophthalmology).

PTOSIS

Causes of unilateral ptosis include:

- Congenital – may be associated with dysmorphic features.
- Horner syndrome (**Figs 8.4–8.7**).
- Third nerve palsy (**Figs 8.8, 8.9**). The ptosis is usually severe (**8.9**). In a complete third nerve palsy (**8.8**), there is associated dilatation of the pupil and the eye will be positioned 'down and out', due to involvement of the superior, inferior and medial rectus and the inferior oblique muscles. See 'Eye movements', page 203, for causes.
- Marcus–Gunn jaw winking (**Figs 8.10, 8.11**).

EXAMINATION IN HORNER SYNDROME

- The ptosis is usually mild and is associated with constriction of the pupil, enophthalmos and decreased sweating (**Figs 8.4, 8.5**).
- Congenital Horner syndrome is accompanied by heterochromia iridis in a brown-eyed child (**Fig. 8.6**).
- Look for lateral scar from cardiac operation.
- Examine the ipsilateral hand:
  - severe clawing in Klumpke paralysis (**Fig. 8.7**).
  - wasting of small muscles if T1 lesion alone (tumour in Pancoast region).
- Examine sensation in the arms:
  - syringomyelia – preserved position and vibration, reduced temperature and pain.
  - reduced sensation in T1 distribution with a T1 lesion.
- Examine sensation in the face:
  - pain and temperature are distributed concentrically from around the mouth.
  - tactile sensation is distributed in the V1,V2 and V3 distributions:
    - any abnormality in brainstem tumour.
    - dissociated in syringobulbia.

Causes of bilateral ptosis include:

- Congenital: may have other dysmorphic features (sometimes associated with syndromes such as Noonan).
- Myasthenia (congenital and myasthenia gravis) (**Figs 8.12, 8.13**)
  - The ptosis may be associated with involvement of the external ocular muscles leading to paralytic squint or even complete ophthalmoplegia. Facial and bulbar weakness may also be prominent and there may be more generalised weakness.
  - Look for evidence of fatiguability by asking the child to look up for a minute, to count to 50 or sing a nursery rhyme, or to hold their arms forward flexed to 90 degrees at the shoulder for 1 minute.
- Neuromuscular diseases such as mitochondrial myopathy, myotonic dystrophy (see Chronic progressive weakness) and some congenital myopathies.

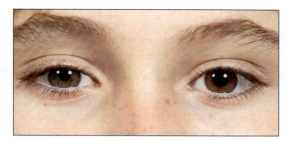

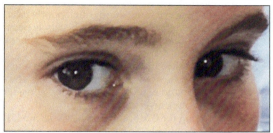

FIGURES 8.4, 8.5 Right Horner syndrome with slight ptosis, enophthalmos and pupillary constriction with decreased sweating and flushing (**8.5**) in a child who had carotid occlusion after a quinsy (see **8.29**).

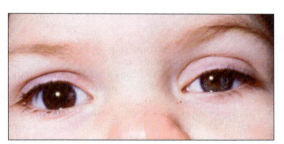

FIGURE 8.6 Unilateral congenital ptosis with heterochromia iridis (left eye is blue; right eye is brown).

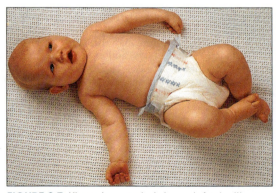

FIGURE 8.7 Klumpke paralysis in an infant with an ipsilateral Horner syndrome.

FIGURES 8.12, 8.13 **8.12**: Right ptosis and partial opthalmoplegia in myasthenia gravis, with improvement after edrophonium (**8.13**).

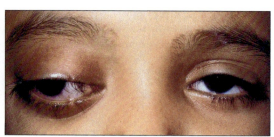

FIGURE 8.8 Third nerve palsy and exophthalmos secondary to an orbital tumour. There is severe ptosis and the eye is 'down and out'; the pupillary dilatation cannot be seen.

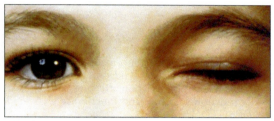

FIGURE 8.9 Third nerve palsy with complete ptosis.

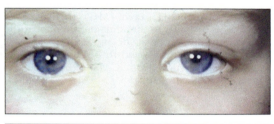

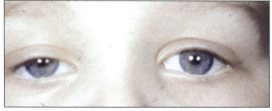

FIGURES 8.10, 8.11 Intermittent ptosis in the Marcus–Gunn jaw winking phenomenon.

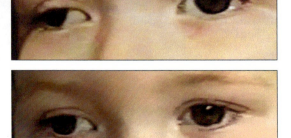

201

MYASTHENIA

Neonatal myasthenia occurs in the infants of mothers with acetylcholine receptor (AChR) or MuSK antibodies and is usually transient.

Congenital myasthenic syndromes (CMS) are inherited (usually recessively except for slow channel syndromes). Mutations in at least 19 genes cause pre- and postsynaptic abnormalities. The commonest are postsynaptic disorders, including:

- AChR deficiency due to mutations in *CHRNE*, encoding the epsilon AChR subunit.
- CMS due to mutations in *RAPSN*.
- 'Limb girdle' CMS due to mutations in *DOK7*.

Rarer causes include:

- Synaptic acetylcholinesterase deficiency (*COLQ* mutations).
- Postsynaptic kinetic abnormalities of the AChR (slow and fast channel syndromes).
- Disorders of glycosylation affecting neuromuscular junction structure and function (e.g. *GFPT1*, *DPAGT1*).
- Presynaptic choline acetyltransferase deficiency (*CHAT* mutations).

Juvenile myasthenia gravis (MG), particularly in adolescents is similar to the adult autoimmune form, but young children may be more likely to have purely ocular symptoms and to be AChR antibody negative. Distinction from CMS is important as management is different.

CLINICAL SIGNS

- Arthrogryposis at birth, which is often subtle (e.g. affecting only the hands) (CMS).
- Repeated apnoeas from infancy (CMS).
- Frequent chest infections (CMS).
- Respiratory failure (CMS and MG).
- Ptosis (may be subtle or absent in some CMS subtypes, unilateral ptosis is more likely in MG) (**Figs 8.12, 8.13**).
- Ophthalmoplegia (often incomplete) (MG and some subtypes of CMS, e.g. *CHRNE*).
- Facial weakness (MG and CMS).
- Bulbar weakness with swallowing difficulty (MG and CMS).
- Generalised weakness (MG and CMS – also a predominant 'limb girdle' weakness occurs in some CMS).
- Fatigue, evident on walking, running, climbing stairs, repeat sit to stand, outstretched arms and upgaze.

DIAGNOSIS

- Pharmacological:
  - Edrophonium (tensilon) – test dose 0.01 mg/kg; full dose 0.15 mg/kg. This is used with caution in CMS (see below). Atropine (0.1–0.4 mg) must be drawn up before the test starts and should be given immediately if there is bradycardia or respiratory depression. Resuscitation trolley must be available and checked before

testing starts. Improvement in ptosis is usually the best end-point. Video monitoring of the test is often useful as improvement is transient and often subtle (**Figs 8.12, 8.13**).
  - A trial of a longer acting anticholinesterase (oral pyridostigmine) may be preferable, but must be given in hospital if CMS is suspected as pyridostigmine (and edrophonium) worsens some forms of CMS.
- Electrodiagnostic studies:
  - Stimulation single fibre electromyography.
  - Repetitive nerve stimulation (often poorly tolerated in young children and may be falsely negative; it is occasionally performed under general anaesthesia if there is diagnostic difficulty).
- AChR antibodies: these may be negative in autoimmune MG in some children. Test for low-affinity AChR and MuSK antibodies and consider CMS in 'seronegative' cases.
- Genetic testing for CMS: this is available in the UK via the NHS Highly Specialised Service national diagnostic service in Oxford. Phenotypic clues may help target the likely gene (e.g. ophthalmoplegia with *CHRNE* and *COLQ* mutations, episodic apnoea with *RAPSN* and *CHAT* CMS, limb girdle weakness with *DOK7*, *GFPT1* and *DPAGT1* CMS).

MANAGEMENT

Autoimmune MG

- Anticholinesterase drugs (e.g. pyridostigmine, or neostigmine in neonates).
- Early thymectomy in cases of AChR antibody-positive disease with generalised weakness, especially with bulbar involvement.
- Immunosuppression with alternate day steroids (+/– azathioprine) for severe symptoms not controlled with pyridostigmine.
- Immunoglobulin or plasma exchange for acute exacerbations.

Congenital myasthenic syndromes

- Pyridostigmine for CMS with mutations causing AChR deficiency, fast channel syndromes, *RAPSN*, *CHAT*, *GFPT1* and *DPAGT1*. Addition of 3,4-diaminopyridine may also help.
- Quinidine or fluoxetine (caution due to psychiatric effects in children) for slow channel syndromes.
- Salbutamol or ephedrine for *DOK7* and *COLQ* CMS.

General

- Awareness of the risk of fulminating bulbar and respiratory insufficiency in myasthenic crises and the need for emergency respiratory support in MG and CMS (especially during chest infections).
- Monitoring for chronic nocturnal respiratory insufficiency in some forms of CMS (e.g. *COLQ*, *DOK7* and slow channel syndromes) that cause progressive weakness with respiratory failure.
- Monitoring bulbar weakness and feeding difficulty in MG and CMS. Timing meals with medication, food texture modification, calorie supplementation and need for temporary nasogastric feeding or gastrostomy (CMS).

DISORDERS OF EYE MOVEMENT

See also Chapter 7 Ophthalmology, page 191.

The mnemonic for innervation of eye muscles is LR6 (SO4)3 (lateral rectus, 6th; superior oblique, 4th; 3rd). **Eye movement testing** (see Chapter 7 Ophthalmology) is easy in young children if a hand puppet is used. The examiner should ask the child to follow eye movements horizontally to right and left and vertically in the midline and to each side. Nystagmus on lateral gaze is usually secondary to a cerebellar or brainstem lesion in childhood.

THIRD NERVE PALSY

At rest the eye is deviated 'down and out' (**Fig. 8.8**), due to involvement of the superior, inferior and medial rectus and the inferior oblique muscles. The eyelid may be completely closed (**Fig. 8.9**).

Causes of third nerve palsy include:

- Space-occupying lesion in the orbit, e.g. tumour (**Fig. 8.8**) or orbital pseudotumour (which responds to steroids).
- Pressure of the third nerve against the tentorium in uncal herniation (see 'Coma', **Fig. 8.109**).
- Inflammation at the base of the skull (e.g. tuberculous meningitis).
- Space occupying lesion in the midbrain (e.g. tumour – pyramidal tract signs are usually present).
- Aneurysm of the posterior communicating artery (extremely rare in childhood).

FOURTH NERVE PALSY

This is extremely rare. It causes paralysis of the superior oblique muscle (SO4). Head tilt is often prominent and the patient has difficulty looking down (e.g. when walking downstairs). It is usually idiopathic but may be due to a pseudotumour of the orbit (see 'Third nerve palsy').

SIXTH NERVE PALSY

The eye is unable to look laterally because of paralysis of the lateral rectus muscle (LR6) (**Fig. 8.14**, see **Fig. 8.65**).

Causes of sixth nerve palsy include:

- False localising sign in intracranial hypertension (see 'Headache') (**Fig. 8.14**, see **Fig. 8.65**) (e.g. tumour with hydrocephalus or pseudotumour cerebri – benign intracranial hypertension). There is papilloedema and other neurological signs may be present if there is a space occupying lesion.
- Local causes in the orbit (e.g. tumour or pseudotumour – see 'Third nerve palsy').
- Lesions in the nucleus in the pons (e.g. tumour) – the seventh nerve is usually involved as well.

OPHTHALMOPLEGIA

Paralysis of third, fourth and sixth nerves.

Causes include tumour or pseudotumour of the orbit (usually unilateral); MG and congenital myasthenic syndromes (bilateral) – see Ptosis, **Figs 8.4–8.13**; mitochondrial disorders and some congenital myopathies; Miller–Fisher variant of Guillain–Barré syndrome (descending paralysis with prominent involvement of the cranial nerves) (bilateral).

UPWARD GAZE PALSY

The child is unable to look upwards (**Fig. 8.15**). This implies pressure on the midbrain.

Causes include pinealoma (**Fig. 8.15**) or severe hydrocephalus (see **Fig. 8.66**) with 'sun setting' sign.

LATERAL GAZE PALSY

The child is able to look to one side but not the other (**Fig. 8.16**). Convergence is preserved (**Fig. 8.17**).

Causes include frontal or brainstem lesion (**Figs 8.16, 8.17**).

INVESTIGATIONS IN OPHTHALMOPLEGIA

- Neuroimaging of the brain and orbits: if any orbital lesion is suspected, MRI is preferred because of the risk of radiation to the lens with CT and the higher diagnostic rate.
- For bilateral ophthalmoplegia, myasthenia (see 'Ptosis', **Figs 8.12, 8.13**), mitochondrial and myopathic disorders must be excluded.
- Nerve conduction studies may be required to exclude the Miller–Fisher variant of Guillain–Barré syndrome (see under 'Acute weakness', page 215, **Fig. 8.39**).

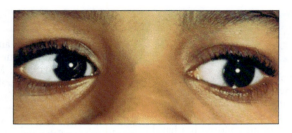

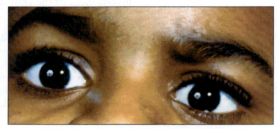

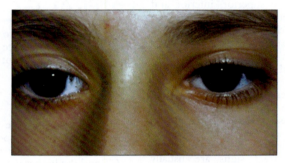

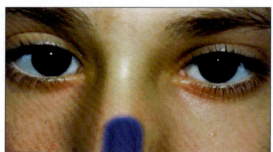

FIGURES 8.14–8.17 Gaze palsies (the blue bar represents the direction of gaze). **8.14**: Left sixth nerve palsy as a false localising sign of intracranial hypertension in a boy who also has an upgaze palsy (**8.15**) in the context of an operable pinealoma; **8.16**: lateral gaze palsy in a girl with an operable brainstem tumour; although she cannot look to the left with either eye on command, the eyes do move to converge (**8.17**).

LOWER MOTOR NEURON FACIAL PALSY

The child is asked to show his/her teeth (**Fig. 8.18**), screw up his eyes voluntarily (**Fig. 8.19**) and against resistance, look surprised (**Fig. 8.20**) and blow his cheeks out (**Fig. 8.21**). The facial expression (e.g. on smiling spontaneously) should also be noted.

A lower motor neuron facial palsy presents as a very obvious weakness of the face with involvement of the eye. It may be unilateral (**Figs 8.18–8.21**) or bilateral (see **Fig. 8.26**).

CAUSES

Unilateral in the newborn
- Trauma to the facial nerve (e.g. due to direct compression against the maternal sacrum or forceps delivery).
- Congenital peripheral abnormalities (usually isolated) or nuclear abnormalities (may be associated with other cranial nerve palsies).

Bilateral in the newborn
- Moebius syndrome (usually with bilateral sixth nerve and lower cranial nerve palsies).

Unilateral in a previously well child (Figs 8.18–8.21)
- Acute otitis media.
- Viral – herpes simplex; herpes zoster, including chickenpox (sometimes without vesicles); parvovirus B19.
- Lyme disease (*Borrelia burgdorferi*).
- *Mycoplasma pneumoniae*.
- Hypertension.
- Trauma.
- Kawasaki disease (see Chapter 3 Infectious Diseases, page 75).
- Sarcoidosis (associated with parotitis).
- Tumour of the pons (children usually also have a sixth nerve palsy).
- Idiopathic (Bell palsy).

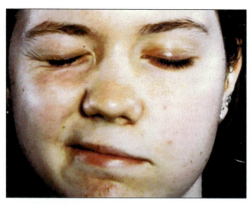
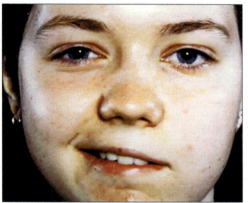
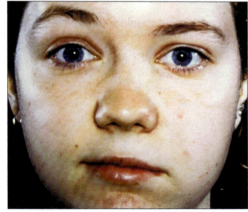
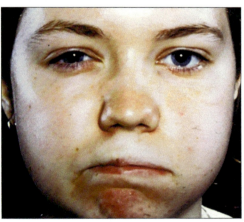

FIGURES 8.18–8.21 Left lower motor neuron facial palsy in a child. **8.18**: Her mouth does not move on the left when asked to show her teeth; **8.19**: she cannot fully close the left eye; **8.20**: her left eyebrow does not move when asked to look surprised; **8.21**: the left cheek does not move when asked to blow out her cheeks. Note the very obvious abnormality involving both upper and lower face. Titres to *Mycoplasma pneumoniae* and *Borrelia burgdorferi* were raised. The facial palsy had almost completely recovered 48 hours after the start of azithromycin and high-dose amoxycillin.

Bilateral in a previously well child

(Often associated with other lower cranial nerve signs – bulbar palsy (see **Fig. 8.29**).

- Guillain–Barré syndrome (see **Fig. 8.39**).
- Myasthenia.
- Mitochondrial disease (ptosis and ophthalmoplegia are often also prominent, see 'Ptosis').
- Bell palsy (and other causes of unilateral facial palsy, including infections) may be bilateral.
- Brainstem lesion.

MANAGEMENT

Newborn

Clinically, it is important to distinguish between facial palsy and hypoplasia of the depressor angularis oris in asymmetric crying facies. EMG and nerve conduction studies may be needed to distinguish between a slowly resolving traumatic lesion and a congenital abnormality. Imaging of the base of the brain may be required. Occasionally, an injured facial nerve may require surgical repair if there is no recovery by 3 months. Cosmetic surgery usually offers a considerable improvement in facial appearance in congenital lesions, but may not be advisable until late childhood.

Previously well child

Lubricating eye drops and patching are important in preventing damage to the cornea.

Antibiotics should be used for otitis media or if there is a suspicion of mycoplasma or Lyme disease; azithromycin and high-dose amoxycillin is typically used. Hypertension should be appropriately investigated and managed. Aciclovir should be considered if a viral aetiology is suspected and immunoglobulins are indicated for Kawasaki disease. Steroids are of no long-term benefit.

PROGNOSIS

There is usually a good recovery.

UPPER MOTOR NEURON FACIAL PALSY

An upper motor neuron facial palsy is often mild (**Fig. 8.22**). The eye is usually not involved because of the bilateral innervation of the upper part of the face (**Fig. 8.23**). The child usually smiles normally (**Fig. 8.24**). Upper motor neuron facial palsies may also be bilateral (**Fig. 8.25**).

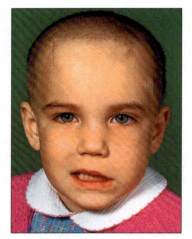

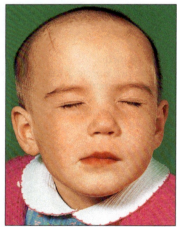

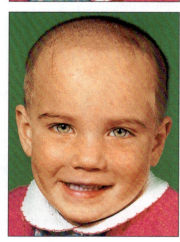

FIGURES 8.22–8.24 Upper motor neuron facial palsy. **8.22–8.24**: Unilateral in a child recovering from a cerebral abscess. The asymmetry of the lower face is obvious when the child is asked to show her teeth (**8.22**), but the upper face is not involved and she is able to close both eyes normally (**8.23**), and the palsy is not obvious with spontaneous emotion (e.g. when she smiles, **8.24**).

UNILATERAL

Causes

- Involvement of the pyramidal tract above the facial nerve nucleus in acute stroke or space occupying lesion (**Figs 8.22–8.24**) (usually in association with a hemiparesis).
- Lesion of the pons (in association with sixth nerve palsy: **Fig. 8.14**).
- An apparently isolated upper motor neuron facial palsy is not uncommon in children with hippocampal sclerosis (see **Fig. 8.93**) causing intractable epilepsy and maybe a useful lateralising sign.

Bilateral

Children with a spastic quadriparesis commonly have bilateral upper motor neuron facial weakness and bulbar palsy (**Fig. 8.25**).

LOWER CRANIAL NERVE ABNORMALITIES

CLINICAL PRESENTATION

These are usually bilateral, almost always involving several cranial nerves with bilateral involvement of the seventh, ninth, tenth, eleventh and twelfth nuclei together (**Figs 8.25, 8.26**). The weakness may be in upper (**Fig. 8.25**) or lower (**Figs 8.26, 8.27**) motor neurons. Sucking, swallowing and speech are commonly affected. There may be deviation of the uvula in a unilateral lesion (**Fig. 8.28**) causing oromotor dyspraxia. A twelfth nerve palsy (**Fig. 8.29**) may be seen if there is a carotid lesion (e.g. occlusion or dissection).

CAUSES

- Lower motor neuron (bulbar palsy, **Fig. 8.26**) – as for bilateral lower motor neuron facial weakness.
- Upper motor neuron (pseudobulbar palsy, **Fig. 8.25**) – as for bilateral upper motor neuron facial palsy. The Worster–Drought syndrome is a form of cerebral palsy (page 225) involving predominantly the bulbar muscles.

TREATMENT/PROGNOSIS

Management of feeding and speech difficulties is required. The problems often improve with careful management and with time, but there are usually residual difficulties.

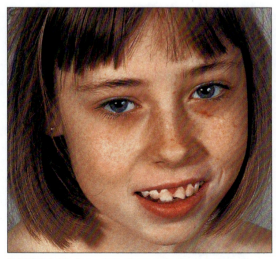

FIGURE 8.25 Pseudobulbar palsy in a child with upper motor neuron cerebral palsy. She had early feeding difficulties and now has bilateral facial weakness and dysarthria.

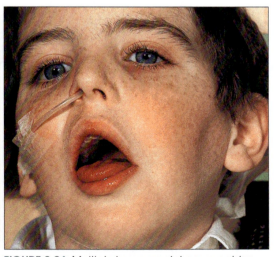

FIGURE 8.26 Multiple lower cranial nerve palsies in a child with a posterior circulation stroke with infarction involving the cerebellum and occipital lobes. There is a bilateral fifth cranial nerve motor weakness evident in the slack jaw, bilateral facial palsy, bulbar palsy (evidenced by the feeding tube) and flaccid tongue weakness.

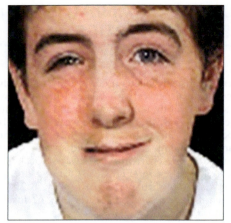

FIGURE 8.27 The same child as in **8.26** made a gradual recovery and had relatively minor difficulties at follow-up 5 years later, although he had an unrecognised visual field defect (see **8.1, 8.2** for testing).

MOTOR SYSTEM

In a child, examination of the motor system is usually performed in the following order:

1. **General observation:** e.g. for wasting (**Fig. 8.30**), immobility, obvious unwanted movements such as ballismus, chorea or tics, or abnormal facial, limb, trunk or tongue movement, such as dyskinesia, dystonia (**Fig. 8.31**) or fasciculation. Observe the pattern of breathing (e.g. diaphragmatic breathing in spinal muscular atrophy [SMA], paradoxical breathing with diaphragmatic weakness).

2. **Gait:** habitually stressed by walking on the toes or heels or running; heel-to-toe test along a line to bring out ataxia. Observe the child hopping (if able) and jumping. Ask the child to sit cross legged or lie supine on the floor, then rise to standing as quickly as possible to examine for proximal weakness (Gowers sign, see **Fig. 8.58**). The following are common:
   - Hemiplegia, with circumduction of affected foot and often dystonic posturing of the hand.
   - Diplegia.
   - Ataxia.

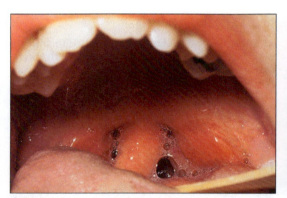

FIGURE 8.28 Deviation of the uvula in a child recovering from a bulbar palsy.

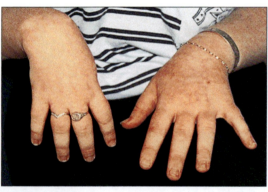

FIGURE 8.30 Wasting of the right hand in a child with a congenital hemiparesis and epilepsy.

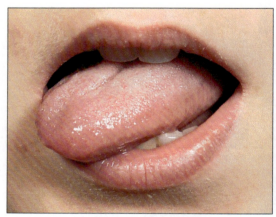

FIGURE 8.29 Twelfth nerve palsy with wasting of the right side and deviation towards that side in a child who had carotid occlusion after a quinsy (see Figs **8.4, 8.5** for associated Horner syndrome).

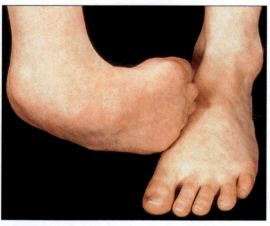

FIGURE 8.31 Severe fixed dystonia of the foot in a teenage girl who disclosed sexual abuse 3 years later.

- A positive Gowers manouevre (see **Fig. 8.58**) (using the hands to 'climb up the legs' when rising from the floor) in neuromuscular disorders such as Guillain–Barré syndrome, Duchenne dystrophy, SMA Type 3, congenital myopathies, spinal cord disorders.

3. **Posture:** ask the child to stand with his feet together, to stretch his arms out with his fingers stretched wide apart and to keep his eyes closed. Even young children can maintain this for a few minutes. The following may be observed:
   - Inability to maintain the posture.
   - Drift downwards and dystonic posturing of one arm in a unilateral pyramidal lesion (hemiparesis).
   - Dyskinetic posturing, e.g. in Wilson disease.
   - Chorea or ballismus.
   - Tremor, e.g. pill-rolling in Wilson disease.
   - Falling over in a child with loss of position sense.

4. **Finger-to-nose testing and heel-to-shin testing:** ask the child to touch his nose and then your finger with the index finger of the same hand to bring out ataxia (with past pointing) or dystonia (usually terminal shake with no past pointing).

5. **Formal examination of all four limbs:** examining for asymmetry, wasting, fasciculation, tone, power, co-ordination and reflexes.

PYRAMIDAL DISORDERS

In a long-standing pyramidal disorder, there is 'clasp-knife' rigidity accompanied by increased tendon reflexes and upgoing plantar responses. For further details, see Cerebral palsy (page 225) – spastic hemiplegia and quadriparesis.

Acutely, hypotonia and hyporeflexia are characteristic (see Stroke, page 246, and Spinal cord disorders, page 217).

EXTRAPYRAMIDAL DISORDERS

The diagnosis of an extrapyramidal disorder is often made simply by observing the posture of the child at rest. Extrapyramidal disorders improve during sleep and examination under anaesthesia may be required to assess whether or not a deformity is fixed. The slow writhing movements of athetosis are a form of dystonia and may be distinguished from the rapid movements of chorea, although the two may occur together. There may be more difficulty in distinguishing some of the other movement disorders (see **Table 8.1**).

TABLE 8.1 Distinguishing between movement disorders

		Tremor	Chorea	Dystonia	Tics	Myoclonus	Ataxia
Action	Rest	+	(+)	(+)	+	(+)	
	Action		+	+		+	+
Speed	Fast	+	+		+	+	
	Slow			+			+
Complexity	Simple	+			+	+	+
	Complex		+	+			
Site	Proximal	+	+	+	+	+	
	Distal		+		+	+	+
Type	Stereotyped	+			+	+	+
	Variable		+	+			

WILSON DISEASE

See also Chapter 14 Metabolic Diseases.

INCIDENCE

One in 30,000. It is an autosomal recessive disease; *ATP78* gene on 13q. Age of onset is 4–50 years (neurological presentation is rare under 8 years, but possible in patients over 4 years of age).

CLINICAL PRESENTATION

- Facial immobility.
- Rigidity.
- Dyskinesia.
- Dysarthria.
- Dysphagia.
- Tremor, especially of the wrist and shoulder (usually pill-rolling).
- Behavioural difficulties with aggression, euphoria, immaturity.
- Kayser–Fleischer ring at the limbus of the cornea(always in patients with neurological presentation) (**Fig. 8.32**).
- Liver disease.
- Haemolytic anaemia.

INVESTIGATIONS

- Serum copper <7.8 mmol/L and caeruloplasmin <100 mg/L.
- 24 hour urinary copper excretion >100 mg.
- Liver biopsy if high clinical index of suspicion and above investigations are normal.
- Neuroimaging may show low density in deep grey matter.

TREATMENT

- D-penicillamine (start slowly, as clinical deterioration is common at the start of treatment).
- Trientine.
- Pyridoxine and zinc supplementation.
- Steroids may be useful if the patient has mild symptoms of hypersensitivity on penicillamine.

SYDENHAM CHOREA AND OTHER POSTSTREPTOCOCCAL MOVEMENT DISORDERS

CLINICAL SIGNS

- Chorea, typically bilateral, and often involving the face and toes as well as the fingers.
- Dystonia (**Fig. 8.33**).
- Behavioural abnormalities – obsessive–compulsive, emotional lability (paediatric autoimmune neuropsychiatric disorders associated with streptococcal infections, PANDAS).

INVESTIGATIONS

- Antistreptococcal titre, anti DNAase B, antibasal ganglia antibodies.
- ECG and ECHO.
- MRI may show abnormality.

TREATMENT

- Long-term penicillin.
- Carbamezepine.
- Haloperidol.
- Trial of steroids in severe cases.
- Psychiatric and psychological support.

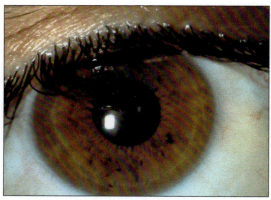

FIGURE 8.32 Wilson disease. Kayser–Fleischer ring in a child.

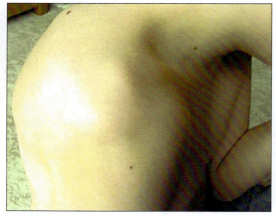

FIGURE 8.33 Severe dystonia of the shoulder causing dislocation in a boy who also had an obsessive–compulsive disorder. He had had previous aseptic meningitis and raised antistreptolysin O titre but negative anti-NMDA antibodies. He responded to penicillin, steroids and psychological input and made a full recovery.

ANTI-N-METHYL-D-ASPARTATE RECEPTOR (NMDAR) ENCEPHALITIS

CLINICAL SIGNS

- Acute encephalopathy with a prominent movement disorder, typically orofacial dyskinesia, dystonia and chorea.
- Psychiatric symptoms include personality change, irritability, anxiety, aggressive behaviour, delusional thoughts, and short-term memory loss.
- Partial or generalised seizure activity may occur.
- Majority are girls, typically presenting after infections.

INVESTIGATIONS

- Anti-NMDAR antibodies in serum.
- Ovarian teratoma is unusual in young girls but must be excluded, especially in teenagers; resolution of movement disorder is common following removal.
- Imaging may show non-specific changes.

TREATMENT

The condition may be self-limiting but typically responds to steroids, immunoglobulin, plasmapheresis and cyclophosphamide.

SANDIFER SYNDROME

Posturing in children with gastro-oesophageal reflux, usually in the context of an underlying movement disorder, is one of the commonest treatable causes of dystonia. Medical treatment may include compound alginate, omeprazole, lanzoprazole or ranitidine. Appropriate seating during and after feeding and passage of a nasojejunal tube may be helpful and fundoplication may be necessary.

SEGAWA SYNDROME (DOPA-RESPONSIVE DYSTONIA)

GENETICS

This syndrome is autosomal-dominant with reduced penetrance. Mutation is in the gene coding for guanosinetriphosphate cyclohydrolase I, the rate-limiting step for tetrahydrobiopterin (cofactor for phenylalanine, tyrosine and tryptophan, mono-oxygenases).

CLINICAL

- Dystonia, often worse in the evening.
- Equinovarus posturing of the foot (see **Fig. 8.37**).
- Gait disturbance.
- Ankle clonus (unsustained).
- Extensor posturing of the big toe (see **Fig. 8.34**).
- Spasticity.

INVESTIGATIONS

- Exclude alternative causes, especially Wilson disease.
- DNA for genetic testing.
- Trial of levodopa.

TREATMENT

Levodopa/carbidopa in doses of up to 100/25 mg tds.

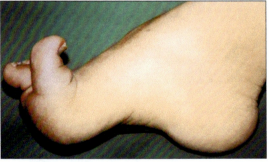

FIGURE 8.34 Extensor toe in a teenager suggests Segawa syndrome.

Causes of dystonia and/or chorea

- Hypoxic–ischaemic damage (may be delayed or worsen after initial stability).
- Bronchopulmonary dysplasia.
- Post cardiopulmonary bypass.
- Intracranial trauma (may be delayed).
- Wilson disease (**Fig. 8.32**).
- Anti-NMDAR antibody encephalitis.
- Extensor toe in a teenager suggests Segawa syndrome (**Fig. 8.34**).
- Poststreptococcal (**Figs 8.33, 8.35**).
- Cerebrovascular disease, e.g. moyamoya (see 'Stroke' page 246, **Fig. 8.125**).
- Ataxia telangiectasia (see 'Ataxia', **Fig. 8.36**).
- GM1 and GM2 gangliosidoses.
- Mitochondrial disease (e.g. Leigh syndrome).
- Pantothenate kinase-associated neurodegeneration (PKAN): an autosomal recessive disorder of coenzyme A homeostasis caused by defects in mitochondrial pantothenate kinase 2 gene (previously known as Hallervordan–Spatz disease).
- Huntington chorea.

Management

- **Clinical:** prepare an accurate description of movement disorder and any associated behavioural manifestation (video and further opinions may be helpful); slit-lamp examination by an ophthalmologist for Kayser–Fleischer rings.
- **Initial investigations:** neuroimaging (including magnetic resonance angiography, MRA), plasma copper and caeruloplasmin, antistreptolysin O titre, plasma amino acids, urine organic acids, plasma lactate, alpha fetoprotein. May need CSF lactate, white cell enzymes, pH studies and barium swallow, DNA testing for Huntington chorea or ataxia telangiectasia if clinically indicated.
- **Long-term:** appropriate treatment of underlying cause (**Table 8.2**), trial of levodopa for dystonia, anticholinergics (e.g. trihexyphenidyl). In severe extrapyramidal disorders, appropriate seating and treatment of Sandifer syndrome, i.e. gastro-oesophageal reflux, may produce improvement and diazepam may reduce dystonic spasms while oral baclofen may reduce associated spasticity. For severe dystonia intrathecal baclofen or deep brain stimulation may be offered in specialist centres.

TABLE 8.2 Treatable causes of extrapyramidal abnormalities

Condition	Diagnostic test	Treatment
Wilson disease	Plasma copper, caeruloplasmin	Penicillamine
Sydenham chorea	Antistreptococcal titre, anti DNAase B	Penicillin
Segawa syndrome	Trial of L-DOPA, guanosine triphosphate cyclohydrolase I gene	L-DOPA
Anti-NMDA encephalitis	Anti-NMDA antibodies	Steroids, immunoglobulin, cyclophosphamide
Systemic lupus erythematosus	Antinuclear antibodies, anti-double-stranded DNA autoantibodies	Immunosuppression
Moyamoya (see 'Stroke')	MR angiography	Revascularisation
Arteriovenous malformation	Contrast CT, MRI, conventional arteriography	Surgery, embolisation, radiotherapy
Tumour	Neuroimaging	Radiotherapy
Glutaric aciduria type I	Urinary organic acids	Protein restriction, carnitine
Homocystinuria	Plasma total homocysteine, methionine	Pyridoxine, methionine restriction, betaine
Infections	Mycoplasma, CMV, HIV	Antimicrobials
Drugs and toxins	Urine and blood screening	Withdrawal
Conversion disorder (hysteria)	Exclusion of alternatives, observation	Rehabilitation
Sandifer syndrome (reflux)	pH studies, barium swallow	Omeprazole, Nissen fundoplication

Although ataxia implies a cerebellar lesion, it may be difficult to distinguish cerebellar ataxia from a peripheral neuropathy, action myoclonus or dystonia in a young child. Horizontal nystagmus and past-pointing suggest involvement of the cerebellum, whereas areflexia indicates a peripheral neuropathy (see also Extrapyramidal disorders).

CAUSES OF ACUTE ATAXIA

- Posterior fossa space occupying lesion (may be accompanied by head tilt) (see **Fig. 8.74**):
  - ○ tumour (e.g. medulloblastoma, astrocytoma, see **Fig. 8.76**);
  - ○ extradural or subdural haematoma;
  - ○ cerebral infarction (**Figs 8.26, 8.27,** see **Figs 8.112–8.125**).
- Acute cerebellitis (e.g. mycoplasma).
- Postinfectious cerebellitis (e.g. chickenpox).
- Guillain–Barré syndrome (see 'Acute weakness' page 215).
- Drugs and toxins (e.g. phenytoin, carbamezepine, lead).

CAUSES OF NON-PROGRESSIVE CHRONIC ATAXIA

- Cerebellar malformations.
- Ataxic cerebral palsy (often accompanied by epilepsy and parietal lesions on neuroimaging).

CAUSES OF PROGRESSIVE ATAXIA

- Ataxia telangiectasia (AT) (**Fig. 8.36**).
- Ataxia–oculomotor apraxia (also abnormality of AT gene).
- Metachromatic leukodystrophy, other leukodystrophies.
- Friedreich ataxia (FA) – abnormality of frataxin gene (**Fig. 8.37**).
- Early onset ataxia with preserved deep tendon reflexes (also abnormality of frataxin gene).
- Hereditary sensory and motor neuropathies (**Fig. 8.38**) (see also Chronic progressive weakness).
- GM1 and GM2 gangliosidoses.

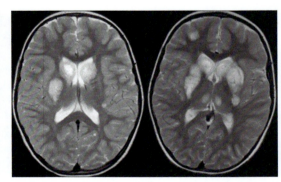

FIGURE 8.35 Relapsing dystonia in a child whose only abnormality was a raised antistreptolysin O titre and who developed progressive basal ganglia abnormality on MRI.

INVESTIGATIONS

See **Table 8.3**.

- Neuroimaging. This should be urgent if there is reduced visual acuity (secondary to raised intracranial pressure), vomiting or headache. It should be avoided if the patient is areflexic and clinically has a peripheral neuropathy or telangiectasia in view of the chromosomal fragility in AT.
- CSF glucose to exclude glut-1 deficiency.
- Biotinidase.
- Nerve conduction studies to diagnose peripheral neuropathy and to distinguish from FA.
- Alpha-fetoprotein and immunoglobulins to screen for AT.
- White blood cell chromosome fragility (AT), DNA for genetic testing if a high index of suspicion of AT or FA; urine amino and organic acids, plasma amino acids; plasma and CSF lactate, biotinidase; phytanic acid; triglycerides and lipoproteins; white cell enzymes.

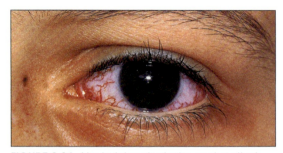

FIGURE 8.36 Ataxia telangiectasia; conjunctival telangiectasia.

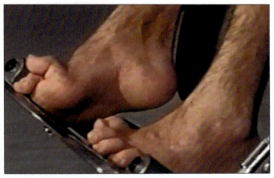

FIGURE 8.37 Pes cavus in Friedrich ataxia.

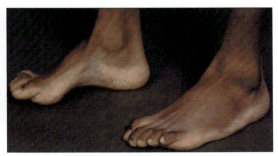

FIGURE 8.38 Pes cavus in hereditary sensory motor neuropathy (CMT).

Ataxia

213

TABLE 8.3 Treatable causes of intermittent or progressive ataxia

Condition	Diagnosis	Treatment
Posterior fossa tumour	Neuroimaging	See 'Brain tumours'
Drugs and toxins	Urine drug screen	Stop drugs
Glucose transporter deficiency	Low CSF glucose	Ketogenic diet
Biotinidase deficiency (see 'Epilepsy')	Urine organic acids Plasma biotinidase	Biotin
Primary vitamin E deficiency	Plasma vitamin E	Vitamin E
Secondary vitamin E deficiency Abetalipoproteinaemia Hypobetalipoproteinaemia Alpha-tocopherol transfer protein	Plasma vitamin E Acanthocytosis Plasma triglycerides Plasma lipoproteins Genetics	Vitamin E (+A+K)
Friedreich ataxia	Frataxin gene	Nicotinamide Erythropoietin
Hartnup disease	Urine amino acids	Nicotinamide
Maple syrup urine disease	Urine amino acids	Thiamine
Hereditary paroxysmal cerebellar ataxia	Gene on 19q	Acetazolamide
Refsum disease	Plasma phytanic acid	Dietary
Pyruvate dehydrogenase complex deficiency	Plasma/CSF lactate Enzyme assay Gene on Xp22	Thiamine may help

ATAXIA TELANGIECTASIA

See also Chapter 16 Immunology, page 494.

AETIOLOGY

AT is autosomal recessive, caused by mutations in the *ATM* gene on 11q22-23. ATM protein is required for DNA repair. The protein is similar to mammalian phosphatidylinositol-3' kinase.

CLINICAL FEATURES

- Oculomotor apraxia.
- Telangiectasia – conjunctiva (**Fig. 8.36**) and upper face.
- Truncal ataxia due to loss of Purkinje cells.
- Dysarthria.
- Choreoathetosis/dystonia.
- Thymic hypoplasia with low IgA, IgG and IgM.
- Recurrent chest infections, bronchiectasis.
- Lymphoma, leukaemia.
- Premature senescence.
- Insulin-resistant diabetes.

DIAGNOSIS

- High alpha-fetoprotein.
- Immunoglobulin deficiency.
- White blood cell chromosome fragility.
- *ATM* gene on 11q22-23.
- MRI shows cerebellar degeneration; may show leukodystrophy.

MANAGEMENT/PROGNOSIS

- Antibiotics are used for infections.
- Avoidance of radiation for diagnosis or treatment of neoplasia.

Prognosis depends on the frequency of infections and/or occurence of neoplasia.

FRIEDREICH ATAXIA

AETIOLOGY

FA occurs in 1 in 8,000. It is autosomal recessive, with reduplication of the GAA sequence in intron 1 of the frataxin gene on 9q. Reduplication reduces frataxin, the protein associated with mitochondrial membranes and crests. It may reduce oxidative stress by preventing iron accumulation. The size of expansion (120–1,700 repeats) is related to the patient's age at onset.

CLINICAL SIGNS

- Ataxia – mixed sensory and cerebellar.
- Speech – scanning dysarthria, then slurred.
- Intention tremor, clumsiness of hands.
- Nystagmus (relatively rare).
- Fatigue.
- Cardiac symptoms secondary to cardiomyopathy.
- Pes cavus (**Fig. 8.37**).
- Loss of position and vibration sensation, particularly in the legs.
- Loss of tendon jerks (classically absent at ankle, brisk at knee).
- Extensor plantar responses (pyramidal involvement, as for brisk knee jerks).
- Scoliosis.
- Diabetes.
- Optic atrophy.
- Deafness.

DIAGNOSIS

- ECG, ECHO.
- Nerve conduction – reduced amplitude sensory nerve action potential; reduced velocity motor and sensory conduction.
- Frataxin gene on 9q.

MANAGEMENT

- Multidisciplinary, treating cardiomyopathy, scoliosis, motor disorder and diabetes.
- Nicotinamide, gamma interferon and erythropoietin may increase frataxin levels.
- Chelation therapies may reduce iron accumulation and improve function in the early stages.

Larger scale clinical trials are awaited to confirm the effectiveness of these therapies.

Death from cardiac complications occurs in early or middle adult life.

ACUTE GENERALISED WEAKNESS IN A PREVIOUSLY WELL CHILD

CAUSES

- Guillain–Barré syndrome (**Fig. 8.39**).
- Cervical cord lesion (e.g. transverse myelitis, stroke, trauma, tumour – **Fig. 8.40**).
- Poliomyelitis (including vaccine-associated; usually asymmetrical weakness.) and other viruses, e.g. non-polio enterovirus such as Coxsackie and Echo, adenoviruses, Japanese B encephalitis virus.
- Dermatomyositis (**Figs 8.41–8.43**).
- Viral myositis.
- MG (see 'Ptosis', **Figs 8.12, 8.13**).
- Botulism – associated with fixed, dilated pupils.
- Other toxins (e.g. lead, vincristine).
- Acute presentation of chronic weakness (e.g. hereditary sensory motor neuropathy, Charcot–Marie–Tooth disease [CMT] – **Fig. 8.38**).

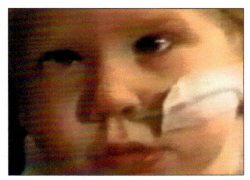

FIGURE 8.39 Obvious left sixth nerve palsy (on formal testing of eye movements, patient had more extensive ophthalmoplegia), bilateral facial nerve weakness and bulbar palsy requiring nasogastric feeding, in a child with the Miller–Fisher variant of Guillain–Barré syndrome.

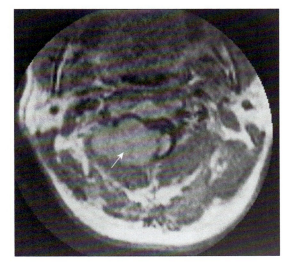

FIGURE 8.40 A neurofibroma at C1 pushing the cord over. This type of lesion can occasionally cause a flaccid quadriparesis and if there is any doubt about the diagnosis of Guillain–Barré, MRI of the neck should be considered, especially if there is bladder involvement.

CLINICAL

- Ascending weakness, starting in feet and legs and progressing to hands and arms and then to respiratory muscles and cranial nerves, strongly suggests Guillain–Barré syndrome.
- Descending weakness starting in cranial nerves strongly suggests the Miller–Fisher variant of Guillain–Barré syndrome (**Fig. 8.39**).
- Spinal cord disease should be excluded as quickly as possible if there is acute flaccid weakness with rapid onset, especially if there is bladder involvement (**Figs 8.40, 8.44–8.46**).
- Asymmetrical flaccid weakness suggests viral infection secondary to polio and non-polio enteroviruses (**Fig. 8.59**).
- Pain suggests myositis in acute viral myositis, polymyositis or dermatomyositis (**Figs 8.41–8.43**) although there may be pain in Guillain–Barré syndrome.

INVESTIGATIONS

- MRI cervical spine if suspicion of cord lesion such a tumour, stroke or transverse myelitis, e.g. if there is bladder involvement (**Fig. 8.40**).
- Creatine phosphokinase (CPK) and EMG to help diagnose dermatomyositis or viral myositis (**Figs 8.41–8.43**).
- Nerve conduction studies to diagnose Guillain–Barré syndrome; may be normal in initial phase of illness and in the Miller–Fisher variant; **Fig. 8.39**); other conditions (e.g. botulism) may have characteristic neurophysiological features.
- Exclusion of myasthenia (see Bilateral ptosis, **Figs 8.8–8.13**).
- CSF is not usually necessary if the clinical diagnosis is clearly ascending weakness consistent with Guillain–Barré syndrome as the protein is not raised until a few days after onset, but should be considered with PCR for a variety of viruses if there are unusual features, e.g. asymmetry suggestive of polio or other viral causes of acute flaccid paralysis.

MANAGEMENT

- Assessment of respiratory function and reserve. Vital capacity using a spirometer should be performed regularly if the child is unventilated and can co-operate.
- Assisted ventilation if there is evidence of increasing respiratory failure, rapid general deterioration or signs likely to be associated with respiratory failure (e.g. ascent of paralysis to cranial nerve involvement in Guillain–Barré syndrome although most children with the Miller–Fisher variant [**Fig. 8.39**] do not require ventilation).
- Treatment of cause (e.g. surgery for spinal cord tumour [**Fig. 8.40**], immunosuppression for dermatomyositis (**Figs 8.41–8.43**), immunoglobulin (and/or plasmapheresis) for Guillain–Barré syndrome if continuing to deteriorate and/or respiratory compromise).
- Physiotherapy and occupational therapy.

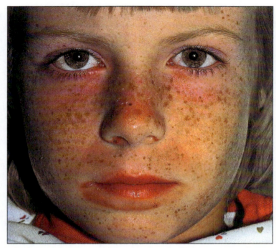

FIGURE 8.41 Dermatomyositis; heliotrope rash in a child. Note the characteristic serious expression.

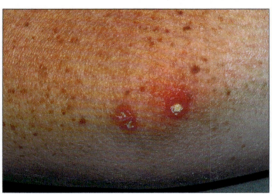

FIGURE 8.42 Dermatomyostis; nodular calcification of the skin over the elbow.

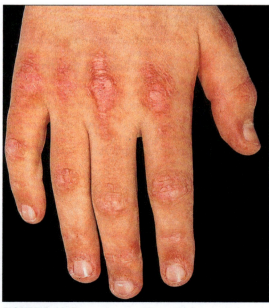

FIGURE 8.43 Dermatomyositis; collodion patches over the finger joints.

Neurology

GUILLAIN–BARRÉ SYNDROME

Incidence is 0.6–1.1/100,000 children.

PATHOLOGY

Inflammatory demyelinating polyradiculoneuropathy in most patients. Preceding infections include *Campylobacter*, CMV, EBV.

CLINICAL SYMPTOMS AND SIGNS

- Pain.
- Ascending weakness.
- Ataxia.
- Respiratory weakness.
- Bulbar weakness.
- Bilateral facial weakness (**Fig. 8.39**).
- Ophthalmoplegia.

MANAGEMENT

- Admission and close observation, particularly of respiratory and cardiac function.
- Intravenous immunoglobulin if there is rapidly ascending weakness, the child is not walking or is likely to require ventilation.
- Plasmapheresis if immunoglobulin does not arrest deterioration or lead to improvement.
- Ventilation for respiratory failure.
- Pacing for cardiac dysrrhythmias.
- Physiotherapy to prevent contractures and aid mobilisation during recovery.

DERMATOMYOSITIS

PRESENTATION

General misery, generalised weakness and pain, heliotrope rash over the eyelids (**Fig. 8.41**), elbows, and knees. Calcinosis over the joints in chronic cases (e.g. the elbow) (**Fig. 8.42**). Collodion patches over extensor surface of the fingers (**Fig. 8.43**).

INVESTIGATIONS

ESR and plasma CK are usually elevated, but not invariably. Muscle biopsy shows increased HLA class I antigen expression. Inflammatory changes may be patchy.

MANAGEMENT

- Immunosuppression with methotrexate or oral steroids, azathioprine and ciclosporin A. Intravenous immunoglobulin.

SPINAL CORD DISORDERS

- Acute spinal cord injury usually occurs in the context of trauma. As there may be no bony injury, all children involved in significant trauma should be nursed flat and in a stiff collar until they are conscious enough to confirm that there is no pain in the neck or back indicative of ligamentous injury and instability.
- Chronic spinal cord injury may occur in children with skeletal deformities and may present with the insidious onset of pyramidal and/or lower motor neuron and sensory signs (**Fig. 8.44**).
- Tumours, e.g. extradural in the context of neurofibromatosis (**Fig. 8.40**), or intradural (extra- or intramedullary) (**Fig. 8.45**), may present with pain, stiffness, focal neurological deficit or bladder symptoms. Diagnosis is usually made with MRI of the spine, which is indicated urgently in

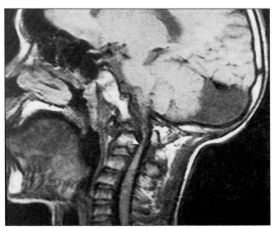

FIGURE 8.44 Conradi syndrome; thinning of the cord in the high cervical region.

a unit where the child can be surgically decompressed if there is recent deterioration.

- Syringomyelia (**Fig. 8.46**) may occur spontaneously or secondary to tumours (**Fig. 8.45**) or in the context of spina bifida (**Figs 8.62, 8.63**).
- Transverse myelitis may be clinically similar, but can be distinguished on MRI. Methyl prednisolone should be given as soon as possible as there is evidence for improved outcome compared with historical controls.
- Discitis is usually painful.

PREDISPOSING SYNDROMES

- Down syndrome.
- Neurofibromatosis (**Fig. 8.40**).
- Mucopolysaccharidoses.
- Achondroplasia.
- Goldenhar syndrome.
- Klippel–Feil syndrome.
- Conradi syndrome (**Fig. 8.44**).
- Coffin–Lowry syndrome.

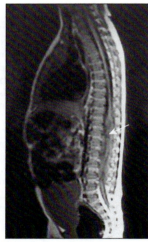

FIGURE 8.45 Cord tumour, probably ependymoma.

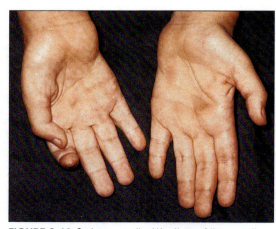

FIGURE 8.46 Syringomyelia. Wasting of the small muscles of the hands, worse on the right.

HYPOTONIA IN INFANCY

CLINICAL SIGNS

- History of maternal illness (e.g. MG, myotonic dystrophy), other family, pregnancy and birth history, fetal movements and presence of poyhydramnios.
- Examination of infant, noting alertness, ability to fix and follow, any distinctive features (e.g. trisomy 21, Prader–Willi syndrome), ptosis, facial (**Fig. 8.47**) and bulbar weakness (difficulty feeding/swallowing secretions), tongue fasciculation (in SMA), posture (**Figs 8.48, 8.51–8.54**), presence of contractures/scoliosis, degree of truncal and limb weakness, reflexes.
- Examination of the mother, for signs of myotonic dystrophy (ability to bury eyelashes (**Figs 8.49, 8.50**), grip myotonia although the ward setting may be too warm to demonstrate difficulty in releasing grip) or myasthenia (**Figs 8.12, 8.13**; ptosis and fatiguable weakness).

Causes of weakness in infancy

- Congenital myotonic dystrophy (**Figs 8.47, 8.48, 8.51, 8.52**).
- SMA types 1 and 2 (**Fig. 8.51**).
- SMARD1 (SMA with respiratory distress due to diaphragmatic weakness).
- Congenital muscular dystrophies: Ullrich (UCMD), merosin deficient (MDC1A).
- Dystroglycanopathies (muscle–eye–brain disease, Walker Warburg syndrome).
- Congenital myopathies:
  - Pompe disease (glycogen storage disease type II).
  - Nemaline myopathy.
  - Myotubular myopathy.
- Congenital and neonatal myasthenia.
- Botulism.
- Congenital hypomyelinating neuropathies.
- Spinal cord disease:
  - Birth trauma (**Fig. 8.52**).
  - Congenital malformation.
- Central:
  - Chromosomal.
  - Down syndrome: trisomy 21.
  - Prader–Willi (**Fig. 8.53**): genomic imprinting with interstitial deletion in paternal 15q1.1-1.3 and uniparental disomy.
  - Metabolic.
  - Peroxisomal: Zellweger syndrome (**Fig. 8.54**), neonatal adrenoleukodystrophy.
  - Amino acidurias.
  - Organic acidurias.
  - Mitochondrial disorders.
  - Structural brain malformation.
  - Cerebral haemorrhage.
  - Sepsis.

Neurology

INVESTIGATIONS

- Genetic studies for characteristic condition, (e.g. myotonic dystrophy – **Figs 8.47–8.50**, SMA – **Fig. 8.51**, Prader–Willi – **Fig. 8.53**).
- Plasma CK.
- ECHO (e.g. for Pompe).
- X-ray of the knee to look for patellar calcification/stippling in peroxisomal disorders, e.g. Zellweger syndrome (**Fig. 8.54**).
- Appropriate biochemistry for metabolic condition (e.g. very long chain fatty acids for peroxisomal disorders [**Fig. 8.54**] or plasma/CSF lactate for mitochondrial disease).
- EMG and nerve conduction studies. Stimulation single fibre EMG +/–repetitive nerve stimulation for myasthenia.
- Neuroimaging of brain to exclude structural brain abnormality, either isolated or in association with muscle disease (e.g. Walker Warburg congenital muscular dystrophy, muscle–eye–brain disease) and of spine to exclude birth trauma (**Fig. 8.52**).
- Muscle biopsy may be needed if diagnosis cannot be secured by an alternative method.
- Stool for clostridium botulinum.

MYOTONIC DYSTROPHY (DM1)

INCIDENCE

DM1 occurs in 1 in 7,500. It is autosomal dominant, inherited from the mother if the neonate is affected. It is due to expansion of a triplet repeat (CTG) in the 3'-untranslated region of the *DMPK* (myotonin protein kinase gene) on chromosome 19q13, disrupting mRNA metabolism.

CLINICAL PRESENTATION

DM1 may present in the neonatal period (congenital myotonic dystrophy) with severe weakness, respiratory insufficiency, facial weakness (**Fig. 8.47**) with characteristic 'tent-shaped' mouth and arthrogryposis (talipes equinovarus is particularly common, **Fig. 8.48**) (maternal inheritance; **Figs 8.49, 8.50**). Limb weakness improves during infancy, but facial weakness persists and these children have learning difficulties, which may be severe. The milder, 'adult' form of myotonic dystrophy (paternal > maternal inheritance) usually presents in later childhood with mild distal limb and characteristic facial weakness,

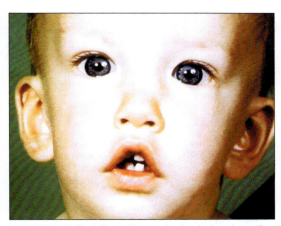

FIGURE 8.47 Toddler with myotonic dystrophy with characteristic myopathic facies.

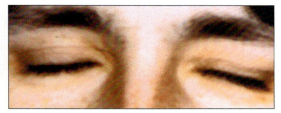

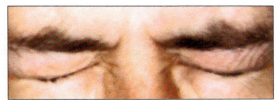

FIGURES 8.49, 8.50 Mother cannot bury her eyelashes (**8.49**), but father can bury his normally (**8.50**).

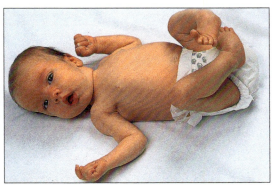

FIGURE 8.48 Infant with myotonic dystrophy with characteristic decreased tone, bilateral talipes and fish-shaped mouth.

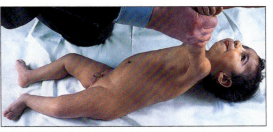

FIGURE 8.51 Infant with spinal muscular atrophy showing truncal and limb hypotonia, bell-shaped chest, frog-legged posture and preserved facial movement with alert expression; tongue fasciculation is also characteristic.

grip myotonia with difficulty releasing the clenched fist – worse in cold weather, early cataracts, cardiac arrhythmias and often mild learning difficulties. In males, frontal balding and testicular atrophy develop in adulthood.

DIAGNOSIS

- DMPK gene analysis should be obtained in characteristic cases.
- EMG shows myopathic features with myotonic discharges ('dive bomber') in older children and adults.

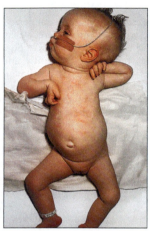

FIGURE 8.52 Infant with hypotonia and abnormal posturing of the hands secondary to a cervical cord lesion.

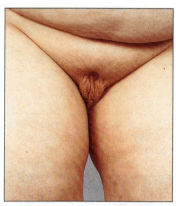

FIGURE 8.53 Microgenitalia in a boy with Prader–Willi syndrome.

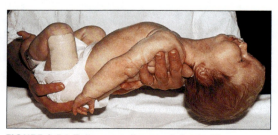

FIGURE 8.54 Zellweger disease: infant with profound hypotonia.

SPINAL MUSCULAR ATROPHY (SMA) TYPE 1 (WERDNIG–HOFFMAN DISEASE)

INCIDENCE

SMA type I occurs in 1 in 20,000. It is autosomal recessive, with deletion of exon 7 of the survival motor neuron (SMN) gene on chromosome 5q13 in 95% of cases. Pathologically there is loss of anterior horn cells.

CLINICAL PRESENTATION

There is progressive proximal weakness of the limbs from birth or soon afterwards (**Fig. 8.51**). Paralysis of the intercostal muscles leads to narrowing of the chest ('bell-shaped' chest) and abdominal breathing. Clinical features include: alert baby with normal eye and facial movement, severe axial and limb weakness (legs > arms, 'frog posture') with small chest, diaphragmatic breathing, tongue fasciculation and areflexia.

DIAGNOSIS

EMG shows neurogenic pattern with reduced activity during maximal effort, increased duration and amplitude of motor unit potentials and increased numbers of polyphasic potentials. Diagnosis is confirmed by SMN genetic testing.

TREATMENT/PROGNOSIS

Trials are in progress of antisense oligonucleotides to redirect SMN2 translation to increase the production of fully functional SMN protein. Previous trials of other treatments, e.g. sodium valproate, have not provided evidence of efficacy.

Respiratory support may prolong life in less severely affected infants, but death usually ensues by 18 months.

SPINAL MUSCULAR ATROPHY (SMA) TYPE 2 AND TYPE 3

SMA type 2 infants are able to sit (unlike infants with SMA type 1 who never sit) but are not able to walk unaided (as in SMA type 3). More mildly affected children with SMA 2 may stand with support and even take some steps with orthoses. Weakness is usually evident in the first year of life. There may be some regression of motor skills at onset, then a relatively stable course with survival to adulthood with optimal surveillance and management of scoliosis, respiratory and nutritional complications. Clinical features include severe axial and limb weakness (legs > arms) with areflexia, tongue fasciculation and hand tremor (very evident as baseline tremor in 12 lead ECG limb leads). SMA2 children are usually of normal intelligence and verbal but have variable bulbar weakness causing feeding difficulty, intercostal weakness with a weak cough, prominent diaphragmatic breathing and susceptibility to chest infections and nocturnal respiratory insufficiency requiring use of non-invasive ventilation.

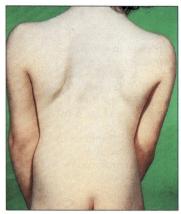

FIGURE 8.55 A child with limb-girdle dystrophy exhibiting scapular winging.

CHRONIC AND PROGRESSIVE WEAKNESS IN THE OLDER CHILD

CLINICAL SIGNS

When there is a history of weakness, enquire about family history and associated features (e.g. learning difficulties, cardiac manifestations, cramps). Examination includes ptosis (**Fig. 8.12**), facial involvement (**Fig. 8.48**), distribution of weakness and wasting (**Figs 8.55, 8.56**), presence or absence of muscle hypertrophy (**Fig. 8.57**), Gowers manoeuvre (**Fig. 8.58**) to demonstrate proximal weakness; additional features may include contractures, scoliosis (**Fig. 8.59**), scapular winging (**Fig. 8.55**), cardiac involvement and learning difficulties. Examination of family members (e.g. both parents in hereditary motor sensory neuropathy [CMT] or dystrophia myotonica **Figs 8.49, 8.50**) can be useful.

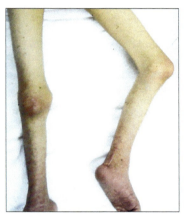

FIGURE 8.56 Severe wasting of both legs in a boy with familial peripheral neuropathy and progressive weakness.

CAUSES OF CHRONIC AND PROGRESSIVE WEAKNESS IN THE OLDER CHILD

Spinal cord disorders (page 217)

Muscle disease

Muscular dystrophies
- Duchenne (DMD) and Becker (BMD) muscular dystrophy (**Fig. 8.57**):
  - X-linked recessive so almost exclusively seen in boys (see below).
  - faulty dystrophin gene on the X chromosome.
  - 'out of frame' mutations – no dystrophin – DMD.
  - 'in frame' mutations – reduced dystrophin – BMD.

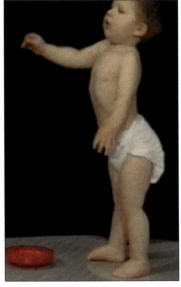

FIGURE 8.57 A boy with Duchenne muscular dystrophy (DMD).

- Limb girdle dystrophies (LGMD) (**Figs 8.55, 8.60**):
  - dominant and recessive forms, many subtypes, some present in adulthood.
  - abnormalities of:
    - lamin A/C (Emery–Dreifuss dystrophy (EDMD)) (**Figs 8.60 C,D 8.26 C,D**).
    - calpain 3 (**Figs 8.60 E,F**).
    - sarcoglycans (**Figs 8.60 A,B,G,D**).
    - FKRP.
    - collagen VI (Bethlem myopathy).
- Fascioscapulohumeral dystrophy (FSHD): D4ZA repeat array on chromosome 4: DUX4.
- Rigid spine muscular dystrophy: selenoprotein N (**Figs 8.60 G,H 8**).

Myotonic dystrophy (Figs 8.47, 8.48)
Congenital myopathies
- Nemaline.
- Central core (**Figs 8.60 I,J**): RYR1.
- Minicore.
- Centronuclear.
- Congenital fibre type disproportion.

Metabolic myopathies
- Mitochondrial disease.
- McArdles disease.
- Fatty acid oxidation defects.

Congenital and autoimmune myasthenia (see under Ptosis, Figs 8.12, 8.13)

Anterior horn cell disease
SMA type 3 (Kugelberg–Welander [see above]).

Neuropathies
Demyelinating and axonal neuropathies: CMT1A, CMT2 (see below).

INVESTIGATIONS
- Plasma CK.
- Genetic studies for: DMD and BMD (**Fig. 8.57**, dystrophin deletion, duplication and point mutation studies), *SMA3* (SMN gene), myotonic dystrophy (*DMPK* gene), CMT1A (duplication of PMP-22 on chromosome 17).
- Muscle MRI: distinctive patterns of selective involvement in congenital myopathies (**Fig. 8.60**) and if appropriate MRI brain and/or spine.
- Muscle ultrasound scan (increased echogenicity in muscular dystrophies and some myopathies).
- EMG and nerve conduction studies. May need to include single fibre EMG studies and repetitive nerve stimulation if initial studies are not diagnostic and myasthenia (**Fig. 8.12**) is likely.
- Edrophonium test and AChR antibodies if autoimmune myasthenia likely, genetic studies if a CMS is suspected.
- ECG and ECHO.
- Muscle biopsy to include detailed histochemistry.

MANAGEMENT
For management of myasthenia, see 'Myasthenia', page 202. Unfortunately, although steroids are of benefit in some muscular dystrophies, no curative treatments exist for the muscular dystrophies, myopathies or the hereditary neuropathies. Management includes physiotherapy to strengthen muscles and reduce contracture formation; maintenance of ambulation with ischial weight-bearing knee/ankle/foot orthoses; treatment of scoliosis by maintaining ambulation, standing, postural management with supportive seating, a polypropylene spinal jacket, and, if necessary surgical stabilisation with spinal fusion. Regular respiratory and cardiac surveillance with nocturnal and/or emergency use of non-invasive ventilation and cardiac drugs as necessary. Maintain bone health including optimising vitamin D and calcium intake.

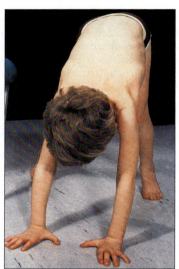

FIGURE 8.58 A boy with DMD executes Gowers manoeuvre, which demonstrates muscular dystrophy and proximal weakness.

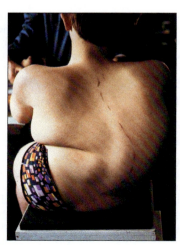

FIGURE 8.59 Asymmetrical flaccid weakness leading to scoliosis in a boy who suffered previously from polio.

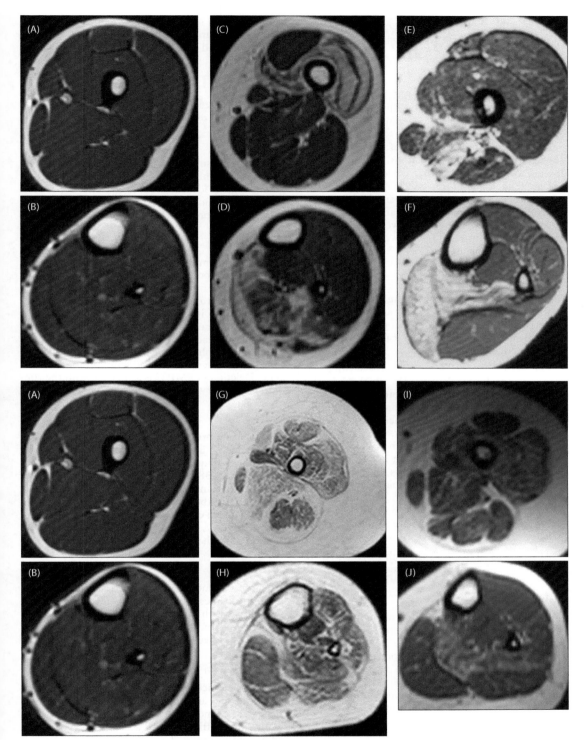

FIGURE 8.60 Axial T1 weighted sections through thigh (A,C,E,G,I) and calf (B,D,F,H,J). Note variable patterns of involvement of various muscle groups in different myopathic conditions.

A, B: Normal scans of a teenage boy.

C, D: Limb girdle muscular dystrophy type IB, autosomal dominant Emery Dreifuss muscular dystrophy, also called laminopathy secondary to LMNA mutation.

E, F: Limb girdle muscular dystrophy type 2A, also called calpainopathy.

G, H: Rigid spine muscular dystrophy1, secondary to mutations in the *SEPN1* gene.

I, J: Central core myopathy secondary to *RYR1* gene mutation.

DUCHENNE/BECKER MUSCULAR DYSTROPHY

INCIDENCE

DMD occurs in 1 in 3,500; BMD in 1 in 30,000 of male births. They are X-linked; a large gene on Xp21 produces a protein, dystrophin, located on the muscle membrane.

DMD (severe) involves 'out of frame' deletions, duplications or point mutations, which lead to absence of dystrophin. BMD (milder, allelic form) has 'in frame' mutations, which result in reduced quantities of abnormal, but partially functional dystrophin. Rarely girls maybe affected, either as manifesting carriers due to skewed X inactivation or Turner syndrome (XO) or have a chromosomal translocation involving Xp21.

CLINICAL PRESENTATION

Children have an abnormal gait aged 3–4 years, are unable to run, have frequent falls and often demonstrate language delay and other cognitive or behavioural problems. Some present earlier with global developmental delay.

- Duchenne: show progressive weakness with loss of ambulation by 8–12 years. The children develop cardiomyopathy (usually asymptomatic) and nocturnal hypoventilation requiring nocturnal non-invasive ventilation (NIV) in their mid teens. Late swallowing difficulty may occur, which may necessitate gastrostomy feeding. With optimum cardio-respiratory management, mean age of survival is now in the late 20s. Survival is likely to be even longer following early oral steroid treatment.
- Becker: usually present later with cramps and/or weakness, with slower progression. Children walk beyond 16 years and often have a normal lifespan. They may develop severe cardiomyopathy.

There is an anaesthetic risk in both DMD and BMD with inhalation anaesthetics and suxamethonium.

MANAGEMENT

- Physiotherapy to maintain full range movements.
- Night ankle/foot orthoses to prevent tendoachilles shortening.
- DMD: oral steroids (prednisolone or deflazacort) either daily, or intermittent 10 day on 10 day off dose.
- Ischial weight-bearing knee–ankle–foot orthoses (KAFOs) to prolong ambulation.
- Once non-ambulant, good postural management is needed in a powered wheelchair with spinal brace or spinal surgery for scoliosis.
- Regular respiratory monitoring with FVC, yearly sleep study and ECHO; nocturnal NIV when there is evidence of sleep hypoventilation and an ACE inhibitor +/– beta-blocker when ECHO shows signs of cardiomyopathy,
- Maintain optimal nutritional status including vitamin D and calcium status for bone health, especially if the child is taking steroids.

- Endocrine referral for osteopenia, delayed puberty or growth restriction.
- Learning and behavioural support as necessary.

HEREDITARY MOTOR AND SENSORY NEUROPATHY (CMT)

CMT comprises demyelinating (CMT1) and axonal (CMT2) subtypes, with autosomal dominant and recessive inheritance. There are currently over 40 CMT genes identified. An X-linked form (CMTX) affects males more than females, with intermediate nerve conduction velocities.

PREVALENCE

CMT1A is the most common form of CMT presenting in childhood, in 1 in 26,000. It is an autosomal dominant mutation; CMT2 and recessive and X-linked forms of CMT1 may be clinically similar. Commonly it involves a 1.5 megabase duplication within band 17p11.2 on chromosome 17. Duplication leads to three copies of the gene encoding peripheral myelinprotein 22 (PMP-22). Occasionally there is point mutation in the PMP-22 gene. Deletion in PMP22 is associated with the condition hereditary liability to pressure palsies (HLPP).

CLINICAL PRESENTATION

CMT usually presents at under 10 years, with gait disturbance – instability, high-stepping, difficulty in running, frequent falls; foot deformity with pes cavus (**Fig. 8.38**; the child may also have hammer toes) or pes planus and valgus deformity, symmetrical wasting of the peroneal muscles, calves or lower thighs, reduced or absent reflexes and subtle sensory abnormalities. Later, weakness and sensory loss may develop in the hands.

DIAGNOSIS

- Nerve conduction: motor and sensory conduction velocities are reduced to <50% of normal in CMT1A with increased distal latencies.
- Genetic studies: PMP22 (CMT1A), GJB2 (CMTX), Neuropathy gene panels (CMT2).

MANAGEMENT

Often none is needed, but includes careful foot care, physiotherapy and orthotic review, occupational therapy assessment for fine motor problems, e.g. handwriting difficulty, with access to keyboard and extra time in exams if necessary. Orthopaedic surveillance and intervention may be needed for progressive foot deformity.

PROGNOSIS

Typically CMT is compatible with a normal lifespan and the child is usually ambulant throughout; however, they may need to use orthoses or walking aids in later life.

CEREBRAL PALSY

See also Chapter 21 Orthopaedics and Fractures, page 645.

Cerebral palsy is a non-progressive movement disorder, caused by an insult to the immature brain occurring prenatally, perinatally or in the first few years of life. It occurs in 1 in 500 live births in Westernised countries. Types of cerebral palsy include:

- Spastic: hemiparesis (**Fig. 8.30**); quadriparesis; diplegia (**Fig. 8.61**).
- Dystonic/dyskinetic: quadriparesis with dystonia or chorea; hemiparesis; diplegia.
- Ataxic: relatively rare; must exclude inherited conditions (see Ataxia).
- Mixed types: commonly dystonic and spastic.

AETIOLOGY

Prenatal factors

Predisposing risk factors:

- Low birth weight for gestational age (dyskinetic; spastic quadriplegia). This may explain the effects of parity, social class and poor reproductive performance.
- Sex: M > F.
- Race: White > Black.
- Multiple birth, twin death, prematurity.
- Complications: bleeding, infection, pre-eclampsia.
- Genetic predisposition (e.g. factor V Leiden).

Specific causes:

- Genetic (e.g. arginase deficiency – diplegia). Also ataxic cerebral palsy (see Ataxia).
- Structural brain malformation (e.g. microcephaly, agenesis corpus callosum, Sturge–Weber syndrome).
- Ischaemia (e.g. porencephaly – often middle cerebral artery, 'fetal stroke', periventricular leukomalacia).
- Teratogens (e.g. alcohol – 8.3% of children with fetal alcohol syndrome have cerebral palsy).
- Deficiencies (e.g. iodine – New Guinea), magnesium.
- Infections (e.g. meningitis, CMV, rubella, *Toxoplasma*).

Perinatal factors

- Prematurity: (**uncomplicated**: diplegia; **complicated**: severe, mixed); intraventricular and intracerebral haemorrhage; periventricular leukomalacia.
- Jaundice (dyskinetic). Kernicterus is now very rare in term infants but hyperbilirubinaemia is a risk factor in the premature.
- Asphyxia (dystonic quadriparesis +/– deafness; spastic quadriparesis +/– dystonia, +/– complications, e.g. learning difficulties, epilepsy). Prenatal factors, especially fetal leanness, are an important risk factor for perinatal asphyxia and cerebral palsy.

Postnatal factors

- Infection – meningitis, encephalitis, gastroenteritis with dehydration.
- Head injury – car accidents, non-accidental injury.

- Hypoxic-ischaemic encephalopathy – near miss sudden infant death syndrome, near drowning, postoperative (e.g. cardiopulmonary bypass).
- Status epilepticus – may be followed by hemiseizure/hemiplegia/epilepsy.
- Cerebrovascular accident (see 'Stroke').

Non-motor features associated with cerebral palsy

- Microcephaly.
- Learning difficulties.
- Speech disorders.
- Epilepsy.
- Disorders of vision and/or hearing.
- Squint.
- Sensory loss.
- Impaired growth – local or general.
- Contractures and deformities.

MANAGEMENT

Cerebral palsy is managed by a therapy team, consisting of physiotherapists, occupational therapists, speech therapists, social workers, community nursing team and community paediatrician. The team is responsible for:

1. Assessment and management of feeding difficulties (the patient may need nasogastric feeding or gastrostomy if the problem is severe); gastroesophageal reflux; management of drooling (hyoscine patches, reimplantation salivary ducts).
2. Diagnosis and management of epilepsy (see 'Epilepsy', page 237).
3. Management of hydrocephalus (see 'Hydrocephalus', page 230).
4. Managing motor disorder and its potential consequences: seating to prevent hip dislocation and scoliosis; standing frame to prevent hip dislocation (**Fig. 8.61**); walking aids (e.g. K-walker);

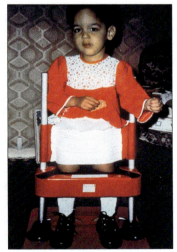

FIGURE 8.61 Child with diplegia in a standing frame. Putting weight through the legs encourages the correct formation and orientation of the head of the femur and the acetabulum, making dislocation less likely.

postural management (e.g. discouraging children with diplegia from sitting between their legs); stretching exercises to keep the full range of movement; ankle-foot orthoses (day and/or night) to keep full range of movement; botulinum toxin to encourage full range movement and prevent shortening; regular x-rays of hips (to exclude dislocation) and spine (if there is concern about progressive scoliosis); orthopaedics or gait laboratory.

5. Language difficulties: comprehension; expression (children with dysarthria may benefit from communication aids); support for family and child; education.

SPINA BIFIDA

See also Chapter 21 Orthopaedics and Fractures, page 647 and Chapter 18 Neonatal and General Paediatric Surgery, page 569.

INCIDENCE/AETIOLOGY

Spina bifida occurs in pproximately 1 in 500, but is very variable geographically. There is reduced incidence since the introduction of folic acid supplementation in pregnancy and antenatal diagnosis with α-fetoprotein and ultrasound.

Genetic factors are important. The risk of having a further affected child if one is already affected is 1 in 30. The risk of having a third child if two are affected is 1 in 6. Environmental factors are also important, particularly poor intake of folic acid in the first trimester.

DEFINITIONS

- Meningocoele (**Fig. 8.62**): cord is usually normal, lesion is covered with skin, neurology is often normal.
- Myelocoele or myelomeningocoele (**Fig. 8.63**): cord is exposed and abnormal, with only a thin covering if any; the risk of neurological impairment is very high.
- Spina bifida occulta: spinal cord is covered with bone and skin, but usually marked with a sacral pit, hairy patch or lipoma. Children usually present later with bladder problems or minor gait disorders.

SITE

The defect most commonly occurs in the lumbosacral area, less commonly in the dorsal region and uncommonly in the cervical region. Ten percent of lesions affect the skull (encephalocoeles).

COMPLICATIONS OF SPINA BIFIDA

- **Loss of sensation**: sensory loss in the skin can lead to ulceration (**Fig. 8.64**) as the child may not know that he has burnt or cut himself. The ability to recognise a full rectum or bladder may also be lost.

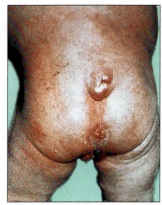
FIGURE 8.62 Meningocoele with relatively normal legs.

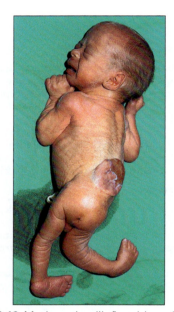
FIGURE 8.63 Myelocoele with flaccid, wasted legs.

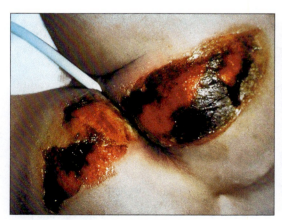
FIGURE 8.64 Pressure sores secondary to poor sensation in spina bifida. Although bladder problems are common, patients now intermittently catheterise rather than having indwelling catheters.

- **Bladder problems**: most children with lumbo-sacral myelomeningocoeles are incontinent to a degree. The bladder sphincters are often inner-vated abnormally and this may lead to a neuro-pathic bladder, which does not empty properly. The pressure inside the urinary tract may be high because of this and the child is also subject to fre-quent urinary tract infections. There is a risk of chronic renal failure in the long term if the blad-der is not appropriately managed.
- **Hydrocephalus**: usually secondary to Arnold–Chiari malformation of the brainstem. It occurs in patients with high lesions – e.g. thoracolumbar myelomeningocoele.
- **Paralysis**: with a lumbosacral lesion, the legs will be partially paralysed (**Fig. 8.63**) to an extent dependent on the site of the lesion and the degree of damage to the spinal cord. Secondary syringo-myelia may lead to deterioration.
- **Limb deformities**: if the limbs are partially para-lysed, there will be muscular imbalance and limb deformities may be present from birth (**Fig. 8.63**) or develop at a later stage.
- **Kyphoscoliosis**: the vertebral column may be abnormal and children are at high risk of kyphoscoliosis.

MANAGEMENT

- Early closure of the spinal defect. Today this is done in the majority of instances although sur-gical treatment may not be appropriate in some children with extensive neurological damage or severe hydrocephalus.
- Management of hydrocephalus: a shunt will usu-ally be inserted.
- Management of the bladder: it is essential that the child has a urodynamic study to examine the nature of the neuropathic bladder. Intermittent catheterisation is usually used to improve conti-nence and prevent infection. Children will need regular urines performed and adequate treat-ment of the urinary tract infections. With care-ful management, it is now unusual for children to develop chronic renal failure.
- Physical management: many children with flaccid limbs can be given appropriate orthoses and can walk. Other children may be wheelchair depen-dent. It is important to prevent kyphoscoliosis with an appropriate spinal brace if indicated.

HEADACHES

Headache is common in children and only rarely sig-nifies serious intracranial pathology (**Table 8.4**).

However, brain tumour is the second commonest form of cancer in childhood and a delay between the onset of symptoms and diagnosis has significant influ-ence on the prognosis. It is impossible to be absolutely certain of the aetiology of a child's headache on the basis of one consultation and for those with onset of headaches less than 6 months previously, if the child does not have neuroimaging after the first consulta-tion, a follow-up appointment is mandatory to check that new neurological signs have not become apparent.

TABLE 8.4 Causes of headache

Monophasic illnesses associated with headache

- Headache associated with acute infections in childhood:
  - *Usually not serious*: associated with fever caused by e.g. otitis media, tonsillitis
  - *Potentially serious*: neck stiffness (?meningitis, subarachnoid haemorrhage)
- Headache after head injury:
  - Usually benign
  - Occasionally associated with microscopic damage to the brain
  - Migrainous triggered by the head injury in a child with a family history – may be associated with hemiplegia or cortical blindness

Recurrent headaches

- Migraine
- Tension
- Intracranial hypertension – space occupying lesion; idiopathic intracranial hypertension; (**Fig. 8.65**)
- Sleep-disordered breathing

HISTORY TAKING

- Headache: timing, site, severity, nature, duration of symptoms.
- Associated symptoms (e.g. nausea, visual disturbance).
- Snoring, sleep apnoea, recurrent tonsillitis, aller-gic rhinitis, sinusitis.

INDICATIONS FOR NEUROIMAGING

- Nocturnal or early morning headaches.
- Headaches associated with nausea or vomiting.
- Any neurological signs.
- Age <6 years or learning difficulties.
- Inability to reassure child and family.

MIGRAINE

CLINICAL CRITERIA

Paroxysmal headache separated by free intervals, with at least two to four of the following: unilateral pain; nausea; visual aura; family history in parents or siblings.

PREVALENCE

The overall prevalence of migraine in childhood is 4%. Girls are affected more than boys in a ratio of 5:1. Onset is typically in the teenage years. A family history is very common.

CLINICAL PRESENTATION

Characteristic features

- Periodic throbbing, severe headaches.
- Gastrointestinal symptoms.
- Visual phenomena (e.g. photophobia or scotomata).

- Pallor, malaise.
- Desire to lie down in a darkened room/inability to continue tasks.

Occasional features
- Hemiplegia (hemiplegic migraine) (see 'Motor system', page 208).
- Aphasia.
- Visual field defects (see 'Cranial nerves', **Figs 8.1, 8.2**).
- Third nerve palsy (ophthalmoplegic migraine) (see 'Cranial nerves', **Figs 8.8, 8.9**).

MANAGEMENT

Full neurological and general examination should be performed on two occasions. A simple analgesic can be prescribed as soon as the child knows the migraine is starting. Reassurance and removal of triggers (e.g. lack of regular food or sleep) with relaxation techniques to combat stress and psychological support and a 3-month trial of a diet free of chocolate, cheese (including pizza) and oranges (including juice) works for the majority of children. Prophylactic medications include pizotifen (but this may cause weight gain), propranolol (contraindicated in asthma), sodium valproate and topiramate. Verapamil may help those with hemiplegic migraine. Rapidly absorbed triptans as nasal spray or buccal wafers may occasionally be taken at the onset of symptoms in children with very severe migraines. Oxygen may be used for cluster headache and indomethacin for hemicrania continua.

PSYCHOGENIC HEADACHES

The distinction between psychogenic (tension) headaches and common migraine is blurred, but psychogenic headaches are typically continuous.

CHARACTERISTIC FEATURES
- Continuous pressure like a tight band or an aching.
- A precipitating cause, such as a family problem or examination pressure.

MANAGEMENT

Full neurological and general examination on two occasions. Reassurance and removal of triggers, relaxation and psychological support as for migraine.

EXAMINATION OF A CHILD WITH HEADACHE
- Level of consciousness.
- Neck stiffness.
- Measure height and weight and compare with previous (?craniopharyngioma).
- Measure child's head circumference.
- Blood pressure with a paediatric cuff.
- Skin for café-au-lait spots of neurofibromatosis (see Chapter 6 Dermatology, page 137).
- Visual fields (**Figs 8.1, 8.2**) (bitemporal loss in craniopharyngioma, homonymous hemianopia or quadrantinopia in temporal/parietal/occipital lesions).
- Visual acuity (**Fig 8.3**, reduced in papilloedema, craniopharyngioma, optic glioma).
- Fundi (for papilloedema) (Chapter 7 Ophthalmology).
- Cranial nerves (?brainstem involvement), nystagmus (?posterior fossa lesion) (**Figs 8.4–8.29**).
- Gait – habitual, on toes, on heels, heel to toe (?ataxia, ?hemiparesis).
- Arms outstretched, eyes closed (?pyramidal drift, ?extrapyramidal movements).
- Finger-to-nose testing or building tower for younger children (?ataxia).

INTRACRANIAL HYPERTENSION

CHARACTERISTIC FEATURES OF RAISED INTRACRANIAL PRESSURE
- Nocturnal, waking the child from sleep.
- Early morning.
- Associated with nausea and/or vomiting.
- Reduced visual acuity (**Fig. 8.3**)
- False localising sign – lateral rectus palsy (**Figs 8.14, 8.65**).
- Focal signs if space occupying lesion.
- Papilloedema (Chapter 7 Ophthalmology).

OCCASIONAL FEATURES OF RAISED INTRACRANIAL PRESSURE
- Continuous headache.
- Headache later in the day.
- Headache increasing in frequency.

MANAGEMENT

Immediate referral for neuroimaging and possible neurosurgical intervention, especially if visual acuity is reduced (see 'Cranial nerves').

CAUSES
- Hydrocephalus.
- Tumours.
- Other space occupying lesions (e.g. abscess, haemorrhage).
- Venous sinus thrombosis (see **Fig. 8.115**).

Neurology

IDIOPATHIC INTRACRANIAL HYPERTENSION ('BENIGN' INTRACRANIAL HYPERTENSION, PSEUDOTUMOUR CEREBRI)

INCIDENCE

This occurs in 0.5 per 100,000 children <18 years.

CLINICAL FEATURES

Features include headaches characteristic of intracranial hypertension and papilloedema (not essential for diagnosis) (see Chapter 7 Ophthalmology). There can be reduced visual acuity (in association with papilloedema) as well as visual field abnormalities (enlarged blind spot, reduced nasal field with papilloedema) and VI palsy (not essential for diagnosis) (**Fig. 8.65**).

MANAGEMENT

Neuroimaging is advised to exclude space occupying lesion and venous sinus thrombosis. A lumbar puncture under sedation is used to measure ICP and remove CSF to reduce it. Medical treatment includes steroids and acetazolamide, as well as anticoagulation for venous sinus thrombosis. Frequent ophthalmological/neurological follow-up is necessary, with ICP monitoring for a decision on lumboperitoneal shunting if headaches are intractable. Optic nerve fenestration may be required if there is visual deterioration.

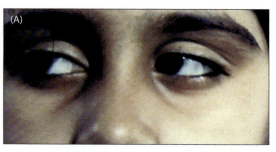
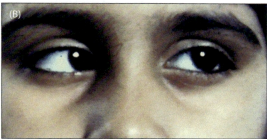
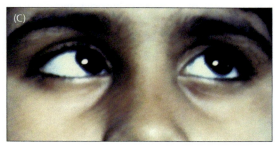
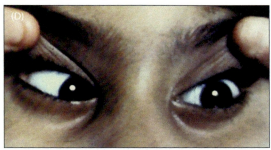

FIGURE 8.65A–D False localizing signs in a child with lateral rectus palsy exhibiting characteristic features of raised intracranial pressure. The lateral rectus muscle pulls the eye away from the nose and when the lateral rectus muscle is weak, the eye crosses inward toward the nose.

MACROCEPHALY

CAUSES

- Familial.
- Ex-premature infant.
- Hydrocephalus (**Figs 8.66, 8.67, 8.70– 8.73**).
- Subdural haemorrhage or effusion (**Fig. 8.68**).
- Glutaric aciduria type I.
- Degenerative (**Fig. 8.69**):
  - Alexander disease.
  - Canavan disease (N-acetylaspartic aciduria).

HYDROCEPHALUS

Hydrocephalus is the presence of an increased amount of CSF under increased pressure, with enlargement of the ventricular system.

ANATOMY

See **Fig. 8.70**. CSF is produced from the choroid plexuses of the lateral ventricles and circulates through the foramina of Monro, the third ventricle, the aqueduct of Sylvius and the foramina of Luschka and Magendie at the exit of the fourth ventricle, entering the subarachnoid space in the cisterna magna, which is continuous with the spinal subarachnoid space. The fluid passes via the basal and ambiens cisterns to reach the subarachnoid space over the surface of the cerebral hemispheres and the spinal cord, where it is absorbed through the arachnoid villi or granulations into the cerebral venous sinuses.

AETIOLOGY

Obstruction to the flow of CSF at any point, failure of CSF absorption, or over-production of CSF.

DEFINITIONS

Communicating hydrocephalus implies that there is no obstruction to CSF flow, but there is either a failure of reabsorption, which is common (e.g. secondary to meningitis or subarachnoid bleeding), or overproduction of CSF (e.g. choroid plexus tumour).

Non-communicating or obstructive hydrocephalus is a term used for hydrocephalus due to mechanical obstruction, occasionally at the foramina of Monro, more commonly at the aqueduct of Sylvius, or at the foramina of Luschka and Magendie.

SPECIFIC CAUSES

Congenital malformations

- Congenital aqueduct stenosis. Usually sporadic, occasionally X-linked with adducted thumbs.
- Chiari or Arnold–Chiari malformation (**Fig. 8.71**). Downward displacement of the medulla and cerebellar tonsils through the foramen magnum, usually associated with open spina bifida.
- Dandy–Walker syndrome (**Fig. 8.72**): The cause is the obstruction of the foramina of Luschka

and Magendie during early cerebral development. The cerebellum is hypoplastic and there is a greatly distended fourth ventricle.

Tumours

Tumours can block the CSF flow at any point, most commonly at the aqueduct of Sylvius, in the fourth ventricle or at the foramen of Monro.

Inflammation

- Infection. Hydrocephalus may occur after severe meningitis, which can cause adhesions, particularly in the subarachnoid space, thus blocking the reabsorption of CSF. Organisms include bacteria (e.g. *Pneumococcus, Haemophilus influenzae, Mycobacterium tuberculosis* and *Toxoplasma*).
- Bleeding. Hydrocephalus is common after intraventricular bleeding in preterm babies, either secondary to blockage at the aqueduct of Sylvius or to blockage of the absorption channels in the subarachnoid space. Hydrocephalus also occurs after subarachnoid bleeding in older children.

CLINICAL PRESENTATION

- Fetus: obstructed labour.
- Neonate: increasing head circumference (**Figs 8.66, 8.67**), separation of the sutures, sunset sign (**Fig. 8.66**).
- Older child: symptoms of raised ICP; nighttime or early morning headache; early morning vomiting; poor visual acuity; papilloedema (see Chapter 7 Ophthalmology); ataxia, deterioration in school performance.

INVESTIGATIONS

- CT scan (**Figs 8.70, 8.72**).
- MRI scan (**Fig. 8.71**) for aqueduct anatomy.
- Skull x-ray and shunt series (**Fig. 8.73**) to exclude disconnection if symptoms of raised intracranial pressure in a child with a shunt.

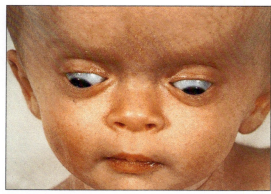

FIGURE 8.66 Hydrocephalus showing 'sunsetting' in an infant.

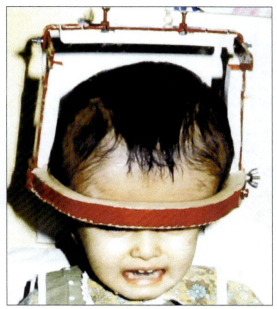

FIGURE 8.67 Hydrocephalus in an older child with a head so large it requires support.

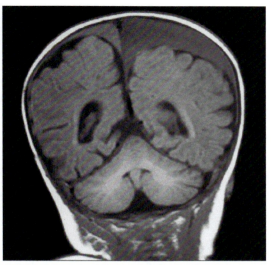

FIGURE 8.69 MRI showing bilateral subdural effusions and communicating hydrocephalus in a baby who was non-accidentally shaken. Cranial ultrasound is not sufficient to exclude this diagnosis. The advantage of MRI over CT is that the likely number and timing of injury(ies) may be established, as effusions of different ages have different densities on the scan.

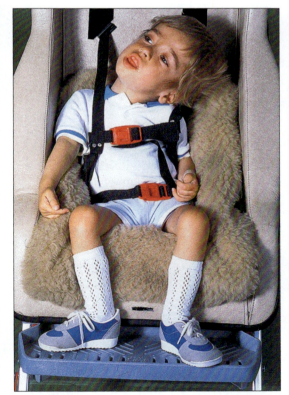

FIGURE 8.68 Macrocephaly in a child with progressive disease.

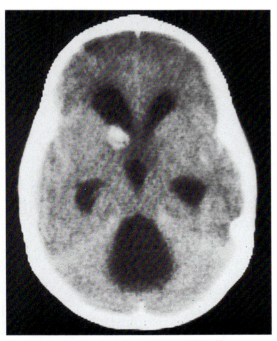

FIGURE 8.70 Hydrocephalus in a child with tuberous sclerosis and vomiting who died a brain death after cerebral herniation from raised intracranial pressure. All four ventricles are demonstrated.

MANAGEMENT

- Medical: osmotic diuretics such as isosorbide or acetazolamide are of no benefit and may be harmful.
- Shunt procedures: various types of shunt have been designed, the majority allowing drainage of CSF from the lateral ventricles via tubing passed underneath the skin, usually into the peritoneum.
- Third ventriculostomy.

SHUNT COMPLICATIONS

- Infection. Low-grade pathogens such as *Staphylococcus epidermidis* commonly colonise the shunt during insertion. They continue to divide very slowly and become protected from the natural host defences and from antibiotics by secreting a slime.

Children may present years after the original insertion of the shunt with fever, vomiting, headache and symptoms of shunt blockage.

- Blockage. The shunt may block either because it is infected, or because the child has grown so much that the tubing no longer reaches the atrium or the peritoneum.
- Disconnection (**Fig. 8.73**).
- Epilepsy.

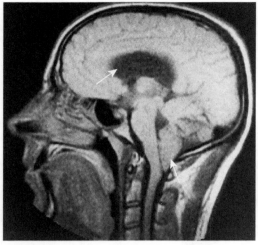

FIGURE 8.71 Chiari malformation with cerebellar tonsillar hernation and hydrocephalus.

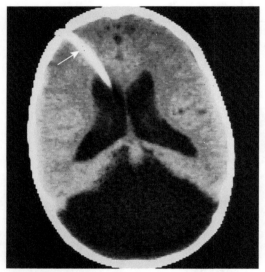

FIGURE 8.72 Dandy–Walker malformation with cerebellar hypoplasia, an enlarged fourth ventricle and hydrocephalus drained by a shunt.

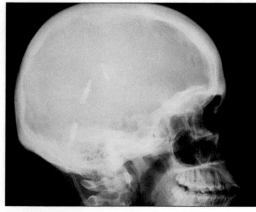

FIGURE 8.73 Skull x-ray showing shunt disconnection.

BRAIN TUMOURS

INCIDENCE/SITE

Brain tumours occur in 1 in 27,000 children. It is the second commonest form of cancer in childhood. 55% are infratentorial (cerebellum or brainstem) in children under 12 years.

CLINICAL PRESENTATION

Raised intracranial pressure

- Headache (classically in the early morning and often mild).
- Vomiting (classically in the early morning).
- Diplopia secondary to VI nerve palsy as a false localising sign (**Fig. 8.65**).
- Reduced visual acuity about which the child may not complain (**Fig. 8.3**; for methods of testing, see 'Cranial nerves', page 199).
- Papilloedema (see Chapter 7 Ophthalmology).

Symptoms and signs directly referable to the tumour

- Head tilt (**Fig. 8.74**) (posterior fossa tumour).
- Reduced visual acuity (**Fig. 8.3**; optic nerve or chiasm glioma; craniopharyngioma; **Fig. 8.75**).
- Visual field defect (**Figs 8.1, 8.2**; craniopharyngioma; occipital glioma).
- Ataxia (posterior fossa tumour – truncal suggests medulloblastoma or brainstem glioma; unilateral suggests cerebellar astrocytoma (**Fig. 8.76**).
- Cranial nerve signs (brainstem glioma, gaze palsy VI+VII; **Figs 8.14, 8.18–8.21**;– diffuse fibrillary pontine glioma: lateral gaze palsy – pilocytic pontine lesion; **Figs 8.16, 8.17**).
- Hemiplegia (thalamic glioma; cortical glioma; brainstem glioma).
- Epilepsy (supratentorial astrocytoma, oligodendroglioma, ependymoma).
- Parinaud syndrome (tumour in the pineal region) – upgaze paralysis (**Fig. 8.15**), retraction nystagmus, dissociation pupillary response to light and accommodation.
- Diencephalic syndrome (**Fig. 8.77**; hypothalamic glioma) – emaciation, accelerated skeletal growth, hypotension, hypoglycaemia, hyperactivity.
- Precocious puberty (hypothalamic glioma).
- Diabetes insipidus (craniopharyngioma; **Fig. 8.75**).

MANAGEMENT

- Surgery: is always undertaken if possible – total excision, partial excision, or biopsy. It may be impossible if the site of the lesion means that surgery would cause extensive brain damage.
- Radiotherapy – local, sometimes using proton beam, or whole craniospinal axis. This may be avoided if the patient is under the age of 3 years because of the neurodevelopmental sequelae but the priority is survival.
- Chemotherapy is useful for very malignant tumours, because drugs kill rapidly growing cells (e.g. medulloblastoma and malignant astrocytoma of the cerebrum). It is used as an adjunct to surgery and radiotherapy if excision is incomplete or there is a relapse. It is also used in the very young (<3 years) to postpone or avoid the need for radiotherapy but survival is not as good as with adjunctive radiotherapy.

COMMON BRAIN TUMOURS IN CHILDREN

See also Chapter 12 Oncology.

Infratentorial (see 'Ataxia' page 213)

Medulloblastoma

A midline tumour presenting with truncal ataxia and signs and symptoms of raised ICP. It seeds down the neuraxis via the CSF, so there may be spinal cord dysfunction at presentation. The 5-year survival rate with surgery, craniospinal irradiation and chemotherapy is about 55%.

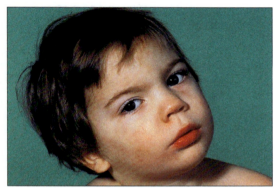

FIGURE 8.74 Head tilt suggests a posterior fossa tumour and a careful examination should be performed to look for evidence of nystagmus, ataxia and cranial nerve signs.

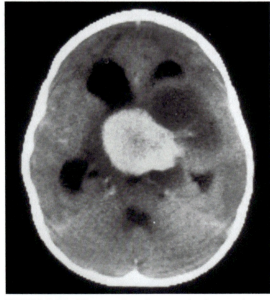

FIGURE 8.75 CT scan showing craniopharyngioma.

Astrocytoma (Fig. 8.76)

This arises in the midline of the cerebellum but usually extends into the cerebellar hemisphere on one side. On imaging the majority have a cyst with a tumour nodule in the wall; histologically these are pilocytic (benign). Management is mainly surgical and prognosis is usually good, with 94% 25-year survival in one series. Diffuse or fibrillary tumours have a less good prognosis and require radiotherapy.

Ependymoma

This arises from the lining of the ventricle, with variable histology. It may spread along CSF pathways and occasionally outside the CNS. It is treated with surgery alone if possible; radiotherapy is required if excision is incomplete or the tumour is malignant.

Brainstem glioma

The prognosis for diffuse fibrillary glioma is very poor indeed, with survival usually less than 1 year. Radiotherapy and chemotherapy offer palliation. Focal pilocytic glioma (**Figs 8.16, 8.17**) may be cured by resection.

Supratentorial

Craniopharyngioma (Fig. 8.75)

This tumour arises from the Rathke pouch (buccal epithelium). It often comprises solid and cystic components. The tumour is slow growing but may be diagnosed late if visual acuity (**Fig. 8.3**) and fields (**Figs 8.1, 8.2**) are not tested in children with headache. Surgical excision is curative if the tumour is not large; radiotherapy is required if complete excision would jeopardise the carotid arteries, optic nerves or hypothalamus. Survival is excellent if total removal is achieved, but children often have endocrine sequelae (e.g. diabetes insipidus, hypothyroidism or inadequate corticosteroid production), requiring appropriate replacement.

Optic glioma

Thirty to forty percent of patients have NF1 (see Chapter 6 Dermatology, page 137). Treatment is controversial. Surgery is usually required for anterior optic nerve tumours with complete visual loss. A conservative approach is warranted if visual loss is minimal. Radiotherapy and/or chemotherapy are then instituted if the vision deteriorates.

Glioma

Surgery alone is sufficient if it is pilocytic (benign; **Figs 8.16, 8.17**) and accessible; radiotherapy and/or chemotherapy if it is fibrillary (malignant) or in eloquent territory (e.g. the thalamus).

Primitive neuroectodermal tumours

These are highly malignant, with a tendency to seed (similar to infratentorial medulloblastoma) and usually present under the age of 5 years (see Chapter 12 Oncology, page 369). Treatment is usually radical surgery plus chemotherapy with or without radiotherapy.

PROGNOSIS

This depends on the site of the lesion, its histology and on whether or not total excision can be performed. Over half of children with brain tumours survive for more than 5 years and are considered to be cured. Quality of life is often compromised by learning difficulties following radiotherapy as well as neurological disability (most commonly ataxia, visual impairment or epilepsy). Endocrine deficits may be the result of tumour, surgery and/or radiotherapy. Abnormalities such as growth hormone deficiency and hypothyroidism may be late effects; careful long-term monitoring is essential.

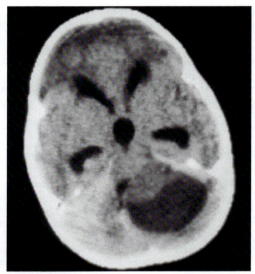

FIGURE 8.76 CT scan showing a cystic astrocytoma in one lobe of the cerebellum.

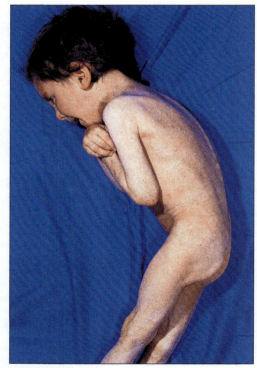

FIGURE 8.77 Extreme wasting in the diencephalic syndrome.

Neurology

LEARNING DIFFICULTIES

The majority of children with learning difficulties make steady progress through their developmental milestones but at a slower speed than normal. Developmental slowing, arrest or regression is more likely to be caused by a treatable condition (e.g. epilepsy, hydrocephalus or sleep apnoea) than by a degenerative disease, although it is important to take a careful history and to perform a full physical examination to exclude the latter.

Certain children with learning difficulties may have cerebral palsy, with implications for aetiology and therapy. Serial measurement of head circumference is important from the diagnostic point of view, as microcephaly recognised at birth is very likely to be genetically determined and recessively inherited (see Chapter 15 Genetics, page 468), while acquired microcephaly may be due to birth asphyxia (**Fig. 8.78**) or Rett syndrome (**Fig. 8.79**).

A detailed developmental assessment should be undertaken to determine the cognitive profile, as the causes of specific learning difficulties (for example, in language) may be different from those causing global delay. In some cases the cognitive profile may be specific for the underlying diagnosis (e.g. relatively well-preserved verbal ability in children with Williams syndrome, **Fig. 8.80**). Parents may find the associated behavioural difficulties (e.g. hyperactivity or behaviour within the autistic spectrum) more difficult to deal with than the learning difficulties.

Some children with learning difficulties have distinctive (dysmorphic) features (**Figs 8.81–8.84**), which may be diagnostic. Those with neurocutaneous stigmata (see sections on Neurofibromatosis, Tuberous sclerosis, Chapter 15 Genetics, pages 473–475) may have other associated problems, such as epilepsy or the risk of malignancy. Epilepsy should be managed carefully, as frequent fits may reduce the child's potential for learning.

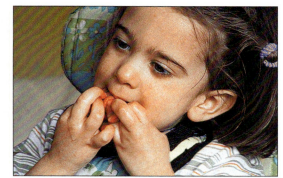

FIGURE 8.79 Child with Rett syndrome, showing characteristic hand involvement.

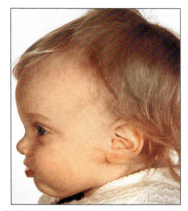

FIGURE 8.80 Williams syndrome in an infant.

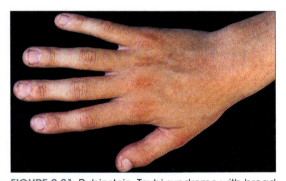

FIGURE 8.81 Rubinstein–Taybi syndrome with broad thumbs.

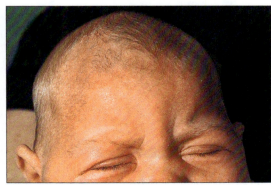

FIGURE 8.78 Acquired microcephaly in a child asphyxiated at birth.

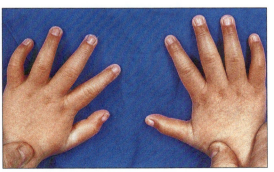

FIGURE 8.82 Coffin–Lowry syndrome with tapering fingers.

ESSENTIAL INVESTIGATIONS

- Chromosome analysis (**Fig. 8.85**), including fragile X. If a diagnosis (e.g. Angelman syndrome – see 'Epilepsy', **Fig. 8.86**) is considered likely clinically, a more specific genetic investigation is often appropriate (e.g. microarray-based comparative genomic hybridisation [array CGH]).
- Metabolic investigations suggested by clinical features (e.g. mucopolysaccharides, **Fig. 8.84**).
- EEG if epilepsy or for confirmation of a specific syndrome, e.g. Angelman.
- Neuroimaging has a low yield unless there is epilepsy or a specific syndrome (e.g. Joubert, **Fig. 8.87**).

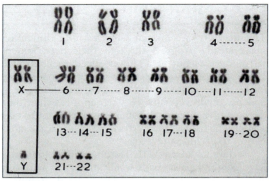

FIGURE 8.85 Klinefelter syndrome. Chromosomes showing an extra X chromosome in a boy who presented with language delay.

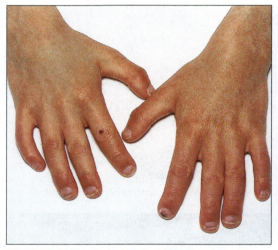

FIGURE 8.83 Smith–Lemli–Opitz syndrome, with broad space between thumb and first finger.

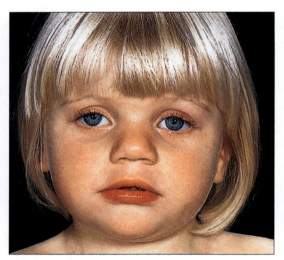

FIGURE 8.86 Angelman syndrome.

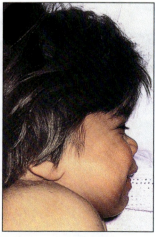

FIGURE 8.84 Hurler syndrome with coarse hair; the diagnosis was confirmed by urinary mucopolysaccharides.

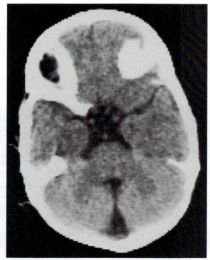

FIGURE 8.87 Joubert syndrome (abnormal eye movements, intermittent hyperpnoea and apnoea, hypotonia, ataxia). CT shows cerebellar vermis agenesis.

EPILEPSY

PREVALENCE

Epilepsy affects 1/200 children; up to 25% is intractable.

CAUSES

Neonate

Hypoglycaemia; hypocalcaemia; hyponatraemia; hypernatraemia; infection – meningitis, systemic; birth asphyxia; birth trauma; intraventricular haemorrhage; drug withdrawal; stroke – venous sinus thrombosis, arterial; structural brain malformations (e.g. lissencephaly), cortical dysplasia; metabolic conditions (e.g. hyperglycinaemia; pyridoxine deficiency/dependency); biotinidase deficiency (see Chapter 14 Metabolic Diseases, **Fig. 14.26**, page 437); peroxisomal disorders; mitochondrial disorders; Menke kinky hair disease (**Fig. 8.88**, see Chapter 14 Metabolic Diseases, page 435).

Child

- Genetic syndromes (e.g. Angelman – **Fig. 8.86**).
- Neurocutaneous syndromes e.g. tuberous sclerosis (see Chapter 15 Genetics), hypomelanosis of Ito (**Fig. 8.89**), linear sebaceous naevus, or incontinentia pigmenti (**Fig. 8.91**); Sturge–Weber syndrome (**Figs 8.90, 8.92**)
- Metabolic (e.g. mitochondrial, glucose transporter deficiency).
- Primary/secondary tumour – glioma; dysembryoblastic neuroepithelial tumour.
- Structural brain abnormality – neuronal migration defects, such as lissencephaly, double cortex, polymicrogyria, or hemi-megalencephaly, hippocampal sclerosis (**Fig. 8.93**).

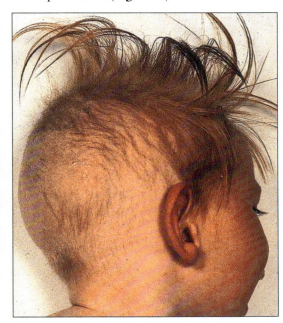

FIGURE 8.88 Menke kinky hair disease diagnosed after a low serum copper in a boy with seizures who improved after copper supplementation.

CLASSIFICATION OF SEIZURES

- Focal.
- Generalised: absence/tonic–clonic/tonic/akinetic/myoclonic.
- Unclassified.

It is usually important to classify syndrome as well as seizures in children (see **Table 8.5**).

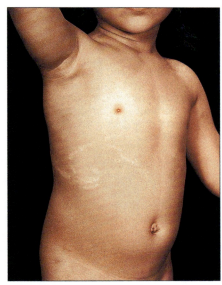

FIGURE 8.89 Hypomelanosis of Ito.

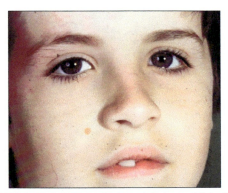

FIGURE 8.90 Subtle port wine stain in a child with epilepsy and a mild hemiparesis consistent with Sturge–Weber syndrome.

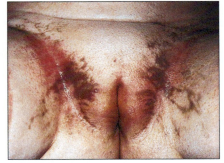

FIGURE 8.91 Blisters in the neonatal period in a child with incontinentia pigmenti.

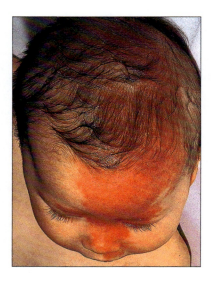

FIGURE 8.92 Capillary haemangioma in the ophthalmic division of the fifth cranial nerve; Sturge–Weber syndrome is diagnosed when there is underlying pial angioma over the surface of the brain. This may lead to epilepsy, contralateral hemiparesis and learning difficulties. Epilepsy surgery (e.g. hemispherectomy) may improve behaviour and learning as well as seizures if epilepsy is severe.

TABLE 8.5 Common seizures syndromes in childhood

Name	Age onset	Seizures	EEG	Treatment
Febrile convulsions	6 m–5 y	Generalised tonic–clonic	Not necessary	Buccal midazolam only
Reflex anoxic	6 m–5 y	Jerking after breath-hold	Not necessary	Iron if deficient
Generalised tonic–clonic	Any	Generalised tonic–clonic	Spike + wave	Valproate, leveteracetam
Partial	Any	Localised manifestations	Ictal focus	Lamotrigine, carbamazepine
Childhood absence	3–12 y	Absence +/– automatism	3Hz spike + wave	Ethosuximide, valproate
Myoclonic absence	1–12 y	Absence+myoclonic jerk	3Hz spike + wave	Valproate, lamotrigine
Absence + eyelid myoclonia	2–5 y	Absence + eyelid myoclonia	High amplitude spikes/slow	Valproate + ethosuximide, zonisamide
Juvenile myoclonic	3–18 y	Absence, myoclonic jerks, generalised tonic–clonic	Multi-spike with fragmentation	Valproate, lamotrigine, topiramate
Benign Rolandic	1–12 y	Focal motor with oropharyngeal manifestation	Rolandic spikes	Lamotrigine, carbamazepine (nocte)
Benign occipital	1–10 y	Nocturnal vomiting, eye deviation, coma	Occipit paroxysms, high amp spike/wave	Lamotrigine, carbamazepine
Infantile spasms	3–18 m	Brief spasms in runs	Hypsarrhythmia	Steroids, vigabatrin
Severe myoclonic of infancy	3–12 m	Early, prolonged, lateralised febrile convulsions, myoclonic, absence		Valproate + clobazam +/– stiripentol
Landau–Kleffner	2–5 y	Loss comprehension, occasional seizures	Generalised abnormality asleep	Prednisolone, valproate
Lennox–Gastaut	2–5 y	Absence, akinetic, tonic, generalised tonic–clonic	1–2.5 Hz spike + wave	Valproate, lamotrigine, topiramate, rufinamide
Myoclonic-astatic	2–4 y	Absence, akinetic	2.5–3 Hz spike/wave	Valproate, lamotrigine

Neurology

CLINICAL EVALUATION

- History taking to establish seizure type and seizure syndrome, family history, pregnancy and birth, development and progress at school.
- Examination, particularly looking for abnormal head size, neurocutaneous syndromes (see Chapter 6 Dermatology), focal signs (e.g. mild upper motor neuron VII – see 'Cranial nerves'; **Figs 8.22–8.24**), or mild hemiparesis (see 'Motor system').
- ECG to exclude cardiac dysrhythmia as a cause of convulsions.
- Iron studies in reflex anoxic seizures.
- EEG – initially while the patient is awake (**Fig. 8.94**) and, if this is not diagnostic, sleep-deprived or asleep. Video telemetry maybe required for surgical candidates, patients who may have non-epileptic seizures and in other cases where the diagnosis of epilepsy is uncertain; seizures may then be documented synchronously on EEG (**Fig. 8.94**) and video.
- Neuroimaging is unnecessary if the child has easily-controlled primary generalised epilepsy or a clinical history and an EEG compatible with a benign partial epilepsy syndrome. MRI (**Fig. 8.93**) is usually preferred as the diagnostic rate is much higher; specific sequences may be required, such as coronal cuts through the temporal lobes. CT is occasionally useful to demonstrate calcification, for example in tuberous sclerosis or Sturge–Weber syndrome (**Fig. 8.92**). Positron emission tomography (PET) and single photon emission tomography (SPECT) (**Fig. 8.95**) are usually reserved for patients who are surgical candidates.
- Biotinidase, vitamin B12 and trial of vitamins including biotin, pyridoxine.
- CSF for glycine (?hyperglycinaemia).
- CSF for lactate (?mitochondrial encephalopathy with ragged red fibres – MERRF).
- CSF glucose to be compared with blood glucose (?glut-1 deficiency).
- Chromosomes to exclude ring chromosome 20, array-CGH.
- Specific genes, e.g. SCN1A (Dravet, generalised epilepsy febrile seizures+ – GEFS+).
- Sulfite oxidase, molybdenum cofactor.

MANAGEMENT

- No regular treatment, e.g. for febrile convulsions or occasional generalised tonic–clonic seizures, but a benzodiazepine, e.g. buccal midazolam, should be available.

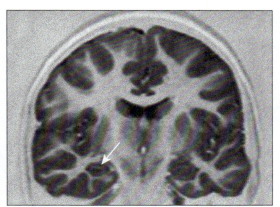

FIGURE 8.93 MRI scan showing R hippocampus with signal change and atrophy compatible with hippocampal sclerosis (arrow). Around 70% are seizure-free after surgery.

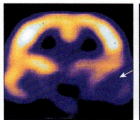 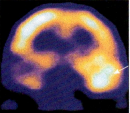

FIGURE 8.95 Interictal (i) and ictal (ii) single photon emission computed tomography (SPECT) scans showing relative hypoperfusion in the ipsilateral temporal lobe interictally and hyperperfusion ictally, demonstrating concordant evidence that the seizure arises in the structurally abnormal temporal lobe.

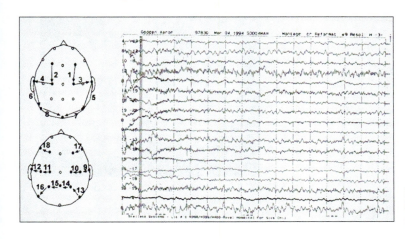

FIGURE 8.94 Electroencephalography (EEG) at the onset of a seizure.

- Iron supplementation for reflex anoxic seizures if iron deficiency.
- Anticonvulsants (see **Table 8.5**).
- Ketogenic diet.
- Surgery:
  - Resection for focal lesions (e.g. temporal lobectomy or amygdalohippocampectomy to remove dysplastic and/or scarred tissue, removal of cortical dysembryoplastic neuroectodermal tumour, hemispherectomy).
  - Vagal nerve stimulation.
  - Corpus callosotomy is usually reserved for intractable drop attacks.
- Appropriate education and family support.

NEUROLOGICAL AND COGNITIVE DETERIORATION

The majority of children who deteriorate neurologically and cognitively do not have a recognisable degenerative disease.

LIKELY CAUSES OF HEMIPARESIS

- Epilepsy, either clinically obvious or unrecognised (see 'Epilepsy'). May be associated with cognitive deterioration, aphasia (Landau–Kleffner syndrome), autistic regression, orhemiparesis.
- Hydrocephalus (**Figs 8.66, 8.67, 8.70–8.73**). May be associated with cognitive deterioration and/or ataxic diplegia.
- Malnutrition.
- Sleep apnoea.
- Psychosocial deprivation.
- Physical or sexual abuse.

CAUSES IN SPECIFIC CONDITIONS

- Sickle cell disease. Subclinical infarction (**Figs 8.124, 8.125**). See 'Stroke', page 246.
- Cerebral palsy, epilepsy, hydrocephalus, cervical cord damage (causes deteriorating pyramidal function) or vertebrobasilar dissection (causes recurrent strokes) in athetoid cerebral palsy with constant head movement.

TESTS FOR CHILDREN WITH PROGRESSIVE CONDITIONS

- Sleep study.
- EEG (awake and asleep).
- Urine for metachromatic granules.
- Blood film to look for evidence of storage in lymphocytes.
- CT and/or MRI head and ?spine, MRA, magnetic resonance venography (MRV).
- Biotinidase and trial of biotin.
- Plasma lactate.
- Plasma amino acids.
- Urine organic acids.
- Plasma ammonia.
- Acyl carnitine.

- CSF lactate, glucose, measles antibodies, neurotransmitters.
- Electroretinogram (ERG), visual evoked potentials (VEPs).
- Nerve conduction studies.
- Very long chain fatty acids.
- White cell enzymes.
- Skin biopsy, e.g. to exclude Nieman–Pick.
- Genetics: chromosomes, array-CGH, DNA for the appropriate mutation.

COMMON CONDITIONS WITH NEUROLOGICAL DETERIORATION

MULTIPLE SCLEROSIS

Multiple sclerosis (MS) is rare in childhood, and uncommon in adolescence (2.7% of all cases present <16 years). Although usually relapsing–remitting, it is occasionally chronic progressive. It presents with sensory symptoms, optic neuritis (but most cases of optic neuritis do not have MS), diplopia and motor disturbance. MS has an unpredictable course.

Diagnosis
- MRI abnormality (**Fig. 8.96**).
- CSF oligoclonal bands in 85% of cases.
- Abnormal visual evoked potentials.
- Elevated myelin basic protein.

Treatment
Intravenous methyl prednisolone is used for acute relapse. Other immune therapies may be considered. β-interferon decreases the frequency of attacks in relapsing–remitting MS.

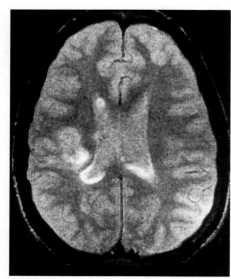

FIGURE 8.96 Patchy demyelination on MRI in multiple sclerosis.

ADRENOLEUKODYSTROPHY

X-linked gene (ABCD1) at Xq28, coding for peroxisomal membrane protein is at fault. Onset is commonly between the ages of 4 and 8 years. The child shows deterioration in gait with cognitive decline and pyramidal, extrapyramidal and cerebellar signs. Adrenocortical insufficiency is present in about 10% of cases (pigmentation is very rare, see **Fig. 8.102**).

Diagnosis
- Neuroimaging – white matter abnormality (**Fig. 8.97**).
- Elevated very long chain fatty acids.
- DNA testing.

Management
- Allogenic bone marrow transplantation (BMT) for early symptomatic cerebral disease (few lesions on MRI and performance IQ >80) or autologous BMT transfected with ABCD1 for advanced cerebral disease.
- Steroid replacement therapy for adrenal insuffiency.
- ?Dietary manipulation for asymptomatic patients.
- Symptomatic management for those with advanced neurological manifestations.

KRABBE (GLOBOID CELL) LEUKODYSTROPHY

This is due to an autosomal recessive gene on 14q coding for α-galactocerebrosidase. The infantile form is commonest but it may present at later ages. Clinical signs include restlessness, irritability, progressive pyramidal and extrapyramidal hypertonia and reduced reflexes.

Diagnosis is from high CSF protein and prolonged nerve conduction velocities. Neuroimaging is often non-specific (usually not a white matter abnormality). White cells enzymes (α-galactosidase) are measured.

METACHROMATIC LEUKODYSTROPHY

Due to an autosomal recessive gene on 22q coding for cerebroside sulfatase. There are infantile and juvenile forms:
- Infantile (0–25 mo): irritability; gait disturbance; spasticity in legs; reduced tendon reflexes.
- Juvenile (4–10 y): mental regression; movement disorder (mixed pyramidal and peripheral neuropathy (**Fig. 8.101**); seizures.

Diagnosis
- Urinary metachromatic granules.
- Nerve conduction velocities are prolonged.
- High CSF protein.
- Neuroimaging shows periventricular white matter abnormality.
- White cell enzymes (e.g. low arylsulfatase A).

CEROID LIPOFUSCINOSES (INFANTILE – SANTAVOURI)

This affects infants aged from 6 to 12 months, causing developmental regression and ataxia. The patient has stereotyped hand movements, with progressive microcephaly and optic atrophy.

Diagnosis
- Extinguished ERG.
- Progressive slowing and flattening on EEG.
- Cerebral atrophy on neuroimaging.
- Autosomal recessive CLN1 gene on chromosome 1p coding for palmitoyl protein thioesterase.

CEROID LIPOFUSCINOSES (LATE INFANTILE – JANSKI–BIELSCHOWSKY)

This affects children between 18 months and 4 years, causing developmental regression, ataxia and eventually epilepsy and macular and retinal degeneration.

Diagnosis
- EEG shows spike in response to photic stimulation synchronous with flash.
- ERG extinguished (not necessarily at presentation).
- Skin shows curvilinear bodies in cytosomes.
- Autosomal recessive CLN2 gene on chromosome 11 codes for a lysosomal peptidase.

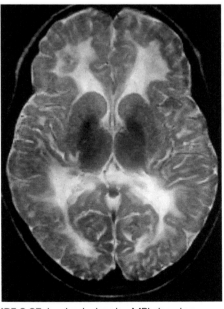

FIGURE 8.97 Leukodystrophy. MRI showing abnormal white matter in a child with a progressive movement disorder.

CEROID LIPOFUSCINOSES
(JUVENILE – BATTEN)

This affects children between 4 and 7 years of age, causing progressive visual loss and behavioural disturbance, with slow cognitive deterioration. Dysarthria, and extrapyramidal, pyramidal and cerebellar signs gradually supervene.

Diagnosis
- Vacuolated lymphocytes in peripheral blood.
- EEG shows pseudoperiodic bursts of slow waves.
- ERG and VEP are decreased.
- Atrophy and calcification on neuroimaging.
- Skin shows fingerprint profiles.
- Autosomal recessive gene on chromosome 16 coding for a novel protein.

Management of all ceroid lipofuscinoses
- Seizure control (lamotrigine, sodium valproate).
- Management of progressive movement disorder (see 'Cerebral palsy'; **Fig 8.61**), visual loss and behavioural problems.
- Antiapoptotic and anti-inflammatory treatments are undergoing consideration.

TAY SACHS DISEASE

Due to an autosomal recessive gene on chromosome 15 causing hexosaminidase A deficiency. It is common in Ashkenazi Jews. The child is startled by loud noises, with developmental regression, hypotonia, then hypertonia and seizures. A cherry-red spot at the macula is a characteristic early sign (**Fig. 8.100**).

Diagnosis is from white cells (hexosaminidase A).

NIEMANN–PICK DISEASE TYPE C

An autosomal recessive disease (95% are homozygous for NCP1 gene on chromosome 18); lysosomal cholesterol storage. Children show poor school progress, ataxia, hepatomegaly and vertical gaze palsy (**Fig. 8.99**).

Miglustat appears to slow the progression of neurological symptoms.

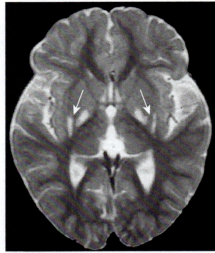

FIGURE 8.98 Leigh disease. MRI showing characteristic basal ganglia involvement.

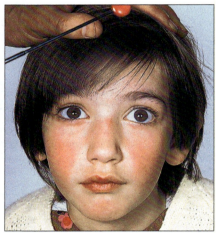

FIGURE 8.99 Difficulty in looking up in a patient with Niemann–Pick type C.

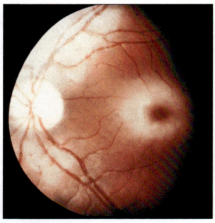

FIGURE 8.100 Cherry-red spot in the fundus of a child with Tay–Sachs disease.

Neurology

LEIGH DISEASE

This is due to mitochondrial disorders (pyruvate carboxylase deficiency, pyruvate dehydrogenase deficiency, respiratory chain enzyme deficiencies). Children show progressive movement disorders, usually extrapyramidal, ptosis and ophthalmoplegia and seizures.

Diagnosis

- Neuroimaging shows low density in the putaminae and caudate (**Fig. 8.98**). Raised blood and CSF lactate.
- Blood for mitochondrial mutations.
- Muscle biopsy for respiratory chain enzyme analysis.
- Skin biopsy for pyruvate dehydrogenase deficiency and respiratory chain enzymes.

Treatment

Early studies report a positive effect of coenzyme Q in particular mutations.

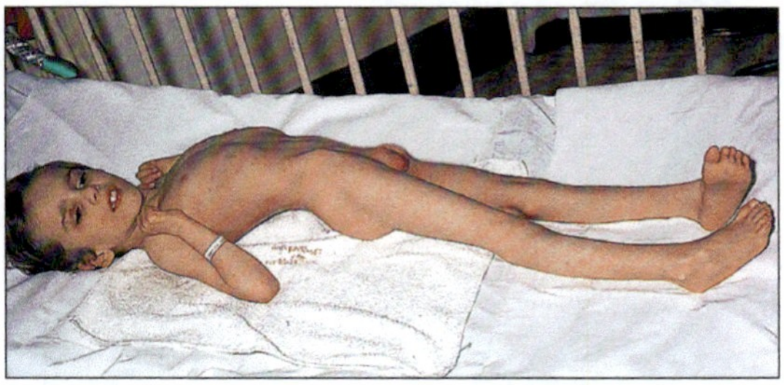

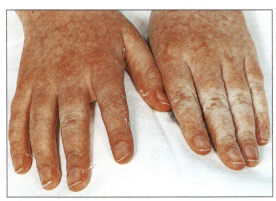

FIGURE 8.101 Metachromatic leukodystrophy. Quadriparesis in a child with peripheral neuropathy.

FIGURE 8.102 Adrenoleukodystrophy: pigmentation of the hands.

COMA AND ACUTE ENCEPHALOPATHIES

CAUSES

- Accidental head injury: extradural haematoma (**Fig. 8.103**); intracerebral haematoma; penetration (e.g. gunshot wound); diffuse brain oedema (**Fig. 8.104**).
- Non-accidental injury: subdural haemorrhage/ effusion (see 'Macrocephaly', **Fig. 8.68**).
- Stroke – spontaneous intracerebral haemorrhage; hemispheric ischaemia secondary to carotid occlusion; posterior fossa stroke; venous sinus thrombosis(see **Fig. 8.117**).
- Infections: meningitis – bacterial: *Pneumococcus*, *Haemophilus*, *Meningococcus* (**Fig. 8.108**) treatable with antibiotics; tuberculosis (**Fig. 8.105**) treatable with triple therapy; encephalitis with

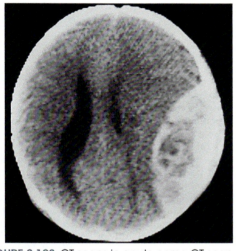

FIGURE 8.103 CT scans in acute coma CT scan showing L extradural haematoma.

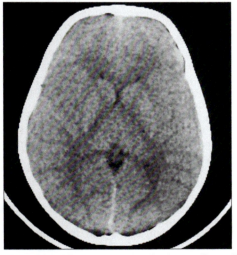

FIGURE 8.104 CT scan showing brain swelling with small ventricles.

243

specific distribution of abnormality on MRI (**Figs 8.111–8.113**), herpes simplex (**Fig. 8.111**) treatable with aciclovir; enteroviruses, mycoplasma; cerebral abscess (**Fig. 8.106**); cerebral malaria (**Fig. 8.107**) treatable with quinine or artemether.

- Shock: meningococcal sepsis (**Fig. 8.108**); toxic shock syndrome (*Staphylococcus*); haemorrhagic shock/encephalopathy.
- Diabetic encephalopathy – ketotic. Diffuse brain oedema may worsen after treatment.
- Drug-induced coma/poisoning.
- Status epilepticus.
- Hypertensive encephalopathy (**Fig. 8.110**) – preceded by visual symptoms and seizures.
- Hypoxic–ischaemic encephalopathy.
- Hepatic encephalopathy. Mild encephalopathy accompanied by foetor/flap. Viral hepatitis.
- Space occupying mass: spontaneous intracerebral haemorrhage (see **Fig. 8.128**; arterial stroke – large hemispheric or brainstem; venous sinus thrombosis; tumour.

EMERGENCY MANAGEMENT

- Secure airway, treat shock, measure and maintain blood pressure, stop seizures.
- Assess level of consciousness using the AVPU scale or paediatric modification of the Glasgow coma scale (GCS) (main differences from adult version are in the verbal scale).
- Patient should be ventilated electively if the GCS score <12 or deteriorating level of consciousness or signs of central or uncal herniation.
- Assess brainstem function for signs of central or uncal herniation: posturing – extensor or flexor; pupillary size, symmetry, reaction to light; oculocephalic (Doll's eye) reflex (provided there is no neck trauma); oculovestibular (caloric) reflex; unilateral ptosis and/or eye down and out and/or large fixed pupil and/or contralateral hemiparesis suggests uncal herniation (**Fig. 8.109**).
- Immediate investigations include blood glucose, chemistry including liver function tests, ammonia, full blood count, blood cultures, urine drug screen.
- Immediate treatment may include antibiotics if fever, aciclovir particularly if there are seizures.
- Emergency neuroimaging and referral to neurosurgical unit if there is a space occupying lesion.
- Establish cause if CT normal. It is safer to delay lumbar puncture if the patient is deeply unconscious (GCS <12) or has signs suggesting cerebral herniation. Bacterial meningitis may be diagnosed by rapid antigen screening at delayed lumbar puncture after antimicrobial therapy; tuberculous meningitis is usually accompanied by communicating hydrocephalus (**Fig. 8.105**) but must be excluded (Ziehl–Nielsen, PCR, interferon-gamma release test) or treated.
- Continue fluids – maintenance post resuscitation; avoid hypo-osmolar fluids and fluid restriction. Mannitol may be given if the patient is not shocked or dehydrated and does not have an intracranial haemorrhage.
- Consider other causes, e.g. metabolic (**Fig. 8.34**) and autoimmune (**Fig. 8.96**).

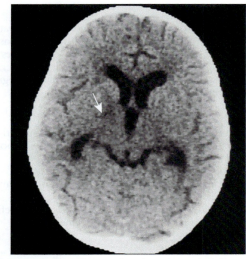

FIGURE 8.105 CT scan showing characteristic hydrocephalus and small right internal capsule lesion (arrow) in a child with tuberculous meningitis and a hemiplegia.

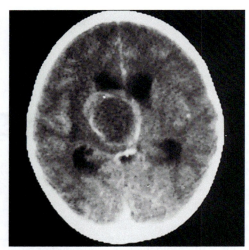

FIGURE 8.106 Contrast CT scan showing ring enhancement in cerebral abscess.

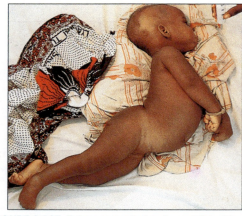

FIGURE 8.107 Extensor posturing in a child with cerebral malaria.

PROGNOSIS

This may be extremely difficult to predict accurately (**Figs 8.26, 8.27, 8.111–8.113**) and should only be attempted by experienced doctors with as many ancillary investigations as possible. Although improving level of consciousness and preserved EEG do not guarantee a good outcome, prolonged deep coma with a low amplitude EEG almost always predicts severe handicap, persistent vegetative state or death. MRI may assist prognosis in encephalitis (**Figs 8.111–8.113**).

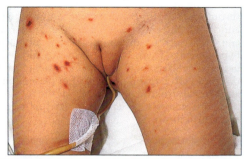

FIGURE 8.108 Purpuric rash in meningococcal septicaemia.

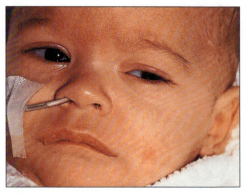

FIGURE 8.109 Left third nerve palsy with ptosis and eye 'down and out' in an infant with left hemispheric swelling in the context of non-accidental injury.

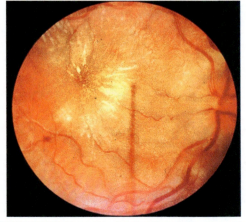

FIGURE 8.110 Hypertensive fundus with a macular star and papilloedema.

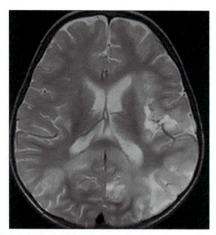

FIGURE 8.111 MRI in herpes simplex encephalitis for which the prognosis is very good if aciclovir is started within 48 hours.

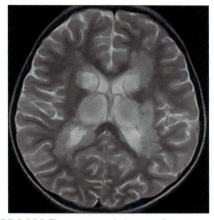

FIGURE 8.112 The prognosis is poor for patients whose MRI shows acute nectrotising encephalomyelitis, which may indicate genetic predisposition to an abnormal response to common infections, e.g. influenza A.

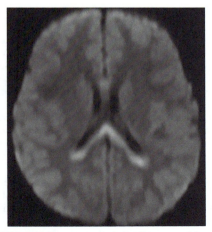

FIGURE 8.113 The prognosis is often good for children with encephalitis with abnormality of the corpus callosum on MRI.

STROKE

INCIDENCE

Stroke occurs in 1 in 15,000 children (half haemorrhagic, half ischaemic).

CONDITIONS PREDISPOSING TO ARTERIAL STROKE

These include sickle cell disease (see **Figs 8.124, 8.125**), cardiac disease and homocystinuria (**Fig. 8.116**). Approximately 50% of children have no previously diagnosed underlying condition.

Fifteen percent of children presenting with acute focal neurological signs suggestive of arterial ischaemic stroke have alternative aetiologies, e.g. cerebral venous sinus thrombosis (**Fig. 8.117**), hemiplegic migraine, metabolic disease (e.g. mitochondrial cytopathy or ornithine carbamoyl transferase deficiency).

RISK FACTORS FOR ISCHAEMIC STROKE IN CHILDHOOD

Infection (chickenpox, tonsillitis, *Mycoplasma* or *Chlamydia*); head or neck trauma (arterial dissection) (**Figs 8.118, 8.120, 8.121**; hyperhomocysteinaemia; prothrombotic disorders (e.g. factor V Leiden, antiphospholipid syndrome – more evidence for role in venous thrombosis); hyperlipidaemia – cholesterol or lipoprotein (a); hypoxaemia and reactive polycythaemia in sickle cell disease and cyanotic congenital heart disease; immunodeficiency (e.g. HIV).

CLINICAL SIGNS

History – rapidity of onset (sudden suggests an embolus, stuttering suggests thrombotic occlusion of underlying cerebrovascular disease), known medical conditions, recent illnesses (e.g. chickenpox, recent head trauma major or minor – predisposes to arterial dissection), family history. Examination – level of consciousness (see 'Coma'), distribution and severity of weakness, facial involvement, associated features.

INVESTIGATIONS

- Neuroimaging. Haemorrhage must be excluded by CT (see **Figs 8.128, 8.129**), which may demonstrate infarction (**Figs 8.114, 8.117, 8.118**), or MRI. MRI detects smaller ischaemic lesions in symptomatic and asymptomatic high-risk patients (**Figs 8.122–8.125**) and is particularly useful for separating ischaemic stroke from alternative pathologies such as posterior reversible encephalopathy syndrome (PRES; **Fig. 8.115**). MRA allows diagnosis of some of the possible underlying cerebrovascular abnormalities (e.g. demonstrating turbulence or occlusion in the distal internal carotid or proximal middle cerebral arteries [**Figs 8.124, 8.125**]). MRV may demonstrate occlusion of the large venous sinuses (e.g. in sagittal or straight sinus thrombosis, **Fig. 8.117**). Arteriography may be used to diagnose arteriovenous malformations (**Fig. 8.129**) or aneurysms

in patients with haemorrhage or to delineate the cause of stroke in ischaemic cases if MRA is normal or not diagnostic (e.g. in arterial dissection [**Fig. 8.119**] or small vessel vasculitis).
- ECG and echocardiography, although relatively few children with stroke have previously unrecognised cardiac abnormalities.
- Iron status.
- Screening for underlying prothrombotic and metabolic disorders which might predispose to recurrent stroke (activated protein C resistance; DNA testing for factor V Leiden, thermolabile methylene tetrahydrofolate reductase and prothrombin 20210; plasma total homocysteine; anticardiolipin antibodies and lupus anticoagulant; cholesterol; immunodeficiency, nocturnal hypoxaemia). There is little evidence for a link between deficiencies of protein C, protein S, antithrombin III, heparin cofactor II or plasminogen and arterial stroke in childhood, but the tests may be worth doing in patients with cerebral venous sinus thrombosis.

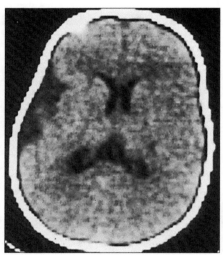

FIGURE 8.114 Residual cortical damage in a child who presented with stroke in the neonatal period.

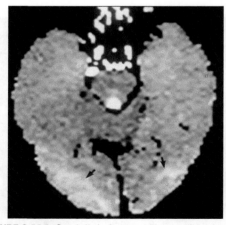

FIGURE 8.115 Occipital abnormality consistent with posterior reversible encephalopathy syndrome (PRES) on MRI in a child with seizures and hypertension.

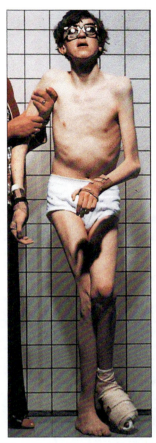

FIGURE 8.116 Homocystinuria with poor vision secondary to eye manifestations, including ectopia lentis, Marfanoid habitus, skeletal abnormalities and L hemiparesis secondary to cerebrovascular disease.

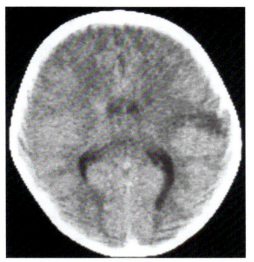

FIGURE 8.118 CT scan showing an infarct in a child who had sustained a head injury the previous day.

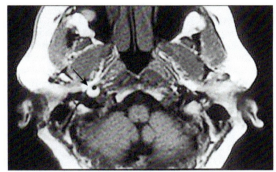

FIGURE 8.119 Axial fat saturated T-weighted MRI of the neck shows blood in the wall (arrow), characteristic of dissection.

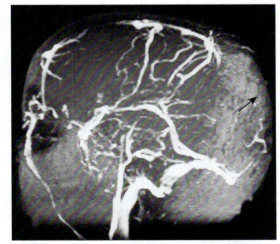

FIGURE 8.117 Magnetic resonance venogram showing sagittal thrombosis in a teenage girl with headache and acute behavioural issues, anaemia and a rash over her nose. She was behaviourally normal after anticoagulation and a diagnosis of systemic lupus erythematosus was made.

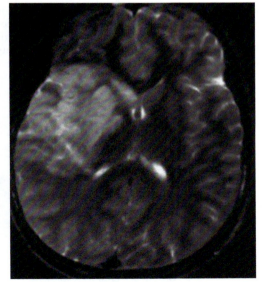

FIGURE 8.120 Large infarct with midline shift in the right middle cerebral territory in a child who sustained a carotid dissection.

Stroke

247

MANAGEMENT

Acute presentation

Urgent transfer to a centre with neurosurgical and paediatric neurological facilities enables rapid decompression of haemorrhage or massive cerebral infarction if necessary, and may also allow emergency management of ischaemic stroke in selected patients after MR imaging (e.g. anticoagulation for venous sinus thrombosis or arterial dissection).

Aspirin reduces early recurrence in arterial stroke in adults and at low dose (5 mg/kg), the risk of Reye syndrome is less than the risk of recurrence, although there are no data on efficacy in childhood. Thrombolysis improves outcome for arterial stroke in adults if commenced within 3 hours and may be worth considering for stroke occurring in hospital (e.g. in the context of congenital heart disease) or secondary to basilar occlusion (**Figs 8.126, 8.127**), although a recent procedure is a contraindication.

Prevention of recurrence

Although there are no population-based data, recurrent stroke occurs in at least 10% of hospital based series of paediatric ischaemic stroke. Folate, B6 and B12 supplementation may reduce homocysteine levels, carries no known risk and is probably a reasonable addition to low-dose aspirin prophylaxis. Anticoagulation with warfarin for 3–6 months may be considered for those with venous sinus thrombosis, arterial dissection or, more controversially, for the relatively few children with factor V Leiden, prothrombin 20210, anticardiolipin antibodies >100 IU or lupus anticoagulant. Regular transfusion to maintain the haemoglobin S percentage below 30% is the only evidence-based method of preventing recurrent stroke in sickle cell disease, and appears to have a role in primary prevention, although it is often poorly tolerated by the patient; evidence that hydroxyurea is of benefit is emerging. Increasing fruit/vegetable intake and exercise, and correction of chronic hypoxaemia (e.g. corrective surgery for cyanotic congenital heart disease, adenotonsillectomy or oxygen supplementation for those with sleep-disordered breathing – for example, patients with sickle cell disease) may be important.

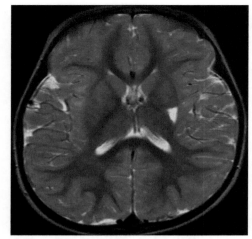

FIGURES 8.122 Small basal ganglia infarct secondary to middle cerebral artery stenosis 6 months after chickenpox.

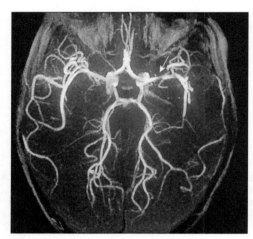

FIGURE 8.123 MRA showing turbulence in the proximal middle cerebral artery (arrow), probably secondary to chicken pox.

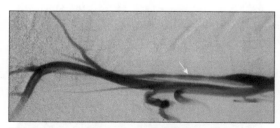

FIGURE 8.121 Arteriogram showing the typical 'rat-tail' dissection of the internal carotid artery in a child who presented in a coma with a very large right middle cerebral artery territory infarct. He had a previous history of hemiplegic migraine but developed this episode of hemiparesis a few days after falling from his skateboard.

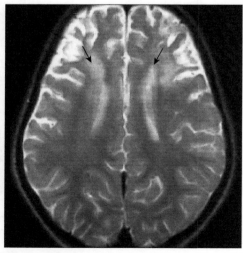

FIGURE 8.124 Bilateral frontal infarction in a child with sickle cell disease.

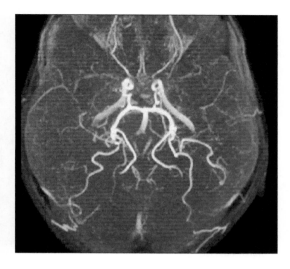

FIGURE 8.125 MRA arteriogram showing bilateral occlusion of the distal internal carotid arteries in a child with sickle cell disease. Moyamoya collateral is not obvious on this scan but may be seen on MRA or conventional angiography in patients with severe stenosis or occlusion.

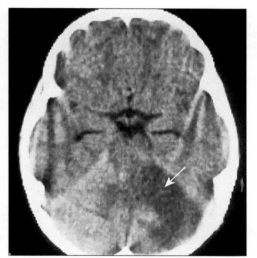

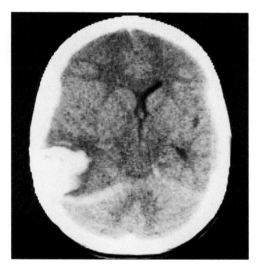

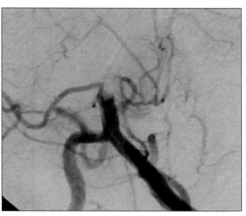

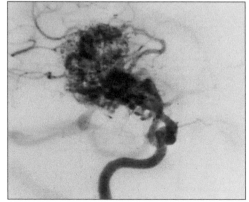

FIGURES 8.126, 8.127 8.126: CT scan of a patient presenting in coma, illustrating the left cerebellar infarct secondary to basilar occlusion (**8.127**) suitable for thrombolysis within 12 hours of presentation.

FIGURES 8.128, 8.129 8.128: CT scan showing acute spontaneous intracerebral haemorrhage with midline shift secondary to an operable arteriovenous malformation shown on a contrast arteriogram (**8.129**).

FURTHER READING

Aicardi J, Gillberg C, Ogier H, Bax M. *Diseases of the Nervous System in Childhood* (3rd edn). London: Wiley, 2009.

Aicardi J, Arzimanoglou A, Guerrini R. *Aicardi's Epilepsy in Children*. Lippincott Williams and Wilkins, 2003.

Alper G, Narayanan V. Friedreich's ataxia. *Pediatr Neurol.* 2003;28:335–41.

Al-Zaidy S, Rodino-Klapac L, Mendell JR. Gene therapy for muscular dystrophy: moving the field forward. *Pediatr Neurol* 2014;51:607e618.

Brewer GJ, Askari FK. Wilson's disease: clinical management and therapy. *J Hepatol* 2005;42(Suppl1):S13–21.

Callenbach PM, van den Maagdenberg AM, Frants RR, Brouwer OF. Clinical and genetic aspects of idiopathic epilepsies in childhood. *Eur J Paediatr Neurol* 2005;9:91–103.

Cohen ME, Kressel P. *Weiner and Levitt's Pediatric Neurology* (House Officer Series), 8th edn, 2008.

Dubowitz V. *A Colour Atlas of Muscle Disorders in Childhood.* London: Wolfe Medical Publications, 1989.

Eyre JA. Coma. *Baillière's Clinical Paediatrics.* London: Baillière Tindall, 1994.

Guerrini R. Genetic malformations of the cerebral cortex and epilepsy. *Epilepsia* 2005;46(Suppl 1):32–7.

Ganesan V, Kirkham F. *Stroke and Cerebrovascular Disease in Childhood.* London International Review of Child Neurology: MacKeith Press, 2011.

Jan MM. Misdiagnoses in children with dopa-responsive dystonia. *Pediatr Neurol* 2004;31:298–303.

Kirkham FJ. Stroke in childhood. *Arch Dis Child* 1999;81:85–9.

Kirkham FJ. Non-traumatic coma. *Arch Dis Child* 2001;85:303–12.

Kirkham FJ, Ganesan V. *Neurology.* In: Stroobant J, Field D (eds). *Paediatric Investigations.* Churchill Livingstone 2002; chapter 12 pp. 331–81.

Kumar A, Agarwal S, Agarwal D, Phadke SR. Myotonic dystrophy type 1 (DM1): a triplet repeat expansion disorder. *Gene* 2013;15:226–30.

Levene M, Chervenak F, Whittle M, Bennett M, Punt J. *Fetal and Neonatal Neurology and Neurosurgery*, 4th edn. London: Churchill Livingstone, 2009.

Maria BL. *Current Management in Child Neurology*, 4th edn. Hamilton, Ontario: BC Decker Inc, 2009.

McKinnon PJ. ATM and ataxia telangiectasia. *EMBO Rep* 2004;5:772–6. Review.

Mercuri E, Pichiecchio A, Allsop J, Messina S, Pane M, Muntoni F. Muscle MRI in inherited neuromuscular disorders: past, present, and future. *J Magn Reson Imaging* 2007;25(2):433–40.

National Institute for Health and Clinical Excellence (NICE). The diagnosis and care of children and adults with epilepsy. www.nice.org.uk/cg137, 2012.

Royal College of Paediatrics and Child Health. *The Management of Children and Young People with an Acute Decrease in Conscious Level.* 2015. http://www.rcpch.ac.uk/system/files/protected/page/Decon%20guidelines%20final%20updated%2015.07.15.pdf

Ryan MM, Ouvrier R. Hereditary peripheral neuropathies of childhood. *Curr Opin Neurol* 2005;18:105–10.

Segawa M, Nomura Y, Nishiyama N. Autosomal dominant guanosine triphosphate cyclohydrolase I deficiency (Segawa disease). *Ann Neurol* 2003;54(Suppl 6): S32–45.

Segawa M, Nomura Y. Rett syndrome. *Curr Opin Neurol* 2005;18:97–104.

Straub V, Carlier PG, Mercuri E. TREAT-NMD workshop: pattern recognition in genetic muscle diseases using muscle MRI: 25–26 February 2011, Rome, Italy. *Neuromuscul Disord* 2012;22(Suppl 2):S42–53.

van de Warrenburg BP, Sinke RJ, Kremer B. Recent advances in hereditary spinocerebellar ataxias. *J Neuropathol Exp Neurol* 2005;64:171–80.

Walker DA, Perilongo G, Punt JAG, Taylor RE. *Brain and Spinal Tumours of Childhood.* London: Arnold Publishers, 2004.

Neurology

9 Gastroenterology

Susan Hill and Keith Lindley

CLINICAL PRESENTATION

ACUTE GASTROENTERITIS

INCIDENCE

Diarrhoea is the commonest cause for hospitalisation in infants aged from 6–24 months and one of the most common childhood diseases world-wide. There are about 0.3–0.8 episodes per child per year world-wide, with more than one episode in many infants. Infective gastroenteritis is by far the most common aetiology of sudden onset of diarrhoea, with or without vomiting in children. Although enteric viruses account for most cases in the developed world, bacterial and protozoal pathogens may also be responsible.

AETIOLOGY/PATHOGENESIS

An acute infectious disease that is usually viral in developed countries. The most common viruses are norovirus – a small round virus and rotavirus (**Fig. 9.1**). Other causes include adenovirus, astrovirus and calicivirus (**Figs 9.2, 9.3**). These infect the small intestine and causes diarrhoea by a number of mechanisms including villus damage and direct (neurogenic) stimulation of water and electrolyte transport. Rotavirus diarrhoea is inevitable by the age of 5 years. Acquisition of immunity makes episodes clinically milder with increasing age.

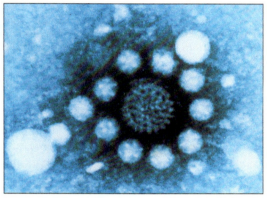

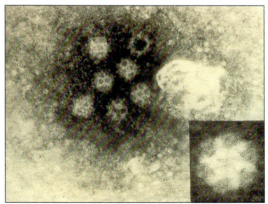

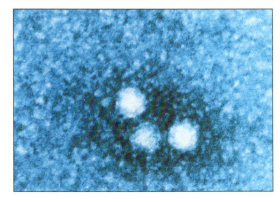

FIGURES 9.1–9.3 Acute gastroenteritis. Electron microscope appearance of enteric viruses (all named after their electron microscope appearances). **9.1**: Rotavirus (centre) and astrovirus (surrounding); **9.2**: calicivirus; **9.3**: small round virus.

CLINICAL PRESENTATION

An acute onset of vomiting then diarrhoea, often with abdominal pain and possible pyrexia. The incubation period is 2–7 days.

DIAGNOSIS

A history of frequency, volume and content of diarrhoea and vomitus should be obtained. Fluid balance (with record of recent fluid intake and urine output) and clinical examination are required to assess risk and current state of dehydration. Clinical examination is performed to assess state of hydration (**Table 9.1**).

TREATMENT

The mainstay of treatment is oral rehydration solution (ORS) (water/balanced electrolyte solution with a low concentration of carbohydrate to drive active electrolyte absorption; hypo-osmolar solutions are generally better). It should be given in small quantities as often as possible (even every 15 or 30 minutes). A nasogastric tube may be needed. If possible intravenous fluids should be avoided (enteral fluids are less likely to cause fluid/electrolyte imbalance). ORS is best absorbed immediately after a vomit. Only commercially available solutions should be given and homemade preparations (approximately one tablespoon sugar, and one teaspoon of salt/pint of water) avoided. ORS is used to rehydrate the child, typically over 4 hours after which attempts should be made to continue with normal feeding.

Where intravenous rehydration is required the type of rehydration solution used and its speed of administration will be dictated by the blood electrolytes.

Food should be continued as tolerated, particularly if the patient is malnourished.

Note: acute gastroenteritis is highly contagious. Careful hand-washing is the most effective way to prevent spread. Rotavirus is resistant to soaps/detergents and more effectively killed with alcohol solutions, whereas norovirus is better killed with detergents.

PROGNOSIS

Full recovery usually occurs within 24–36 hours, but symptoms can persist for 10–14 days. The patient can excrete the virus and remain infectious even after clinical recovery. In the immunocompromised, symptoms may persist for more than 2 weeks. Rarely children go on to develop a more chronic diarrhoea (postenteritis syndrome) in which an acquired immunologically-mediated sensitivity to dietary food proteins might be implicated. Highly efficacious rotavirus vaccines are recommended by the World Health Organisation in infants world-wide: live attenuated two-dose oral monovalent vaccine are given with other routine vaccines by 4 months of age in the UK (www.dh.gov.uk/health/2012/11/rotavirus).

TABLE 9.1 Clinical features of dehydration

Percentage weight loss	Severity	Clinical	Signs
<5%	Mild	Not unwell	Dry mucous membranes, thirst
5–10%	Moderate	Unwell	Apathetic, Sunken eyes and fontanelle (infants)
			Reduced skin turgor, oliguria, tachypnoea
10–15%	Severe	Shocked	Poor peripheral circulation, hypotension, tachycardia
>15%	Critical	Moribund	Severely shocked

FALTERING GROWTH/ FAILURE TO THRIVE

CLINICAL PRESENTATION

The child demonstrates failure to gain weight at the expected rate/according to the weight percentile (**Table 9.2**), for example below the 0.4 centile for weight (and possibly height), not explained by parental size (**Fig. 9.4**), or a child whose parents claim he/she has not gained weight or grown for several months or the weight is more than 2 centiles below the height centile.

'Catch down' growth is the term used for slow, but normal growth during the first year of life. It occurs when the birth weight centile (that is most closely related to maternal nutritional state) is a higher centile than the genetically defined centile for an appropriately nourished infant. Over the first 12 months of life the infant's length and weight will gradually fall through the centiles to the genetically-defined centile for the infant. Large babies at birth are more likely to have slower weight gain and smaller babies greater weight gain during the first year of life. Growth in a healthy, appropriately nourished infant is largely genetically dependent whereas in the older child it is growth hormone driven.

DIAGNOSIS

The history of feeding, diet, bowel motions, family, behaviour/activity/energy level should be obtained and investigations performed as guided by the clinical presentation.

TABLE 9.2 Gastrointestinal causes of failure to thrive

- Poor calorie intake:
  - Protein-calorie malnutrition
  - Feeding problems
- Vomiting:
  - Gastro-oesophageal reflux
- Malabsorption:
  - Small intestinal enteropathy
    - a Coeliac disease
    - b Food sensitive enteropathy
    - c Small intestinal Crohn disease
    - d Eosinophilic gastroenteropathy
    - e Autoimmune enteropathy
    - f Other less common enteropathies
    - g Protein-losing enteropathy
    - h Lymphangiectasia
  - Pancreatic insufficiency
    - a Shwachma–Bodian–Diamond syndrome
    - b Cystic fibrosis
- CHO intolerance
  - Lactose

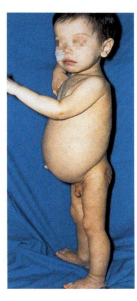

FIGURE 9.4 Failure to thrive. Typical appearance of patient, secondary to severe malabsorption, with short stature, distended abdomen, and wasting of buttocks.

CONSTIPATION

INCIDENCE/GENETICS

Constipation can be defined as either the difficult or infrequent passage of stool. It is common, affecting up to 20% of children at some stage of their life although there is marked global variation in prevalence. It can be subclassified into functional, the most common variety, and to subtypes with a physical basis. It can also be subclassified into slow transit constipation with ileo-colonic inertia or defaecatory disorders where the basis is at or near the rectal outlet.

AETIOLOGY

A variety of pathologies/causes are implicated. In infants with difficulty passing stool from birth with/without delayed passage of meconium, physical/anatomical causes need to be carefully considered including Hirschsprung disease, anal stenosis and primary enteric neuromuscular diseases. In infants with normal passage of meconium and normal stool pattern for a few weeks followed by difficult defaecation, atopy related anal spasm needs consideration. In older children with normal passage of stool until after the first year of life functional faecal retention syndromes are prevalent, with a variety of primary causes including anal fissure and behavioural disturbances. Allergy and inflammation are able to alter intestinal transit, sometimes dramatically, and diseases such as gastrointestinal food allergy, celiac disease and Crohn disease can present with constipation over a wide age range.

In functional constipation a primary event, such as poor fluid and/or calorie intake resulting in a small amount of hard stool that is ultimately expelled with painful defaecation (possibly with an anal fissure adding to the pain), leads to efforts to hold stool in and avoid the pain of defaecation. These young children will often adopt stereotypical postures to contract the pelvic floor in an effort to retain stool. If this persists an acquired megarectum with poor faecal sensation and a retained faecal mass may ensue with subsequent overflow faecal incontinence and soiling. Psychological factors such as fear, confusion, shame, guilt, anger, despair, withdrawal, dissociation and abdication of responsibility may ensue.

CLINICAL PRESENTATION/DIAGNOSIS

Presentation is generally age and cause specific. Examples of functional constipation include:

- Abnormally hard and often large stool with increased length of time between defaecation causing distress to the child when bowels are opened.
- Wilful fecal retention with posturing at the time of the urge to defaecate.
- Soiling – escape of stool into underclothing.

Diagnosis should include:

- Examination of spine, sacrum and lower limb reflexes to exclude neuropathic bowel.
- Abdominal x-ray with radio-opaque markers swallowed on each of 3 consecutive days, and x-rayed on the fourth day (**Fig. 9.5**) to estimate whole bowel transit time and to distinguish defaecatory disorders from slow transit constipation.
- Blood tests to exclude hypothyroidism and coeliac disease.
- Rectal biopsy (to look for the presence of increased acetylcholinesterase-positive nerve fibres in the mucosa and an absence of ganglion cells in the submucosa) is necessary to exclude Hirschsprung disease (see Chapter 18 Neonatal and General Paediatric Surgery, page 544).
- Blood specific IgE for foods (including milk, egg, wheat, soya) and skin-prick tests for cow's milk, egg, wheat and soya, if there is a personal or family history of atopy for non-IgE-mediated, atopic-related food allergy.
- Colonoscopy with histological examination of mucosal biopsies in atopic children may demonstrate underlying eosinophilic/allergic colitis or other inflammatory disorders.
- Other investigations as clinically indicated (e.g. sweat test, anorectal manometry etc).

TREATMENT

Treatment is cause specific. General guidance for the management of functional constipation is largely consensus based rather than evidence based. Early treatment is important if a longer-term habit, including fear of defaecation from a painful anal fissure, has developed.

Initial medical treatment

- Soften and evacuate retained stool. A variety of agents are available including polyethylene glycol (PEG)/electrolyte solutions, lactulose and, sodium docusate.
- Prokinetics may be necessary to ensure evacuation in some individuals. Sennokot, sometimes with added sodium picosulphate is generally efficacious.
- Resistant cases will sometimes require nasogastric polyethylene glycol solution to achieve disimpaction (**Fig. 9.6**).
- Micro or phosphate enemas are often effective in evacuating rectal masses, but the child needs to understand and co-operate with treatment, or fear and discomfort of defaecation may be heightened.

Maintenance drug treatment

- Daily PEG/electrolyte solution is commonly efficacious.
- In other children a combination of osmotic laxative and stimulant laxative is necessary (**Table 9.3**). Initial treatment may be with lactulose (5–10 ml tds) or methylcellulose tablets for an osmotic effect along with a stimulant laxative such as

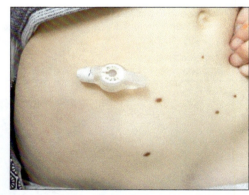

FIGURE 9.6 Button gastrostomy inserted into the colon for antegrade colonic enema (ACE) for bowel washout in severe constipation.

TABLE 9.3 Laxatives

Osmotic	Stimulant
Lactulose	Senna
Methylcellulose	Docusate sodium
Phosphate enemas	Sodium picosulphate
Sodium citrate enemas	Bisacodyl
	Microlax enema

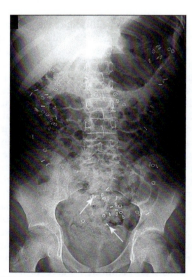

FIGURE 9.5 Plain abdominal x-ray demonstrating three different positions of the three different shaped radio-opaque markers swallowed on 3 consecutive days and now situated in different parts of the left side of the colon.

senna (infants and older children). Docusate can be added from preschool age to soften stool, with intermittent sodium picosulphate elixir as a stimulant providing an osmotic load if maintenance laxatives fail (it may be regularly given at weekends in a school age child).

- Once-daily senna to prevent reaccumulation of faeces (effect for 12–14 hours post dose).
- Parallel psychological treatment for both the child and family may be needed for school age children (around 50%).
- Appropriate dietary exclusions for atopic-related food allergic colitis (see 'Food allergic enteropathy' page 262).

PROGNOSIS

Treatment with stimulant laxatives will usually be required for 12 months or longer in order to prevent relapse. Patients with dependence on medical treatments beyond this time require specialist assessment as a proportion of 'treatment failures' will have generalised or segmental intrinsic neuromuscular disease of the large intestine.

INFANTILE COLIC

INCIDENCE/AETIOLOGY

Infantile colic is common. Cows' milk and/or other dietary proteins appear to be associated with the prevalence of infantile colic in a significant number of cases. Transient lactose malabsorption has been implicated in others.

CLINICAL PRESENTATION/DIAGNOSIS

Excessive crying or fussing in an otherwise healthy, thriving infant less than 3 months of age can be the presenting problem. Symptoms usually start from about 4 weeks. The episodes of crying usually occur in the evening and persist for more than 3 hours a day more than 3 days per week for at least 3 weeks. Other causes, such as too hot, too cold, inappropriate feeding or discomfort, should be discounted. The condition can be very stressful for the whole family.

TREATMENT

Parents should be reassured. Exclusion of cow's milk from the diet should be tried, with a hypoallergenic formula given as a milk substitute (usually an extensively hydrolysed infant formula). Many infants are or become symptomatic with soya milk as well. If the infant is breast-fed, the mother can exclude cow's milk from her own diet (ensuring she has adequate calcium). It can also be helpful to reduce stimulation. Supportive counselling and continuing reassurance should be provided.

PROGNOSIS

Infant colic resolves spontaneously by 4–5 months of age.

RECURRENT ABDOMINAL PAIN

INCIDENCE/AETIOLOGY

This affects up to 1 in 10 children. Improvement in gastrointestinal investigation techniques has led to more frequent organic diagnoses although many cases remain 'functional'. The differential diagnosis is very wide with almost any disorder that can cause abdominal pain, including pancreatic and gall bladder disease as well as intermittent testicular torsion having been implicated.

DIAGNOSIS

Diagnosis is made on a history of more than three attacks of abdominal pain over more than 3 months, sufficiently severe to interfere with normal activities. A thorough clinical history and examination are essential to check for non-specific presentations of a range of diseases. Where the physical findings are inconsistent (for example extreme abdominal tenderness on superficial palpation yet an ability to move in an unrestricted pattern), a functional cause is more likely.

Investigations depend on symptoms. It is helpful to examine the patient during an attack. Initial investigations, such as urine culture, full blood count and ESR, stool microscopy and culture and faecal occult blood, may be helpful. Abdominal ultrasound might provide evidence of bowel wall thickening, pancreatobiliary disease, ovarian disease, urinary tract disease, etc. If pain persists and is not resolving, upper and/or lower gastrointestinal endoscopy can be carried out.

A psychosocial history will be important if functional disease seems likely.

TREATMENT

As for the underlying cause. Functional abdominal pain usually responds better to cognitive behavioural therapy and hypnotherapy than to pharmacological approaches. Rehabilitation is key in individuals in whom the pain has resulted in social withdrawal from school and their peers.

PROGNOSIS

Long-term follow-up indicates improvement with age, although a high proportion of patients report symptoms continuing into adult life.

TODDLER'S DIARRHOEA

INCIDENCE/GENETICS

Toddler's diarrhoea is common. It affects males more than females and has a familial predisposition, with a parent with a history of irritable bowel or sibling with similar symptoms in about 80%.

AETIOLOGY

Clinical manifestations are a result of fast intestinal transit, with adequate absorption of most nutrients. In many this is the result of rapid gastric emptying due to a failure of induction of a postprandial motility pattern after a meal. Dietary fruit sugars (fructose) that are absorbed slowly in health may be incompletely absorbed and exacerbate the symptoms due to the osmotic effects of the sugar and its fermentation products within the colon. IgE-mediated reactions to food protein allergens (food allergy) can also cause rapid transit.

DIAGNOSIS

A history of loose, frequent, foul-smelling, daytime stool (usually with mucus) in children aged from about 1–6 years. Affected children frequently need to defaecate in the middle of a meal. Stool microscopy and culture should be performed routinely. Specific IgE to dietary food proteins may be measured to screen for immediate reactions. Non-IgE-mediated/slow onset food allergic reactions should be excluded with oral food challenges. Gastrointestinal mucosal biopsy for histological examination is indicated if weight gain is compromised, or diarrhoea occurs during sleeping hours or if blood is present in the stool.

TREATMENT

Dietary review by a paediatric dietitian and appropriate manipulation – for example, advice on reducing intake of fruit juices if excessive. If there is a positive food specific IgE test, particularly in non-atopic children, the identified food should be excluded from the diet (see Allergic colitis). Trial of diet free from cow's milk, egg and wheat (the most common offending foods) may be tried without initial colonoscopy or if the histological appearance of eosinophilic colitis is detected on colonoscopic biopsies. Some children benefit from Calogen (long-chain triglyceride [LCT]) given with a meal to delay gastric emptying or loperamide treatment.

PROGNOSIS

Diarrhoea improves with age, although milder symptoms commonly persist into adulthood.

CHRONIC INTRACTABLE DIARRHOEA

INCIDENCE/GENETICS

This is a rare condition. It has a familial occurrence with apparent X-linked inheritance in some cases.

AETIOLOGY

Patients can be divided into three groups, with:

- Specific diagnosis, but no known therapy (microvillus inclusion disease, phenotypic diarrhoea, and 'tufting' enteropathy) (**Fig. 9.7**).
- Specific diagnosis, but partial resistance to therapy (some cases of autoimmune enteropathy and immunodeficiency, e.g. immune dysregulation, polyendocrinopathy, enteropathy, X-linked (IPEX) syndrome.
- No specific diagnosis.

DIAGNOSIS

It is defined as four or more loose stools per day for more than 2 weeks, with associated faltering growth (**Figs 9.8, 9.9**) and at least three negative stool cultures (m.c.&s, ova,cysts and parasites) and virology.

- Watery stool may be mistaken for urine.
- **Intractable** if prolonged, despite extensive medical treatment trials and hospital investigations.
- Essential investigations include:
  - stool for malabsorption: fat globules, reducing substances and sugar chromatography (osmotic diarrhoea), alpha-1 antitrypsin.
  - stool electrolyte levels: Na >80 mmol/l if secretory diarrhoea.
  - stool elastase to screen for pancreatic insufficiency (beware of false positive/low results with watery diarrhoea).
- Upper and lower intestinal endoscopy with mucosal biopsies for histological examination (to detect possible enteropathy and colitis):
  - periodic acid Schiff (PAS) staining to detect abnormal brush border in microvillus atrophy (**Figs 9.10, 9.11**).
  - electron microscopy of mucosal biopsies to detect microvillus involutions and inclusion bodies in microvillus atrophy (**Figs 9.12–9.14**) or other less specific abnormalities.
  - peripheral blood immune studies to detect an underlying systemic immunodeficiency that might also involve the intestine.
  - immunological staining of intestinal mucosa if an inflammatory infiltrate is found in the lamina propria.

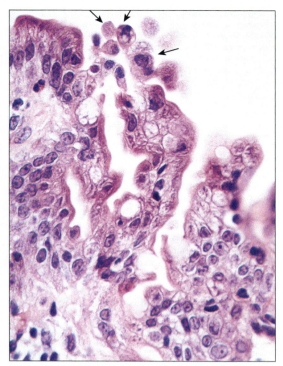

FIGURE 9.7 Tufting enteropathy. Histological appearance of small intestine with 'grape-like' tufts at the villus tip (×25).

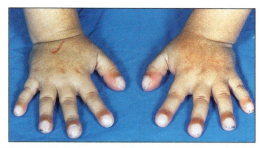

FIGURE 9.9 Anaemia and clubbing of fingers in a child with chronic intractable diarrhoea and malabsorption, with underlying tufting enteropathy.

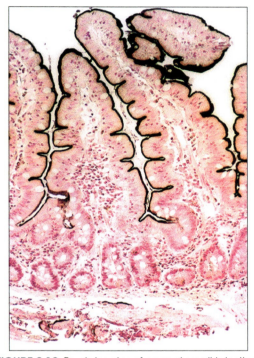

FIGURE 9.10 Brush border of normal small intestine stained with PAS (×40).

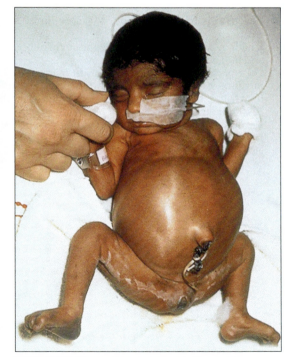

FIGURE 9.8 Neonate presenting with severe, intractable, watery diarrhoea and failure to thrive, with abdominal distention and excoriation of the nappy area.

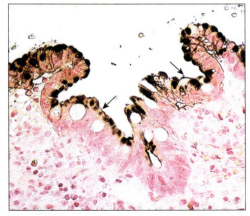

FIGURE 9.11 Brush border stained with PAS in microvillous atrophy, illustrating disruption of the microvilli (×100).

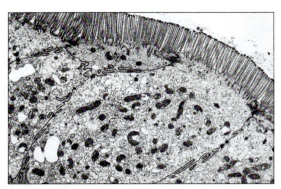

FIGURE 9.12 Electron microscope appearance of normal microvilli on a small intestine enterocyte (×13,000).

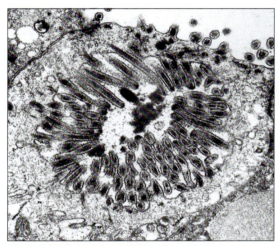

FIGURE 9.13 Electron microscope appearance of distorted microvilli within and on an enterocyte surface in microvillous atrophy (×13,000).

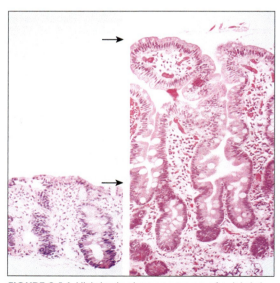

FIGURE 9.14 Histological appearance of subtotal villous atrophy (severe enteropathy) compared with normal small intestine.

Additional investigations include:

- Examination of hair to look for trichorrhexis nodosa in potential syndromic diarrhoea, e.g. trichohepato-enteric syndrome.
- Genetic confirmation of diagnosis may be possible with some aetiologies (e.g. tufting enteropathy, IPEX, trichohepatoenteric syndrome/syndromic diarrhoea).

TREATMENT

- Trial of immunosuppressive treatment if excessive inflammatory cells in intestinal mucosa.
- Gradual reintroduction of enteral feed as tolerated, usually as semi-elemental continuous feed.
- Immunoglobulin replacement therapy or other definitive treatment in primary immunodeficiencies.
- May need elemental or modular feed.
- Supportive therapy with parenteral nutrition (PN) (improving nutrition will frequently ameliorate the diarrhoea).
- Long-term home PN by parents is the best option if the child fails to respond adequately to treatment.
- A multidisciplinary ethical review with parents, before deciding whether to commence long-term home PN, is helpful to establish an appropriate treatment regime.
- Early intestinal transplantation may be appropriate in some instances (for example severe microvillus disease with rapidly progressive PN-associated liver disease).

PROGNOSIS

- Recent improvement with advances in PN treatment.
- Children can now survive throughout childhood and into adult life.
- Poor prognosis in most patients with microvillus inclusion disease: these children usually develop liver failure by 2 years of age.
- Risk of inducing suffering with no eventual recovery needs to be assessed prior to sending the child home on treatment with PN, particularly if child also has failure of another major organ.

CHRONIC INTESTINAL FAILURE

AETIOLOGY/PATHOGENESIS

The three major causes are:

- Severe enteropathy (see 'Intractable diarrhoea').
- Major abnormality of the intestinal neuromusculature.
- Short bowel syndrome.

DIAGNOSIS

The child has an inability to maintain weight or grow despite adequate nutrition. They may present with chronic diarrhoea with or without vomiting. Essential investigations are shown in **Table 9.4**.

TREATMENT

There are two main aims:

- To make the best possible use of any intestinal absorptive capacity (to prevent PN-associated liver disease and to promote intestinal adaptation).
- To maintain normal weight gain and growth with PN (see treatment for short bowel syndrome).

Intestinal transplant with or without liver/other organ transplant is currently reserved for patients with a poor prognosis on long-term PN, e.g. severely reduced central venous access, end-stage intestinal failure-associated liver disease/failure, excessive intestinal fluid losses and poor quality of life.

Complications are largely related to post-transplant immunosuppressive treatment and include systemic infections and lymphoproliferative disease.

PROGNOSIS

Prognosis is dependent on careful administration of over-night PN by formally trained parents at home, with appropriate support from a specialist intestinal failure rehabilitation team. There are fewer complications of PN at home (less frequent septicaemic episodes).

Children on home PN can grow and develop normally and survive into adult life attending school then university, successfully transitioning to adult care. Over 50% of cases wean off PN, successfully developing enteral autonomy with time.

TABLE 9.4 Essential investigations for chronic intestinal failure

- Stool microscopy and culture
- Stool-reducing substances and sugar chromatography for sugar malabsorption (osmotic diarrhoea)
- If liquid stool, check sodium content (>80 mmol/l secretory diarrhoea)
- Peripheral blood immunoglobulin levels and specific IgE for foods
- Upper and lower gastrointestinal endoscopy with mucosal biopsies for histological examination for mucosal inflammation
- Radiological gastrointestinal contrast study to detect structural abnormalities and, if previous intestinal resection, length of remaining small and large intestine
- If there is evidence of abnormal intestinal motility, investigate transit time with marker (such as carmine red dye) or radio-opaque pellets (see constipation), and intestinal motility studies to detect abnormal peristalsis: initially an electrogastrogram – EGG, antroduodenal manometry
- Trial of gradual introduction of appropriate enteral feeds (elemental or semi-elemental liquid feeds) administered in the most appropriate manner (taken orally, via a nasogastric tube or gastrostomy directly into the stomach, or via a jejunostomy or nasojejunal tube into the jejunum)

GASTROINTESTINAL DIAGNOSES

FABRICATED AND INDUCED ILLNESS

INCIDENCE/AETIOLOGY

See Chapter 2 Child Protection, page 36. Males and females are equally affected.

The reason for the perpetrator's actions is often poorly understood. Many are lonely and isolated. Up to half have nursing training or some extra medical knowledge (such as medical receptionist), and some have a previous history of falsifying their own symptoms. The perpetrator is most commonly the mother.

There are several degrees of manifestation of the syndrome. At its least severe, the perpetrator embellishes a history in the hope that the child will have more medical attention. The next stage is the perpetrator who simulates illness without harming the child (for example by contaminating specimens). At its most severe, the perpetrator directly harms the child, for example sabotaging a central venous catheter or giving harmful treatment, such as laxatives when the child already has diarrhoea, or adding excessive salt to infant feeds (**Fig. 9.15**).

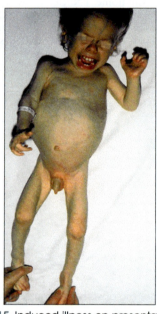

FIGURE 9.15 Induced illness on presentation, aged 20 months, with severe wasting and developmental delay due to starvation. The mother claimed the child had an enormous appetite.

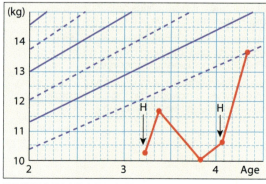

FIGURE 9.16 Weight plotted on weight centile chart for a child aged 3–4 months who gained weight when in hospital (H) and failed to thrive at home.

DIAGNOSIS

Common gastrointestinal symptoms are vomiting, diarrhoea and gastrointestinal bleeding. There is usually a mild underlying gastrointestinal disorder (for example atopic-associated cow's milk protein allergy) with worsening of existing symptoms and development of new symptoms when the mother is with the child. The mother usually appears appreciative, co-operative and pleasant, is close to the child, reluctant to leave the hospital and, whenever possible, forms close relationships with the professional staff caring for the child. The father is usually distant (although the syndrome has been described in fathers). The average time from onset to diagnosis is 15 months.

The closest possible observation of mother and child is necessary. 24-hour individual observation of the patient is often necessary. There is controversy over the use of video surveillance. All staff must meticulously record all observations (**Fig. 9.16**). Toxic screening of urine and vomit specimens and blood group of blood specimens are necessary. A multidisciplinary team should be involved, including a social worker and psychiatrist.

TREATMENT

If the mother is unwilling to confess when presented with all the evidence, she may need to be directly confronted. She should be told that the paediatrician and child psychiatrist are trying to help her and that the social worker has legal responsibilities.

PROGNOSIS

There is a mortality rate of about 9% with the greatest risk among children under 3 years old. Child victims may become perpetrators themselves. Often more than one child in a family is affected at different times.

COELIAC DISEASE

INCIDENCE/GENETICS

Coeliac disease is a permanent chronic autoimmune small bowel enteropathy that is associated with the ingestion of gluten in genetically predisposed individuals. It resolves on exclusion of gluten from the diet. It occurs in 2–3% of Caucasian populations with a high wheat intake, such as Europeans, North and South Americans and Australians. Patients are to all intents and purposes always either HLA- DQ2 or DQ8 positive.

AETIOLOGY

Coeliac disease is an autoimmune disease. Tissue transglutaminase (tTg) has been identified as the major autoantigen. Ingestion of wheat, barley or rye initiates immunologically-mediated tissue injury. This injury is stimulated in subjects with particular HLA genes (see above). An environmental trigger is also necessary (identical twin concordance rates are approximately 70%), as are several non-HLA genes.

Coeliac disease is associated with other autoimmune diseases especially insulin-dependent diabetes and hypothyroidism.

DIAGNOSIS

Symptoms and signs of a 'classical' presentation of coeliac disease are anorexia, vomiting, abdominal distension, diarrhoea, irritability, failure to thrive and buttock wasting in a postweaning infant/young child. Other presentations can include constipation, non-specific abdominal pain, recurrent apthous ulceration of the oral mucosa, anaemia, growth failure or even asymptomatic (**Figs 9.17, 9.18**). Presentation can be at any age throughout life, although roughly 2/3 of cases present in childhood. Autoimmune diseases such as diabetes mellitus and thyroid disease are associated, and it occurs with increased frequency in Down, Turner and Williams syndromes. Coeliac disease should also be considered in epilepsy with intracranial calcification and unexplained neurological conditions, e.g. palsies, neuropathies, migraine. In adults, dermatitis herpetiformis, splenic atrophy and neoplasia (in particular, T-cell lymphoma of the small intestine) may develop.

The revised European Society of Paediatric Gastroenterology, Hepatology and Nutrition (ESPGHAN) criteria for the diagnosis of coeliac disease were published in 2012 and The British Society of Paediatric Gastroenterology, Hepatology and Nutrition (BSPGHAN) criteria in 2013.

According to these criteria, which were established before the availability of serological screening, diagnosis requires proximal small intestinal biopsy. Morphological change within the intestine can be patchy and hence a variety of histological abnormalities may be found. These include villus atrophy, which can be severe, crypt hyperplasia, inflammation within the lamina propria, abnormalities of the surface epithelium and the presence of increased numbers of intraepithelial lymphocytes. Where all of these changes are seen together the diagnosis is fairly secure (**Fig. 9.19**). According to the ESPGHAN

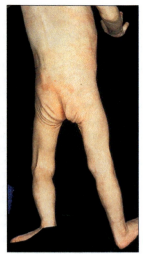

FIGURE 9.17 Coeliac disease, showing severe wasting of buttocks and thighs.

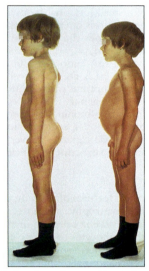

FIGURE 9.18 Coeliac disease. The twin on the right shows the signs of distended abdomen and short stature.

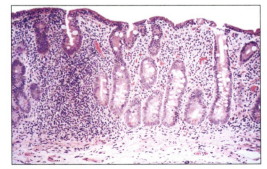

FIGURE 9.19 Coeliac disease. Proximal small intestine histology (×400). Subtotal villous atrophy with villous shortening, crypt hypertrophy, increased numbers of intraepithelial lymphocytes and lamina propria plasma cells.

criteria, if there is full clinical remission when gluten is excluded from the diet, it is only necessary to take one biopsy on presentation. More than one biopsy is required if:

- At presentation the child is under 2 years old.
- There is an atypical histology (in which case rebiopsy off gluten and then following a gluten rechallenge is necessary).

Detection of plasma tTg and/or endomysial antibodies are excellent screening tests for the presence of coeliac disease. Both IgA and IgG antibody screening kits are available, and IgG anti-tTG appears excellent in children with IgA deficiency. In children under the age of 3 years antideaminated tTG may be a better screening test, although this is not widely available. There is little place anymore for the measurement of IgG and IgA antigliadin antibodies. Persistently positive antibodies, or their reappearance, indicate gluten ingestion, but the absence of tTG does not confirm that no gluten is being ingested.

The diagnosis is made when there is a positive blood test for IgA tTG and typical histological appearance of a small intestinal biopsy. However, in some cases the diagnosis can now be established if the blood tTG is **>10 times the upper limit of normal** in a symptomatic child, providing further blood sample are positive for IgA-endomysial antibody (EMA) and HLA-DQ2 or HLA-DQ8 are positive and there is a resolution of symptoms with a gluten-free diet.

Iron-deficiency anaemia, low red cell and serum folate, low plasma albumin and prolonged prothrombin time are non-specific findings in coeliac disease. Stool elastase can also be very low due to secondary pancreatic exocrine insufficiency.

PATHOLOGY

Major histological features of jejunum are hyperplastic subtotal villous atrophy, with increased numbers of lamina propria plasma cells and increased ratio of intraepithelial lymphocytes to surface epithelial cells.

Immunological abnormalities include an increased proportion of intraepithelial lymphocytes with gamma/delta T-cell receptors, reduced lamina propria suppressor cell numbers and increased antibody (including antigliadin antibody) production. Gluten-specific CD4 positive T-cells are restricted by the HLA-DQ DQ2 heterodimer. There is aberrant HLA-DR expression by immature crypt enterocytes, reduced enterocyte survival time and increased intestinal permeability.

DIFFERENTIAL DIAGNOSIS

Wheat sensitive enteropathy and atopy-associated wheat allergy are not autoimmune diseases and have a very different immunological pathology to coeliac disease. Both are transient. They are commonest in infants and preschool children (see 'Food sensitive enteropathy').

TREATMENT

Dietary exclusion of gluten in wheat, rye and barley is advocated. Oats are normally tolerated as these are gluten free when in pure form. Reintroduction of certified wheat free oats can be tried after 1 year if the child is well, but should be excluded again if any symptoms develop.

PROGNOSIS

Coeliac disease is lifelong, but normally controlled with a gluten free diet. There is an association with small intestinal lymphoma in later life, possibly more commonly in patients who continue to ingest a gluten containing diet.

Easy access to paediatric dietitian(s) must be ensured. Parents and patients should be advised to join Coeliac UK: website www.coeliac.co.uk and/or other international support organisations.

FOOD ALLERGIC ENTEROPATHY

INCIDENCE/GENETICS

A disorder, often associated with a family and/or personal history of atopic disease, or immunodeficiency. Gastrointestinal symptoms precipitated by cow's milk may affect 1 in 200 infants.

AETIOLOGY/PATHOGENESIS

Food allergic enteropathy is normally the consequence of a cell-mediated immunological reaction, which leads to the lack of tolerance of a food by the intestinal immune system. Patients usually have a major or minor (often atopic-associated) immunodeficiency. IgA deficiency is common. The enteropathy most frequently occurs with cow's milk (the major dietary constituent in bottle-fed infants), also with egg, soya and wheat or almost any food, e.g. rice, chicken and fish allergies have been described. The enteropathy is of variable severity and rapidly resolves when the offending food is excluded from the diet.

Hypothetically a 'slow onset' food allergy may develop when intestinal immunity is compromised, e.g. during acute gastroenteritis or due to a long-term immunodeficiency that may predispose to excessive antigen absorption.

DIAGNOSIS

It is usually associated with vomiting, diarrhoea, faltering growth, irritability and abdominal pain. Children usually dislike the offending food. For example, children with associated cow's milk allergy may only ingest milk on cereal, in tea or as milkshakes.

The diagnosis may be made when symptoms resolve on excluding the offending food from the diet for 6–8 weeks. If dietary exclusion fails or is inappropriate, upper intestinal endoscopy with duodenal mucosal biopsy should be performed (**Fig. 9.20**). Histologically, there is thinning of intestinal mucosa with a patchy, partial villous atrophy and increased lamina propria cellularity (**Fig. 9.21**). There may be an eosinophilic infiltration of the small intestinal lamina propria. Food specific IgE antibodies in peripheral blood (radioabsorbent [RAST] test) and skin-prick test for dietary allergen may be positive, although these tests are of little diagnostic relevence.

The definitive diagnosis is made if a repeat small intestinal biopsy is histologically normal after a minimum of 8 weeks dietary exclusion (**Fig. 9.22**) – not usually clinically indicated.

DIFFERENTIAL DIAGNOSIS

Food-sensitive enteropathy should be distinguished from immediate hypersensitivity, IgE-mediated, allergic response to food, in which there is usually a reaction to the food within an hour and no underlying enteropathy. The enteropathy is less severe than in coeliac disease and is histologically distinct.

TREATMENT

Removal of the offending food from the diet for a minimum trial period of 6–8 weeks, with advice from a dietitian, simultaneously treats the patient and confirms the identity of the offending food/s. Long-term total exclusion is not essential in all older children who may tolerate certain foodstuffs with traces of the offending food. Gradual reintroduction can be attempted after several weeks or months of full health.

PROGNOSIS

Food allergic enteropathies usually improve as the intestinal-associated immune tissue matures from about 18 months to 2 years of age or later, but can persist throughout childhood and even into adult life. Some patients can tolerate a food in cooking; for example, some children with cow's milk allergy can tolerate milk as cheese and yogurt, but not neat milk in a cup of tea.

AUTOIMMUNE ENTEROPATHY

INCIDENCE/GENETICS

A rare disorder, recognised in European, Arab, North American and Japanese children. There is evidence of a genetic predisposition with both a high incidence of autoimmune disease in first-degree relatives and, in some families, apparent X-linked, recessive inheritance (overall male to female ratio 2:1). IPEX syndrome is one inherited form, characterised by the association of autoimmune enteropathy with polyendocrinopathy and immunodysregulation (linked to dysfunction of the transcriptional activator FoxP3).

AETIOLOGY/PATHOGENESIS

The enteropathy is of variable severity, with lymphocytic infiltration of the lamina propria (**Fig. 9.23**). The three main immunological features are:

- Circulating antienterocyte antibodies.
- In some patients, antibodies have been shown to fix complement.
- Aberrant HLA-DR staining of enterocytes in affected small intestine.

DIAGNOSIS

Protracted diarrhoea with faltering growth that may commence in infancy after the neonatal period, or,

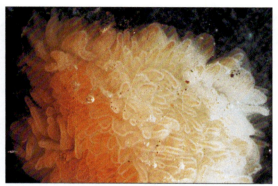

FIGURE 9.20 Food sensitive enteropathy. Dissecting microscope appearance of normal small intestine showing villi when on an appropriate diet.

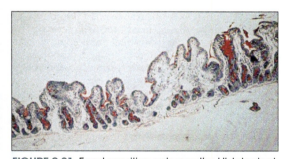

FIGURE 9.21 Food sensitive enteropathy. Histological appearance of proximal small intestinal biopsy in a food sensitive patient, showing partial villous atrophy with mucosal thinning (×250).

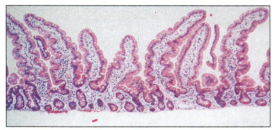

FIGURE 9.22 Food sensitive enteropathy. Normal mucosa on exclusion diet.

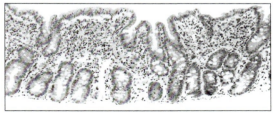

FIGURE 9.23 Sub-total villous atrophy of duodenum with crypt hyperplasia and lymphocytic and plasma cell infiltration in autoimmune enteropathy.

less commonly, at any age throughout childhood. The onset often appears to be after acute infectious gastroenteritis with rapid resolution of symptoms in other affected family members. It is associated with organ specific autoimmune diseases of the thyroid, parathyroid, liver, kidney and pancreas. Peripheral blood should be tested for antienterocyte antibodies. Histological examination of small intestinal mucosal biopsy demonstrates a lamina propria lymphocytic and plasma cell infiltrate. There is frequently an associated colitis.

TREATMENT

Dietary antigen ingestion should be reduced, with specific dietary exclusions. The child may require liquid enteral tube feeds and in severe cases, PN. Patients who do not respond to dietary management are treated with immunosuppressive agents. In most patients prednisolone and azathioprine are effective and, in others, ciclosporin and tacrolimus have been of benefit.

PROGNOSIS

Enteropathy ranges in severity from a form of postenteritis syndrome, i.e. protracted episode of diarrhoea that resolves spontaneously over a few weeks, to a relentless disease process with intestinal failure and survival dependent on PN. Patients may require immunosuppressive treatment for months or years.

EOSINOPHILIC GASTROINTESTINAL DISEASE

This involves a spectrum of disorders grouped together as eosinophilic gastrointestinal diseases. They may be dependent or independent of allergic reaction to specific food proteins. Symptoms depend on the underlying disease, which may be:

- Mucosal with malabsorption or gastrointestinal bleeding.
- Muscle layer disease affecting intestinal motility, typically with vomiting or constipation.
- Subserosal disease with eosinophilic ascites.

There is commonly a family history of atopy.

EOSINOPHILIC OESOPHAGITIS

INCIDENCE/GENETICS

A characteristic set of genes termed the 'EE transcriptome' are expressed.

AETIOLOGY/PATHOGENESIS/DIAGNOSIS

The histological appearance of a minimum of 15 eosinophils per high-power field on oesophageal mucosal biopsy obtained at oesophagogastroduodenoscopy. Eosinophilic degranulation and infiltration of the epithelium may be detected.

Macroscopically, at endoscopy there maybe ridging furrowing or oesophageal rings and, in some cases, a whitish oesophageal exudate (**Fig. 9.24**). Multiple rings have been termed 'corrugated oesophagus'. Upper intestinal radiological contrast study may also detect a 'ringed oesophagus'. Associated problems include psoriasis, seborrhoeic dermatitis, asthma and allergic rhinitis.

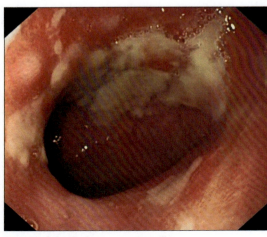

FIGURE 9.24 Reflux oesophagitis.

DIFFERENTIAL DIAGNOSIS

Gastro-oesophageal reflux disease (GORD) (see section below). In contrast to GORD, patients may not respond to proton pump inhibitors treatment. GORD patients may have a lower infiltrate of oesophageal eosinophils.

TREATMENT/PROGNOSIS

- Swallowed steroid aerosol.
- Dietary antigen avoidance.
- In some cases H2 blockers and proton pump inhibitors.

Oesophagitis improves with age. A minority of cases have recurrent oesophageal stricturing.

EOSINOPHILIC ENTEROPATHY

CLINICAL PRESENTATION/DIAGNOSIS

This is a rare enteropathy. Clinical presentation is wide and can include a variety of diverse symptoms. These include abdominal pain, nausea, vomiting, poor weight gain and diarrhoea. Symptoms of intestinal pseudo-obstruction and ascites may develop. Essential investigations include gastrointestinal panendoscopy with mucosal biopsy of oesophagus, stomach, small intestine, ileum and colon.

Histologically there is an eosinophilic infiltration of affected mucosa/submucosa/muscle layer. Plasma albumin, globulins and haemoglobin may be low. Peripheral blood eosinophilia may be present.

DIFFERENTIAL DIAGNOSIS

Non- eosinophilic food allergic enteropathy and autoimmune enteropathy may present with similar symptoms and respond to similar treatment.

TREATMENT/PROGNOSIS

Treatment will depend upon severity of presentation. Exclusion of potentially offending foods from the diet may be tried. Usually a therapeutic trial of prednisolone will be instigated early and if this is efficacious a tailored treatment plan formulated to include steroid sparing agents (for example azathioprine).

Prognosis is good if symptoms are controlled with treatment.

EOSINOPHILIC DISEASE OF THE COLON (EDC) ALLERGIC COLITIS

INCIDENCE/GENETICS

This is the commonest cause of non-infectious diarrhoea in infancy, with a higher incidence in males. There is a family history of atopy, particularly in the mother. It is increasingly recognised in older children.

DIAGNOSIS

There is onset of diarrhoea, often with blood and mucus in the neonatal period or infancy in an otherwise healthy, thriving baby. It occurs in breast-fed as well as bottle-fed babies and may present as toddler's diarrhoea (see page 256). Investigations include colonoscopy with mucosal biopsies. Macroscopically, there is colonic erythema (often patchy) and, histologically, an inflammatory infiltrate of the colonic lamina propria with eosinophils and plasma cells. Specific IgE RAST tests for specific foods, and skin-prick tests for allergens, may indicate offending foods. Plasma immunoglobulin levels may demonstrate immunodeficiency, most commonly a low IgA and/or IgG subclass levels.

TREATMENT

This involves dietary exclusion of offending foods. Cow's milk, soya, egg and wheat are most common, but many other foods have been implicated, including fish, pork and beef.

PROGNOSIS

This improves with age, but there is often persistent intolerance to a large amount of the offending food. Most children cannot drink cow's milk, but may tolerate it in cooking or when boiled.

CLASSIC INFLAMMATORY BOWEL DISEASE

Crohn disease (CD) and ulcerative colitis (UC) are termed idiopathic inflammatory bowel disease (IBD) (**Table 9.5**). They are chronic inflammatory disorders of unknown aetiology, primarily involving the gastrointestinal tract, but with some systemic features. The major features distinguishing UC from CD are the site and type of inflammation and histology. UC affects the colon, although non-specific inflammatory reactions are common in other regions of the gastrointestinal tract. The inflammation is normally limited to the mucosa.

CD may affect any area of the gastrointestinal tract from the mouth to the anus and involves the full thickness of the bowel wall. The immunological mechanisms implicated in the pathogenesis of these disorders differ significantly. Early in the course of the disease the histological and clinical phenotype might be indeterminate, although it is usually apparent within 2 years of presentation which of the clinical phenotypes the child is suffering from.

Genetic and environmental factors are important in the pathogenesis of IBD. More than 100 genetic loci have been identified to contribute to the risk of developing IBD although for the majority the relative risk of developing the disease with one of the mutations is marginal. Exceptions are the nucleotide binding oligomerisation domain protein 2 (NOD2), and IL23R. Homozygous NOD2 mutants have a 5% risk of developing CD and specific mutants of IL23R (Arg381Gln) reduce the risk approximately three-fold.

A number of single gene disorders have been associated with IBD. These are distinct from idiopathic

IBD and include chronic granulomatous disease (mutations in the β-polypeptide of cytochrome b-245), glycogen storage disease type 1b (mutations in the glucose-6-phosphatase transporter SLC37A4) and the phenotype of intractable ulcering enterocolitis of infancy (IL-10 receptor/receptor ligand deficiency). IL-10 is an anti-inflammatory cytokine that is essential for immunoregulation in the intestinal tract. IL-10 deficiency or alpha- or beta-receptor deficiency is associated with early onset intractable IBD affecting the colon with onset within the first 3 months of life. The colitis only partially responds to immunosuppression. It can be effectively treated with haematopoietic stem cell transplant.

ULCERATIVE COLITIS

INCIDENCE/GENETICS

The incidence of UC ranges from 1 in 25,000 to 1 in 50,000 in childhood. Fifteen percent have an affected first-degree relative. Association with -DR2 has been recognised and also a weak association with HLA-B27 and HLA-Bw35 in Caucasians. However, affected patients in the same family may be of different HLA types. Monozygotic twins are frequently discordant for UC with only 15% concordance.

Many of the genetic loci associated with UC are also associated with CD. The types of genes implicated include those involved in microbial recognition, cytokine signalling, lymphocyte activation and intestinal epithelial defence. The strongest association with UC is that with HLA.

AETIOLOGY/PATHOGENESIS

The aetiology is unknown, but appears to be multifactorial. Immunological mechanisms are involved. Autoimmunity is a feature and in 80% of cases there is an IgG1 antibody to a colonic polypeptide, specific to ulcerative colitis. Positive perinuclear anticytoplasmic antibody (p-ANCA) is associated with an increased risk of developing primary sclerosing cholangitis and 'pouchitis'.

Inflammation is normally confined to the intestinal mucosa although will exceptionally become transmural in toxical dilatation of the colon where perforation is imminent. While the colon is affected most severely, inflammation in other regions of the gastrointestinal tract including the stomach and small intestine, is common. Colonic inflammation is continuous, although occasionally the rectum can be spared. At colonoscopy the colon will often have a granular haemorrhagic appearance, with friability and loss of vascular markings (**Fig. 9.25**). Histologically there is vascular congestion, crypt branching and abscesses, loss of goblet cells and Paneth cell metaplasia with mucosal inflammatory cell infiltration.

DIAGNOSIS

UC most commonly presents with bloody diarrhoea and mucus, often having diarrhoea both by day and by night. Other features are lower, colicky abdominal pain, anorexia, weight loss, and urgency of stool.

TABLE 9.5 Extraintestinal manifestations of classic inflammatory bowel disease

- Growth failure
- Arthritis and arthralgia:
  - 20–25% ulcerative colitis and 11% Crohn
- Sacroilitis and ankylosing spondylitis associated with HLA-B27
- Erythema nodosum in approximately 5% of patients with Crohn (commoner in Crohn)
- Pyoderma gangrenosum in 0.5–5% of ulcerative colitis and 0.1% of Crohn
- Liver disease:
  - sclerosing cholangitis
  - chronic active hepatitis and cholelithiasis may rarely occur and can be severe
- Ocular manifestations:
  - uveitis is acutely symptomatic in less than 3% of patients
  - episcleritis and conjunctivitis may develop
- Renal manifestations:
  - usually formation of calcium oxalate stones in up to 5% of children with Crohn disease (associated with ileal disease)

A minority present with severe/fulminating colitis, often with toxic megacolon when vomiting, pyrexia, tachycardia, severe abdominal pain and hypoalbuminaemia; distension and tenderness may occur with reduced bowel sounds and bloody diarrhoea (>5 stools over 24 hours). Extraintestinal manifestations include arthralgia and arthritis, delayed growth and sexual maturation (less severe than in CD) and, rarely, liver disease (in particular primary sclerosing cholangitis). Gastrointestinal panendoscopy is an essential investigation.

Paediatric UC activity Index (PUCAI) for children and young people includes scoring of the presence and severity of abdominal pain, rectal bleeding, stool consistency of most stools, number of stools per 24 hours, stools causing wakening at night and level of activity. Details can be found in the NICE guideline.

TREATMENT

There are two phases – remission induction followed by maintenance. In very mild disease a 5-aminosalicylate preparation that is anti-inflammatory can be used. This generally takes 15–18 days to work. In more severe disease first-line treatments are usually oral corticosteroids, which are reduced slowly over 8–12 weeks. Patients who relapse when the steroids are reduced/stopped will usually require azathioprine or another steroid sparing agent. In patients starting azathioprine thiopurine methyltransferase (TPMT) activity should be measured before starting the thiopurine so that patients likely to be intolerant of regular dose azathioprine can be identified. Ciclosporin has been effective in remission induction in resistant disease, but long-term use of ciclosporin is generally not indicated. With the widespread introduction of monoclonal antibody therapies there is now a place for monoclonal anti-TNFα antibodies in acute disease. Intravenous broad-spectrum antibiotics might be used as an adjunct. Surgical management with usually a total colectomy with ileostomy formation is indicated for disease unresponsive to medical therapies. Subsequent ileoanal pull-through with pouch formation may be undertaken.

Up to 30% may develop antibodies to cow's milk and patients in this group might exhibit an improvement in residual symptoms if cow's milk is removed from the diet.

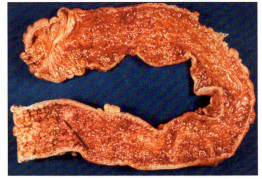

FIGURE 9.25 Ulcerative colitis showing extensive colonic involvement with inflammation and bleeding.

Annual colonoscopy is desirable if pancolitis continues for over 10 years, as surveillance for possible malignancy.

PROGNOSIS

UC has a chronic relapsing disease course. Most children lead a normal lifestyle, but up to 20% have incapacitating disease. The risk of colonic malignancy increases if there is active pancolitis or left-sided colitis for 10 years or more. The disease can be cured by total colectomy, but inflammation or pouchitis of the surgically-fashioned ileal pouch occurs in up to one-third of patients, usually those who manifest an ileitis prior to colectomy.

CROHN DISEASE

INCIDENCE/GENETICS

The incidence of CD has increased since the 1950s to approximately 1 in 25,000 children. Almost one-third of patients present in late childhood. Both sexes are affected equally. North European, Anglo-Saxon and European and North American Jew peoples classically develop the disease although it is being seen with increasing frequency in other populations, such as those from the Middle East. There is a suggestion that improvement in living standards antedates the increment in disease prevalence. Approximately 35% of patients have a first-degree relative affected by CD or UC. Concordance in monozygotic twins is stronger than with UC (30%) and there is a much weaker association with HLA. Many of the genetic loci associated with CD are similarly seen with UC. CD predominant associations include NOD2 and genes that regulate autophagy (autophagy is important in the degradation of damaged subcellular organelles and in the clearance of pathogens, which is required for immunity to many pathogens).

AETIOLOGY/PATHOGENESIS

Genetic and environmental factors are important. The fact that NOD2 mutations are a major genetic factor predisposing to CD (homozygous carriage of an at risk NOD2 allele increases the risk of CD nearly 20-fold) underlines the important of bacterial signalling to the immune system in the pathogenesis of CD. The intestinal immune system has to maintain a state of tolerance to normal bacterial commensals but nevertheless be able to react to intestinal pathogens. This delicate balance of pro- and anti-inflammatory influences may be perturbed in CD. Both T helper (Th) 1 cytokines and Th17 cytokines are upregulated in CD, whereas the functioning of anti-inflammatory regulatory T-cells (Tregs) is impaired. IL-23 is an important activator of Th17 cells and genes encoding proteins involved in IL-23 signalling and Th17 cell differentiation (for example IL23R, IL12B, CCR6 and TNFSF15) are associated with susceptibility to CD.

CD is phenotypically heterogeneous, with the clinical presentation depending upon which areas of the gut are predominantly involved and the presence or absence of stricturing and fistulae. Individuals with two disease associated NOD2 mutations are more likely to have ileal disease and stricturing disease.

DIAGNOSIS

Insidious onset with loss of appetite, weight loss, abdominal pain, diarrhoea and poor growth occurs. Children can present with short stature, delayed puberty or with an abdominal mass, perianal inflammation, aphthous mouth ulcers and extraintestinal problems, such as fever, arthritis, uveitis, erythema nodosum and liver disease. Over 50% of cases have an ileocolitis; at least 30% have small bowel disease alone and 10–15% colonic disease alone. The disease may affect any part of the gastrointestinal tract (**Figs 9.26–9.29**).

Colonoscopy with biopsy of terminal ileal and colonic mucosa should be carried out, along with upper intestinal endoscopy. Macroscopically at colonoscopy there is patchy inflammation with aphthous ulceration (**Fig. 9.30**), sometimes with 'snail track' ulcers and 'cobblestone' appearance. The presence of non-caseating epitheloid granulomata on histological examination is diagnostic. The mucosal inflammatory infiltrate consists of monocytes, macrophages, lymphocytes and plasma cells with neutrophils when acutely inflamed. Often a clinicopathological correlation is necessary to make a clinical diagnosis as pathology alone may not be diagnostic.

Blood platelet and haemoglobin level, ESR/CRP and plasma albumin are used for monitoring disease activity. Barium contrast studies (**Fig. 9.31**) can be undertaken to investigate for strictures (and mucosal oedema and ulceration), although increasingly MRI scanning using either locust bean gum or mannitol solution to increase intraluminal water can be undertaken. MRI can provide information about strictures, wall thickness and mucosal disease when appropriate contrast agents are used. Liver enzymes, bone age and bone density should be checked. Ophthalmological examination is required to investigate for disease involvement and steroid-associated cataract formation.

Paediatric Crohn Disease Activity Index (PCDAI) should be calculated on each clinic visit.

TREATMENT

As with UC, remission induction followed by maintenance therapy is appropriate. The gold standard of remission induction is mucosal healing (as opposed to clinical remission).

- Liquid enteral nutrition as a sole source of nutrition for 6–8 weeks is highly efficacious, especially with ileal disease. Inflammatory markers fall within a few days of starting therapy and mucosal healing can be achieved. Elemental and polymeric feeds are both effective with full (over two-thirds of cases) or partial remission. 'Nutritional' therapies have the added advantage of correcting nutritional deficiencies and facilitating 'catch up' weight gain and growth.

- Immunosuppression: prednisolone produces a clinical remission in many but does not achieve mucosal healing and has negative effects upon bone health. Prednisolone is no longer used as a first-line treatment and its use should be kept to a minimum (for example symptomatic treatment of strictures while awaiting definitive therapy).

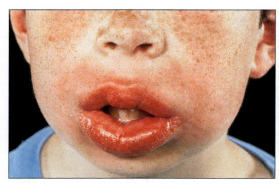

FIGURE 9.26 Crohn disease of the lip.

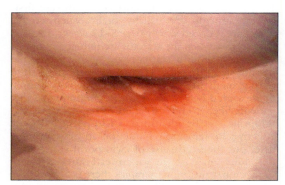

FIGURE 9.27 Crohn disease affecting the perianal region.

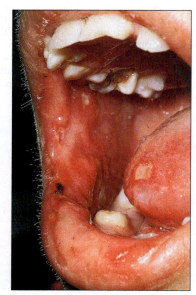

FIGURE 9.28 Crohn disease. Aphthous ulceration of the mouth.

Gastroenterology

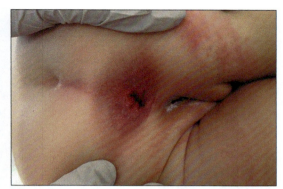

FIGURE 9.29 Crohn disease: perianal erythema and fissuring.

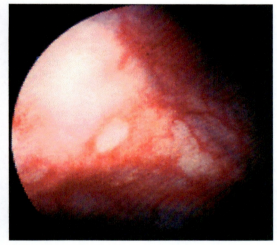

FIGURE 9.30 Crohn disease. Appearance of the colon at colonoscopy, showing aphthous ulceration and loss of normal vascular pattern.

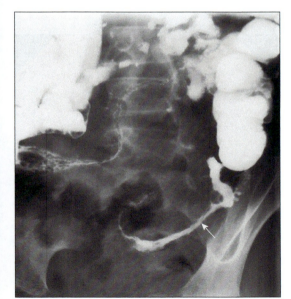

FIGURE 9.31 Crohn disease. Radiological contrast studies demonstrating intestinal stricturing.

- Methotrexate can induce remission but is rarely used as a first-line treatment.
- Azathioprine/mercaptopurine are used as disease modifying drugs. There is little place for these agents in remission induction but once this has been induced they can help prevent recurrence.
- Ciclosporin and tacrolimus are usually not efficacious in CD therapy and their use is usually limited to drug resistant/recalcitrant disease.
- Thalidomide can be effective in some resistant cases.
- Biological therapies including infliximab and adalimumab (anti-TNF antibodies) are now widely used. Anti-TNF therapies can induce remission and achieve mucosal healing and may close fistulae. These therapies are also effective in maintenance, although a percentage of patients appear to lose responsiveness to these agents over time.
- 5-aminosalicylic acid derivative is given to treat colitis. There is little evidence that this approach is efficacious.
- Antibiotics: metronidazole and ciprofloxacin will often improve mucosal inflammation and perianal sepsis.
- Surgery is reserved principally for the relief of chronic strictures, although increasingly these are being treated in paediatric practice with balloon dilatation in the first instance.

PROGNOSIS

There is usually a chronic relapsing disease course. If the disease is controlled with aggressive medical treatment, there is a reduced need for surgery. About 5% of children have an initial presentation, then remain in remission, and about 5% have disease that is resistant to treatment, requiring aggressive medical treatment and possible surgery.

LYMPHANGIECTASIA

INCIDENCE/GENETICS

This is a rare pathological dilatation of lymhatic vessels of the small intestine. Children may also have extraintestinal manifestation such as limb or lung involvement. Hennekam syndrome is a rare autosomal recessive form of intestinal lympangiectasia with lymphoedema, characteristic facial appearance and developmental delay affecting < 1 in 1000,000 (**Fig. 9.32**).

DIAGNOSIS

There is characteristic histological appearance of dilated intestinal lymphatics with diffusely swollen mucosa and enlarged villi on small intestinal biopsy taken at upper intestinal endoscopy.

If the lesion is beyond the duodenum, enteroscopy with biopsy or video-capsule examination is needed. Macroscopically there are dilated lymphatics with diffusely swollen mucosa and enlarged villi.

CLINICAL PRESENTATION

Presentation is with diarrhoea, usually with oedema, most commonly in a child less than 3 years old, but it can develop in adolescence. Lymphangiectasia is associated with faltering growth and increased frequency of infections. Low serum albumin globulin and plasma lymphocytes are found. Untreated lymphangiectasia leads to chronic 'protein-losing enteropathy'. Low blood cholesterol, calcium and fat soluble vitamins may occur.

The condition may also develop secondary to elevated lymphatic pressure in congestive heart failure. Small intestinal mucosal biopsy should be carried out, with histological examination for dilated lacteals and distorted villi. Plasma lymphocytes are $<1.5 \times 10^9/l$.

TREATMENT

A low-fat, high-protein, medium-chain triglyceride (MCT) diet is advised, with fat soluble vitamin supplements. Regular albumin infusions may be required and in severe cases long-term PN support. If a limited area is affected, surgical resection should be considered. In extreme cases small intestinal transplant may be needed.

PROGNOSIS

Severity is in proportion to the extent of intestinal disease.

ULCERS

GASTRIC ULCER

INCIDENCE/AETIOLOGY

Gastic ulcers are rare in children. They are usually secondary to other disorders, such as acute stress, including burns, intracranial pathology, salicylates and other NSAIDs in children under 10 years old. It is still not certain whether *Helicobacter pylori* is associated with gastric ulcer in children.

DIAGNOSIS

Peptic ulcers in the neonatal period commonly present with life-threatening haemorrhage or perforation and secondary ulcers in older children frequently present in a similar manner. Abdominal pain may occur in older children. Gastroscopy should be carried out (**Fig. 9.33**).

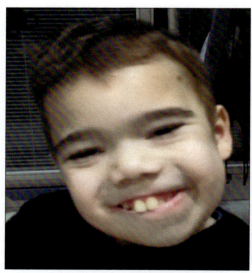

FIGURE 9.32 Lymphangiectasia: facial features of Hennekam disease.

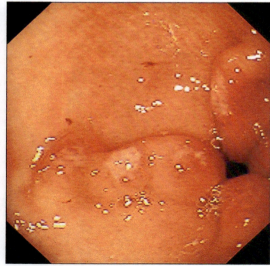

FIGURE 9.33 Endoscopic appearance of gastric ulcers and erosions adjacent to pylorus.

TREATMENT/PROGNOSIS

Treatment is with H2 receptor antagonists or proton pump inhibitors. Secondary ulcers usually resolve completely after the acute episode.

DUODENAL ULCERS

INCIDENCE/AETIOLOGY

Duodenal ulcers are associated with *Helicobacter pylori* infection (see page 273).

CLINICAL PRESENTATION/DIAGNOSIS

Clinically there is usually episodic epigastric pain, often awakening the patient at night. They are associated with recurrent vomiting; haematemesis may occur. Endoscopy should be carried out, with mucosal biopsy for histological examination. Mucosal sections should be stained with a substance, such as Giemsa, to detect *H pylori*.

TREATMENT/PROGNOSIS

As for *H pylori*. Prognosis is excellent, with lack of recurrence if *H pylori* is eradicated.

POLYPS

ISOLATED INFLAMMATORY/JUVENILE POLYP

INCIDENCE/GENETICS

These polyps occur in 1% of preschool/school age children and up to 4% in those under 21 years. Male to female ratio is 3:2, with sporadic occurrence.

AETIOLOGY/CLINICAL PRESENTATION

An inflammatory colonic polyp, with more than one in over 50% of cases. Polyps may occur in any area of the colon. About 60% of polyps are proximal to the sigmoid colon.

Children present with painless rectal bleeding with/without faeces and/or mucus in 90%. Abdominal pain, pain after defaecation and polyp prolapse (dark beefy red mass) may occur. Sloughing of a larger polyp can develop.

DIAGNOSIS

Colonoscopy with polypectomy and histological examination should be conducted (**Fig. 9.34**). Macroscopically, polyps are rounded with a slender stalk; histologically, they are hamartomatous.

TREATMENT/PROGNOSIS

Endoscopic polypectomy is performed via colonoscope. There is low recurrence and no subsequent problems such as malignancy.

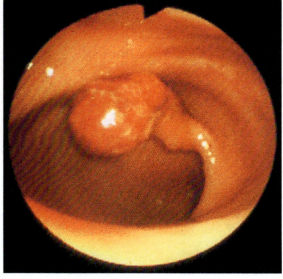

FIGURE 9.34 Isolated inflammatory/juvenile polyp.

JUVENILE POLYPOSIS SYNDROME

INCIDENCE/GENETICS

Polyposis syndrome may be familial or sporadic. Between 1:6,000 and 1:100,000 children are affected. It is autosomal dominant with a mutation in the *BMPR1A* or *SMAD4* gene in some cases.

The syndrome is suspected when there are more than five juvenile polyps of the colon and/or rectum, multiple juvenile polyps throughout the digestive tract or at least one polyp and a family history of juvenile polyps.

AETIOLOGY

Multiple inflammatory polyps occur throughout the colon. The stomach and small intestine may also be affected. Histologically polyps are hamartomatous.

DIAGNOSIS

Most commonly patients present with painless rectal bleeding and prolapse. The rectal haemorrhage is rarely life threatening and can be asymptomatic. Faltering growth, diarrhoea and intussusception may occur. Symptoms usually start from 5 years of age in sporadic cases and from 9 years in familial cases. Colonoscopy (**Fig. 9.35**) with polypectomy and histological examination of polyp should be conducted.

TREATMENT/PROGNOSIS

Polypectomy at colonoscopy should be performed, with regular colonoscopic surveillance.

In generalised juvenile polyposis there is an increased incidence of gastric, duodenal, pancreatic and colonic adenomata and adenocarcinoma (usually in adult life), which has not been seen when polyps are limited to the colon.

FAMILIAL POLYPOSIS COLI AND GARDNER SYNDROME

INCIDENCE/GENETICS

Incidence of familial polyposis coli, also known as familial adenomatous polyposis varies from 1 in 7,000 to 1 in 22,000. It is autosomal dominant with mutations in the *APC* gene or autosomal recessive with mutations in the *MUTYH* gene. Gardner syndrome affects 1:14,025 with an autosomal dominant familial polyposis coli gene (*APC*) on chromosome 5.

AETIOLOGY

Multiple (thousands) of adenomatous colonic polyps occur (**Fig. 9.36**). Gastric and small intestinal polyps also occur in Gardner syndrome.

CLINICAL PRESENTATION/DIAGNOSIS

Diarrhoea, abdominal pain and rectal bleeding occur, usually from about 10 years of age. Patients with Gardner syndrome also develop bony abnormalities (particularly osteomas of frontal and mandibular bones), dental abnormalities, CNS, thyroid and desmoid tumours and, in over 90% of cases, hypertrophy of retinal pigment epithelium. Colonoscopy should be carried out, with polypectomy of larger polyps and histological examination.

TREATMENT/PROGNOSIS

Regular endoscopic examination and eventual colectomy should be performed. There is a 100% malignancy risk with time.

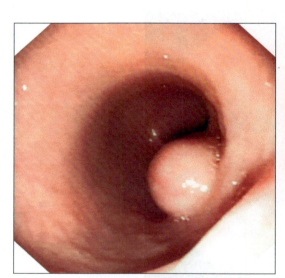

FIGURE 9.35 Juvenile polyposis syndrome: juvenile polyp in duodenum,

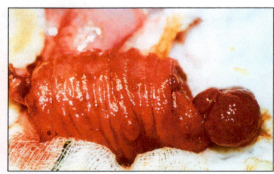

FIGURE 9.36 Colon showing multiple polyposis.

PEUTZ–JEGHER SYNDROME

INCIDENCE/GENETICS

Peutz–Jegher is an autosomal dominant genetic disease with an incidence of approximately 1 in 50,000–200,000 births. It is an autosomal dominant condition associated with the *STK11* gene on chromosome 19 – a possible tumour suppressor gene.

AETIOLOGY

Also known as hereditary intestinal polyposis syndrome, it is characterised by benign hamartomatous polyps in the small intestine and, in some cases, the colon with characteristic hyperpigmented macules on the lips and oral mucosa.

DIAGNOSIS

Abnormal pigmentation of lips is found, extending onto the facial skin and in the buccal mucosa (**Fig. 9.37**). The most common symptom is abdominal pain due to intussusception/mechanical intestinal obstruction by a polyp. It may present with iron deficiency anaemia due to bleeding from an intestinal polyp. Investigations include a small intestinal radiological contrast study and colonoscopy. Video-capsule examination is useful if a suspected polyp is not detected with other investigations.

Differential diagnosis of oral pigmentation includes Addison disease and McCune–Albright syndrome (see pages 393, 399).

TREATMENT/PROGNOSIS

Treatment is conservative, with removal of those polyps causing excessive bleeding or intussusception at endoscopy (or via an enterotomy at laparotomy if otherwise inaccessible).

Prognosis is usually good, but a few patients develop intestinal and, rarely, gastric malignancy.

INFECTIONS AND INFESTATIONS

BACTERIAL ENTERIC INFECTIONS

HELICOBACTER PYLORI

Incidence/ Pathogenesis

H pylori infection is rare in children under 14 years in developed countries, but common world-wide. *H pylori* is a gram-negative, spiral, motile organism (**Fig. 9.38**). It produces a large amount of urease; this may lead to gastritis by producing ammonia that may be toxic to the gastric mucosa. It is probable that spread is by person to person.

Diagnosis

Patients may present with symptoms of duodenal ulcer, epigastric pain and vomiting, often waking the patient at night. Infection with *H pylori* is associated with gastritis, but the gastritis is often asymptomatic. Gastrointestinal symptoms, such as recurrent abdominal pain, are not associated with an increased incidence of *H pylori* gastritis. Upper gastrointestinal endoscopy with biopsy should be conducted. Gastric antral colonisation can be detected on histological appearance (with special staining, such as Giemsa), urease testing and culture.

Treatment/Prognosis

A 2-week course of triple therapy with an H_2 receptor antagonist or proton pump inhibitor, plus antibiotics such as metronidazole and amoxicillin (or clarithromycin) is given.

Duodenal ulcers do not recur after eradication of *H pylori*.

CAMPYLOBACTER JEJUNI

Incidence/Aetiology

Infection is usually sporadic and the source is not identified, but it can be transmitted from undercooked chicken and other meat and untreated water. Currently, it is the most frequently reported cause of

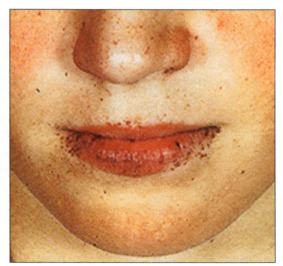

FIGURE 9.37 Peutz–Jegher syndrome, showing brown pigmentation of lips and surrounding facial skin.

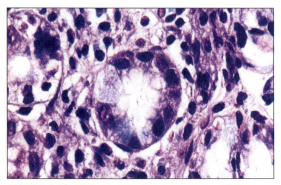

FIGURE 9.38 *Helicobacter*-like organisms within gastric glandular epithelium in sagittal cross-section.

acute bacterial diarrhoea in children world-wide and in the UK. Young children are most commonly affected.

Diagnosis

Onset is with malaise, headache and fever and, within 24 hours, nausea, abdominal pain and diarrhoea. The diarrhoea may be mild, profuse and watery or bloody (especially in young children). Infection is associated with Guillain–Barré syndrome. Stool culture in a low oxygen and high carbon dioxide environment will detect the presence of typical gram-negative curvilinear rods.

Treatment

Infection is usually self-limiting. Erythromycin is given in severe or persistent infection, or the patient is under 2 years old.

CLOSTRIDIUM DIFFICILE

Aetiology

C difficile and toxin can be detected in the healthy newborn and 10–50% of asymptomatic infants, but in less than 5% by 1 year of age. It is a gram-positive anaerobic bacterium that produces a cytotoxin and an enterotoxin.

Diagnosis

Acute or chronic mild diarrhoea occurs, or severe pseudomembranous colitis. Stool testing for cytotoxin, toxigenic *C difficile* or toxin A should be conducted. Colonoscopy will reveal raised, adherent yellow-white mucosal plaques and erythematous friable colonic mucosa (**Fig. 9.39**).

Treatment

Any antibiotic the patient is taking when diagnosed should be stopped and the patient treated with vancomycin or metronidazole. The incidence of clostridial infection can be reduced by treatment with probiotics.

SALMONELLA

Incidence/Aetiology

Peak incidence of infection is in infancy and early childhood. *Salmonella* is a gram-negative, motile, aerobic bacillus (**Fig. 9.40**), acquired from contaminated food or drink. There are three types of *Salmonella: enteritides* (described here) *choleraesius* and *typhi* (typhoid fever).

Diagnosis

The incubation period for *S enteritides* is usually 12–72 hours (longer periods have been described in neonates). Onset is usually accompanied by nausea and fever, then diarrhoea, which can be watery or bloody. Bacteraemia and systemic infection with meningitis, osteomyelitis and pneumonia is most common in infancy.

Treatment

The mainstay of treatment is replacement of fluid and electrolyte losses by oral therapy if possible and, if not, intravenous fluids. Antibiotics are not recommended, except in infants less than 3 months of age or those who are bacteraemic and have signs of systemic infection.

PATHOGENIC ESCHERICHIA COLI

Incidence/Aetiology

Infection with *E coli* is a common, world-wide problem, particularly in developing countries. It is from faecal–oral transmission. *E coli* are gram-negative motile bacilli, which are some of the most common flora of the healthy large intestine. The pathogenic organisms each have one of four properties that the organisms in the normal flora do not possess. These are intestinal wall invasion, enterotoxin and cytotoxin production, or adherence to the bowel wall.

- Enterotoxin producing *E coli* (ETEC) produce heat labile (similar to cholera toxin) and heat stable toxins, which result in profuse diarrhoea.
- Enteroadherent (EPEC) *E coli* (tEPEC and aEPEC) infection with its attaching and effacing (A/E) lesions is a major agent in infantile diarrhoea.
- Enteroinvasive *E coli* (EIEC) produce the same toxin as the shiga toxin from *Shigella dysenteriae*. They are spread through contaminated food and water, but can also pass from person to person.
- Enterohaemorrhagic *E coli* (EHEC) such as *E coli* 0157 produce cytotoxin. They are transmitted from cattle, and are often acquired from undercooked fast food.

Diagnosis

There are at least four different mechanisms of virulence (see Aetiology above), each of which presents in a different way.

- ETEC – 'traveller's diarrhoea', nausea, vomiting, cramping abdominal pain and watery diarrhoea.
- Enteroadherent (EPEC) *E coli* infection presents with a fever and a more prolonged illness, which can persist for many weeks in children, with the same symptoms as ETEC.
- EIEC presents with fever and bloody diarrhoea that is clinically indistinguishable from *Shigella* (**Fig. 9.41**).
- EHEC causes bloody diarrhoea with haemolytic uraemic syndrome often developing about 1 week after the onset, particularly in young children (**Fig. 9.42**). Thrombocytopenic purpura may also develop.

A newly emerging pathotype is the enteroaggregative *E coli* (EAEC). Recognised virulence factors have included adhesins, toxins and associated proteins. No single factor has been associated with virulence in EAEC isolates [Estrada-Garcia T, Navarro-Garcia F 2012].

Investigations should include stool culture and antibiotic sensitivities of organisms. In severe infection in small children, possible haemolytic uraemic syndrome (particularly with 0157:H7 infection) or thrombocytopenia should be monitored for.

Treatment/Prognosis

Children should be rehydrated and hydration maintained (see 'Acute gastroenteritis', page 251). Appropriate antibiotic should be given if there is severe infection, immunosuppressed or in infancy.

Full recovery can be expected with appropriate treatment apart from some cases of haemolytic uraemic syndrome.

GIARDIA LAMBLIA

Incidence/Pathogenesis

G lamblia is a flagellate protozoan, which infects in cyst form and becomes a motile trophozoite. It occurs virtually world-wide. Childhood prevalence increases with age.

Food and water, and person-to-person spread occur and may be transmitted by animals. The organism infects the small intestine and may cause an enteropathy of variable severity.

Diagnosis

Acute infection may present as watery diarrhoea, anorexia and abdominal distension. More frequently chronic diarrhoea develops with nausea, foul smelling flatulence, poor appetite and malabsorption (steatorrhoea) and in some cases there are minimal symptoms only. Microscopy of stool detects only some 80% of cases, even when several specimens are investigated (**Fig. 9.43**). Organisms can be detected on microscopy of duodenal fluid and/or proximal small intestinal mucosal biopsy.

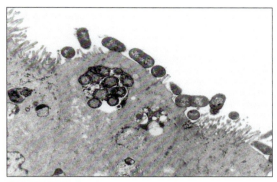

FIGURE 9.41 Electron microscopic appearance of enteropathogenic *Escherichia coli* with patchy loss of microvilli and invasion of cell.

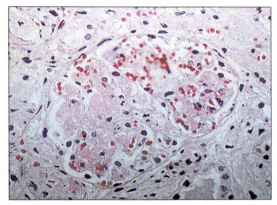

FIGURE 9.42 Renal biopsy of haemolytic uraemic syndrome showing microthrombi, swelling and destruction of glomerular capillaries.

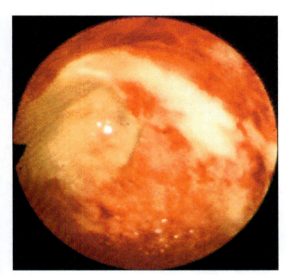

FIGURE 9.39 Macroscopic colon appearance at colonoscopy in pseudomembranous colitis, demonstrating severe erythema and yellow-white plaques.

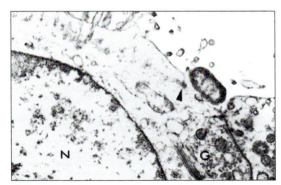

FIGURE 9.40 Electron microscopic appearance of *Salmonella* infection (×15,000).

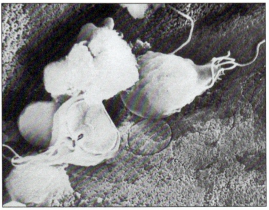

FIGURE 9.43 *Giardia lamblia.* Electron micrograph of trophozoites in the small intestine.

Symptoms may be suggestive of coeliac disease, IBD or anorexia nervosa (anorexia and weight loss).

Treatment/Prognosis
Metronidazole, 30 mg/kg/day is given as a single dose for 3 days, or a single dose of tinidizole, 30 mg/kg.

Chronic infection is associated with immunoglobulin deficiency. If *Giardia* remains untreated, growth of the child may be impaired.

YERSINIA ENTEROCOLITICA
Aetiology
Outbreaks occur from contaminated milk and food.

Diagnosis
Most commonly, children present with acute self-limiting diarrhoea. *Υ enterocolitica* can cause fever and cramping abdominal pain, mimicking acute appendicitis. It is the commonest bacterial aetiology of intussusception. Ultrasound examination can differentiate between them. Chronic diarrhoea may ensue, possibly with erythema nodosum and arthritis. Infection may mimic CD. Isolation of *Yersinia* has been difficult, but a PCR-based assay may be feasible. Colonoscopy findings may mimic CD with mucosal thickening of the terminal ileum, aphthous ulcers and nodularity.

CRYPTOSPORIDIUM
Incidence/Pathogenesis
Cryptosporidium is a coccidian parasite that becomes incorporated in the intestinal epithelial cell, but outside the cytoplasm. Distribution is world-wide with 10% or more prevalence in developing countries. It is spread by water and person-to-person contact.

Pathogenesis may be due to disruption of the microvillous membrane. An enteropathy of variable severity may develop. *Cryptosporidium* may infect small and/or large intestine (**Figs 9.44, 9.45**). It reproduces both sexually and asexually.

Diagnosis
Children present with acute, watery diarrhoea with fever, nausea, vomiting and abdominal discomfort after an incubation period of 1 to 7 days. Prolonged symptoms may occur in immunodeficiency, including post transplant. The stool should be examined for oocytes, which can also be detected in duodenal juices and sputum with suitable staining techniques.

Treatment
There is partial response to macrolide antibiotics (erythromycin, azithromycin, spiramycin, clindamycin). Hyperimmune bovine colostrum may reduce symptoms in the immunocompromised. Boiling tap water/using bottled water is recommended if the child is immunocompromised/post transplant.

ASCARIS LUMBRICOIDES (ROUNDWORM)
Incidence/Aetiology
Ascaris lumbricoides is one of the commonest human parasitic infections world-wide. It is not common in the UK. Larvae hatched from ingested eggs enter the venous system and migrate through the lungs to the oesophagus. Fertilised eggs from adult worms in the intestine are passed with faeces to contaminate soil; the cycle recurs when they, in turn, are ingested.

Diagnosis
Most infected people are symptom free. Respiratory symptoms (cough, wheeze), fever and eosinophilia occur during the pulmonary phase. Anorexia, abdominal cramps and even intestinal obstruction may occur with heavy infestation. Worms can migrate to obstruct the biliary system (causing jaundice), pancreatic ducts (causing pancreatitis), appendix (causing appendicitis), and lead to volvulus, intussusception, intestinal perforation and peritonitis. The faeces should be examined microscopically for ova and adult worms, and sputum and gastric washings should be used to detect larvae.

Treatment
Mebendazole, albendazole, flubendazole or piperazine can be used. Endoscopy is performed to relieve biliary and pancreatic duct obstruction. Intestinal obstruction may be relieved by antihelminthic drug with intravenous fluids and nasogastric suction, but surgery may be necessary.

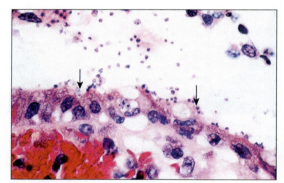

FIGURE 9.44 Cryptosporidiosos: intestinal specimen (×250).

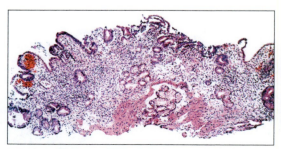

FIGURE 9.45 Cryptosporidiosos: *Cryptosporidium* visible on small intestinal mucosa (×16).

Gastroenterology

ENTEROBIUS VERMICULARIS (PINWORM/THREADWORM)

Incidence/Pathogenesis

E vermicularis is most common in temperate and cold climates, but also occurs world-wide. Although pinworm infection can affect all people, it most commonly occurs among children, institutionalised persons, and household members of persons with pinworm infection.

Aetiology

Pinworms are spread through human-to-human transmission, by ingesting pinworm eggs and/or by anal insertion. Eggs can remain viable in a moist environment for up to 3 weeks.

The sticky eggs are laid near the anus, and are readily transmitted to other surfaces usually through contamination of fingernails, hands, night-clothing and bed linen.

Diagnosis

Children show anal pruritis, particularly at night when the adult female lays eggs in the perianal region. Rarely, other symptoms may develop; for example, symptoms of appendicitis when worms enter the appendix lumen or if adult worms migrate through the intestinal wall to invade other organs. The 'Sellotape test' involves placing a piece of clear adhesive tape over the perianal region at night, then removing it in the morning and examining it for small white specks/ova.

Treatment/Prognosis

Mebendazole is the drug of choice (except for children under 1 year of age, for whom it is not recommended), or piperazine. The whole family should be treated and treatment repeated 2–4 weeks later to eradicate any worms hatched since first treatment.

Reinfection occurs easily and should be prevented, e.g. by treating household contacts as above.

FEEDING DIFFICULTIES

INCIDENCE/AETIOLOGY

Feeding difficulties are common. The aetiology is diverse. They may be caused by poor feeding technique, incorrect feed (for example, powdered milk made up to the wrong strength) or inappropriate type of feed. Gastro-oesophageal reflux disease (GORD) is considered a common underlying/associated disorder. There may be a 'slow onset' food allergy (see **Table 23.2**), or psychosocial deprivation. Poor feeding may also occur with neuromuscular disease, cardiac, respiratory, renal or hepatic failure and inter-current infection. A child who has had a prolonged period of parenteral or enteral feeding may have lost or never developed feeding skills. Poor feeding frequently becomes a secondary behavioural problem, which may persist even if the underlying aetiology has resolved or improved.

DIAGNOSIS

The infant is unwilling to ingest sufficient calories for normal weight gain and growth. Affected children often gag on food or fluids. Food refusal commonly occurs with the child turning their head away from the spoon or teat when fed. Vomiting and poor weight gain are common. There should be close observation of feeding by an experienced nurse (e.g. health visitor). Appropriate advice may resolve the problem. If symptoms persist the patient should have a careful medical examination (to look for evidence of underlying organ failure) and have possible underlying infection excluded (urine culture is essential). If it still continues, appropriate investigations should be performed, which might include oesophageal pH-impedance studies, video-fluoroscopy of swallowing and upper gastrointestinal contrast studies and on occasions high resolution oesophageal impedance manometry.

TREATMENT

Advice should be given by a specialist feeding nurse, speech therapist or other professional with specialist feeding knowledge. Referral to a multidisciplinary feeding clinic is required in more resistant cases. A child unable to feed orally needs cautious stimulation to 'desensitise', initially just touching the face around the mouth, then introducing a variety of shapes and textures to suck and mouth.

Any associated disease should be treated. If unable to ingest sufficient calories despite appropriate treatment, the child may benefit from a commercially available liquid enteral feed administered via an artificial feeding device. The feed may need to be given as daytime bolus feeds, or an overnight continuous feed while the underlying aetiology is investigated and treated.

Artificial feeding devices used are:

- Initially nasogastric tube.
- Gastrostomy may be inserted if support is likely to be needed for several months or years (**Fig. 9.46**).
- Nasojejunal tube if the patient is unable to tolerate feeding via the stomach.
- Gastrojejunostomy.
- Jejunostomy for longer-term small intestinal feeding.

Problems with artificial feeding (**Fig. 9.47**) include local infection at the site of insertion with gastrostomy or jejunostomy devices; dislodgement is also common with gastrojejunostomy and a nasojejunal tube.

PROGNOSIS

As for underlying aetiology. If there is a significant underlying medical disorder the child may need continuous overnight feeds for months or years. Psychological dependence on an artificial feeding device commonly occurs. It is important to 'wean off' the device as soon as possible.

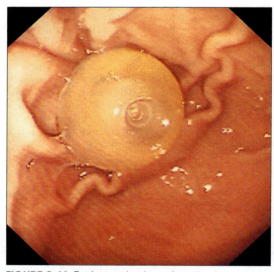

FIGURE 9.46 Endoscopic view of gastrostomy water inflated balloon *in situ*.

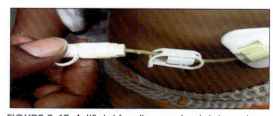

FIGURE 9.47 Artificial feeding gastrostojejunostomy demonstrating the connectors at the two distal lumen ports.

GASTRO-OESOPHAGEAL REFLUX

INCIDENCE/AETIOLOGY

GORD is the commonest cause of chronic 'vomiting' in infancy. It also presents in prepubertal children prior to their growth spurt when they have gained weight but not grown.

GORD commonly occurs in neurodevelopmental disorders such as cerebral palsy and is found in increased frequency in children with other gastrointestinal disease. Mechanisms of reflux include transient lower oesophageal sphincter relaxations (TLESRs – relaxations not associated with swallowing), hiatus hernia, lax lower oesophageal sphincter, chronic cough and increased transdiaphragmatic pressure gradient (for example with wheeze).

DIAGNOSIS

Children present with excessive regurgitation/posseting, oesophagitis or respiratory disease. They may present with poor feeding, poor weight gain or chronic cough. Prolonged crying/colic and nocturnal screaming is not usually due to primary GORD. Onset is usually in the neonatal period, with excessive posseting and regurgitation of milk after and/or between feeds. The refluxate does not contain bile, but can be bloodstained (due to oesophageal excoriation). If reflux is severe there may be associated apnoeic episodes. Older infants are reluctant to ingest lumpy food and may have gagging and choking episodes. Symptoms in the older child include small appetite (frequently do not finish meals), epigastric pain and dysphagia. The child may chew food for a prolonged length of time and 'store' it in the cheeks due to a reluctance to swallow. It is important to distinguish reflux (which is passive movement of gastric contents up the oesophagus) from true vomiting/emesis, which is a centrally-mediated motor event as the aetiologies and treatments will be different.

Investigations should be reserved for those children who do not respond to initial medical treatment and include:

- FBC.
- 24-hour oesophageal impedance/pH study.
- Upper gastrointestinal radiological contrast study in more severe cases (to exclude underlying structural disorder, e.g. intestinal malrotation).
- Upper gastrointestinal endoscopy if anaemic (possible oesophagitis) or faltering growth that does not resolve with treatment. Mucosal biopsy of oesophagus to detect oesophagitis, stomach for gastritis, or small intestine to investigate for enteropathy.
- High-resolution oesophageal impedance/manometry if hiatus hernia is suspected.
- In children with suspected aspiration sputum should be examined for fat laden macrophages.

DIFFERENTIAL DIAGNOSIS

- Hypertrophic pyloric stenosis, urinary tract or other infection.
- Feeding mismanagement.
- Non-IgE-mediated cow's milk protein/other food allergy is frequently associated (particularly in atopic families).

TREATMENT

In healthy infants who are thriving only symptomatic treatments are appropriate. These can include:

- Placing the infant in left lateral position or with the head elevated.
- Thickened feeds with carobel or if growth faltering consider using vitaquik to supplement calorie intake as well as thickening feed.
- Gaviscon.

More severe/complicated reflux may require:

- Prokinetic agents to improve gastric emptying (e.g. domperidone) are used frequently, although the evidence base is poor.
- H2 antagonist (e.g. ranitidine) – withdraw when reflux is well controlled with a prokinetic agent.
- Proton pump inhibitor if poor response to H2 antagonist.
- Baclofen can be used to inhibit TLESRs.
- Manage associated disease, for example exclude offending food(s) from diet (see 'Non-IgE-mediated food allergic enteropathy', **Table 23.2**).
- Surgical management with fundoplication if aspiration episodes or chronic oesophagitis despite maximal medical therapy, or complications such as oesophageal stricture. Individuals with hiatus hernia are usually better treated with fundoplication and repair of the diaphragmatic hiatus.
- Earlier surgery for the neurologically impaired child who fails to respond to medical treatment.

PROGNOSIS

Infantile reflux usually becomes asymptomatic by the second year of life. In some cases more prolonged medical treatment is necessary.

CYCLICAL VOMITING

INCIDENCE/AETIOLOGY

Cyclic vomiting syndrome (CVS) is a rare abnormality of the neuroendocrine system that affects 2% of children. It is associated with a family history of migraine in about one-third of patients.

DIAGNOSIS

Onset is usually between 3 and 7 years of age, with three or more episodes per year of vomiting with/without nausea that lasts less than 1 week with return to full health between episodes. The average is of about 9.6 episodes/year lasting for 3.4 days.

It is a frequently missed diagnosis in the emergency department and may require a number of emergency department visits before the diagnosis is made.

Over 40% of patients have headaches/migraines, with associated anxiety and depression in approximately 30% of cases.

DIFFERENTIAL DIAGNOSIS

Other causes of vomiting must be excluded, including urinary tract infections. Imaging of the brain may be required to exclude a space occupying lesion. Upper intestinal radiological contrast study may be needed to exclude intestinal malrotation with volvulus.

TREATMENT

Some cases respond to avoidance of certain dietary antigens (most commonly milk, egg, wheat, soya). Prophylactic treatment with propranolol or if ineffective, tricyclic antidepressants may reduce the frequency and severity of episodes in about two-thirds of cases.

INTESTINAL PSEUDO-OBSTRUCTION

INCIDENCE/GENETICS

This is very rare. It is congenital, inherited (X-linked or autosomal recessive) or acquired.

AETIOLOGY

There is a lack of normal intestinal motility due to a neuromuscular pathology of the intestine. Pathologies affect either the nerves, muscles or the interstitial cells of Cajal. Examples include the presence of additional muscle layers (for example with X-linked FLNA mutations), abnormalities of smooth muscle contractile proteins and of myocyte phenotype, qualitative and quantitative abnormalities of enteric nerves and inflammatory pathologies including infectious and autoimmune disease. Hollow visceral myopathy is a myopathic variant that affects the urinary tract as well as the intestine. Megacystis, microcolon hypoperistalsis syndrome is a more severe rare form of pseudo-obstruction.

DIAGNOSIS

Abdominal distension, constipation, vomiting and failure to thrive (**Fig. 9.46**) are common presentations. Intermittent more severe obstructive episodes occur. There should be histological examination of full thickness intestinal biopsy to assess abnormalities of intestinal smooth muscle and nerve plexuses. This is obtained either at the time of ileostomy formation (see below) or by laparoscopically assisted full thickness jejunal biopsy. Small bowel manometry might help in the selection of patients for full thickness biopsy.

TREATMENT/PROGNOSIS

Treatment is supportive. Children may need overnight continuous liquid enteral feeds to absorb sufficient nutrients. The most severely affected patients require PN (**Figs 9.48, 9.49**). The only surgical procedure shown to be of benefit is ileostomy formation, which can result in improved feed tolerance (**Fig. 9.50**).

Intestinal pseudo-obstruction is a chronic relapsing disorder. Muscle disease is usually a more severe phenotype than neural disease.

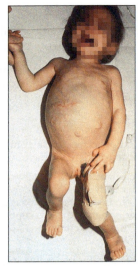

FIGURE 9.48 Intestinal pseudo-obstruction. Abdominal distension and failure to thrive.

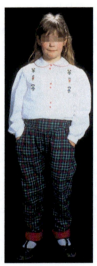

FIGURE 9.49 Intestinal pseudo-obstruction. The same child as in **9.48** growing and developing normally, solely on parenteral nutrition.

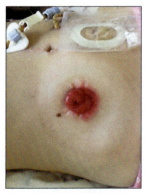

FIGURE 9.50 Ileostomy, gastrostomy and temporary peritoneal drain post abdominal surgery for intestinal pseudo-obstruction.

Gastroenterology

SHORT BOWEL SYNDROME

INCIDENCE/AETIOLOGY

There is malabsorption in the presence of a shortened small intestine resulting in failure of adequate weight gain or growth. The condition is increasing in frequency with improved survival in neonates after intestinal resection for severe necrotising enterocolitis.

Shortening of the small intestine may either be due to a congenital problem or more commonly is acquired during childhood. The syndrome is most commonly associated with intestinal resection in infancy (usually necrotic intestine in necrotising enterocolitis removed from premature infants), or resection of necrotic bowel following volvulus (usually with associated malrotation) at any age. Rarely, congenital short bowel occurs, usually in association with other congenital abnormalities, such as gastroschisis or multiple small intestinal atresias resulting in 'apple peel' or 'Christmas tree' deformities.

DIAGNOSIS

Diarrhoea and faltering growth occurs in association with a short intestine. Watery stool can be caused by osmotic diarrhoea secondary to sugar malabsorption, and steatorrhoea may occur. Symptoms can be exacerbated if there is loss of the ileocaecal valve, which acts as a barrier preventing colonic bacteria invading the small intestine and, more importantly, a 'brake' for the passage of luminal contents along the small intestine.

Investigations include:

- Upper gastrointestinal radiological contrast study to exclude underlying anatomical abnormalities (strictures, malrotation) and estimation of small intestinal length (if not already done at laparotomy).
- Gastrointestinal panendoscopy to rule out coincident inflammatory pathologies.
- Intermittent monitoring for bacterial overgrowth, which is a greater risk if there is loss of the ileocaecal valve. Microscopy and culture of stool and duodenal juices and indirect evidence from detection of bacterial matabolites in urine or hydrogen breath test.
- Nutritional investigations, plasma electrolytes and urea (low if poor protein intake), trace elements (including zinc, copper, selenium), fat soluble vitamins, A, E (most likely to be low)

and K (prothrombin time) and haemoglobin, ferritin and folate. Vitamin B_{12} deficiency is particularly likely to develop subsequent to terminal ileal resection, but may not be evident for even several years after resection. Oxalate may be raised in individuals with steatorrhoea due to the absorption of calcium oxalate – fatty acid soaps from the large intestine.

- Trace elements and fat soluble vitamins need to be monitored at least annually.

TREATMENT

Immediately postresection, total PN is necessary to replace all nutrient, electrolyte and fluid losses. Enteral feeds should be introduced at the earliest opportunity in order to maintain intestinal and liver function. Longer-term management is to aim to gradually reduce the volume of PN, with a corresponding increase in enteral feeds as adaption occurs.

- Once enteral feeds are established on a reasonable volume of enteral feed, it is best given continuously overnight with small daytime boluses.
- Once about 50% of nutrition is tolerated enterally, an attempt can be made to reduce the number of nights per week on parenteral feeds.
- If long-term PN is required, management at home by parents should be organised (fewer complications than in hospital).

PROGNOSIS

Children can survive for many months and even years with PN support at home with care by formally trained parents. However, over 75% patients sent home on PN are able to wean off this treatment within 4–5 years. Intestinal function continues to improve over the first 4–5 years. Adaption is often sufficient for PN to be withdrawn, providing there is about 25–30 cm of small intestine. The patient is unlikely to cope without PN if still receiving it at 5 years of age, despite good management.

If less than 30 cm of small intestine remains, many patients continue to be dependent on PN for normal growth (extreme short stature if PN is withdrawn). Small intestinal transplantation should be considered when international transplant criteria are met (loss of more than two central venous access sites, two or more serious episodes of septicaemia within 12 months or poor quality of life on PN treatment). Prognosis post-transplant is approximately 70% 2-year survival (with intestinal graft survival about 50%).

CONGENITAL CHLORIDE DIARRHOEA

INCIDENCE/GENETICS

This is a rare, (1 in 43,000 in Finland) autosomal recessive disease.

AETIOLOGY

There is a defect in the intestinal epithelial apical membrane chloride/bicarbonate exchanger molecule associated with mutations in the *SLC26A3* gene (solute carrier family 26).

DIAGNOSIS

Children present with maternal polyhydramnios (**Fig. 9.51**), often premature birth, lack of passage of meconium (instead watery stool often mistaken for urine) with distended abdomen. Secretory diarrhoea continues when the child is fasted. There is rapid hyponatraemic, hypochloraemic dehydration with mild metabolic alkalosis (and hypokalaemia). Children may lose more than 10% of birth weight in 24 hours (up to 300 ml/kg/d stool losses). Referral to a renal unit with secondary prerenal renal failure may be required. There should be investigations of plasma electrolytes and acid:base balance. Small bowel biopsy will be morphologically normal and should always be performed as part of the diagnostic work-up.

TREATMENT

Intravenous fluid resuscitation with adequate sodium chloride replacement is first-line treatment.

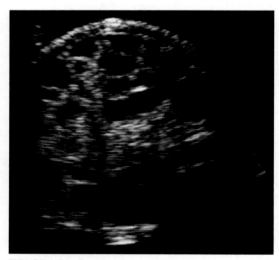

FIGURE 9.51 Congenital chloride diarrhoea: antenatal ultrasound for polyhydramnios showing dilated loops of bowel due to *in utero* diarrhoea.

When stable, the child can be switched to oral supplementation with sodium chloride and potassium. Sodium, chloride and potassium maintenance requirement may be as much as 6 mmol/kg/d chloride in infancy, but less with increasing age. Ratio of Na:K Cl typically 2:1 in infancy and 6:5 in older children). Butyrate therapy might reduce stool electrolyte losses, probably by stimulating colonic butyrate/chloride absorption.

PROGNOSIS

If diagnosed early in neonatal life and adequately treated, there will be normal growth and development. It is essential to give adequate electrolyte replacement to avoid secondary hyperaldosteronism and eventual secondary chronic renal failure. Therefore it is of paramount importance to monitor urine sodium and blood pressure at least twice a year. Intercurrent episodes of acute diarrhoea require admission to hospital and IV fluids as early as possible.

GLUCOSE–GALACTOSE MALABSORPTION

INCIDENCE/GENETICS

This is a rare, autosomal recessive condition, with about 200 recognised cases world-wide.

AETIOLOGY

A selective defect occurs in the intestinal sodium coupled glucose–galactose cotransporter. The gene, *SGLT1* is on chromosome 22. Phenotype varies depending upon the 'severity' of the gene mutation. At least 10% of the general population has glucose intolerance, which maybe a milder form of the disease.

DIAGNOSIS

Severe osmotic diarrhoea occurs from the first glucose/galactose-containing feed, which stops when fasted. Therefore, there is no hydramnios and normal passage of meconium. Stools are positive for reducing sugars when the child is fed glucose/galactose-containing sugars. Stool sugar chromatography confirms the diagnosis.

TREATMENT/PROGNOSIS

Glucose and galactose should be excluded from the diet, substituting a fructose-based feed. In older children and adults a small amount of glucose and galactose may be tolerated requiring colonic salvage of malabsorbed sugars. Hence dietary intake in adults is altered according to symptoms.

Clinical tolerance of offending carbohydrates improves with age. If diagnosed and treated early, the child shows normal growth and development.

SUCROSE–ISOMALTASE DEFICIENCY

INCIDENCE/GENETICS

A rare condition that is inherited as an autosomal recessive trait.

AETIOLOGY

There is total or almost complete lack of sucrase activity with reduced maltase activity on the small intestinal brush border. Phenotypic variation of the disease is wide with severe and mild phenotypes. The gene is *EC 3.2.1.48* on chromosome 3q25-q26.

DIAGNOSIS

Frothy, watery diarrhoea is present, possibly with secondary dehydration, malnutrition, some vomiting and even steatorrhoea. Onset of symptoms occurs when sucrose is added to the diet – usually at the time of weaning.

TREATMENT/PROGNOSIS

During the first year of life, diet excludes sucrose, glucose polymers and starch. The patient can usually tolerate variable amounts of starch after the age of 2 or 3 years.

Adult patients adjust their diet according to symptoms.

LACTOSE MALABSORPTION

INCIDENCE/AETIOLOGY

In most of the world's population, lactose intolerance develops in adult life due to a reduction in expression of the intestinal brush border enzyme lactase. This, exceptionally, is not seen in most Caucasians.

Low or absent mucosal lactase is normal in non-Caucasians over 5 years old, with activity falling to 5–10% of the childhood level (**Figs 9.52, 9.53**). Primary hypolactasia is extremely rare (Gene *LCT*, chromosome 2q21). Secondary lactose intolerance may occur when the small intestinal enterocyte brush border is damaged during infectious gastroenteritis and other enteropathic disorders in which villus morphology is damaged.

DIAGNOSIS

Loose, watery, frothy stools are produced following ingestion of milk, with perianal excoriation. It may develop following an acute infectious episode of gastroenteritis. Stool sugar chromatography identifies lactose in the stool.

TREATMENT/PROGNOSIS

Treatment is avoidance of the offending sugars. Non-Caucasian adults avoid symptoms with a low-lactose diet.

Secondary hypolactasia following infectious gastroenteritis usually rapidly resolves. Congenital deficiencies are lifelong, but are asymptomatic if an appropriate diet is adhered to.

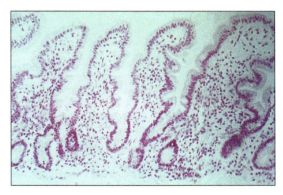

FIGURE 9.52 Absence of lactase in inherited lactose intolerance. Note the histologically normal small intestine (×40).

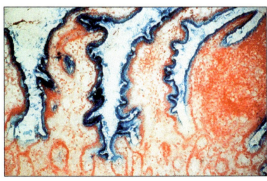

FIGURE 9.53 Normal small intestinal mucosa with positive brush border staining for lactase.

PANCREATIC DISEASE

CYSTIC FIBROSIS

See also Chapter 4 Respiratory Medicine, page 79.

INCIDENCE/GENETICS

Cystic fibrosis (CF) is a disorder of epithelial cell chloride transport. At 1 in 2,000–3,000 live births, CF is the commonest autosomal recessive disease in Caucasians. Carrier frequency is about 5%. The CF gene was discovered in 1989 and over 400 mutations are known. Disease severity correlates with mutation type; there is concordance for disease severity within families. The ΔF508 mutation (a severe mutation) accounts for about 70% of cases in Caucasians. Patients with two 'severe' mutations have worse pancreatic failure.

AETIOLOGY

CF is caused by mutations in the transmembrane conductance regulator protein (CFTR) gene on chromosome 7, which encodes a cyclic-AMP regulated chloride and bicarbonate channel.

Defective CFTR leads to altered electrolyte transport in epithelial cells of the gastrointestinal tract and tracheobronchial tree. The major gastrointestinal defect is malabsorption due to steatorrhoea, because of greatly reduced pancreatic exocrine secretions. Liver disease develops due to damage to intrahepatic biliary epithelial cells. Mutations in CFTR are not infrequently associated with mucosal inflammation within the gastrointestinal tract, which can result in an enteropathy.

DIAGNOSIS

Diagnosis is highly variable depending upon the nature of the disease-causing gene mutation. It may present in the neonatal period or later in childhood with failure to thrive and/or recurrent chest infections. Gastrointestinal abnormalities involve the intestine, pancreas and liver.

- Over 85% of patients have fat malabsorption and failure to thrive. They may present in infancy with oedema, hypoalbuminaemia and anaemia. Patients have a large appetite (unless severe chest disease or other disorder such as GORD has developed) in association with poor weight gain.
- Meconium ileus occurs in ± 10% of cases.
- Distal intestinal obstruction syndrome (DIOS) affects about 10% of cases. Patients have intermittent episodes of intestinal obstruction with inspissated faecal contents (meconium ileus equivalent) in the terminal ileum and right colon. Intussusception may occur. The aetiology of this is probably a secondary neuropathy consequent upon transmural lymphocytic inflammation of the intestine.
- Rectal prolapse occurs in up to 20% of cases (in 10% prior to diagnosis). This is probably related

to poor nutrition. Onset is from 1–2.5 years of age and spontaneous remission usually occurs by the age of 5 years.

- Cow's milk protein intolerance occurs in about 8% of patients under 3 years old.
- 20–25% of patients develop liver disease, progressing to cirrhosis in about 5% (see page 288).
- Virtually all males are infertile.

Investigations include:

- Sweat test: pilocarpine iontophoresis of a small area on the forearm to induce sweating and analysis for chloride and sodium content. Normally, for individuals older than 6 months of age, a chloride level of:
  - ○ 0–39 mmol/l = CF is very unlikely.
  - ○ 40–59 mmol/l = indicates that CF is possible.
  - ○ ≥ 60 mmol/l = CF is likely.

For reliable results, especially in the neonatal period, care has to be taken to collect at least 50 mg or, preferably, 100 mg of sweat. This may be difficult in very young infants.

- Serum trypsinogen: high level in early infancy. May be elevated in normal infants following abdominal surgery.
- Stool elastase: screening test for pancreatic insufficiency. Children with fecal elastase < 200μg/g should be treated with pancreatic exocrine replacement therapy (PERT).
- Pancreatic function tests: low volume of secretions with low bicarbonate but usually relatively normal enzyme levels. The test is now rarely used.
- Genetic markers include the ΔF508 gene mutation.
- Nasal potential difference, which can measure chloride and bicarbonate secretion in the nasal epithelium, is sometimes used as a confirmatory diagnostic test in reference centres.
- In older children chest CT might provide supportive evidence of CF with the finding of bronchiectasis (see also Chapter 4 Respiratory Medicine, page 80).

Other investigations:

- Plain abdominal x-ray in meconium ileus: ground glass appearance (due to air bubbles trapped in meconium). Intraperitoneal calcification is seen if meconium peritonitis is present.
- Barium enema in meconium ileus: microcolon (**Fig. 9.54**).
- Nutritional monitoring: includes serum fat soluble vitamin levels (particularly vitamin E).

TREATMENT

See also Chapter 4 Respiratory Medicine, page 80 for non-gastroenterological treatments.

- High calorie intake, including increased fat, should be encouraged. Pancreatic enzyme (enteric-coated) and fat soluble vitamin supplements should be given to all patients with stool elastase <200μg/g. Doses of PERT should generally be <10,000 IU/kg/d. In individuals with persisting significant steatorrhoea on this dose of PERT, other causes of fat malabsorption should be sought (for example CF-related enteropathy). Medium-chain triglyceride (MCT)-containing milks might be absorbed more efficiently as post lipolytic absorption of long-chain triglyceride (LCT) is impaired in CF.

- Simple meconium ileus is treated with a hypertonic enema (gastrografin or hypaque) with intravenous fluid support.
- Distal intestinal obstruction syndrome can be relieved with a mild laxative (if mild), oral N-acetylcysteine, gastrografin enema or intestinal lavage. Ensure appropriate dose of pancreatic supplements is prescribed.
- Psychological support if needed.
- Combined heart–lung transplants have been given with a similar success rate to transplants given for other diseases.
- Preliminary gene therapy studies are in progress using viral vectors to introduce normal CFTR DNA.

PROGNOSIS

Morbidity and early mortality are usually secondary to chronic pulmonary disease. Today many people with CF are living into their late 30s and beyond. It is estimated that about 8 in 10 of today's children with CF should live into their mid 40s or 50s. If a patient has a less severe genetic mutation with relatively good pancreatic function (hence less steatorrhoea and a better nutritional state), presentation is later and prognosis better.

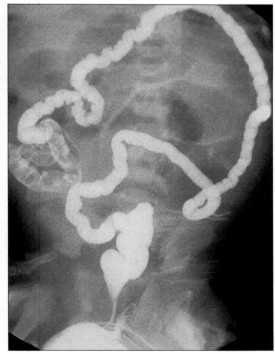

FIGURE 9.54 Cystic fibrosis. Barium study showing extensive microcolon in a child presenting with meconium ileus.

SHWACHMAN–BODIAN–DIAMOND SYNDROME

INCIDENCE

Shwachman–Bodian–Diamond syndrome (SDS), is a rare autosomal recessive disorder characterised by exocrine pancreatic insufficiency hematopoietic dysfunction and neurocognitive deficiency, which is caused by mutations in the Shwachman–Bodian–Diamond syndrome (SBDS) gene. It is an inherited bone marrow failure syndrome that affects multiple organ systems.

AETIOLOGY

The mutations in the SBDS gene are found in >90% of individuals with clinical manifestations of SDS. The SBDS protein is involved in several key cellular functions including ribosomal function, and hence mutations involve multiple organ systems.

DIAGNOSIS

The clinical manifestations of SDS are wide and varied. Essential elements for the clinical diagnosis comprise the presence of haematological cytopenia of any lineage in conjunction with exocrine pancreatic insufficiency. Supportive evidence of SDS is provided by the presence of bony abnormalities including short stature, delayed ossification and metaphyseal widening, hepatomegaly and learning and behavioural difficulties.

Feeding difficulties with failure to thrive, diarrhoea and recurrent infections usually develop within the first few months of life. There is exocrine pancreatic insufficiency associated with bone marrow and haematological abnormalities.

Investigations include:

- Pancreatic function tests: reduced lipase, trypsin and amylase secretion, with relative normal fluid volume and bicarbonate level in comparison to CF.
- Ultrasound: may demonstrate a small pancreas. The main pancreatic ducts are normal. Pancreatic lipomatosis might be present.
- Haematology: cyclical neutropenia and neutrophil mobility tests demonstrate an abnormal response to standard bacterial stimulation in over 90% of all cases. A cyclical thrombocytopenia occurs in two-thirds and anaemia in 50% of patients.
- Bone marrow aspiration: may demonstrate marrow replacement by fibrous tissue or fat or myeloid arrest.
- Skeletal x-rays: metaphyseal chondrodysplasia of the femoral neck, short ribs with anterior flaring, vertebral wedging, clinodactyly and long bone changes.
- Hepatomegaly may occur and raised serum aminotransferase levels.
- Rarely, cardiac, respiratory, renal and testicular abnormalities may occur.
- Mutations in the SBDS gene are present in up to 90%.

DIFFERENTIAL DIAGNOSIS

CF can be excluded with a sweat test, as patients with SDS have normal sweat electrolytes. Other causes of malabsorption, such as food sensitive enteropathy or coeliac disease, are excluded with small intestinal biopsy (histologically normal small intestinal mucosa in SDS). Other immunodeficiencies not associated with pancreatic insufficiency and bony abnormalities should be considered.

TREATMENT

Pancreatic enzyme is replaced. The initial dose should be 2,000 units of lipase/kg/d in divided doses according to the fat content of the meal(s). Blood concentrations of fat soluble vitamins should be measured 6 monthly and supplements started if necessary. Prophylactic antibiotics may reduce the frequency of intercurrent infections. Severe haematological manifestations may warrant bone marrow transplantation. Anaemia might require repeated blood transfusions with a subsequent need for iron chelation therapy. Children with recurrent invasive bacterial/fungal infections in the presence of neutropenia might benefit from granulocyte colony stimulating factor (G-CSF) therapy. In children developing a myelodysplastic syndrome, haematopoetic stem cell transplantation (HSCT) is required on an urgent basis. The criteria for HSCT include severe cytopenia, myelodysplastic syndrome with excessive blasts and overt leukaemia. Regular dental surveillance is essential.

PROGNOSIS

The majority of patients enjoy relatively good health. Poor growth persists, despite pancreatic enzyme replacement. Recurrent infections continue and were the cause of death in up to 20% of cases in the past. Cases of leukaemia have been reported.

ACUTE PANCREATITIS

INCIDENCE/GENETICS

Inflammation of the pancreas is uncommon. Acute pancreatitis may develop after a penetrating abdominal injury.

AETIOLOGY

About 30% of cases are associated with severe multisystem disease, such as sepsis, shock, systemic infection, collagen vascular diseases, IBD and Reye syndrome. About 25% are related to trauma (blunt abdominal injury, including child abuse) or mechanical obstruction, others to metabolic disorders (hyperlipidaemia, hypercalcaemia, CF, malnutrition, renal disease, hypothermia, diabetes mellitus, organic acidaemias). Reaction to any medication should be considered. In up to 25% of cases there is no known predisposing factor.

PATHOLOGY

The pathology is poorly understood. Pancreatic inflammation can be induced by overstimulation of the gland, obstruction, increased permeability or overdistension of the duct, drugs, toxins and certain metabolic abnormalities.

DIAGNOSIS

Abdominal pain of sudden onset occurs, usually epigastric, with increasing severity over a few hours and continuing for just a few hours or as long as several weeks (average 4 days). In about one-third of cases, pain radiates – usually through to the back. Attacks can be pain free. Also, the child frequently vomits, particularly with food, may exhibit anorexia and may develop greasy stool.

Investigations include:

- Contrast-enhanced CT scan is the most useful investigation. It can be normal in mild pancreatitis. Abnormalities include changes in pancreatic size and texture, and visualisation of complications such as pseudocyst, abscesses, calcification, duct enlargement, oedema, exudate and bowel distension. CT is probably best carried out on day 4 to look for evidence of pancreatic necrosis. Secretin stimulated MRI will be useful at a later date.
- Serum amylase: raised level for 2–5 days. Diagnostic if amylase level is raised to more than three times normal, but may not be increased at all. Serum lipase remains elevated for longer.
- Abdominal ultrasound may demonstrate an enlarged pancreas with reduced echogenicity. Causative pathologies (for example gall stones) might be seen although intra-abdominal gas might interfere with visualisation.

DIFFERENTIAL DIAGNOSIS

Other causes of abdominal pain and vomiting; for example, food sensitivity, intestinal malrotation, hepatitis.

TREATMENT

Treatment is supportive, according to symptoms and complications. If pancreatitis severe, full monitoring in intensive care is necessary. The aim is to rest the pancreas, but controlled trials have not usually demonstrated benefit. The usual treatment is to stop oral intake, give intravenous fluids, jejunal feeds (i.e. beyond the pancreatic duct) or PN, analgesia and antibiotics if infection is suspected (**Figs 9.55, 9.56**). Octreotide is anecdotally helpful in reducing pancreatic pain.

PROGNOSIS

Prognosis is variable, ranging from mild self-limiting abdominal discomfort to fulminant disease, progressing to multiorgan failure and, in some cases, a fatal outcome in hours or days.

CHRONIC PANCREATITIS

INCIDENCE/GENETICS

Chronic pancreatitis is idiopathic or has autosomal dominant inheritance with variable penetrance (40–80%). Recognised genetic associations include cationic trypsinogen (PRSS1), SPINK 1, CFTR and chymotrypsinogen C (CTRC) mutations.

DIAGNOSIS

Usual onset is around 10 years of age, but can begin as early as 1 year. Episodes of abdominal pain lasting from 2 days to 2 weeks occur from monthly to yearly. Attacks can be precipitated by large, fatty meals, alcohol and stress. Frequency of attacks usually decreases with age. There is severe epigastric pain that may radiate to the back and is lessened by adopting the fetal position. Epigastric tenderness and, in some cases, reduced bowel sounds and abdominal distension occur (**Figs 9.57, 9.58**). Helpful investigations include blood pancreatic enzyme levels, abdominal ultrasound and MRI.

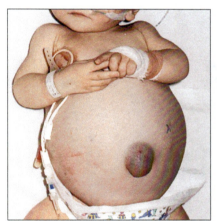

FIGURE 9.55 Acute pancreatitis: abdominal distension with blood stained ascetic fluid, positive Cullen's sign (bruising around the umbilicus).

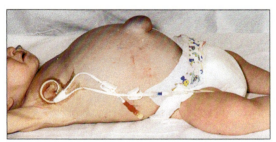

FIGURE 9.56 Management, including parenteral feeding with nasogastric drainage.

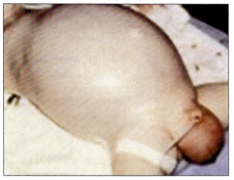

FIGURE 9.57 Severe abdominal distension with everted umbilicus and scrotal oedema in a child with chronic pancreatitis.

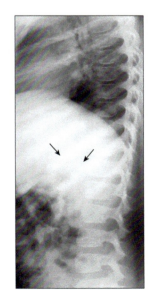

FIGURE 9.58 Chronic pancreatitis: lateral x-ray of abdomen and chest demonstrating pancreatic calcification.

Endoscopic retrograde cholangiopancreatography (ERCP) should be performed when an anatomical cause is suspected.

TREATMENT

Treatment is symptomatic and supportive (see 'Acute pancreatitis' above). Pain relief can be difficult even with strong analgesics. Somatostatin, oral pancreatic supplements and daily vitamin A and E can be helpful. Surgical treatment should be considered if there is intractable pain or complications.

PROGNOSIS

Long-term complications such as pancreatic exocrine insufficiency or diabetes mellitus may develop. If the pancreatic duct is dilated or pseudocyst or pancreatic ascites develops, pancreaticojejunostomy is beneficial. Other patients lead normal lives without surgery.

LIVER DISEASE

PRIMARY SCLEROSING CHOLANGITIS

INCIDENCE/GENETICS

This condition is rare, but increasingly recognised with improved investigatory techniques. There is a family history of autoimmune disease. It can be hereditary, presenting in the neonate.

AETIOLOGY

It is most commonly associated with IBD in about 70% of cases, in particular with UC and occurs with other autoimmune disease (including autoimmune enteropathy), or may develop with immunodeficiency, CF, psoriasis, reticulum cell sarcoma and sickle cell disease.

PATHOGENESIS

Primary sclerosing cholangitis is a chronic cholestatic disorder of unknown aetiology. There is chronic inflammation and fibrosis with beading (dilatation) and stenosis of affected intra- and/or extrahepatic bile ducts and obliteration of peripheral ducts.

DIAGNOSIS

An insidious onset occurs with intermittent jaundice, pruritis, hepatomegaly, pyrexia, weight loss and lethargy. On examination hepatomegaly +/− jaundice and splenomegaly may be present. Abdominal ultrasound may be normal or bile duct wall thickening or focal bile duct dilataion may be detected. Magnetic resonance cholangiography (MRC) is used to discover any bile duct changes (**Fig. 9.59**); non-organ-specific autoantibodies are associated (antinuclear antibody [ANA] and ANCA). Liver biopsy may detect small duct disease and autoimmune/immune-mediated parenchymal disease.

Overlap syndrome with autoimmune hepatitis is commoner in children than adults.

TREATMENT/PROGNOSIS

Children are responsive to immunosuppressive therapy if the condition is autoimmune associated. The condition progresses to cirrhosis, portal hypertension and liver failure over about 10 years, with eventual need for liver transplant.

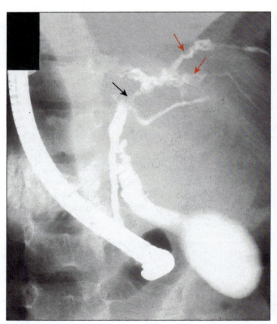

FIGURE 9.59 Sclerosing cholangitis. Endoscopic retrograde cholangiogram demonstrating dilatation, stenosis (black arrow) and irregularity of bile ducts (red arrows).

CHRONIC HEPATITIS

This may present either when jaundice continues for more than 3 months after an acute hepatitis or develops insidiously.

Currently diagnosis is moving towards an aetiological classification.

INCIDENCE/AETIOLOGY

Chronic hepatitis is rare. Aetiology includes:

A: Hepatitis surface antigen-positive hepatitis.
B: Hepatitis surface antigen-negative hepatitis.

- Viral infection:
  - hepatitis C (HCV).
  - CMV.
  - EBV.
- Autoimmune chronic hepatitis:
  - primary biliary cirrhosis.
- Metabolic/genetic abnormalities:
  - Wilson disease.
  - Alpha-1 antitrypsin deficiency.
  - CF.
- Drugs such as isoniazid.

CHRONIC ACTIVE HEPATITIS

Pathogenesis
Autoimmune damage to the liver with defective supressor T-lymphocytes.

Diagnosis
An acute onset of jaundice occurs in most patients. It may present insidiously with malaise, fatigue, anorexia and nausea. Hepatosplenomegaly is found in up to 80% of patients. Patients may develop symptoms secondary to other organ-specific autoimmune disorders (see 'Autoimmune enteropathy', page 263) or IBD.

Diagnosis is made on the histological appearance of percutaneous liver biopsy. Patchy hepatocellular necrosis with destruction of lobular architecture and regenerating hepatocytes with multiple nuclei are all seen.

Raised serum transaminases and bilirubin almost always occur. Frequently there are several other circulating autoantibodies, including ANA in up to 75% of cases, with smooth muscle (SMA) or liver/kidney microsomal antibodies and multiple organ-specific autoantibodies.

Treatment/Prognosis
Immunosuppressive therapy with prednisolone and azathioprine is used for autoimmune disease. Interferon therapy is given if there is hepatitis B.

Patients usually have a good response to immunosuppressive therapy (usually prednisolone then agathioprine), preventing progression to serious liver damage and cirrhosis.

ACUTE HEPATITIS

AETIOLOGY

Acute hepatitis can be caused by viral infection such as hepatitis A, B,C, D, E, CMV and EBV. It may also be drug-related.

DIAGNOSIS

Usual onset is with flu-like symptoms. Jaundice, nausea, vomiting, loss of appetite, fever, tenderness in the right hypochondrium, muscle and joint pain, and pruritis with erythmatous macular rash may also occur. Investigations include viral screening and liver function tests.

TREATMENT/PROGNOSIS

Any drug treatment that may cause hepatitis should be withdrawn.

Prognosis depends on aetiology. There is full recovery in the vast majority of cases. Approximately 5% of cases of hepatitis B and 50% of hepatitis C develop chronic disease.

ALAGILLE SYNDROME

INCIDENCE/AETIOLOGY

The major inherited biliary disorders are those affecting the intrahepatic ducts. Alagille syndrome is the most common. It is a rare, autosomal dominant multisystem disorder, characterised by reduced bile duct number and function and caused by mutations in the *JAG1* gene and in < 1% the *NOTCH2* gene.

The incidence is about 1:70,000 live births.

DIAGNOSIS

Alagille syndrome sually presents in the first 2 years of life. Typical facial features of deep set eyes, straight nose, pointed chin and wide forehead are not usually recognisable until older. There is intrahepatic bile duct paucity and vascular anomalies. Other abnormalities may occur in the development of the heart (most commonly pulmonary stenosis), eyes, vertebrae and the craniofacial region.

TREATMENT

Children should be given a low fat diet with increased intake of MCT and best possible carbohydrate and protein intake, with fat soluble vitamin supplements.

Over 75% affected people live until at least 20 years of age. Death related to liver failure, heart problems and blood vessel abnormalities. Liver transplant may be required.

MINERAL DISORDERS (DEFICIENCIES, HIGH LEVEL POISONING)

ZINC DEFICIENCY

INCIDENCE/GENETICS

Acrodermatitis enteropathica is a rare autosomal recessive disorder due to a selective defect in the intestinal absorption of zinc (see also Chapter 6 Dermatology, page 144).

AETIOLOGY

Zinc deficiency may also develop in protein-energy malnutrition, short bowel syndrome and other malabsorptive states.

DIAGNOSIS

A scaly, erythematous skin rash with bullae and pustules develops around the mouth and anus. It may occur symmetrically in interdigital areas and over the buttocks, hands, feet and elbows. Alopecia, dystrophic nails, photophobia, conjunctivitis and glossitis may also develop (**Figs 9.60–9.63**). Diarrhoea with malabsorption, psychological and behavioural disturbances and susceptibility to infection may develop.

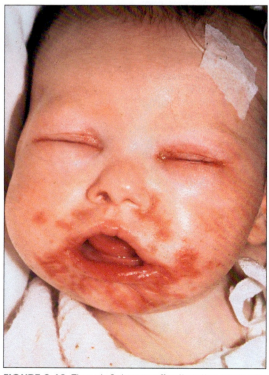

FIGURE 9.60 Zinc deficiency affecting the perioral area and face.

Plasma copper and zinc levels are inversely proportional to each other; other trace elements may also be deficient.

TREATMENT

Oral zinc supplementation is given. If possible, the underlying malabsorptive disorder should be treated.

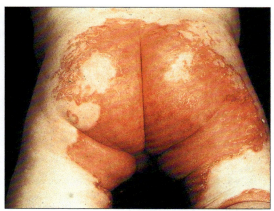

FIGURE 9.61 Zinc deficiency: skin rash on the buttocks.

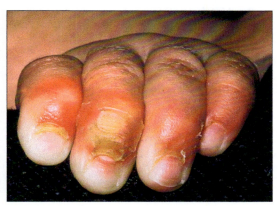

FIGURE 9.62 Zinc deficiency affecting the fingers.

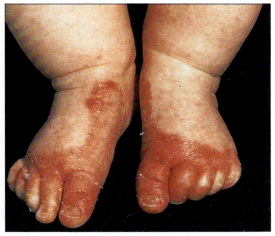

FIGURE 9.63 Zinc deficiency: appearance of the feet.

IRON DEFICIENCY

INCIDENCE/AETIOLOGY

Iron deficiency is common in infancy and adolescents. There is increased frequency in Asian children, vegetarians and vegans.

Deficiency may result from poor intake, malabsorption or excessive loss. Poor nutritional intake usually occurs in the preschool child, particularly if the child has a high milk intake. It can result secondary to overt or occult gastrointestinal or other blood loss. For example, severe GORD, gastritis or UC.

DIAGNOSIS

Children are lethargic with poor exercise tolerance. Pica, poor appetite and poor concentration span are evident. The children also have lowered resistance to infection and poor thermoregulation and anaemia.

Investigations include: haemoglobin; haematocrit; red blood cell indices demonstrate a normocytic, or microcytic, hypochromic anaemia; rarely, a bone marrow aspirate is required. Plasma ferritin level indicates adequacy of iron stores.

TREATMENT

The child should be given an improved diet or treatment of the underlying cause of blood loss. Oral iron supplements may also be required. If unable to absorb iron, an infusion or blood transfusion may be needed.

COPPER DEFICIENCY

INCIDENCE/GENETICS

Copper deficiency is rare. Menke disease is an X-linked recessive disease with poor copper absorption and metabolism, affecting 1 in 50,000–100,000.

AETIOLOGY

Copper deficiency can result from unsupplemented, long-term, total PN, severe malabsorption or administration of high-dose zinc. In Menke disease, there is a defect of intracellular copper transport.

DIAGNOSIS

Anaemia and neutropenia are present. Bony abnormalities, skeletal fragility and skin depigmentation occur. Microscopically, pili torti of hair is seen in Menke disease (**Fig. 9.64**).

TREATMENT

Treatment is with copper supplements and parenteral supplements in Menke disease.

COPPER EXCESS: WILSON DISEASE

INCIDENCE/GENETICS

Wilson disease is a rare autosomal recessive disorder, found in 1 in 10,000–30,000 world-wide. Carrier frequency is 1 in 90. The gene identified is on chromosome 13 – 13q14.3 (MIM277900).

AETIOLOGY

It is a disorder of copper balance in which there is inadequate biliary excretion of copper.

DIAGNOSIS

- **Hepatic disease:** seen from 5 years of age, variable manifestation ranging from an acute self-limiting hepatitis with full recovery, to fulminant hepatic failure. Chronic liver failure and cirrhosis occur in older patients.
- **CNS:** seen from 6 years of age, but more commonly in teens and 20s. It is a motor, not sensory disease. Initially tremor, inco-ordination, dystonia, fine motor difficulties occur. Later drooling, dysarthria and gait disturbance present.
- **Ophthalmological:** Kayser–Fleischer rings.
- **Psychiatric:** poor school performance, anxiety, depression, compulsive behaviour, even psychosis.
- **Cardiac:** arrythmia, myocardial disease.
- **Renal:** proximal tubular dysfunction. Renal stones are common.
- Investigations: increased 24-hour urinary copper excretion, usually decreased caeruloplasmin level.

TREATMENT

Chelation therapy is given to remove excess copper (see Chapter 8 Neurology, page 210).

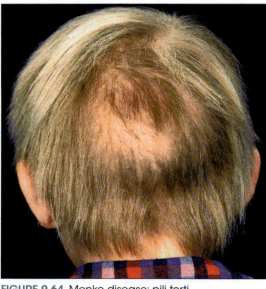

FIGURE 9.64 Menke disease: pili torti.

SELENIUM DEFICIENCY

INCIDENCE/AETIOLOGY

Selenium deficiency is rare. It occurs in children on unsupplemented long-term PN or with severe malabsorption.

DIAGNOSIS

Cardiomyopathy, myositis and macrocytic anaemia are present. Measurement of plasma level and glutathione peroxidase activity is helpful.

TREATMENT

Oral/enteral/parenterel selenium supplements are administered as tolerated.

VITAMIN DEFICIENCIES

Vitamins are organic food substances that are not synthesised by the body. Small amounts are essential for normal body metabolism. The B group vitamins and vitamin C are water soluble. Vitamins A, D, E and K are fat soluble.

SCURVY, VITAMIN C/ ASCORBIC ACID DEFICIENCY

INCIDENCE/AETIOLOGY

Scurvy rarely occurs in famines. Citrus fruit and green vegetables contain ascorbic acid. It is essential for collagen synthesis for bone, cartilage and dentine. Ascorbic acid is an important antioxidant. It is also required for adrenal gland function and iron absorption.

DIAGNOSIS

There is bleeding of gums and around hair follicles and capillaries. Children show irritability and painful limbs causing 'pseudoparalysis'. Investigations include: the response to supplements; plasma and white cell ascorbic acid level; bone x-ray: calcification of subperiosteal haematoma with 'ground glass' appearance of metaphyses and dense rim and 'smoke-ring' of cortical bone around epiphyses.

TREATMENT/PROGNOSIS

Ascorbic acid 500 mg per day for a week is given, and dietary source investigated.

The patient should be treated immediately or is at risk of sudden death. There is a rapid response to treatment, apart from bone remodelling, which takes some months.

BERIBERI, VITAMIN B$_1$/ THIAMIN DEFICIENCY

DIAGNOSIS

Beriberi manifests in two forms – 'wet' and 'dry'.

- India and the Far East: 'wet' beriberi occurs with acute high output cardiac failure in breast-fed infants of mothers with a diet of polished rice. Coughing, choking and aphonia with laryngeal oedema occurs. Children show drowsiness and meningism.
- Developed countries and older children: 'dry' beriberi/Wernicke's encephalopathy presents as encephalopathy in children on long-term total PN given without B supplements. In older children with a diet based on polished rice, it presents with sensory and motor neuropathy.

Patients can become comatose just 2 weeks after stopping vitamin supplements in PN, if there is no oral intake. Investigations include a trial of supplements. The blood should be examined for transketolase activity.

TREATMENT

Parenteral (intravenous or intramuscular) vitamin B (50–100 mg) preparation is given, then oral supplements. Dietary intake of nuts, peas, beans, pulses and brewer's yeast should be increased. Rice should be enriched with thiamin.

PELLAGRA, NIACIN DEFICIENCY

INCIDENCE/AETIOLOGY

Pellagra is endemic in parts of Africa, where diet is based on maize. There is poor bioavailability of nicotinic acid and low tryptophan in maize. Pyridoxine deficiency may also result in pellagra – it is an essential cofactor for nicotinic acid synthesis from trypyophan.

DIAGNOSIS

- Skin: photosensitive dermatitis with scaling and pigmentation (**Fig. 9.65**).
- Gut: angular stomatitis and diarrhoea.
- Neurological: depression, dementia, delerium, peripheral neuropathy.
- Investigations: there is a rapid response to supplements. Measurement of N1methyl nicotinamide and pyridone derivatives in urine.

TREATMENT

Orally, parenteral vitamin B (100 mg) preparation is given 4-hourly. Pulses, wholemeal cereals, meat or fish should be added to the diet.

RIBOFLAVIN/VITAMIN B$_2$ DEFICIENCY

AETIOLOGY

Pyridoxine is antagonised by isoniazid, hydralazine, penicillamine and oestrogens.

DIAGNOSIS

Cheilosis, magenta coloured tongue (**Fig. 9.66**) and nasolabial seborrhoea occur. If deficient, *in vitro* addition of flavin adenine dinucleotide increases erythrocyte glutathione reductase activity by more than 30%.

TREATMENT

Riboflavin 20 mg/d is given. Milk, eggs, liver, pulses or legumes should be added to the diet.

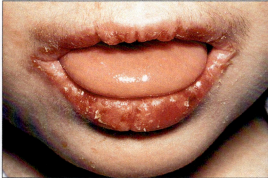

FIGURE 9.66 Angular stomatitis and cheilosis (inflammation and cracking of the lips) and magenta tongue with B-group vitamin deficiency.

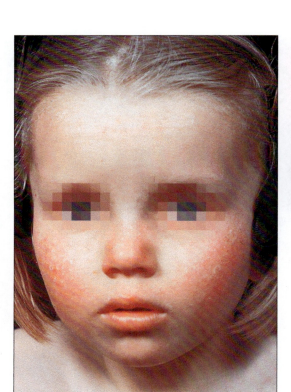

FIGURE 9.65 Pellagra patient showing associated dermatitis.

PYRIDOXINE/VITAMIN B₆ DEFICIENCY

- Aetiology: deficiency may occur iatrogenically when treated with isoniazid, hydralazine, penicillamine or oestrogens since they antagonise pyridoxine.
- Diagnosis: convulsions, depression and peripheral neuropathy are seen.
- Investigations: there is a rapid response to supplements; serum pyridoxal 5-phosphate; *in vitro* increase in red cell aspartate and alanine aminotransferases in the presence of pyridoxal 5-phosphate.
- Treatment; oral pyridoxine 10 mg/d is given. Whole grains, bananas, liver and peanuts are dietary sources.

CYANOCOBALAMIN/ VITAMIN B₁₂ DEFICIENCY

INCIDENCE/AETIOLOGY

Vitamin B₁₂ deficiency is rare although it is common in patients following ileal resection. A vegan diet or intrinsic factor deficiency or abnormality can also result in deficiency. B₁₂ is derived solely from animal products.

DIAGNOSIS

Anaemia, a yellow tint to the skin, glossitis, paraesthesia, ataxia and dementia can occur. Investigations include blood B₁₂ level; Schilling test – give vitamin B₁₂ radioactive isotope orally, then a non-radioactive intramuscular dose. Collect urine for 24 hours. If < 10% of oral dose is detected there is malabsorption. Repeat the same test with intrinsic factor to exclude intrinsic factor deficiency as the cause for malabsorption.

TREATMENT

Vitamin B₁₂ 1,000 μg twice-weekly is given until normal haemoglobin is achieved, then every 6 weeks.

VITAMIN K/ NAPTHAQUINONE DEFICIENCY

INCIDENCE/AETIOLOGY

Vitamin K deficiency is rare and occurs in newborn infants and in children with fat malabsorption.

DIAGNOSIS

Children may present with coagulopathy or haemorrhagic disease of the newborn. Deficiency may affect bone formation. Prothrombin time is prolonged. The normal intestinal flora can manufacture quinones with vitamin K activity. Antibiotics may lead to deficiency by supressing intestinal flora.

TREATMENT

Oral Vitamin K supplements are given.

RETINOL/VITAMIN A DEFICIENCY

- Incidence/aetiology: an estimated 250 million preschool children are vitamin A deficient worldwide. Poor dietary intake is responsible or deficiency is secondary to fat malabsorption.
- Diagnosis: xerophthalmia: conjunctival xerosis with Bitot spots, keratinisation and necrosis of cornea (**Figs 9.67, 9.68**). Vitamin A blood level is <200 μg/l.
- Treatment: vitamin A is given orally with an IM supplement as well if severely deficient. Dietary intake of yellow or orange fruit and green leafy vegetables, liver, milk, butter, cheese, eggs is augmented.
- Prognosis: an estimated 250,000–500,000 vitamin A-deficient children become blind every year, half of them dying within 12 months of losing their sight.

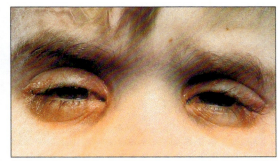

FIGURE 9.67 Vitamin A deficiency in a child with short gut and steatorrhoea.

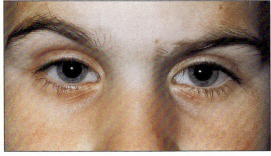

FIGURE 9.68 The child in **9.67** after treatment.

TOCOPHEROL/VITAMIN E DEFICIENCY

- Incidence/aetiology: rare. Fat malabsorption is responsible. This is the most common vitamin deficiency in children with long-term intestinal failure.
- Diagnosis: presents with steatorrhoea and haemolysis in premature neonates. Neurological changes: wide-based gait, spinocerebellar degeneration, ocular palsy. Investigations: serum vitamin E level or red cell susceptibility to haemolysis by hydrogen peroxidase.
- Treatment: oral or intramuscular tocopherol supplements.

VITAMIN D DEFICIENCY

INCIDENCE/GENETICS

Vitamin D deficiency is common in the general population, with highest incidence in individuals who avoid sunlight and/or avoid ingestion of dairy products. Rarely, children have autosomal recessive vitamin D-dependent rickets or X-linked dominant hypophosphataemic rickets.

AETIOLOGY

- Poor dietary intake, e.g. vegan diet.
- Renal disease (low 1,25 dihydroxy vitamin D – the most active form).
- Vitamin D deficiency in the absence of metabolic defect may develop in children who are not exposed to sunlight, e.g. institutionalised children or those with clothing covering the whole body.
- Increased frequency in obesity since vitamin D is taken up into fat cells.
- Children with fat malabsorption, e.g. coeliac disease, CF, small intestinal CD may develop rickets due to vitamin D and calcium malabsorption. Black children are most susceptible.
- Anticonvulsants induce hepatic enzymes; 10 μg/d vitamin D should be administered.
- Vitamin D could play a role in the prevention and treatment of a number of different conditions, including type 1 and type 2 diabetes, hypertension, glucose intolerance and multiple sclerosis.

DIAGNOSIS

- Rickets: genu valgum, epiphyseal swelling (especially distal radii) and growth retardation.
- Skull: craniotabes, delayed closure of fontanelles and bossing of frontal and parietal bones.
- Chest: 'pectus carinatum', rickety rosary (enlarged costochondral junctions) and Harrison's sulci (rib cage depression where the diaphragm is inserted) (**Fig. 9.69**).
- Teeth: delayed dentition.
- Additionally, irritability, hypotonia, respiratory failure, tetany, laryngospasm, convulsions, aminoaciduria may be present.
  ○ Increased risk of severe asthma in children.

Investigations: blood – plasma alkaline phosphatase is raised with low phosphate and/or calcium; x-ray – wide metaphyseal plate and concave diaphyseal ends (**Fig. 9.70**); plasma vitamin D level. The severity of rickets is proportional to the amount of specific vitamin D metabolites and calcium and phosphate ion product.

TREATMENT

Vitamin D 1,000–5,000 μg IV/d is given until normal alkaline phosphatase is achieved, then 10 μg/d and 500 ml/d of milk for calcium requirements. The child should be exposed to sunlight (ergocalciferol is the most important source). Dietary sources include oily fish and fortified margarine.

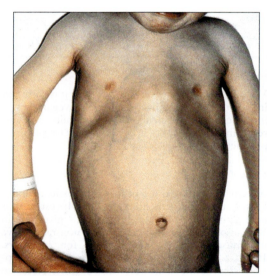

FIGURE 9.69 Nutritional rickets. Pectus carinatum and Harrison's sulci.

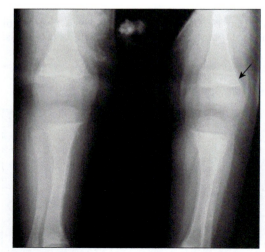

FIGURE 9.70 Rickets: x-ray of knee demonstrating splaying (arrow) and irregularity of femoral and tibial metaphyses.

FURTHER READING

Acute gastroenteritis
Guarino A, Dupont C, Gorelov AV, *et al.* The management of acute diarrhea in children in developed and developing areas: from evidence base to clinical practice. *Expert Opin Pharmacother* 2012;13:17–26.

Faltering growth
Taal HR, Vd Heijden AJ, Steegers EA, Hofman A, Jaddoe VW. Small and large size for gestational age at birth, infant growth, and childhood overweight. *Obesity* (Silver Spring). 2013;21:1261–8.

Infantile colic
Iacovou M, Ralston RA, Muir J, Walker KZ, Truby H. Dietary management of infantile colic: a systematic review. *Matern Child Health J* 2012;16:1319–31.

Constipation
Constipation in Children and Young People: Diagnosis and Management of Idiopathic Childhood Constipation in Primary and Secondary Care NICE Clinical Guidelines - National Collaborating Centre for Women's and Children's Health (UK). Version: 2010.

Recurrent abdominal pain
Berger MY, Gieteling MJ, Benninga MA. Chronic abdominal pain in children. Br Med J 2007;334:997–1002.

Cyclical vomiting
Lee LY, Abbott L, Mahlangu B, Moodie SJ, Anderson S. The management of cyclic vomiting syndrome: a systematic review. *Eur J Gastroenterol Hepatol* 2012;24(9):1001–6.

Toddler's diarrhoea
Di Lorenzo C, Rasquin A, Forbes D, *et al.* Childhood functional gastrointestinal disorders: child/adolescent. In: Drossman DA (ed). *Rome III: The Functional Gastrointestinal Disorders*, 3rd edn. Lawrence: Allen Press, 2006, p. 739.

Intractable diarrhoea
Hannibal MC, Torgerson T. IPEX Syndrome. [Updated 2011 Jan 27]. In: Pagon RA, Adam MP, Ardinger HH, *et al.* (eds). GeneReviews® [Internet]. Seattle (WA): University of Washington, Seattle; 1993–2015. Available from: http://www.ncbi.nlm.nih.gov/books/NBK1118/
Pezzella V, De Martino L, Passariello A, Cosenza L, Terrin G, Berni Canani R. Investigation of chronic diarrhoea in infancy. *Early Hum Dev* 2013;89:893–7.

Chronic intestinal failure
Fishbein TM. Special Issue: Focus on small bowel transplantation: selected works from the XII International Small Bowel Transplant Symposium. *Am J Transplant* 2012;12:S1.

Fabricated and induced illness
Bass C, Glaser D. Early recognition and management of fabricated or induced illness in children. *Lancet* 2014:383:1412–21.

Coeliac disease
Mooney PD, Hadjivassiliou M, Sanders DS. Treating coeliac disease. *Br Med J* 2014;348(1561):30–4.
Murch S, Jenkins H, Auth M, *et al.*; BSPGHAN. Joint BSPGHAN and Coeliac UK guidelines for the diagnosis and management of coeliac disease in children. *Arch Dis Child* 2013;98:806–11.

Food allergic gastrointestinal disease
Fox AT, Lloyd K, Arkwright PD, *et al.*; Science and Research Department, Royal College of Paediatrics and Child Health. The RCPCH care pathway for food allergy in children: an evidence and consensus based national approach *Arch Dis Child* 2011;96(Suppl 2):i25–9.

Eosinophilic oesophagitis
Soon IS, Butzner JD, Kaplan GG, Debruyn JC. Incidence and prevalence of eosinophilic esophagitis in children. *J Pediatr Gastroenterol Nutr* 2013;57:72.

Eosinophilic gastroenteropathy
Ruffner MA, Ruymann K, Barni S, *et al.* Food protein-induced enterocolitis syndrome. *J Allergy Clin Immunol Pract* 2013;1:343–9.

Crohn disease
National Institute for Health and Clinical Excellence (NICE). Crohn disease: management in adults, children and young people. London (UK): National Institute for Health and Clinical Excellence (NICE); 2012. (NICE clinical guideline; no. 152).

Ulcerative colitis
Turner D, Levine A, Escher JC, *et al.* European Crohn and Colitis Organization; European Society for Paediatric Gastroenterology, Hepatology, and Nutrition. Management of pediatric ulcerative colitis: joint ECCO and ESPGHAN evidence-based consensus guidelines. *J Pediatr Gastroenterol Nutr* 2012;55(3):340–61.

Duodenal ulcer
Guariso G, Gasparetto M. Update on peptic ulcers in the pediatric age. *Ulcers* vol. 2012, Article ID 896509, 2012. doi:10.1155/2012/896509.
Erdman SH, Barnard JA. Gastrointestinal polyps and polyposis syndromes in children. *Curr Opin Pediatr* 2002;14:576–82.

Bacterial enteric infections
Chao HC, Chen CC, Chen SY, Chiu CH. Bacterial enteric infections in children: etiology, clinical manifestations and antimicrobial therapy. *Expert Rev Anti Infect Ther* 2006;4:629–38.

Helicobacter pylori
Koletzko S, Jones NL, Goodman KJ, *et al.*; H pylori Working Groups of ESPGHAN and NASPGHAN. Evidence-based guidelines from ESPGHAN and NASPGHAN for Helicobacter pylori infection in children. *J Pediatr Gastroenterol Nutr* 2011;53(2):230–43.

Campylobacter jejuni
Lehours P, Aladjidi N, Sarlangue J, Mégraud F. Campylobacter infections in children. *Arch Pediatr* 2012;19:629–34 (French).

Clostridium difficile
Hickson M. Probiotics in the prevention of antibiotic-associated diarrhoea and *Clostridium difficile* infection. *Therap Adv Gastroenterol* 2011;4(3):185–97.
Tamma PD, Sandora TJ. Clostridium difficile infection in children: current state and unanswered questions. *J Pediatric Infect Dis Soc* 2012;1:230–43.

Pathogenic Escherichia coli
Estrada-Garcia T, Navarro-Garcia F. Enteroaggregative *Escherichia coli* pathotype: a genetically heterogeneous emerging foodborne enteropathogen. *FEMS Immunol Med Microbiol* 2012;66:281–98.

Yersinia enterocolitica
May AN, Piper SM, Boutlis CS. *Yersinia* intussusception: Case report and review. *J Paediatr Child Health* 2014;50:91–5.

Giardia lamblia
Escobedo AA, Cimerman S. Giardiasis: a pharmacotherapy review. *Expert Opin Pharmacother* 2007;8:1885–902.

Cryptosporidium
Jex AR, Smith HV, Nolan MJ, *et al.* Cryptic parasite revealed improved prospects for treatment and control of human cryptosporidiosis through advanced technologies. *Adv Parasitol* 2011;77:141–73.

Helminth infections

Awasthi S, Bundy DAP, Savioli L. Helminthic infections. *Br Med J* 2003;327:431–3.

Gastro-oesophageal reflux

Lightdale JR, Gremse DA; Section on Gastroenterology, Hepatology and Nutrition. Gastroesophageal reflux: management guidance for the pediatrician. *Pediatrics* 2013;131(5):e1684–95. http://pediatrics.aappublications.org/content/early/2013/04/24/peds.2013-0421

Congenital diarrhoea

Terrin G, Tomaiuolo R, Passariello Elce A, *et al*. Congenital diarrheal disorders: an updated diagnostic approach. *Int J Mol Sci* 2012;13:4168–85.

Pancreatitis

Chapman R, Fevery J, Kallooo A, *et al*. Diagnosis and Management of Primary Sclerosing Cholangitis; AASLD Practice Guidelines. *Hepatology* 2010;51:660–78.
Nydegger A, Couper RT, Oliver MR. Childhood pancreatitis. *J Gastroenterol Hepatol* 2006;21:499–509.

Chronic active hepatitis
Wilson disease

Ferenci P, Caca K, Loudianos G. Diagnosis and phenotypic classification of Wilson disease. *Liver Int* 2003:139–42.

Iron deficiency

Wang B, Zhan S, Gong T, Lee L. Iron therapy for improving psychomotor development and cognitive function in children under the age of three with iron deficiency anaemia. *Cochrane Database Syst Rev* 2013.
De-Regil LM, Jefferds ME, Sylvetsky AC, Dowswell T. Intermittent iron supplementation for improving nutrition and development in children under 12 years of age. *Cochrane Database Syst Rev* 2011;7:CD009085.

Nutritional deficiencies

Shaw V, Lawson M (eds). *Clinical Paediatric Dietetics*. Wiley-Blackwell 2007.
Thomas B, Bishop J (eds). *Manual of Dietetic Practice*. Blackwall Publishing 2007.

10 Renal Diseases

Stephen D. Marks

ACUTE KIDNEY INJURY

INCIDENCE

Acute kidney injury (AKI) is a sudden decline in glomerular filtration rate (GFR) with urine output less than 0.5 ml/kg/h, resulting in salt and water retention, together with metabolic abnormalities.

AETIOLOGY

Prerenal AKI has a history or signs of circulatory collapse (**Table 10.1**). There is peripheral vasoconstriction, a low blood pressure and central venous pressure (CVP) and a fractional excretion of sodium of less than 1%. If AKI is due to renal causes, there is salt and water retention with blood, protein and casts in the urine, and symptoms specific to an accompanying disease (e.g. Henoch–Schönlein purpura and nephritis, now called IgA vasculitis). Acute kidney injury in a patient with undiagnosed chronic kidney disease (CKD) is suggested by a poorly grown child with long-standing symptoms typical of CKD.

INVESTIGATIONS

An ultrasound is the most important investigation, in order to identify obstruction of the renal tract that may require intervention, small kidneys of CKD, or large echobright kidneys with loss of corticomedullary differentiation, typical of an acute process (**Table 10.2**). Percutaneous renal biopsy is indicated

TABLE 10.1 Causes of acute kidney injury

Prerenal

Hypovolaemia and/or hypotension

(e.g. gastroenteritis, dehydration, sepsis, burns, cardiac failure, cardiac tamponade)

Renal

Arterial (e.g. haemolytic uraemic syndrome, arteritis, embolic)

Venous (e.g. renal venous thrombosis)

Glomerular (e.g. glomerulonephritis)

Interstitial (e.g. tubulointerstitial nephritis, pyelonephritis)

Tubular (e.g. acute tubular necrosis, ischaemic, toxic, obstructive)

Acute on chronic kidney disease

Postrenal

Congenital obstruction

Acquired obstruction

TABLE 10.2 Investigation of acute kidney injury

- Blood tests:
  - full blood count, blood film, coagulation screen
  - ESR, CRP and blood culture
  - sodium, potassium, chloride, bicarbonate, urea, creatinine, glucose, blood gas
  - calcium, phosphate, magnesium, albumin
  - alkaline phosphatase, albumin, liver function tests, urate
  - ASO titre and antiDNase B
  - Complement C3, C4, serum immunoglobulins IgG, IgA and IgM
  - ANA, anti-dsDNA, ANCA and anti-GBM antibody
- Urine tests:
  - dipstick (blood and protein), microscopy and culture,
  - sodium, urea and creatinine
- Throat swab
- Stool culture
- Doppler renal ultrasound
- Percutaneous renal biopsy (if unknown cause of acute kidney injury)
- X-ray hand and wrist, chest x-ray, ECG, ECHO and PTH if acute on chronic kidney disease

if the diagnosis is unclear, in order to exclude a crescentic nephritis that would require treatment with immunosuppression (**Fig. 10.1**).

TREATMENT

Conservative management is by attention to fluid balance and diet (controlled protein, high calorie, low phosphate and potassium) and attention to fluid balance. Hypovolaemia should be corrected with normal saline or plasma. Fluid overload may respond to furosemide and fluid restriction to insensible losses, although some children may require dialysis (**Table 10.3**).

TABLE 10.3 Indications for dialysis

- Failure of conservative management
- Hyperkalaemia
- Severe hypo- or hypernatraemia
- Fluid overload resistant to medical therapy with pulmonary oedema and/or hypertension
- Severe acidosis
- Multisystem failure

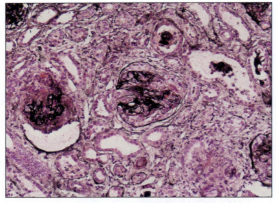

FIGURE 10.1 Histopathology of percutaneous renal biopsy showing a crescentic nephritis causing acute kidney injury with rapidly progressive glomerulonephritis.

HAEMOLYTIC URAEMIC SYNDROME

INCIDENCE/AETIOLOGY

Haemolytic uraemic syndrome (HUS) is one of the commonest causes of AKI in childhood. It is classified into diarrhoea-associated (D+ HUS) or typical HUS, and non-diarrhoea associated (D− HUS) or atypical HUS. However, nomenclature may be confusing, since diarrhoea may be present in first presentation of D− HUS and be mislabelled as D+ HUS until relapse.

- D+ HUS occurs mainly in childhood but also in the elderly population, sporadically in summer months or in epidemics. Infective causes vary in different countries across the world, but Shiga-toxin producing *Escherichia coli* (STEC) 0157 H7 and other serotypes and *Shigella dysenteriae* type 1 are the commonest aetiological organisms. Infections have been isolated from various sources from ingestion of unpasteurised milk and apple juice, unwashed vegetables, uncooked meat to contaminated water supplies.

- D− HUS accounts for 10% of cases, affects all ages without seasonal pattern. Infective causes are neuraminidase-producing *Streptococcus pneumoniae* and HIV. Inherited forms of this life-threatening disease, characterised by chronic uncontrolled complement activation, may have identifiable complement gene mutations (such as factor H and factor I mutations) in 60–70% of patients. Our genetics knowledge is evolving with autosomal dominant or recessive forms as well as neonatal presentation of inborn errors of cobalamin metabolism. The incidence is approximately 2 per million population, of which nearly 60% present in children, although the oldest patient has presented at age of 83 years, and can be associated with relapses with worsening hypertension, proteinuria and/or renal dysfunction. Deficiency of complement factor H-related (CFHR) proteins and CFH autoantibody-positive HUS (DEAP-HUS) represents a unique subgroup of complement-mediated atypical HUS. Autoantibodies to the C-terminus of CFH block CFH surface recognition and mimic mutations found in the genetic form of CFH-mediated atypical HUS. CFH autoantibodies are found in 10–15% of atypical HUS patients and occur almost exclusively in patients with CFHR1 or CFHR3/CFHR1 deletions.

Drug-induced causes of HUS are rare but have been reported with calcineurin inhibitors (ciclosporin and tacrolimus), chemotherapeutic agents, antiplatelet agents and oral contraceptive pills. Other causes include bone marrow and solid organ transplantation, malignancy, pregnancy, systemic lupus erythematosus (SLE) and glomerulonephritis.

CLINICAL PRESENTATION

HUS should always be considered in children who present with diarrhoea (often bloody), vomiting and severe abdominal pain with associated pallor, lethargy, jaundice, petechiae, bleeding, oliguria, anuria, fluid overload, oedema, hypertension, convulsions, coma, pancreatitis and pneumonia.

DIFFERENTIAL DIAGNOSIS

There is an overlap with thrombotic thrombocytopenic purpura (TTP), which is also characterised by thrombocytopenia, microangiopathic haemolytic anaemia and abnormalities in renal function. However, neurological symptoms and signs, and associated fever, are much more prominent in TTP.

DIAGNOSIS

A triad of Coombs' negative microangiopathic haemolytic anaemia (**Fig. 10.2**) with fragmented red cells, thrombocytopenia and acute kidney injury is found. Investigations include: full blood count; differential white cell count; blood film; reticulocyte count; ferritin; Coombs' tests; group and save; urea; creatinine; serum electrolytes; glucose; amylase; lipase; lactate dehydrogenase; haptoglobin; liver function tests; serology; Thomsen–Friedenreich antigen (T-Ag); antistreptolysin O titre (ASOT); urine dipstick and urine albumin to creatinine ratio; stool culture; and Doppler renal ultrasound. Percutaneous renal biopsy is not routinely indicated in D+ HUS but may show predominant glomerular or arteriolar involvement and acute cortical necrosis.

TREATMENT

Overall treatment of HUS is similar to any cause of AKI therapy, with optimal fluid and electrolyte management, diuretic therapy, other antihypertensive agents and dialysis. There is no role for antibiotics, except when there is proven streptococcal infection, which may exacerbate HUS. Peritoneal dialysis is the preferred renal replacement modality. Unregulated complement leads to progression of symptoms so there should be consideration for plasma infusions and/or exchange using Octaplas® in patients with atypical HUS (**Fig. 10.3**). Eculizumab is a humanised anti-C5 monoclonal antibody that may overcome the lack of complement regulation and subsequently reduce the symptoms of C5 activation. Eculizumab blocks terminal complement activation and binds with high affinity to C5 so the proximal functions of complement remain intact (**Fig. 10.4**). Eculizumab has superseded previous treatments of corticosteroids, intravenous immunoglobulin, vincristine and splenectomy for poorly responsive or resistant forms of atypical HUS. Fluid overload with severe hypertension can exacerbate the clinical situation and bilateral nephrectomies have been anecdotally advocated in malignant hypertension. Renal replacement therapy with peritoneal and haemodialysis can be offered with consideration of prophylactic or therapeutic eculizumab for prevention or treatment of recurrence of HUS post-transplantation in those at higher risk (such as with a defined genetic mutation).

PROGNOSIS

D+ HUS results in complete recovery in the majority of cases without relapses, but can lead to chronic kidney disease. There is reduced morbidity and mortality during epidemics by prompt recognition, identification and isolation of individuals to prevent spread, and elimination of the source with removal of contaminated food and water. The prognosis in D− HUS is worse, with a progressive course and 25% relapse rate, with potentially improved clinical outcomes now with new therapeutic interventions.

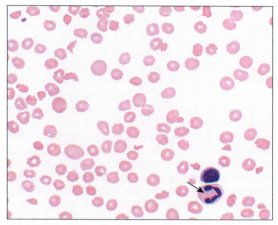

FIGURE 10.2 May Grünwald–Giemsa stained peripheral blood smear showing a reactive lymphocyte above a neutrophil (arrow) with evidence of microangiopathic haemolytic anaemia. There are numerous red blood cell fragments, thrombocytopenia, few spherocytes and polychromasia in a case of diarrhoea-associated haemolytic uraemic syndrome.

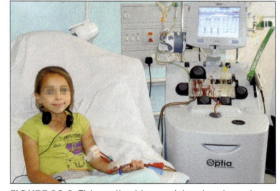

FIGURE 10.3 This patient is receiving treatment with immunoadsorption prior to ABO incompatible living related renal transplantation for atypical haemolytic uraemic syndrome. Plasmapheresis has also been advocated for the glomerulonephritides (either primary renal diseases such as membranoproliferative glomerulonephritis and idiopathic, rapidly progressive glomerulonephritis, or secondary to vasculitis or systemic lupus erythematosus).

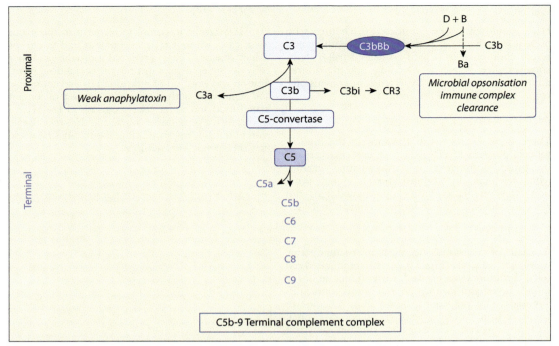

FIGURE 10.4 Eculizumab is a humanised anti-C5 monoclonal antibody that may overcome the lack of complement regulation and subsequently reduce the symptoms of C5 activation. Eculizumab blocks terminal complement activation and binds with high affinity to C5 so the proximal functions of complement remain intact.

GLOMERULONEPHRITIS

INTRODUCTION

The commonest cause of glomerulonephritis is a postinfectious glomerulonephritis where patients develop AKI after having an infection (typically streptococcal throat or skin infection) associated with bacterial growth on throat or skin swab, positive ASO titre and anti-DNase B and evidence of hypocomplementaemia (with low complement C3). Clinically, children present with features of nephritic syndrome with haematuria, proteinuria, fluid overload, hypertension and oliguric renal failure (see 'AKI'). However, some patients may present with features of mixed nephritic and nephrotic syndrome (see nephrotic syndrome).

Some children present with features of systemic disease, suggestive of SLE (with American College of Rheumatology and/or Systemic Lupus International Collaborating Clinics classification criteria [see also Chapter 17 Rheumatology, page 525]) with lupus nephritis. The International Society of Nephrology and Renal Pathology Society working groups published the histopathological classification of lupus nephritis (**Fig. 10.5**).

Other patients may present with vasculitis. The Chapel Hill consensus criteria nomenclature update on the classification of vasculitis from 2012 distinguishes large vessel vasculitis from medium vessel vasculitis and immune complex and anti-neutrophil cytoplasmic antibody (ANCA)-associated small vessel vasculitis (**Fig. 10.6**).

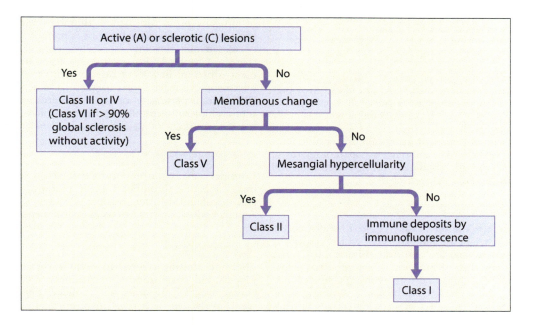

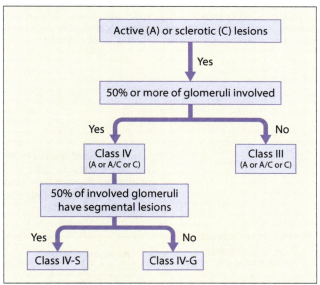

FIGURE 10.5 International Society of Nephrology/Renal Pathology Society working group classification of lupus nephritis (modified from original source *JASN and Kidney Int* 2004).

IgA VASCULITIS

INCIDENCE/AETIOLOGY

Henoch–Schönlein purpura or IgA vasculitis is a relatively common small vessel vasculitis, often preceded by upper respiratory tract infection, peaking at 4–6 years of age. Its cause is unknown; it is rarely associated with underlying C2 or C4 deficiency but an infectious trigger of genetically susceptible individuals is likely. Skin and renal histopathology reveal a leucocytoclastic vasculitis, with IgA deposition and IgA nephropathy respectively.

CLINICAL PRESENTATION

All patients develop a rash (required for diagnosis), typically symmetric and gravity dependent, especially on forearms, legs and buttocks (**Figure 10.7**). The rash is petechial or purpuric in nature, often palpable, non-blanching and with evolving colours (pink, yellow, green and then brown), although some children have macular or urticarial rashes initially. They may have oedema, especially of hands, feet, face and/or scrotum. Gastrointestinal tract involvement is present in 65% of cases, with bowel wall haemorrhage causing dull periumbilical abdominal pain, vomiting, and tenderness, but also melaena or intussusception with typical 'thumb-printing' on barium enema. Transient arthritis is present in 65% of cases in multiple joints, especially knees and ankles (see also Chapter 17 Rheumatology). Renal involvement is present in 50% of cases, which varies from microscopic or macroscopic haematuria to nephrotic syndrome, hypertension or rapidly progressive crescentic glomerulonephritis. Patients may have non-specific symptoms of malaise, fever and headaches.

DIFFERENTIAL DIAGNOSIS

Consider causes of thrombocytopenia (sepsis, leukaemia, idiopathic thrombocytopenic purpura, HUS) and vasculitis (SLE, microscopic polyangiitis, polyangiitis nodosa, postinfectious glomerulonephritis).

DIAGNOSIS

FBC and clotting screen (to exclude thrombocytopenia and coagulation abnormalities); urea; creatinine; electrolytes; urinalysis (to detect significant renal involvement). If renal involvement is severe, consider complement C3, C4, antinuclear antibody (ANA), ANCA, ASOT and anti-DNase B, renal ultrasound and percutaneous renal biopsy. If intussusception is suspected, abdominal ultrasound should be performed.

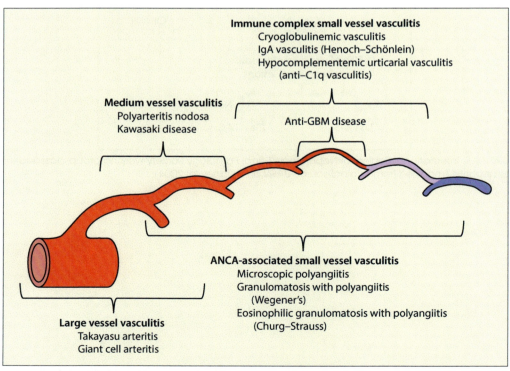

FIGURE 10.6 Chapel Hill consensus criteria nomenclature update on the classification of vasculitis from 2012. ANCA: anticytoplasmic antibody; GBM: glomerular basement membrane.

Renal diseases

TREATMENT

General treatment is with symptomatic pain relief, explanation and reassurance although nutritional supplementation may be required in prolonged episodes. Oral prednisolone 1–2 mg/kg/d may be given for severe gastrointestinal involvement (this has also been suggested for severe joint or skin involvement), and NSAIDs for joint pain. Consider intravenous methylprednisolone, oral prednisolone, plasma exchange, cyclophosphamide, dipyridamole and aspirin for rapidly progressive glomerulonephritis. Follow-up for renal dysfunction, hypertension and proteinuria for at least 1 year, or longer if these problems persist.

PROGNOSIS

The prognosis is very good as it is usually self-limited with complete resolution by a mean of 1 month, but can recur, more rarely after years. Microscopic haematuria may persist, or macroscopic episodes occur after subsequent upper respiratoray tract infections. One to five percent have long-term renal problems, with hypertension, proteinuria or renal dysfunction. This is more likely if there has been hypertension, significant proteinuria, or rapidly progressive crescentic glomerulonephritis at presentation. It uncommonly recurs in renal transplants.

NEPHROTIC SYNDROME

INCIDENCE

Idiopathic nephrotic syndrome (NS) consists of heavy proteinuria (at least 3+ proteinuria on urinary dipstick) and albuminuria (early morning urine albumin to creatinine ratio above 200 mg/mmol), hypoalbuminaemia (below 25g/l) and oedema, usually associated with hyperlipidaemia (**Fig. 10.8**). It is the commonest chronic glomerular disease in children with an incidence of 2–4 cases per 100,000 children in the UK. It may be primary or secondary to an overt systemic disorder and is associated with atopy. The commonest type of NS in children is characterised by minimal histological changes in the glomeruli. This is called minimal change nephrotic syndrome (MCNS) (**Fig. 10.9**) and is mostly responsive to corticosteroid therapy (steroid-sensitive nephrotic syndrome [SSNS]) (**Table 10.4**).

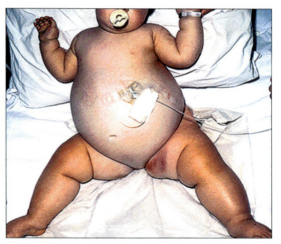

FIGURE 10.8 An infant aged 3.5 years with evidence of oedema due to nephrotic syndrome. The oedema is dependent in nephrotic syndrome, accumulating in low pressure areas around the eyes, in the legs and as ascites.

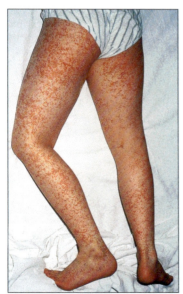

FIGURE 10.7 Classical purpuric rash on bilateral lower limbs of patient with Henoch–Schönlein purpura.

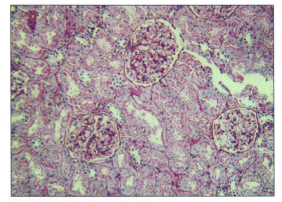

FIGURE 10.9 Minimal histological changes in the glomeruli from a percutaneous renal biopsy of a child with minimal change nephrotic syndrome.

INCIDENCE OF MCNS

MCNS usually presents in children aged 2–6 (median age of onset of 2.5) years, is commoner in boys and has greater prevalence in Asian children. It is associated with atopy. There is heavy, highly selective proteinuria that responds to corticosteroid therapy. Microscopic (usually not macroscopic) haematuria may be present in up to 25% of cases (**Table 10.5**).

DIAGNOSIS

Hypoalbuminaemia causes oedema because of a disturbance of the Starling equilibrium in the capillary bed, and rapid albumin loss results in hypovolaemia with abdominal pain, shock and risk of thrombosis.

Venous thrombosis is multifactorial, with sluggish peripheral circulation, relative polycythaemia, hyperlipidaemia, platelet hyperaggregability, hyperfibrinogenaemia and loss of control proteins such as antithrombin-III, all contributing to the procoagulant state. Loss of IgG and complement components, particularly factor B of the alternative pathway, predisposes to infection, typically pneumococcal septicaemia and peritonitis.

TREATMENT

The primary treatment objective is to achieve remission, alleviate symptoms and prevent and treat acute risks such as infection, thrombosis and hypovolaemia with minimisation of long-term

TABLE 10.4 Glomerular histology and corticosteroid responsiveness in primary nephrotic syndrome in children

Glomerular histology	% Children	% Steroid sensitive
Minimal change	78	95
Focal and segmental glomerulosclerosis	8	2
Membranoproliferative glomerulonephritis	6	1
Diffuse mesangial sclerosis	4	4
Glomerulonephritis	2	0
Membranous nephropathy	2	0

TABLE 10.5 Clinical and laboratory features in children with primary nephrotic syndrome

Percentage of cases	MCNS	FSGS	MPGN
Total	78	8	6
Age under 8 years	80	50	3
Male	60	69	36
Hypertension*	21	49	36
Microscopic haematuria #	23	48	51
Hypocomplementaemia $	1	4	74
Renal dysfunction ^	33	41	50

Definitions

*: Hypertension is defined as systolic blood pressure above the 95th centile and/or requiring antihypertensive agents.

#: Microscopic haematuria is defined as the presence of red blood cells in the urine (≥3 red blood cells per high power field) on urine microscopy.

$: Hypocomplementaemia is defined as low complement C3 level (below the normal laboratory reference range).

^: Renal dysfunction is defined as plasma creatinine above the 98th centile for age and sex.

Renal diseases

complications, such as bone disease, hypertension, Cushing syndrome, obesity, growth retardation, striae, cataracts and a variety of psychological, social and behavioural disturbances. The initial treatment is corticosteroids prior to the use of other immunosuppressive agents (**Table 10.6**). Percutaneous renal biopsy should be considered in atypical presentations (in infants under 12 months or adolescents over 12 years of age). Familial nephrotic syndrome, macroscopic haematuria, significant renal dysfunction or hypertension and steroid resistant nephrotic syndrome after 4 weeks of high-dose corticosteroids without response to intravenous methylprednisolone pulses are also an indication for a biopsy (**Table 10.7**). If the child is steroid sensitive, minimal change histology can be presumed and does not need to be confirmed by biopsy. Prophylactic penicillin should be prescribed when young patients are clinically nephrotic.

PROGNOSIS

Children presenting with initial onset of NS have a 24-month sustained remission rate of 49% with a frequent relapse rate of 29%. One-third of children with MCNS have only a single episode, one-third relapse occasionally and one-third become steroid-dependent frequent relapsers. Relapses eventually cease and the development of steroid resistance is unusual; end-stage kidney disease almost never occurs (unless MCNS on initial biopsy is focal segmental glomerulosclerosis [FSGS] on subsequent biopsies).

TABLE 10.6 Modern treatment of primary nephrotic syndrome

Level	Relapse	Treatment
1	Initial episode	Prednisolone 60 mg/m^2/d for 28 days with subsequent alternate day regimen (current trial of 8 versus 16 weeks total of corticosteroids)
2	Infrequent relapse therapy	Prednisolone 60 mg/m^2/d until remission with subsequent 40 mg/m^2 alternate day regimen for 4 weeks
3	Frequent relapse therapy	Prednisolone 60 mg/m^2/d until remission with subsequent 40 mg/m^2 alternate day regimen for 4 weeks weaning to 0.5–1.0 mg/kg alternate days for at least 6 months
4	Steroid sparing agents	Levamisole 2.5 mg/kg alternate days Cyclophosphamide 3 mg/kg/day for 8 weeks Calcineurin inhibitor (ciclosporin/tacrolimus) Mycophenolate mofetil Intravenous rituximab

TABLE 10.7 Definitions

1.	Nephrotic syndrome	Proteinuria >40 mg/m^2/h, hypoalbuminaemia <25 g/l and oedema
2.	Remission	Proteinuria <4 mg/m^2/h or no or trace of proteinuria on urine dipstick testing for 3 consecutive days irrespective of loss of oedema
3.	Relapse	Proteinuria >40 mg/m^2/h or at least 3+ proteinuria on urine dipstick testing for 3 consecutive days
4.	Frequent relapses	Two relapses within 6 months of initial response or four or more relapses within any 12 month period
5.	Steroid sensitive	Remission achieved within 28 days of corticosteroid therapy
6.	Steroid resistance	Failure to achieve remission despite at least 4 weeks of high-dose corticosteroids (prednisolone 60 mg/m^2/d) and three pulses of intravenous methylprednisolone
7.	Steroid dependence	Relapse on or within 2 weeks of corticosteroid therapy discontinuation or as tapering of corticosteroid therapy

CHRONIC KIDNEY DISEASE

INTRODUCTION

The commonest cause of irreversible kidney failure or CKD is congenital anomalies of the kidney and urinary tract. CKD is divided into the severity from Stage I, II, III, IV and V, corresponding to GFR of >90, 60–89, 30–59, 15–29 and <15 ml/min/1.73 m^2, respectively. Renal replacement therapy is usually required for Stage V chronic kidney disease and the gold standard therapy is pre-emptive living related renal transplantation prior to the requirement of dialysis (assuming patients present before requiring renal replacement therapy with dialysis).

PATHOGENESIS

Renal osteodystrophy is the term used to describe the disturbance of bone formation in CKD, secondary to abnormalities of vitamin D metabolism and secondary hyperparathyroidism. Reduced activity of the renal 1-α hydroxylase enzyme, with progressive renal failure, causes decreased production of the active hormone 1,25-dihydroxyvitamin D$_3$. This results in increased bone resorption (i.e. osteitis fibrosa due to secondary hyperparathyroidism) and impaired mineralisation of osteoid (i.e. rickets). Parathyroid hormone (PTH) secretion is stimulated by a fall in ionised calcium due to reduced calcium absorption mediated by 1,25-dihydroxyvitamin D$_3$ and hyperphosphataemia secondary to phosphate retention.

DIAGNOSIS

Children with early changes of renal osteodystrophy are usually asymptomatic but if untreated they may develop bone pain with or without fractures or slipped epiphyses, skeletal deformities and weakness secondary to proximal myopathy (**Fig. 10.10**).

A raised level of intact PTH is indicative of active bone disease. Measurements of intact PTH can be used to monitor treatment in conjunction with measurement of plasma phosphate, total calcium and ionised calcium. Indirect assessments of PTH activity (i.e. alkaline phosphatase, bone radiographs and biopsies and tubular resorption of phosphate) are less reliable.

TREATMENT

The principles of management of renal osteodystrophy are:

- Correction of acidosis using sodium bicarbonate.
- Phosphate restriction by control of dietary intake and the use of a phosphate binder (e.g. calcium carbonate to maintain plasma phosphate within the normal range for age).
- Supplements of oral 1-α-hydroxycholecalciferol or 1,25 dihydroxycholecalciferol to maintain the PTH within normal range, if not achieved by control of plasma phosphate. This may require the total calcium to be maintained at the upper end of the normal range. Total calcium is a measurement of bound, ionised and complexed calcium. The proportion may increase in CKD, reflected by total hypercalcaemia. However, if the ionised calcium is within the normal range, treatment with vitamin D analogues may continue.

PROGNOSIS

With medical management and adherence to medications, this can be controlled with linear growth maintained, but progression may occur with deteriorating renal function.

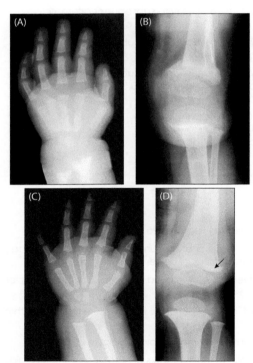

FIGURE 10.10 Bone radiographs of wrist and knee in a boy who presented aged 10 months with severe chronic kidney disease secondary to posterior urethral valves and bilateral renal dysplasia. (A,B): Pre-treatment. Coarse trabecular pattern with wide irregular metaphyseal plates and subperiosteal bone resorption, with periosteal reaction in the lower femur; (C,D): post-treatment. Resolution of bone changes with the appearance of a dense white line indicating normal bone formation at the zone of provisional calcification (arrow).

CYSTIC KIDNEY DISEASES

CLASSIFICATION AND GENETICS

- Autosomal recessive polycystic kidney disease (ARPKD). Caused by mutations in *PKHD1* on 6p21.
- Autosomal dominant polycystic kidney diseases (ADPKD). Commonest mutation is in *PKD1* on 16p13. The gene codes for a cell signalling molecule. A minority of ADPKD cases are caused by PKD2 on 4q, which encodes a calcium channel.
- Nephronophthisis. Caused by homozygous or compound heterozygous mutation in or deletion of the gene encoding nephrocystin on chromosome 2q13 (*NPHP1* with latest genetics research identifying multiple genes, now at *NPHP16*).
- Renal cysts and diabetes syndrome (RCAD) caused by mutations and deletions in hepatocyte nuclear factor-1-beta (*HNF1B*) gene, which maps to chromosome 17q12.
- Glomerulocystic disease. Autosomal dominant with increasing understanding on underlying genetics (including *HNF1B*).
- Tuberous sclerosis. Autosomal dominant, with mutations of *TSC2* on 16p13 (adjacent to *PKD1*).
- von Hippel–Lindau disease. Autosomal dominant inheritance with mutation of gene on 3p25-26.
- Orofaciodigital syndrome type 1. X-linked dominant.
- Acquired cystic kidney disease. Secondary to chronic hypokalaemia or uraemia.

INCIDENCE

The incidence of ARPKD and ADPKD is 1 in 10,000 and 1,000 respectively in paediatric and adult populations together. The former accounts for the majority of cases in childhood but it is increasingly recognised that ADPKD is not uncommon in paediatric practice. Nephronophthisis is an autosomal recessive cystic kidney disease that is the most frequent genetic cause of renal failure in childhood and adolescence. There are genetics advances in the other, rare causes that are listed above.

CLINICAL PRESENTATION

ARPKD may present antenatally, with abnormal renal ultrasound (including enlarged, echogenic kidneys), or neonatally with nephromegaly, hypertension and/or renal dysfunction. Less severe cases have hypertension and renal dysfunction in infancy whereas, in later childhood, mild renal disease can coexist with liver fibrosis and portal hypertension. ADPKD can present with loin pain, urinary tract infections (UTIs), mild renal dysfunction or hypertension in childhood but is generally clinically silent until adulthood. Some patients with ADPKD are diagnosed in childhood due to incidental findings on abdominal ultrasound or familial requests for ultrasound screening. This can be debated ethically as there are no proven therapies known, although some asymptomatic children could be recruited to clinical trials. There is a rare and severe early onset variety of ADPKD with tuberous sclerosis due to contiguous mutations of *PKD1* and *TSC2*. Nephronophthisis can be combined with extrarenal manifestations, including situs inversus, cardiac malformations, hepatic fibrosis, cerebellar vermis hypoplasia (Joubert syndrome), retinitis pigmentosa (Senior–Loken syndrome) and multiple developmental and neurological abnormalities (Meckel–Gruber syndrome).

DIAGNOSIS

Prenatal genetic diagnosis of ADPKD or ARPKD is feasible, especially if DNA from affected relatives is available. Severe ARPKD may be detected in the last trimester by ultrasound scan showing enlarging kidneys and oligohydramnios. Due to the different types of cystic kidney diseases, historically an intravenous urogram postnatally was utilised if renal failure was not severe, to delineate the characteristic dilatation of the medullary collecting ducts of ARPKD.

Abdominal ultrasound scans (**Fig. 10.11**) may not always reliably distinguish between ARPKD and early ADPKD, with cysts enlarging considerably in the course of ADPKD. Although renal cysts are seen well on CT scanning, this form of imaging is not routinely advocated in paediatric practice due to the radiation burden and as this is not superior to the less costly and less invasive ultrasound (**Fig. 10.12**). It is always prudent to investigate the parents with renal ultrasound scans as they may be affected in ADPKD as new mutations are unusual. Liver cysts may be present in ADPKD and periportal liver fibrosis in ARPKD can be diagnosed by biopsy or suggested by isotope ^{99}Tc-hepatobiliary iminodiacetic acid (HIDA) scans.

PATHOLOGY

Many cystic diseases are caused by ciliopathies, which are genetic disorders of the cellular cilia or the cilia anchoring structures. The basal bodies of ciliary function PKHD1 and PKD182 are expressed in the primary cilium, whereas OFD1 protein is expressed

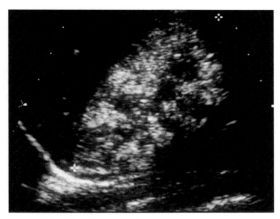

FIGURE 10.11 Ultrasound scan image demonstrating the large bright kidney of autosomal recessive polycystic kidney disease (ARPKD).

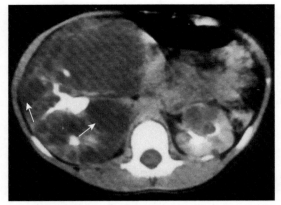

FIGURE 10.12 Computerised tomography scan of autosomal dominant polycystic kidney diseases (ADPKD). Note the asymmetrical involvement with visible cysts (arrows).

in the centrosome/basal body of the primary cilium. ARPKD cysts arise from collecting ducts while ADPKD cysts arise from all nephron segments. There are aberrations of cell proliferation, apoptosis, epithelial cell polarity and the extracellular matrix.

TREATMENT

Controlled trials in adults with ADPKD show that low protein diets, control of hypertension and cyst surgery have little, if any, significant influence on progression to renal failure. However, hypertension in PKD should be vigorously treated to reduce cardiovascular damage and possibly slow progression. Renal transplantation is effective, although native nephrectomy may be required for nephromegaly or recurrent UTIs. Some children with ARPKD develop hepatic fibrosis and portal hypertension, which may require sequential or combined liver–kidney transplantation. Hepatic cysts and Berry aneurysms in patients with ADPKD may also require treatment.

PROGNOSIS

A significant proportion of ARPKD patients develop renal failure soon after birth and a small subset of ADPKD patients have a severe infantile presentation. Half of ARPKD patients develop end-stage kidney disease by adolescence, whereas only half of ADPKD patients develop uraemia in a lifetime. The rate of disease progression is highly variable even in single PKD kindreds.

CONGENITAL ANOMALIES OF THE KIDNEY AND URINARY TRACT

CLASSIFICATION/GENETICS

Renal agenesis and dysplasia represent malformations in which the fetal organs have failed to undergo a normal pattern of differentiation. In renal agenesis, no renal tissue can be detected. Dysplastic kidneys contain undifferentiated and metaplastic elements, while multicystic dysplastic kidneys contain large cysts; their excretory function is often absent or considerably reduced. Most are sporadic, although some are associated with other defects in multiple organs (e.g. CHARGE and VACTERL associations).

Rarely, families have been reported with definite inheritance of agenesis or dysplasia. These can occur in isolation or be syndromal (e.g. X-linked Kallmann syndrome with renal agenesis and infertility; autosomal dominant branchio-otorenal syndrome with renal dysplasia and deafness; renal cysts and diabetes syndrome).

INCIDENCE

The incidence of bilateral renal agenesis is highly variable, depending on the study. Unilateral disease is often clinically silent and the estimated incidence is 1 in 1,000–10,000. The incidence of multicystic dysplastic and renal hypoplasia/dysplasia is about 1 in 5,000.

CLINICAL PRESENTATION

Unilateral multicystic dysplastic kidneys classically present as an abdominal mass in infancy although, increasingly, these malformations are detected by antenatal ultrasound scanning. About 20–30% of such children have contralateral abnormalities, including pelviureteric or vesicoureteric junction obstruction. Bilateral renal malformations can result in oligohydramnios, premature delivery and the Potter sequence (oligohydramnios, oliguria, pulmonary hypoplasia and limb deformities). Renal dysplasia is very commonly associated with abnormalities of the lower urinary tract including obstructive lesions (e.g. posterior urethral valves in boys and ureteroceles in girls).

DIAGNOSIS

Renal dysplasia is suggested on ultrasound scanning by the visualisation of irregular-shaped organs with loss of corticomedullary differentiation (**Fig. 10.13**). Cysts, where present, can be identified but these cases need to be distinguished from PKD or hydronephrosis.

Technically, the diagnosis of dysplasia can only be made by histology but this is rarely clinically indicated. If ultrasound suggests unilateral agenesis, a dimercaptosuccinic acid (DMSA) isotope renogram can be performed to exclude the possibility of an ectopic kidney.

PATHOLOGY

Dysplastic kidneys contain immature ducts that are considered to be branches of the ureteric bud surrounded by fibromuscular and undifferentiated cells (**Fig. 10.14**). There may also be metaplastic tissue including cartilage.

TREATMENT

When bilateral malformations are associated with severe oligohydramnios, termination may be considered due to the poor prognosis associated with pulmonary hypoplasia. A subgroup with large bladders and urinary obstruction have been treated with vesicoamniotic shunts. Although this procedure may increase the amount of liquor, it is unproven whether lung growth is accelerated. Those with bilateral renal dysplasia require lifetime follow-up for the detection and treatment of CKD.

Unilateral multicystic dysplastic kidneys probably do not require any specific treatment, but prophylactic antibiotics should be considered until associated urological contralateral abnormalities can be excluded. There is evidence that many of these organs involute spontaneously over months or years (**Fig. 10.15**). Some authorities, however, recommend removal of these kidneys because of a (disputed) risk of renal malignancy and hypertension.

PROGNOSIS

Bilateral renal agenesis or severe dysplasia may cause neonatal death if associated with pulmonary hypoplasia. With advances in dialysis and transplantation, renal failure can be adequately treated although some of these children die in the first year from malformations of other organs (e.g. lung, heart, brain and gut). Unilateral renal agenesis may be clinically silent throughout life and has minimal increased morbidity if the contralateral kidney is normal, although deterioration in renal function may occur with age if there is associated contralateral renal dysplasia. Vesicoureteric reflux and contralateral kidney abnormalities occur in 30–50% of patients with unilateral dysplasia.

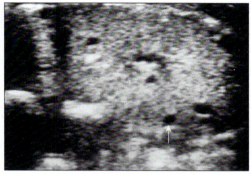

FIGURE 10.13 Renal ultrasound scan shows loss of corticomedullary differentiation in a dysplastic kidney. Note the small subcortical cysts (arrow).

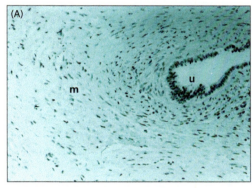

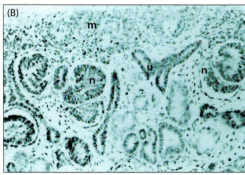

FIGURE 10.14 (A) Histology of a dysplastic kidney. Note the lack of tissue differentiation versus a human fetal kidney (B), which contains primitive nephrons (n) in addition to mesenchyme (m) and branches of the ureteric bud (u).

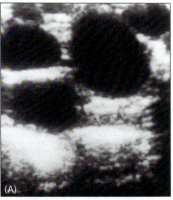

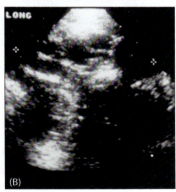

FIGURE 10.15 Renal ultrasound demonstrating multicystic dysplastic kidney, which partially involuted over 2 years.

VESICOURETERIC REFLUX

See also Chapter 22 Urology, page 663.

CLASSIFICATION

Vesicoureteric reflux (VUR) is the retrograde passage of urine from the bladder into the ureter and/or the renal pelvis, calyces and collecting ducts. It can be secondary to high bladder pressure due either to anatomical lesions of the urethra (e.g. posterior urethral valves) or to neuromuscular incoordination of bladder emptying (e.g. neurogenic bladder). It can occur in children who have either normal or abnormal kidneys with congenital anomalies of the kidney and urinary tract (CAKUT) (e.g. bilateral renal dysplasia with VUR) and 'reflux nephropathy' denotes the presence of primary VUR when associated with renal disease.

GENETICS

Isolated primary VUR is an autosomal dominant disorder with incomplete penetrance and variable expression; the genetic defect is unknown. Rarely primary VUR can be inherited (although several candidate loci have been defined) as part of a syndrome (e.g. with optic nerve colobomata when mutations of *PAX2* have been described).

INCIDENCE

Estimates of the incidence of VUR in children range between 1 in 50 to 1 in 200. The risk of primary VUR in a sibling approaches 50% when screened with micturating cystourethrography (MCUG) before the age of 2 years.

CLINICAL PRESENTATION

When VUR is associated with other abnormalities the clinical presentation is determined by the primary disease (e.g. poor urinary stream with posterior urethral valves). Primary VUR may be clinically silent and many of the milder cases regress over years. The commonest presentation is with UTI and indeed VUR is frequently diagnosed when investigating children for UTI. Recurrent pyelonephritis in the first years of life may lead to hypertension or CKD in later childhood or adulthood.

DIAGNOSIS

Severe antenatal VUR can be detected as hydronephrosis on ultrasound scanning in the second trimester. In this case, a MCUG soon after birth will confirm the presence and define the extent of VUR, and will also diagnose any coexisting urethral pathology. It is important to exclude posterior urethral valves in boys as they need surgical resection. In younger children with UTI, MCUG is the investigation of choice to detect VUR (**Fig. 10.16**), while in older children VUR can be diagnosed by indirect radionucleotide cystogram (**Fig. 10.17**).

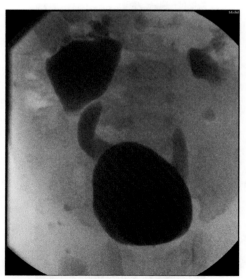

FIGURE 10.16 Micturating cystourethrography demonstrating bilateral vesicoureteric reflux.

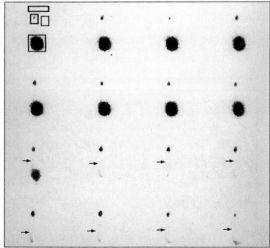

FIGURE 10.17 Indirect radionucleotide cystogram shows a small amount of isotope in the left kidney after injection of MAG3, which is filtered by the glomerulus. On sequential views, the urinary bladder empties upon voiding with reflux of isotope up the left ureter (arrows).

In addition, the kidneys should always be imaged to assess the presence of coexisting renal malformations (by ultrasound scan) or scarring (by DMSA isotope renography; **Fig. 10.18**). Given the high familial incidence of primary VUR, screening of young siblings of index cases should be considered, especially if symptomatic there are febrile UTIs.

PATHOLOGY

There is an anatomical defect in primary VUR at the vesicoureteric junction. Renal histopathology can demonstrate either immature tissues (dysplasia) or scarring (chronic interstitial fibrosis).

TREATMENT

All neonates with severe antenatal hydronephrosis should be commenced on prophylactic antibiotics pending definitive diagnosis. Posterior urethral valves should be resected and other associated defects treated. Management of primary VUR involves prompt diagnosis and management of febrile UTIs to prevent renal damage caused by recurrent pyelonephritis. There is controversy regarding the effectiveness of either medical (long-term antibiotic prophylaxis) or surgical interventions (antireflux surgery) in affected children.

PROGNOSIS

The long-term prognosis of primary VUR depends on the presence and severity of the associated nephropathy.

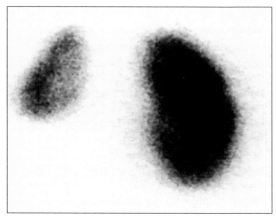

FIGURE 10.18 DMSA isotope is taken up by functional kidney tubules. In this posterior view, the left kidney is small after scarring from pyelonephritis.

RENOVASCULAR HYPERTENSION

INTRODUCTION

The incidence of hypertension is increasing in children due to screening programmes, earlier detection of hypertension and the obesity epidemic. However, it is important to distinguish those patients with secondary forms of hypertension, such as renovascular hypertension.

INCIDENCE

Renovascular disease accounts for 10% of children with hypertension and is often due to fibromuscular dysplasia. In some patients, this may be associated with neurofibromatosis, William syndrome, mid-aortic syndrome, Marfan syndrome and Klippel–Trenaunay–Weber and Feuerstein–Mims syndromes. The prevalence is estimated to be approximately 1 in 10,000 children.

DIAGNOSIS

One-quarter of patients are diagnosed on routine blood pressure screening. Many have symptoms such as headache (50%), lethargy (39%), cardiac failure, failure to thrive, and weight loss at presentation. A significant number (10–15%) present with neurological features alone, such as facial palsy, hemiplegia and convulsions. Patients should have full examination to exclude coarctation of the aorta, neurocutaneous stigmata and evidence of hypertensive retinopathy with fundoscopy.

INVESTIGATIONS

Patients require 24-hour ambulatory blood pressure monitoring (unless present with severe or malignant hypertension when this is required to monitor response to therapy as opposed to confirming hypertension). The most useful diagnostic tests include blood and urine tests (to see if hypokalaemic metabolic alkalosis and evidence of hyperreninaemic hyperaldosteronism, renal dysfunction, haematuria and/or proteinuria), echocardiography (to exclude target organ damage with left ventricular hypertrophy but excluding coarctation of the aorta), Doppler renal ultrasound, DMSA scan prior to proceeding with renal vein renin and digital subtraction angiography. However, the vascular disease may involve intrarenal vessels and other organs (particularly the brain). Therefore, investigations should also be directed to identify these, especially if there are cerebral symptoms.

TREATMENT

Children in hypertensive crisis should be treated with an intravenous antihypertensive agent such as labetalol or sodium nitroprusside initially, with very careful and slow reduction of blood pressure over 48–72 hours. Calcium channel blockers and beta-blockers are the most useful oral pharmacological agents in the treatment of renovascular disease-associated hypertension. Furosemide can be used if there is evidence of fluid overload. ACE inhibitors are normally contraindicated; however, they may be necessary in the management of patients with difficult to control blood pressure or in subjects with severe intrarenal vascular disease.

Digital subtraction renal angiography and angioplasty (**Fig. 10.19**) is the treatment of choice for cases with unilateral, main or branch artery stenoses. Some patients may need vascular reconstructive procedures. Approximately one-third of these achieve complete cure and most of the others show a reduction in drug therapy requirement after surgery.

PROGNOSIS

Children require follow-up to ensure that their blood pressure is treated to reduce longer-term complications.

RENAL FANCONI SYNDROME

INCIDENCE

The renal Fanconi syndrome consists of generalised proximal tubular dysfunction (aminoaciduria, glycosuria, bicarbonaturia, phosphaturia) and rickets or osteomalacia. Most cases occur as part of a metabolic disorder or are secondary to drugs/toxins, renal or other diseases (**Table 10.8**).

DIAGNOSIS

Children present with both symptoms of the underlying cause and features of proximal tubular dysfunction: polyuria, polydipsia, recurrent dehydration, poor growth, vomiting and rickets. Children with cystinosis (the commonest inherited cause of Fanconi syndrome) often have a characteristic appearance with sparse, blond hair and a pale complexion, but the condition can occur in any racial group and non-Caucasian patients have a complexion appropriate to their racial group.

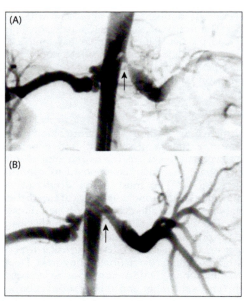

FIGURE 10.19 Digital subtactration renal angiography demonstrating left renal artery stenosis before (A) and after angioplasty (B).

TABLE 10.8 Causes of renal Fanconi syndrome

Inherited (specific investigation)
Cystinosis (leukocyte cystine concentration)
Tyrosinaemia (plasma amino acids, urine organic acids)
Galactosaemia (galactose 1-phosphate uridyl transferase)
Fructosaemia (fructose-1-phosphate aldolase B)
Lowe syndrome (X-linked, cataracts, hypotonia)
Mitochondrial disorders (lactate, pyruvate)
Wilson disease (copper, caeruloplasmin)
Glycogen storage disease (hepatomegaly, hypoglycaemia)
Dent disease (X-linked, hypercalciuria, nephrocalcinosis)
Idiopathic: autosomal dominant/recessive/X-linked
Acquired
Drugs: ifosfamide, aminoglycosides, valproate cisplatin, azathioprine
Heavy metals: lead, cadmium, mercury
Nephrotic syndrome (rare)
Renal transplant
Tubulointerstitial nephritis
Amyloidosis
Myeloma

INVESTIGATIONS

Urinalysis may reveal glycosuria and proteinuria but this is not invariable. Plasma biochemistry usually shows hypokalaemia, hypophosphataemia, a hyperchloraemic metabolic acidosis (e.g. normal anion gap) and sometimes hyponatraemia and hypocalcaemia. The urine is usually alkaline but will acidify in the presence of severe acidosis (bicarbonate <15 mmol/l) since it is a proximal renal tubular acidosis. Generalised aminoaciduria together with a low tubular reabsorption of phosphate confirm a Fanconi syndrome. Radiographs may demonstrate rickets. Specific investigations to determine the cause are listed in **Table 10.8**.

TREATMENT

In the acute situation, patients need rehydration with 0.9% saline usually with added potassium. Supplements of bicarbonate, potassium and phosphate are required. Vitamin D is used to treat the rickets. Specific treatments are required for the causative metabolic conditions.

PROGNOSIS

The outlook depends on the cause of the Fanconi syndrome. In addition, several of the causes lead to CKD (especially cystinosis, Lowe syndrome, tyrosinaemia and 'idiopathic' cases), although this occurs at a variable rate.

FURTHER READING

General

Avner ED, Harmon WE, Niaudet P, Yoshikawa N. *Pediatric Nephrology*, 6th edn. Berlin; Springer–Verlag, 2009.

Geary DF, Schaefer F. *Comprehensive Pediatric Nephrology*, 1st edn. Philadelphia: Mosby Elsevier, 2008.

Rees L, Brogan PA, Bockenhauer D, Webb NJA. *Oxford Specialist Handbooks in Paediatrics: Paediatric Nephrology*, 2nd edn. Oxford: Oxford University Press, 2012.

Webb NJA, Postlethwaite RJ. *Clinical Paediatric Nephrology*, 3rd edn. Oxford: Oxford University Press, 2003.

Haemolytic uraemic syndrome

Ariceta G, Besbas N, Johnson S, *et al.* Guideline for the investigations and initial therapy of diarrhoea-negative hemolytic uremic syndrome. *Pediatr Nephrol* 2009; 24(4):687–96.

Elliott EJ, Robins-Browne RM, O'Loughlin EV, *et al.*; Australian Paediatric Surveillance Unit. Nationwide study of haemolytic uraemic syndrome: clinical, microbiological, and epidemiological features. *Arch Dis Child* 2001;85:125–31.

Taylor CM. Hemolytic-uremic syndrome and complement factor H deficiency: clinical aspects. *Semin Thromb Hemost* 2001;27(3):185–90.

Chronic kidney disease

Kemper MJ, van Husen M. Renal osteodystrophy in children: pathogenesis, diagnosis and treatment. *Curr Opin Pediatr* 2014;26(2):180–6.

Rees L, Mak RH. Nutrition and growth in children with chronic kidney disease. *Nat Rev Nephrol* 2011;7(11):615–23.

Cystic kidney diseases

Igarashi P, Somlo S. Genetics and pathogenesis of polycystic kidney disease, *J Am Soc Nephrol* 2002;13(9):2384–98.

Waters AM, Beales PL. Ciliopathies: an expanding disease spectrum. *Pediatr Nephrol* 2011;26(7):1039–56.

Woolf AS, Feather SA, Bingham C. Recent insights into kidney diseases associated with glomerular cysts. *Pediatr Nephrol* 2002;17(4):229–35.

Congenital anomalies of the kidney and urinary tract

de Bruyn R, Marks SD. Postnatal investigation of fetal renal disease. *Semin Fetal Neonatal Med* 2008;13(3):133–41.

Woolf AS, Winyard PJD. Molecular mechanisms of human embryogenesis: developmental pathogenesis of renal tract malformations. *Pediatr Dev Pathol* 2002;5(2):108–29.

Woolf AS, Price KL, Scambler PJ, Winyard PJD. Evolving concepts in human renal dysplasia. *J Am Soc Nephrol* 2004;15(4):998–1007.

Vesicoureteric reflux

Feather SA, Malcolm S, Woolf AS, *et al.* Primary, nonsyndromic vesicoureteric reflux and its nephropathy is genetically heterogeneous, with a locus on chromosome 1. *Am J Hum Genet* 2000;66(4):1420–5.

Lambert HJ, Stewart A, Gullett AM, *et al.* Primary, nonsyndromic vesicoureteric reflux and nephropathy in sibling pairs: a United Kingdom cohort for a DNA bank. *Clin J Am Soc Nephrol* 2011;6(4):760–6.

Glomerulonephritis

Bertsias GK, Tektonidou M, Amoura Z, *et al.* European League Against Rheumatism and European Renal Association-European Dialysis and Transplant Association. Joint European League Against Rheumatism and European Renal Association-European Dialysis and Transplant Association (EULAR/ERA-EDTA) recommendations for the management of adult and paediatric lupus nephritis. *Ann Rheum Dis* 2012;71(11):1771–82.

Marks SD, Tullus K. Modern therapeutic strategies for paediatric systemic lupus erythematosus and lupus nephritis. *Acta Paediatr* 2010;99(7):967–74.

McCarthy HJ, Tizard EJ. Clinical practice: diagnosis and management of Henoch–Schonlein purpura. *Eur J Pediatr* 2010;169(6):643–50.

Tullus K, Marks SD. Vasculitis in children and adolescents: clinical presentation, etiopathogenesis and treatment. *Paediatr Drugs* 2009;11(6):375–80.

Weening JJ, D'Agati VD, Schwartz MM, *et al.*; International Society of Nephrology Working Group on the Classification of Lupus Nephritis; Renal Pathology Society Working Group on the Classification of Lupus Nephritis. The classification of glomerulonephritis in systemic lupus erythematosus revisited. *J Am Soc Nephrol* 2004;15(2):241–50; *Kidney Int* 2004;65(2):521–30.

Nephrotic syndrome

Eddy AA, Symons JM, Nephrotic syndrome in childhood. *Lancet* 2003;362(9384):629–39.

Samuel S, Morgan CJ, Bitzan M, *et al.* Substantial practice variation exists in the management of childhood nephrotic syndrome. *Pediatr Nephrol* 2013;28(12):2289–98.

Renovascular hypertension

Marks SD, Tullus K. Update on imaging for suspective renovascular hypertension in children and adolescents. *Curr Hypertens Rep* 2012;14 (6):591–5.

Marks SD, Tullus K. Do classification criteria of Takayasu arteritis misdiagnose children with fibromuscular dysplasia? *Pediatr Nephrol* 2010;25(5):989–90.

Tullus K, Roebuck DJ, McLaren CA, Marks SD. Imaging in the evaluation of renovascular disease. *Pediatr Nephrol* 2010;25(6):1049–56.

Haematology

Owen P. Smith and Ian Hann

NON-HODGKIN LYMPHOMA

CLINICAL PRESENTATION

Non-Hodgkin lymphomas (NHL) are haematological malignancies whose clinical presentation can resemble those of acute leukaemia with or without features of a solid tumour. These lymphomas tend to spread along lymphoid tissue distibutions, namely: lymph nodes, thymus, Waldeyer ring, Peyers patches and bone marrow. Abdominal and intrathoracic disease presentations occur in approximately 35% and 25% of cases, respectively.

COMMON SUBTYPES

The majority of childhood and adolescents NHL are high-grade and clinically aggressive. The range of histological subtypes is much narrower than seen in the adult population. There are essentially three subgroups: (i) precursor lymphoid neoplasms (T-cell lymphoblastic lymphoma [15–20%] and B-cell lymphoblastic lymphoma [3%]); (ii) mature B-cell neoplasms (Burkitt lymphoma [35–40%], diffuse large B-cell lymphoma [15–20%] and primary mediastinal B-cell lymphoma [1–2%]); and (iii) mature T-cell neoplasms (anaplastic large cell lymphoma, ALK positive [15–20%]).

Burkitt lymphoma

In Western countries the commonest presentation for the so called sporadic form of Burkitt lymphoma (BL) is abdominal, bone marrow, lymph nodes (especially head and neck/nasopharyngeal) (**Fig. 11.1**) and ovaries, while in the endemic form seen in Equatorial Africa, New Guinea, Amazonian Brazil and Turkey, the jaw (**Fig. 11.2**), abdomen, CNS and CSF have a higher frequency of involvement.

Over 90% of cases of endemic BL are positive for Epstein–Barr virus (EBV) DNA in the tumour cells, this falling to only 15% in sporadic BL. In both types of BL, the MYC oncogene locus on chromosome 8q24 is deregulated as it is juxtaposed to one of the imunoglobulin gene loci, the commonest

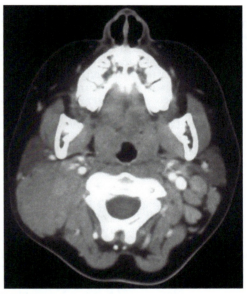

FIGURE 11.1 Sporadic Burkitt lymphoma: large multilobular heterogeneous solid mass in the right side of the neck.

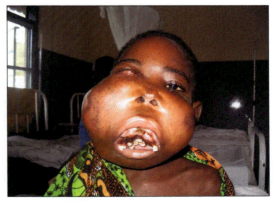

FIGURE 11.2 Endemic Burkitt lymphoma: extensive jaw tumour involving the mandible and surrounding soft tissues.

translocation being t(8;14)(q24;q32), which involves the IgH gene locus in 80% of cases. Sporadic and endemic BL show similar typical morphological features (**Fig. 11.3**).

Primary mediastinal B-cell lymphoma (PMBCL)

This is a rare, clinically distinct mature B-cell lymphoma that originates from thymic B-cell and is characterised by diffuse proliferation of large cells and sclerosis (**Fig. 11.4**). It can be difficult to distinguish it from Hodgkin lymphoma (HL) and although cell surface markers are more in keeping with a mature B-cell lymphoma, gene expression profiling suggests it to be more similar to HL.

T-cell lymphoblastic lymphoma

Up to 70% of children with T-cell lymphoblastic lymphoma (T-LL) present with mediastinal involvement and respiratory symptoms, cervical and supraclavicular adenopathy or superior vena cava syndrome (**Fig. 11.5**). Haemodynamic compromise due to pericardial effusions may occur. Lymphoblastic lymphoma is distinguished from acute lymphoblastic leukaemia (ALL) on the percentage of blasts in the marrow – ALL being diagnosed if there are greater then 25% blasts. Numerous chromosomal translocations have been described in T-LL, the majority involving T-cell receptor rearrangements with proto-oncogenes. Recently, deletions in chromosome 6q (del[6q]) have been reported to have an adverse prognostic impact.

Anaplastic large cell lymphoma

Anaplastic large cell lymphoma (ALCL), a large T-cell lymphoma is the most common peripheral T-cell lymphoma in children. ALCL is subdivided into two groups based on deregulation of the *ALK* (anaplastic lymphoma kinase) gene on chromosome 2p23, with greater than 90% of paediatric ALCL being ALK positive. *ALK*-positive patients are predominantly male with a bimodal age distribution. Approximately 70% of patients have disseminated (stage III/IV) disease at diagnosis. Unlike cutaneous ALCL (**Figs 11.6, 11.7**), the systemic and more common form of ALCL usually has a variable set of clinical presenting features that often includes constitutional symptoms of fever and weight loss. ALCL tends to present in lymph nodes and extranodal sites, especially in the skin, soft tissues and bone.

DIAGNOSIS AND STAGING

As a significant number of patients with NHL will present with a rapidly growing tumour with potential life-threatening complications, tissue procurement using the least invasive procedure and staging evaluation should be carried out as soon as possible. The most challenging clinical scenario is usually a massive mediastinal mass in association with respiratory distress and/or superior vena cava obstruction. It may be necessary to induce tumour shrinkage and thus clinical stability with corticosteroids prior to

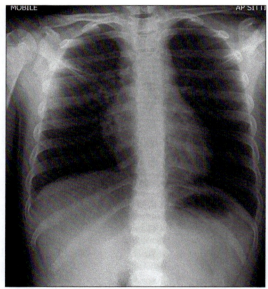

FIGURE 11.4 Primary mediastinal B-cell lymphoma: lobular widening of the superior mediastinum with no axillary or hilar adenopathy.

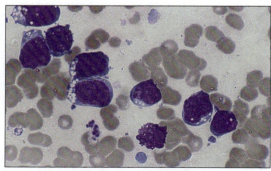

FIGURE 11.3 L3 (Burkitt) lymphoblasts.

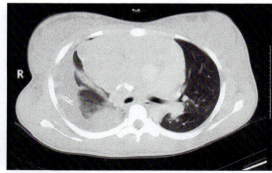

FIGURE 11.5 T-cell lymphoblastic lymphoma: mass with mediastinal shift, pericardial effusion and right pleural effusion.

tissue biopsy. Blood, bone marrow, ascites and pleural fluid may also be helpful in making the diagnosis. Although morphology and immunophenotyping of NHL material provide the cornerstone for making the diagnosis, cytogenetic and molecular studies usually add prognostic information.

CT and/or MRI of the primary site is the norm. The role of PET in paediatric NHL has yet to be determined. The St. Jude staging system for paediatric NHL has been widely accepted (**Table 11.1**).

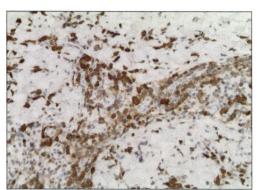

FIGURE 11.7 Classic pattern of anaplastic lymphoma kinase (ALK) staining of anaplastic large cell lymphoma with a t(2;5) containing tumour with nuclear and cytoplasmic staining.

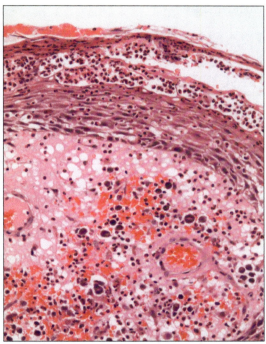

FIGURE 11.6 Dermal infiltrate of classic variant anaplastic large cell lymphoma with numerous large tumour cells multilobulated and wreath-like forms.

TABLE 11.1 St. Jude staging system for paediatric non-Hodgkin lymphoma

Stage I
A single tumour (extranodal) or single anatomic area (nodal) with the exclusion of thoracic or abdomen

Stage II
A single tumour (extranodal) with regional node involvement
Two or more nodal areas on the same side of the diaphragm
Two single (extranodal) tumours with or without regional node involvement on the same side of the diaphragm
A primary gastrointestinal tract tumour that is resectable, usually in the ileocaecal area, with or without involvement or associated mesenteric nodes

Stage III
Two single (extranodal) tumours on opposite side of the diaphragm
Two or more nodal areas above and below the diaphragm
All the primary intrathoracic tumours (mediastinal, pleural, and thymic)
All extensive primary intraabdominal disaese
All paraspinal or epidural tumours, regardless of other tumour site(s)

Stage IV
Any of the above with initial central nervous system and/or bone marrow involvement.

TREATMENT

Treatment is based on clinical staging, localised versus disseminated disease and histologic subtype. Surgery and radiotherapy have a very limited role in modern treatment strategies. Multiagent chemotherapy is the treatment of choice in childhood and adolescent NHL, which should be considered as a systemic malignancy even when the disease is localised. These tumours often respond dramatically to induction therapy (**Fig. 11.8**), but there is a high risk of tumour lysis syndrome, and careful monitoring for hyperphosphataemia, hypocalcaemia, hyperkalaemia and ECG monitoring is warranted. All patients should receive hyperhydration and allopurinol or uricozyme, although some patients may require haemodialysis. In general children and adolescents with localised disaese have an excellent outcome with approximately 90–95% long-term survival. Those with dissseminated NHL, long-term survival rates for the different subgroups would include: BL – 80–90%; T-LL and B-LL – 80–90%; DLBCL – 85–90%; PMBCL – 65–70%; and ALCL – 70–75%.

HAEMATOLOGICAL DISORDERS AND DOWN SYNDROME

Down syndrome (DS), the most common syndrome-associated chromosomal anomaly in humans, affecting 1 in 800–1,000 live born infants, is associated with a number of distinct haematological disorders occurring at different ages.

TRANSIENT MYELOPROLIFERATIVE DISORDER

Children with DS have a predilection to develop transient myeloproliferative disorder (TMD). This is a rare clonal 'pre-leukaemic' condition that is characterised by circulating megakaryoblasts (indistinguishable from acute megakaryoblastic leukaemia (AMKL) in the blood (**Fig. 11.9**) and spontaneous resolution within 3–6 months of life in the majority of cases. It occurs in approximately 5–10% of infants with DS.

CLINICAL PRESENTATION

The striking haematological finding is an elevated white cell count (WCC) with circulating blasts, relatively well preserved haemoglobin and a moderate thrombocytopenia. Other haematological associations with this syndrome include: (i) a peak incidence of myeloid leukaemia (DS-ML) occurring under 4 years of age in 10–20 % of TMD cases; (ii) the association of myelodysplasia and subsequent acute myeloid leukaemia (AML) development; and (iii) the propensity of megakaryoblastic subtype (AMKL) of AML with or without marrow fibrosis in over 90% of ML-DS cases.

Physical findings include; hepatosplenomegaly, pleural/pericardial effusions, ascites and rash (**Fig. 11.10**). A significant number will die *in utero*

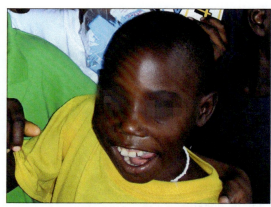

FIGURE 11.8 Endemic Burkitt's lymphoma: rapid response following 6 weeks of cyclophosphamide based chemotherapy (see **11.2**).

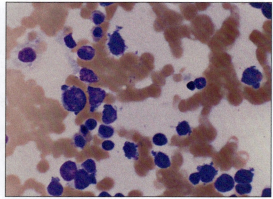

FIGURE 11.9 Transient myeloproliferative disorder: circulating megakaryoblast with classic cytoplasmic blebbing.

or will be born in extremis from severe hydrops, massive hepatosplenomegaly, liver failure with direct hyperbilirubinaemia secondary to release of platelet derived growth factor from megakaryoblasts that reside in the liver and fulminant consumptive coagulopathy.

MOLECULAR PATHOGENESIS

Acquired somatic mutations in exon 2 of the haematopoietic transcription factor gene *GATA1* (Xp11.23) are present is almost all DS children who develop TMD and AML-MK and therefore the *GATA1* assay can be very informative in making the diagnosis of TMD and AMKL. Although *GATA1* mutations are necessary for the development of DS AMKL from TMD they are not felt to be the initial event leading to AMKL.

FOLLOW-UP AND TREATMENT

The majority of infants with TMD do not require treatment. However, close follow-up, over the first 4 years of life is required as up to 20% of cases will develop AMKL that will need polychemotherapy. Low-dose cytosine arabinoside may be life-saving in those who develop hepatic, renal and cardiac involvement.

MYELOID LEUKAEMIA AND DS

Myeloid leukaemia develops in approximately 1% of children with DS corresponding to an annual instance of approximately 0.6–1 per million children. Clinical and biological features of ML-DS are very different from those of AML in children without DS. Both platelet and WCC are usually lower than in non-DS patients and this is in contrast to the very high WCC seen in TAM. Many (20–60%) patients have a relatively indolent course characterised by a period of thrombocytopenia (the commonest presenting cytopenia) and myelodysplasia (MDS) in association with marrow fibrosis with relatively few blasts in the bone marrow (**Fig. 11.11**). Meningeal involvement at diagnosis is rare. There is a strong age-related increased risk with the vast majority of patients presenting during the first 4 years of life (very few presenting before the age of 1 year).

The blast cells in the majority (~90%) of cases presenting within the first 4 years of life are of megakaryocytic-erythroid origin (**Fig. 11.11**) and have similar phenotype to the TAM, namely: CD45+, CD34+, CD33+, CD38+, CD36+, CD56+, HLA-DR+, CD7+ and at least one of the specific megakaryocytic markers CD41, CD42a or CD61. The other cases comprise other subtypes of AML, namely: FAB M0, M2 and M6. The cytogenetic findings usually seen non-DS AML, such as t(8;21), t(15;17), 16q22 and 11q23 rearrangement, and t(1;22) and t(1;3) as associated with non-DS AMLK, are rarely seen in ML-DS.

PATHOGENESIS

As leukaemia in children with trisomy 21 mosaicism selectively involves the trisomic cells it is now generally accepted that trisomy 21 represents the 'first hit' and subsequent acquisition of *GATA1s* mutations representing the 'second hit' in the development of ML-DS. Transformation to frank ML-DS however, requires further altered expression or mutations in other pathways. *GATA1s* mutations are not found in acute megakaryoblastic leukaemia in non-DS or in other AML patients.

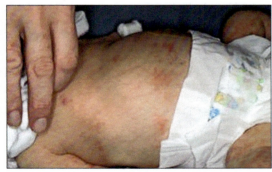

FIGURE 11.10 Transient myeloproliferative disorder: TMD cutis.

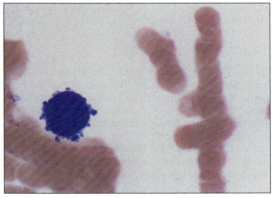

FIGURE 11.11 Down syndrome myeloid leukaemia: leukaemic blast cells of megakaryocytic-erythroid origin.

AML in DS children older than 4 years tend to be *GATA1s* negative and have a worse prognosis.

TREATMENT/PROGNOSIS

In contrast to TAM, ML-DS is fatal if untreated. Children with ML-DS have a superior outcome (>80%) compared to non-DS children with AML (~60%) when treated with standard AML protocols. Although this improved survival rate in the ML-DS patients is due to a lower relapse rate, a significant number of these patients experience an increased risk of side-effects related to chemotherapy dose and intensity timing of remission induction courses.

ACUTE LYMPHOBLASTIC LEUKAEMIA AND DS

The incidence of acute lymphoblastic leukaemia in children with DS (DS-ALL) is approximately 30-fold higher than in the general population and accounts for approximately 3% of all cases of ALL. Unlike in ML-DS, a 'pre-leukaemic' phase is not clearly observed and there is no survival advantage when compared with non-DS ALL patients.

CLINICAL PRESENTATION

Although there is no difference in the common clinical risk factors such as age and WCC at presentation, gender (NCI risk grouping) and leukaemic blast phenotype (CD10+, CD19+ and CD79a+) when compared with non-DS Bp-ALL (common ALL), the following clinical features are almost exclusively seen in DS-ALL patients: (i) it is rarely, if ever, seen in infants; (ii) the leukaemic blast count at diagnosis rarely exceeds 50×10^9/l; (iii) meningeal involvement is almost never present; and (iv) the incidence of T-cell ALL is markedly reduced or absent. Also, the commoner leukaemic karyotypes such as t(12;21)(p13;q22), associated with the *ETV6-RUNX1* fusion and hyperdiploidy (>50 chromosomes) that are seen in approximately 60% of Bp-ALL and associated with favourable outcomes are much less frequently encountered in ALL-DS. There is also a lower incidence of Philadelphia chromosome-positive ALL and MLL-rearranged ALL in children with DS.

TREATMENT/PROGNOSIS

As stated above, unlike for ML-DS, which is uniquely sensitive to chemotherapy, the presence of an extra copy of chromosome 21 does not improve the prognosis of DS-ALL. Several recently published studies from the US and Europe reported an inferior event-free survival and overall survival compared with children with non-DS ALL. The inferior survival is most likely multi-factorial encompassing different host and leukaemic blast characteristics.

Children with DS have an exquisite sensitivity to methotrexate (Mtx) that is most likely due to excess activity of the reduced folate carrier (RFC) encoded by a gene on chromosome 21. The overexpressed RCF is responsible for transporting increased amounts of Mtx into DS cells and therefore it is not surprising that these children experience higher rates of morbidity (mucositis, myelosuppression, transaminitis and infections) and mortality, especially following high-dose Mtx courses. Individuals with DS-ALL also experience a higher incidence of hyperglycaemia and long-term cardiotoxicity secondary to corticosteroids/asparaginase and anthracyclines, respectively.

ACUTE PROMYELOCYTIC LEUKAEMIA AND THROMBOSIS

Acute promyelocytic leukaemia (APL), is a specific type of AML characterised by the morphology of blast cells (M3 in the French–US–UK classification of AML), the t(15:17) translocation that fuses the promyelocytic leukaemia (PML) gene on chromosome 15 to the retinoic acid receptor-alpha (RARα) gene on chromosome 17, and a coagulopathy (mostly haemorrhagic) that occurs in most patients and is often life threatening. Although APL represents approximately 4–8% of paediatric AML, its incidence is higher in children of Hispanic and Mediterranean origin. The median age at presentation is probably similar to that of other AML subtypes (7–9 years), but APL has rarely been reported in the first year of life.

While the outcome of APL patients with the PML-RARα fusion treated with extended courses of all-trans retinoic acid (ATRA) in combination with anthracycline-based chemotherapy is generally favourable, paediatric patients appear to more commonly present with high WCC, as compared to their adult counterparts. Approximately 35–40% of children with APL fall within a high-risk group defined by a presenting WCC $\geq 10 \times 10^9$/l. This is due both to an increased risk of induction death, particularly as a result of haemorrhage, as well as a significantly higher rate of relapse. Thrombotic complications including arterial and venous events (**Figs 11.12, 11.13**) have been reported to occur in 10% of patients at presentation, thus making APL the commonest subtype of leukaemia to be associated with inappropriate clot formation. Increased risk of thrombosis has also been associated with so-called M3 variant leukaemic blast morphology, the expression of CD2, bcr3 *PML-RARA* transcript and the presence of *FLT3*-internal tandem duplication (*FLT3-ITD*). As the majority of these patients will also have evidence of ongoing consumptive coagulopathy antithrombotic therapy is difficult as it can increase the bleeding risk significantly.

Using ATRA and anthracycline-based chemotherapy protocols followed by maintenance with ATRA, 6-MP and Mtx, relapse rates for patients with a WCC $<10 \times 10^9/l$ at diagnosis are typically 10% or less, while rates may exceed 20% for patients with a WCC $\geq 10 \times 10^9/l$.

More recently the combination of ATRA and arsenic trioxide as induction and consolidation therapy (no maintenance) has been shown to be at least not inferior and possibly superior to ATRA plus chemotherapy in adults with acute promyelocytic leukaemia.

CONGENITAL (MONOCYTIC AND MYELOMONOCYTIC) LEUKAEMIA

CLINICAL PRESENTATION

Rarely, leukaemia can present in the newborn period (congenital leukaemia) and, if so, it usually presents as a monocytic variety of leukaemia with leukaemia cutis in approximately two-thirds of patients, the so-called 'blueberry muffin' appearance (**Fig. 11.14**).

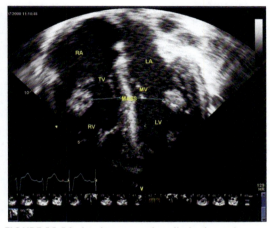

FIGURE 11.12 Acute promyelocytic leukaemia: thrombi in left and right ventricles with associated decreased myocardial contractility. LA: left atrium; LV: left ventricle; MV: mitral valve; RA: right atrium; RV: right ventricle; TV: tricuspid valve.

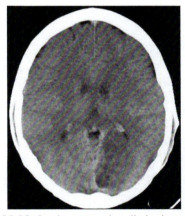

FIGURE 11.13 Acute promyelocytic leukaemia: CT brain showing extensive areas of ischaemia and infarction with minimal evidence of haemorrhage.

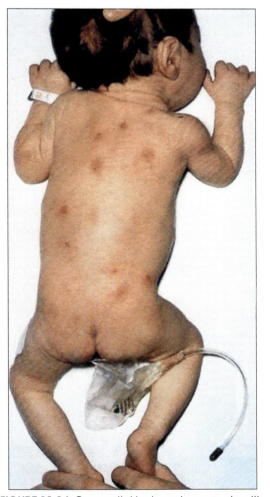

FIGURE 11.14 Congenital leukaemia: neonate with 'blueberry muffin' appearance.

These neonates usually have marked hepatosplenomegaly and lymphadenopathy and CNS involvement is seen in approximately 50% of cases. Occasionally, monocytic/myelomonocytic leukaemia can present with skin lesions in older children (**Fig. 11.15**). There is also a predisposition to gum hypertrophy and for involvement of other extramedullary sites, such as pericardium (**Fig. 11.16**) and testes.

DIAGNOSIS

The bone marrow in myelomonocytic leukaemia (**Fig. 11.17**) shows a mixture of myeloblasts and monocytes (French–US–UK classification, AML-M4 subtype). Figure **11.18** shows the features of monocytic leukaemia (AML-M5) (monomorphic population of monoblasts). A significant proportion of the neonatal leukaemias have 11q23 chromosomal abnormalities.

TREATMENT

Treatment of all types of AML includes intensive combination chemotherapy, with or without an allogeneic stem cell marrow transplant. In neonates, AML-directed therapy should have dosing adjustments for size, as treatment-related mortality is a significant contributor to failure in this group of patients.

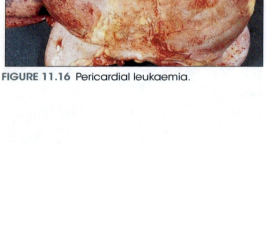

FIGURE 11.16 Pericardial leukaemia.

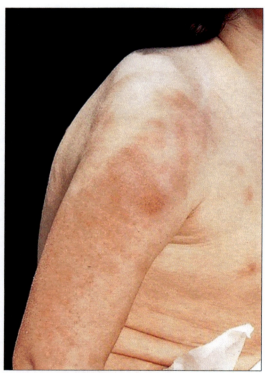

FIGURE 11.15 Leukaemia cutis in an older child.

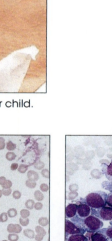

FIGURE 11.17 Myelomonocytic leukaemia (FAB M4 subtype).

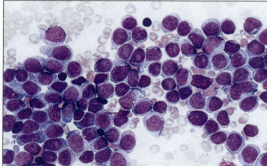

FIGURE 11.18 Monocytic leukaemia (FAB M5 subtype).

Haematology

324

OPHTHALMIC EXTRAMEDULLARY LEUKAEMIC DEPOSITS

Occult ocular involvement can be picked up in approximately one-third of newly diagnosed children with acute leukaemia following careful ophthalmologic examination. It can manifest as retinal haemorrhage, leukaemic infiltration of the orbit, optic nerve, retina, iris, cornea or conjunctiva; or hypopyon (layering of white cells in the anterior chamber of the eye) in association with blurred vision, photophobia or ocular pain. While haemorrhage and leukaemic infiltration of the retina and optic nerve are not an unusual initial manifestation in ALL, overt leukaemic infiltration of the eye (such as oculomotor palsies in association with periorbital chloromas or hypopyon) is uncommon at presentation and is usually seen in the setting of relapse of either acute lymphoblastic or myeloid leukemia. About one-half of children with overt leukaemic eye infiltration present with overt CNS relapse.

GRANULOCYTIC SARCOMA

A 9-year-old boy presented with a 2-day history of left-sided facial nerve palsy and proptosis (**Fig. 11.19**). CT brain showed a retro-orbital lesion. He was pancytopenic; haemoglobin 8.1 g/dl, WCC $4.5 \times 10^9/l$, neutrophils $1.0 \times 10^9/l$ and platelets of $93 \times 10^9/l$, with circulating moderate sized myeloperoxidase positive agranular blasts expressing CD34+,CD13+,CD33+ and CD117+.

Granulocytic sarcoma of the orbit, although a rare presenting feature of AML, primarily occur in children from non-Western industralised countries, for unknown reasons. They are usually unilateral and may precede other evidence of AML as was the case here. They are usually associated with t(8;21) often in association with –Y. These masses tend to arise from bones with intense haematopoietic activity and a delicate periosteum, such as orbital floor and vertebral bodies. Granulocytic sarcoma can sometimes be the only manifestation of leukaemia.

HYPOPYON

A 6-month-old Nigerian infant presented with cloudiness in his left pupil. He was otherwise well and examination and blood count were normal. Ophthalmic examination showed an intraocular mass and fluid in the anterior chamber – hypopyon (**Fig. 11.20**). The differential diagnosis included: leukaemia, juvenile xanthogrannulare, endogenous endopthalmitis or infection with tuberculosis, *Toxocara* or toxoplasmosis. Fluid aspiration of the anterior chamber showed monocytic blasts expressing CD13+,14+,33+,64+,117+ and HLA DR+ with normal karyotype.

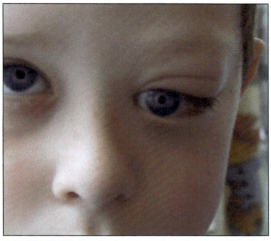

FIGURE 11.19 Proptosis secondary to granulocytic sarcoma.

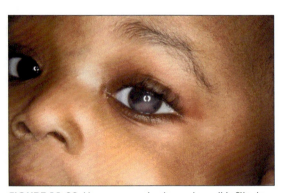

FIGURE 11.20 Hypopyon – leukaemic cell infiltrate in the anterior chamber of the eye.

SEVERE APLASTIC ANAEMIA

CLINICAL PRESENTATION

Severe aplastic anaemia (SAA) is characterised by pancytopenia with a hypocellular, often called 'empty' bone marrow (**Fig. 11.21**). The clinical onset is usually insidious with the initial symptom complex related to the pancytopenia, namely: (i) anaemia leads to fatique, weakness and lassitude; (ii) thrombocytopenia produces mainly mucosal bleeding, petechiae of the skin and mucous membranes, epistaxis and gum bleeding; and (iii) infection

may occur at presentation in the setting of neutropenia (**Figs 11.22, 11.23**). SAA is uncommon in Western countries, its incidence in Europe is about two cases per million of the population.

DIAGNOSIS

Bone marrow aspirate and trephine biopsy together with marrow cytogenetics is essential in making the diagnosis. Differential diagnosis includes; inherited bone marrow failure syndromes, myelodysplastic syndrome – especially hypocellular refractory cytopenia of childhood, aplastic presentation of acute lymphoblastic leukaemia, NHL, HLH and infection (e.g. herpes group of viruses, HIV, parvovirus B19, and leishmaniasis).

TREATMENT

Bone marrow as a source of haematopoietic stem cells from an HLA-matched family donor (MFD) is the treatment of choice for SAA. If a MFD is not available, immunosuppressive therapy (IST) with antithymocyte globulin and ciclosporin represents a very good alternative; however, relapse and clonal evolution to paroxysmal nocturnal haemoglobinuria (PNH) and AML/MDS remain a lifetime risk. If IST fails, matched unrelated haematopoietic stem cell transplantation (HSCT) is a reasonable second-line approach.

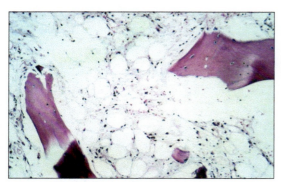

FIGURE 11.21 Severe aplastic anaemia: bone marrow biopsy showing hypocellular marrow with less that 5% cellularity, so called 'empty' marrow.

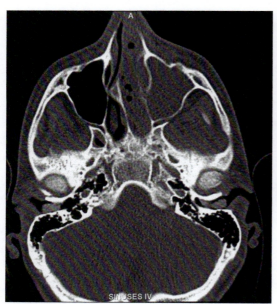

FIGURE 11.22 Fungal sinusitis: extensive soft tissue opacification of the left maxillary sinus with early bony destruction involving the posterior wall of the sinus.

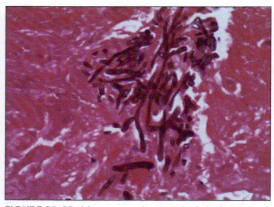

FIGURE 11.23 *Mucor* species was isolated.

Haematology

326

JUVENILE MYELOMONOCYTIC LEUKAEMIA

CLINICAL PRESENTATION

Juvenile myelomonocytic leukaemia (JMML) is a rare disorder of early childhood (0.7 per 1 million children) characterised by uncontrolled proliferation of monocytes and granulocytes, as well as myelodysplastic features of anaemia and thrombocytopenia. The usual clinical presentation is splenomegaly (**Fig. 11.24**), maculopapular rash (**Fig. 11.25**), lymphadenopathy, fever, high WCC (**Fig. 11.26**) and an absolute monocytosis ($>1 \times 10^9/l$) (**Table 11.2**). Café-au-lait spots (**Fig. 11.27**) and bowing of the tibia (**Fig. 11.28**) are not uncommon clinical associations, especially when there is neurofibromatosis-1 (NF1) involvement.

MOLECULAR PATHOGENESIS

JMML is a heterogeneous myeloproliferative disorder. Germline or somatic mutations of four genes of the RAS signal transduction pathway (Rasopathy), namely: PTPN11, CBL, NF1 and RAS play a pivitol role in its pathogenesis. These RAS pathway mutations represent major somatic events that contribute to oncogenesis. In addition, monosomy occurs frequently in JMML but its significance is not known.

TREATMENT

Allogeneic HSCT is the only curative therapy in the majority of children, especially those who harbour NF1 or somatic PTPN11 mutations with overall survival rates of 40–50%. There is a suggestion that mutations in *NRAS* are not sufficient to cause a lethal variant of JMML.

Azacitidine, an inhibitor of DNA methylation, may have a role in 'bridging' to HSCT or indeed in prolonging survival for children with MDS/JMML in a palliative setting following relapse after HSCT.

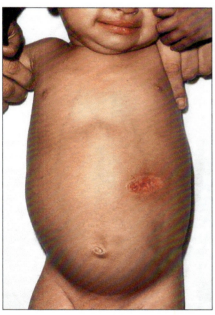

FIGURE 11.24 Juvenile myelomonocytic leukaemia: massive splenic enlargement.

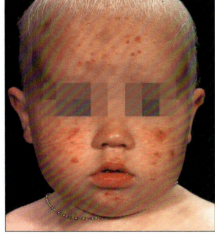

FIGURE 11.25 Juvenile myelomonocytic leukaemia: erythematous maculopapules on the face.

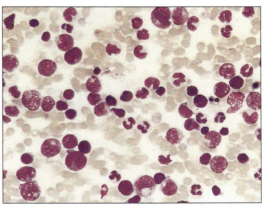

FIGURE 11.26 Juvenile myelomonocytic leukaemia: bone marrow morphology showing dysplastic change in the myeloid lineage.

327

TABLE 11.2 World Health Organisation criteria of juvenile myelomonocytic leukaemia

1. Peripheral monocytosis ($>1 \times 10^9/l$)
2. Absence of $t(9;22)$ or BCR-ABL (not CML)
3. Bone marrow or blood with <20% blasts (not AML)
4. And any 2 of the following:
   Myeloid precursors in the blood
   White cell count $10 \times 10^9/l$
   Increased haemoglobin F for age
   GM-CSF hypersensitivity
   Cytogenetic abnormality

CML: chronic myelogenous leukaemia; GM-CSF: granulocyte monocyte colony stimulating factor.

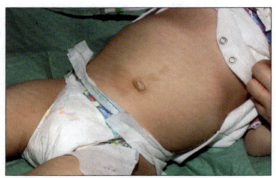

FIGURE 11.27 Juvenile myelomonocytic leukaemia: café-au-lait spots.

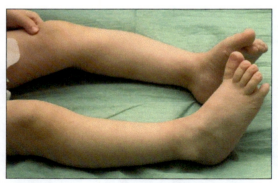

FIGURE 11.28 Juvenile myelomonocytic leukaemia: bowing of the tibia.

PAEDIATRIC MYELODYSPLASTIC SYNDROMES

CLINICAL PRESENTATION

Myelodysplastic syndromes (MDS) are rare diseases of childhood. MDS is associated with ineffective haematopoiesis, characterised by abnormal dysplastic cells and cytopenias. They represent a group of clonal myeloid stem cell disorders characterised by abnormal differentiation, increased apoptosis, varying degrees of dysplasia or leukaemic blasts and a high risk of progression to AML (**Table 11.3**). MDS can be primary (*de novo* or idiopathic) or secondary, as seen in various syndromes (e.g. DS, Fanconi anaemia, Shwachman–Bodian–Diamond and Diamond–Blackfan) or to previous treatment (e.g. IST in SAA or chemotherapy for cancer).

DIAGNOSIS

The majority of children with MDS have marrow cytogenetic abnormalities, which have an important effect on evolution to AML and on overall prognosis. In some cases it is almost impossible to distinguish hypocellular MDS (refractory cytopenia of childhood – RCC) from severe aplastic anaemia. The blood smear may be helpful – showing neutrophils with so called pseudo-Pelger–Huët nuclei and hypogranular cytoplasm (**Fig. 11.29**) making MDS the most likely diagnosis.

Monosomy 7 (**Fig. 11.30**) is present in approximately 30% of primary childhood MDS cases and approximately 50% of therapy-related MDS cases. It is important to distinguish between primary MDS, secondary MDS and SAA. Hypocellularity is more commonly seen in childhood MDS than in its adult equivalent. Almost 75% of RCC shown considerable hypocellularity and therefore it can be challenging to differentiate RCC from other bone-marrow failure syndromes including acquired SAA. Hypercellular bone marrow with trilineage dysplasia (**Fig. 11.31**) with fibrosis (**Fig. 11.32**) is associated with a less favourable outcome.

TREATMENT

Allogeneic stem cell transplantation is the only curative therapeutic modality. RCC is the most common subtype of childhood MDS. The risk of relapse following HSCT is negligible and therefore HSCT with reduced intensity conditioning (thiotepa/fludarabine) is a very attractive approach, albeit there appears to be a significant risk of graft failure and delayed platelet engraftment.

TABLE 11.3 World Health Organisation classification of paediatric myelodysplasia

	Blood findings	Marrow findings
RCC	Sustained unexplained cytopenia with <2% blasts	Morphologic dysplasia with <5% blasts
RAEB 1	2–4% blasts	5–9% blasts
RAEB 2	5–19% blasts	10–19% blasts
RAEB t	20–29% blasts	20–29% blasts, no AML-related recurrent cytogenetic changes

AML: acute myeloid leukaemia; RCC: refractory cytopenia of childhood; RAEB: refractory anaemia with excess of blasts; RAEB-t: refractory anaemia with excess of blasts in transformation.

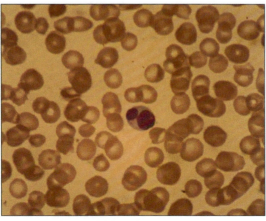

FIGURE 11.29 Myelodysplasia: dysplastic neutrophil, so called pseudo Pelger–Huët form.

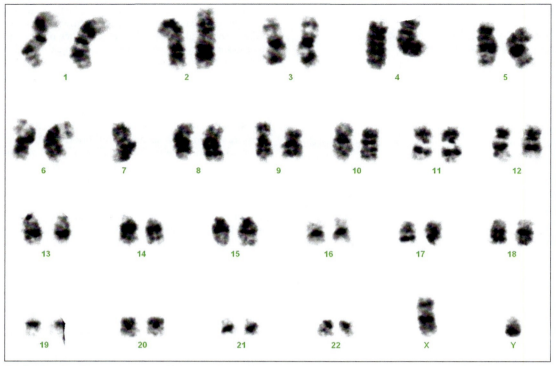

FIGURE 11.30 Myelodysplasia: G-banded karyotype of bone marrow from a patient with RAEB1 showing the abnormality: 45,XY,-7 (monosomy 7).

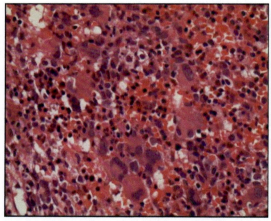

FIGURE 11.31 Myelodysplasia: hypercellular bone marrow with dyserythropoiesis, dysgranulopoiesis and bizarre megakaryocytic forms.

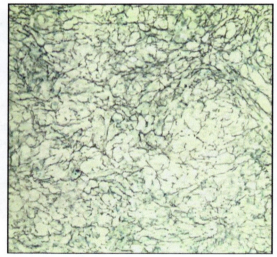

FIGURE 11.32 Myelodysplasia: reticulin staining showing moderate to severe bone marrow fibrosis.

FANCONI ANAEMIA

CLINICAL PRESENTATION

Most children with Fanconi anaemia (FA) are diagnosed between 6 to 9 years, with boys presenting earlier. However, it should be remembered that the condition presents with a variable phenotype and it is being increasingly recognised in the adult population. In paediatrics the diagnosis is usually suspected when the child presents with hyper- or hypopigmented skin lesions, short stature, anomalies of the upper limb or thumb (**Fig. 11.33**), microcephaly and characteristic facial features (**Fig. 11.34**). Other somatic abnormalities involve the genitourinary, gastrointestinal and central nervous systems. The first symptomatic cytopenia is usually thrombocytopenia, followed by anaemia, which is usually macrocytic and reticulocytopenic. Serum alpha-fetoprotein levels are elevated.

DIAGNOSIS

At the cellular level FA is characterised by increased cross-linker sensitivity and G2 arrest in the cell cycle, in particular in response to genotoxic stress.

Diagnosis is made with a chromosomal breakage test that involves the DNA cross-linkers, diepoxybutane or mitomycin C. It should be noted these tests do not pick up carriers.

CANCER PREDISPOSITION

FA is an inherited disease with congenital and developmental malformation, bone marrow failure and a cancer predisposition with relative risk of 40-fold, 500-fold and 7000-fold for solid tumours, AML and MDS, respectively. FA results from a defect in a DNA damage response pathway in which the products of 15 FA genes have been identified. Several of the FA genes link this condition to familial breast and ovarian cancer (BRACA) syndromes.

TREATMENT

Treatment of bone marrow failure is initially with supportive use of blood products. HSCT is the only curative treatment for the BMF. Follow-up care, especially after HSCT should be multidisciplinary as squamous cell carcinoma becomes the life-threatening and limiting complication.

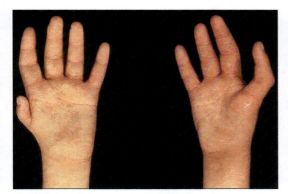

FIGURE 11.33 Fanconi anaemia: thumb abnormalities.

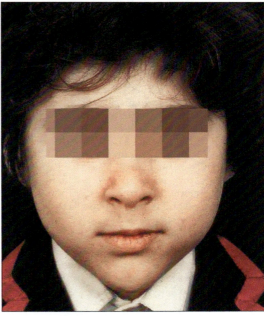

FIGURE 11.34 Fanconi anaemia: facial appearance.

DYSKERATOSIS CONGENITA AND *TINF2* MUTATIONS

CLINICAL PRESENTATION

Clinical manifestations in dyskeratosis congenita (DC) often appear during childhood, although there is a wide age range most likely reflecting the type of mutation causing DC. Skin pigmentation and nail changes (**Fig. 11.35**) typically appear first with bone marrow failure occuring a number of years later. The clinical complexity of the disease has expanded in recent years to include: idiopathic aplastic anaemia +/− MDS; (ii) idiopathic pulmonary fibrosis; (iii) the Hoyeraal–Hreidarrson syndrome, characterised by microencephaly, cerebellar hypoplasia, growth retardation, enteropathy and immunodeficiency with or without aplastic anaemia; (iv) a presentation overlapping Revesz syndrome or Coats plus, with retinopathy and intracranial calcifications.

MOLECULAR PATHOGENESIS

DC is a clinically and genetically heterogeneous disorder, showing X-linked, autosomal dominant and recessive inheritence. Several genes have been shown to cause DC, all of whom have clear roles in teleomere maintenence. These include the telomerase complex (*TERC, TERT, DKC1, NHP2, NOP10*), the shelterin complex (*TINF2*), telomerase trafficking (*TCAB1*) and the telomere capping complex (*CTC1*).

TINF2, the second most commonly mutated gene in DC encodes *TINF2*, a member of the telomere-associated shelterin complex, which plays integral roles in the structure and function of telomeres. *TINF2* mutations are usually associated with extremely short telomeres, earlier onset of disease and bone marrow failure that usually occurs prior to manifestation of any signs of the classic triad of DC (**Fig. 11.36**). All reported mutations are heterozygous and most arise *de novo*. Retinal abnormalities are seen in about 20% of patients with DC (**Figs 11.37, 11.38**). In Revesz syndrome (Mendelian Inheritance in Man #268130), a severe DC variant caused by *TINF2* mutations, bilateral exudative retinopathy is a defining feature along with intrauterine growth retardation, intracranial calcification and cerebellar hypoplasia.

TREATMENT

As with FA, oxymetholone can produce durable haematologic responses in over 40% of patients. HSCT using low intensity conditioning protocols is the only curative modality.

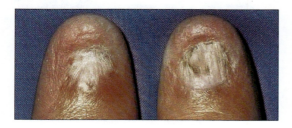

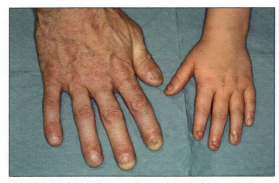

FIGURE 11.36 Autosomal dominant dyskeratosis congenita: dystrophic nails in father and son secondary to *TINF2* mutation.

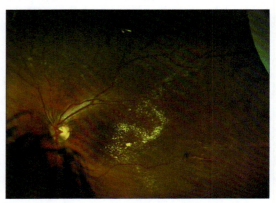

FIGURE 11.37 Autosomal dominant dyskeratosis congenita: vitreous haemorrhage in the right eye and the left eye with a large circinate exudate encroaching on the macula. In the left temporal retina, areas of retinal haemorrhage and extensive areas of arterial occlusion and vascular sheathing are seen.

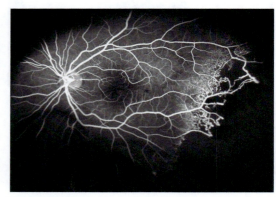

FIGURE 11.38 Fluorescein angiography shows extensive and profound vascular shut down in the temporal retina and choroid. At the junction of perfused and non-perfused retina there were numerous arteriovenous shunts.

FIGURE 11.35 Nail dystrophy in a 12-year-old female.

HYPEREOSINOPHILIC SYNDROME AND T(5;12)

CLINICAL PRESENTATION

The hypereosinophilic syndrome (HES) is rare in children and can occur at any age. The presenting features vary from non-specific complaints like fatigue, cough, rhinitis, dyspnoea, skin infiltration (**Fig. 11.39**) to life-threatening cardiac and neurological events.

DIAGNOSIS

HES is defined as blood eosinophilia ($>1.5 \times 10^9/l$) (**Fig. 11.40**) on at least two occasions, or evidence of prominent tissue eosinophilia associated with symptoms and marked blood eosinophilia after exclusion of secondary causes of eosinophilia. HES results from sustained overproduction of eosinophils in the bone marrow (**Fig. 11.41**), eosinophilia, tissue infiltrates and organ damage. Part of the investigative work-up is marrow morphology and cytogenetics looking for marked expansion of the eosinophil compartment and abnormalities at 4q12 and 5q33 that involve platelet derived growth factor receptor-alpha (PDGFRα) and PDGFRι respectively.

TREATMENT

Marrow cytogenetics in this case show a balanced chromosomal translocation involving chromosomes 5 and 12 exhibiting an abnormality of the imatinib-responsive tyrosine kinase, PDGFRß at 5q31-33. Not surprisingly he had an exquisite response to the first generation tyrosine kinase inhibitor, imatinib. Other therapeutic options for HES include: hydroxyurea, interferon-alpha, mepolizumab (anti-IL5) and alemtuzumab (anti-CD52). The role of HSCT in HES has yet to be defined.

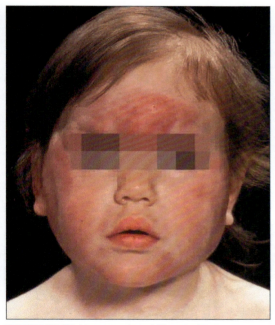

FIGURE 11.39 Hypereosinophilic syndrome: urticarial facial rash.

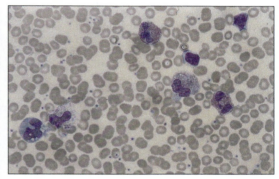

FIGURE 11.40 Hypereosinophilic syndrome: absolute blood eosinophilia.

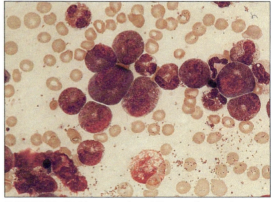

FIGURE 11.41 Hypereosinophilic syndrome: bone marrow showing expansion of the eosinophil compartment.

ACUTE FEBRILE NEUTROPHILIC DERMATOSIS – SWEET SYNDROME

CLINICAL PRESENTATION

Sweet syndrome (SS) or acute febrile neutrophilic dermatosis is chracterised by fever, painful erythematous papules, nodules and plaques usually over the trunk, face and upper limbs usually in association with a neutrophil leucocytosis. It can present in several clinical settings: classical (idiopathic) SS, malignancy-associated SS, and drug-induced SS, especially following G-CSF administration.

CASE STUDY

A 14-year-old boy with newly diagnosed normal karyotype, NPM1(-)/FLT3(-) AML developed a hot tender erythematous swelling over the tunnel area of his central venous catheter on day 6 of induction chemotherapy. Empiric combination antibacterials for a presumed cellulitis were commenced. Over the next 4 days despite line removal, escalating empiric antibacterials to cover potential resistant gram-negative, gram-positive and anaerobic bacteria and the addition of empiric antifungal treatment, he remained pyrexial. Blood cultures and imaging studies were negative. Ten days into his febrile neutropenic episode while clinically unstable requiring intensive care support he developed a diffuse painful erythematous rash that occurred in clusters with papules coalescing into plaques. Also, areas of erythema spontaneously regressed while new lesions appeared with a skipping migratory pattern. The distribution of papules and plaques was largely confined to arms (**Fig. 11.42**) and upper torso with sparing of the face and lower limbs. A skin biopsy showed a diffuse inflammatory infiltrate of neutrophils in the dermis (**Fig. 11.43**).

DIFFERENTIAL DIAGNOSIS

The pathogenesis of SS has not been fully elucidated. SS is extremely rare in children and adolescents; however, when it does occur it is often associated with haematological malignancies especially AML. Interestingly, the first report of malignancy-associated SS was in a 16-year-old girl with AML. SS should be considered in the differential diagnosis of unexplained prolonged fever with cutaneous involvement in patients with haematological malignancy, especially AML.

TREATMENT

Clinical and laboratory evidence suggests the SS is a hypercytokinaemic state. Systemic corticosteroids are the gold standard. In the case above methylprednisolone was commenced and his pyrexia and rash resolved within 48 hours.

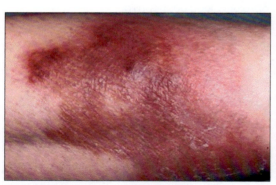

FIGURE 11.42 Sweet syndrome: well-circumscribed painful extensive nodular lesion on the forearm.

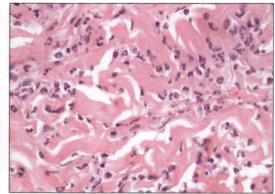

FIGURE 11.43 Sweet syndrome: skin biopsy showing a diffuse inflammatory infiltrate of neutrophils in the dermis.

MYELOFIBROSIS AND SYSTEMIC LUPUS ERYTHEMATOSUS

CLINICAL PRESENTATION

A 15-year-old girl presented with a 4-week history of increasing fatigue, generalised myalgia and a facial rash. Blood count showed her to be pancytopenic (haemoglobin 9 g/dl, platelets 10×10^9 /l, WCC 1.1×10^9 /l and neutrophils 0.5×10^9 /l). Her creatinine was elevated at 112 μmol/l and chest x-ray showed bilateral pleural effusions. Bone marrow biopsy showed hypercellularity with hypolobulated megakaryocytes. Myelopoeisis was left-shifted without any increase in blast cells and reticulin was markedly increased (**Fig. 11.44**). A strongly positive anti-double stranded DNA antibody titre and low serum complement C3 and C4 levels confirmed a diagnosis of systemic lupus erythematosus (SLE) with renal, pleural and myelofibrosis involvement.

DIFFERENTIAL DIAGNOSIS

Myelofibrosis (MF) is a rare childhood disorder characterised by progressive fibrous tissue replacement in the bone marrow. Primary MF, a myeloproliferative disorder is exceedingly rare in children. Most cases are secondary to other disorders such as neoplasia: leukaemias (especially megakaryoblastic), lymphomas, myeloproliferative disorders (see **Fig. 11.22**) metastatic solid tumours (especially neuroblastoma), systemic mastocytosis and Langerhans cell histiocytosis. Benign aetiologies include vitamin D-dependent rickets, granulomatous disease, osteopetrosis, primary hyperthyroidism, renal osteodystrophy, haemophagocytic lymphohistiocytosis and SLE.

TREATMENT

Treatment involves treating the underlying cause. The girl in the case history developed worsening acute renal and respiratory failure necessitating haemodialysis and ventilation. She was treated with a combination of high-dose methylprednisolone, intravenous immunoglobulin, daily 3 litre plasma exchange ($3 l/d \times 5$) and intravenous cyclophosphamide ($500 mg/m^2$) depending on kidney involvement and neutrophil count, e.g. at 2 weekly intervals. Her clinical condition improved and after 4 weeks her full blood count had returned to normal. Repeat bone marrow biopsy 2 months later showed trilineage haematopoiesis with normal megakaryoctes and normal reticulin pattern (**Fig. 11.45**).

Haematological problems can figure prominently in patients with SLE; however, pancytopenia secondary to myelofibrosis is a rare phenomenon. Improvement in blood counts and bone marrow fibrosis with steroid therapy has also been reported. This case demonstrates the dramatic resolution of bone marrow fibrosis and megakaryocyte dysplastic change in association with normalisation of peripheral blood counts following intensive immunosuppressive treatment.

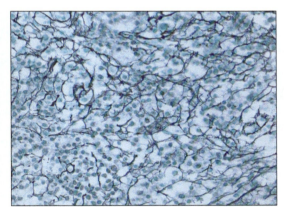

FIGURE 11.44 Systemic lupus erythematosus: left-shifted myelopoiesis without any increase in blast cells and reticulin is markedly increased.

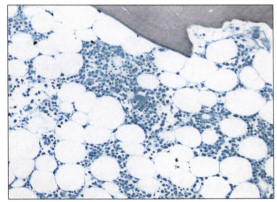

FIGURE 11.45 Systemic lupus erythematosus: trilineage haematopoiesis with normal megakaryoctes and normal reticulin pattern after 2 months of treatment.

INFANT MEGALOBLASTIC ANAEMIA: TRANSCOBALAMIN II DEFICIENCY

CLINICAL PRESENTATION

Patients usually present within the first few months of life with megaloblastic anaemia that may be accompanied by neurological complications, such as hypotonia (**Figs 11.46, 11.47**) and occasionally pancytopenia. Other manifestations include: failure to thrive, weakness, diarrhoea, vomiting and recurrent infections due to hypogammaglobulinaemia.

DIAGNOSIS

Serum vitamin B_{12} levels are normal because it is transported in the plasma by transcobalamin I (TCI). The bone marrow is severly megaloblastic (**Fig. 11.48**) and the blood smear shows oval macrocytes and other features of megaloblastic anaemia. Due to the absence of TCII, vitamin B12 cannot enter cells and this results in homocystinuria and methyl malonic aciduria. Absence of the protein capable of binding radiolabelled cobalamin and migrating with TCII can be detected by chromatography or gel electrophoresis. TCII is an autosomal recessive disorder. The TCII gene was found by linkage analysis to lie close to the P blood group system on chromosome 22q12-q13.

TREATMENT

Serum vitamin B_{12} levels must be kepy high and titrated to the clinical response. Oral hydroxyocobalamin or cyanocobalamin (500–1000 μg twice weekly) or systemic (intramuscular) hydroxyocobalamin (1000 μg weekly) is given. The prognosis for neurological complications depends upon whether or not treatment is instituted early and patients must be monitored for any deterioration in neurological status, at which stage the vitamin B12 injections should be increased in dosage.

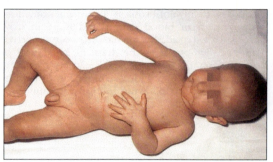

FIGURE 11.46 Transcobalamin II deficiency: hypotonia.

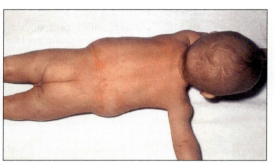

FIGURE 11.47 Transcobalamin II deficiency: hypotonia.

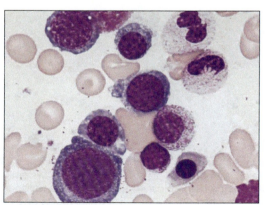

FIGURE 11.48 Transcobalamin II deficiency: megaloblastic change in the bone marrow.

CONGENITAL ERYTHROPOIETIC PORPHYRIA

CLINICAL PRESENTATION

Congenital erythropoietic porphyria (CEP), also known as Gunther disease is a rare form of porphyria. The diagnosis may be suspected when pink or brown stains are noted in the nappy (due to large amounts of porphyrins in the urine). Other clinical manifestations can range from mild to severe. Porphyrins are photosensitisers and hence chronic damage to the skin occurs following exposure to sunlight. Initial subepidermal bullous lesions progress to crusted erosions (**Figs 11.49–11.51**), which heal with scarring and (usually) increased pigmentation. Hypertrichosis and alopecia are frequent and erythrodontia (red fluorescence under ultraviolet light) (**Fig. 11.51**) are virtually pathognomic of the disease. Damage to cartilage and bone can cause mutilating consequences.

Discolouration of the teeth can occur (**Fig. 11.52**). Haemolytic anaemia can be mild or severe and in the latter, splenomegaly is usually present.

DIAGNOSIS

CEP is caused by a deficiency of uroporphyrinogen III, a key enzyme in heme metabolism and leads to increased production of porphyrins in the bone marrow. The diagnosis of CEP is confirmed by finding high levels of porphyrins in the urine (elevated levels of uroporphyrin 1 and coproporphyrin 1), faeces (elevated levels of coproporphyrin 1) and circulating red cells.

TREATMENT

Sunlight exposure and trauma to the skin should be avoided. Topical sunscreens may be of help, as may oral treatment with beta-carotene. Haemolysis may warrant blood transfusion and splenectomy. HSCT may be curative.

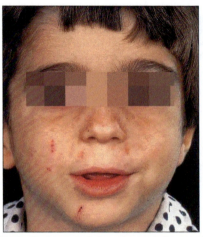

FIGURE 11.49 Congenital erythropoietic porphyria: skin erosions as a result of photosensitivity.

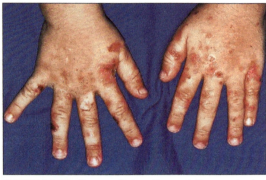

FIGURE 11.51 Congenital erythropoietic porphyria: blistering of the hands.

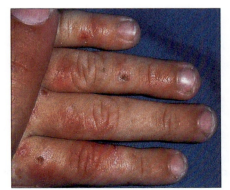

FIGURE 11.50 Congenital erythropoietic porphyria: phototoxic damage to the hands.

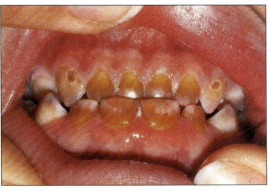

FIGURE 11.52 Congenital erythropoietic porphyria: discolouration of the teeth.

KASABACH–MERRITT SYNDROME

CLINICAL PRESENTATION

The child usually presents in the neonatal period with a massive haemangioma (**Fig. 11.53**), which may be clinically obvious, as in this case, or may be occult (e.g. primary splenic haemangioma or gut haemangioma). Bleeding manifestations are frequently preceded by enlargement and hardening of the haemangioma. This phenomenon most likely reflects intralesional platelet activation with adherence to the activated endothelium resulting in thrombus and new vessel formation. The net result is an ongoing consumptive coagulopathy with further dropping in circulating platelets, fibrinogen and prolongation in coagulation parameters.

DIAGNOSIS

Imaging confirms the vascular nature of the lesion. MRI is the imaging technique of choice. The blood smear usually (but not always) shows evidence of microangiopathic haemolytic anaemia, with red cell fragmentation and a low platelet count, as in this case (**Fig. 11.54**).

TREATMENT

Current treatment options remain controversial. Surgical excision is the most effective treatment; however, resection is often not feasible, due to direct invasion of adjacent structures, particularly in visceral lesions, or in the presence of severe refractory coagulopathy. Therapy is usually multimodal and includes combination of supportive measures such as fresh frozen plasma (FFP), cryoprecipitate and fibrinogen and treatment with corticosteroids, cytotoxic agents, antiplatelet and antifibrinolytic agents, interferon and arterial embolisation. Historically, radiotherapy has been used with success; however, long-term iatrogenic complications, including reports of malignancy and limb shortening, preclude its routine use.

PLATELET TRANSFUSION CONTRAINDICATION

In spite of the degree of thrombocytopenia, catastrophic haemorrhage occurs relatively infrequently, and thus management should not focus on correction of haematological parameters. Platelet transfusions are contraindicated, unless in the presence of an acute or anticipated haemorrhage or preoperatively, as transfusion *in vivo* and *in vitro* causes an increase in the size of the tumour due to a combination of sequestration of platelets within the tumour mass, and degranulation causing release of platelet derived growth factors. Additionally, transfused platelets are consumed rapidly by the tumour, with a significantly reduced half-life of between 1 and 24 hours. The risk–benefit ratio of transfusion in each clinical scenario must therefore be carefully measured.

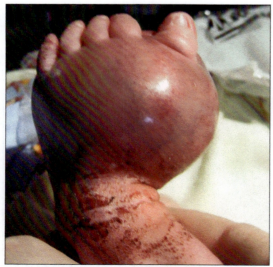

FIGURE 11.53 Kasabach–Merritt syndrome: massive Kaposiform haemangioendothelioma of the foot.

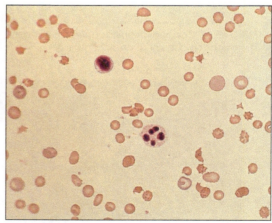

FIGURE 11.54 Kasabach–Merritt syndrome: peripheral blood film showing microangiopathic change.

THROMBOCYTOPENIA ABSENT RADIUS

CLINICAL PRESENTATION

The diagnosis of thrombocytopenia absent radius (TAR) is usually made at birth because of the characteristic physical appearance combined with thrombocytopenia. The pathognomonic physical finding is bilateral absence of the radii with thumbs present (**Fig. 11.55**), which can distinguish TAR from FA in which thumbs may be absent and the radii are present (**Fig. 11.56**).

DIAGNOSIS

Clinical observation and blood count showing severe thrombocytopenia. There may be other associated findings, including hand anomalies and abnormalities of the shoulder, neck and lower limbs. Skin haemangiomas also occasionally occur. Females are more often affected than males, as opposed to FA where there is a male predominance. The diagnosis must be distinguished from idiopathic thrombocytopenic purpura (ITP) and from megakaryocytic thrombocytopenia (other than ITP) because this latter condition has a propensity to the development of marrow aplasia and MDS.

TREATMENT

If patients survive the first 2 years the life expectancy is normal. The main cause of death is a haemorrhage. In the past, mortality was approximately 25%, the majority of deaths occurring in the first year. Platelet transfusions should be used during bleeding episodes or operations, including those to correct the deformities. Occasional transient responses to splenectomy have occurred and tranexamic acid may be useful for mucosal bleeding, but must not be used when haematuria (macroscopic or microscopic) occurs. There are also anecdotal reports of responses to immunoglobulin therapy.

PROGNOSIS

If the patient survives the first year the prognosis is excellent.

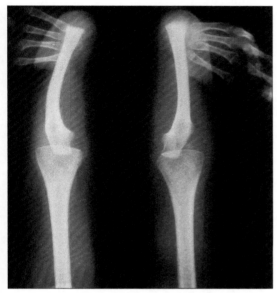

FIGURE 11.55 Thrombocytopenia absent radius: x-ray showing absent radii.

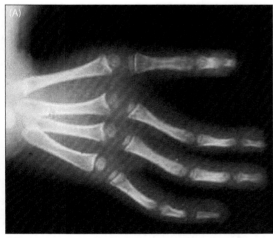
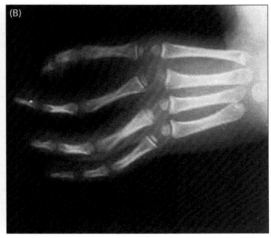

FIGURE 11.56 Thrombocytopenia absent radius: x-ray showing that thumbs are absent in Fanconi anaemia.

BERNARD–SOULIER SYNDROME

CLINICAL PRESENTATION

Children present usually with epistaxis and mucocutaneous bleeding within the first year of life. Bleeding into joints and muscles does not occur.

DIAGNOSIS

The main diagnostic pointer is the presence of reduced numbers of platelets ($40–80 \times 10^9/l$) that are usually large in size. The glycoproteins are usually quantified on the platelet surface via fluorescence-activated cell sorting (FACS) analysis using specific antibodies.

Bernard–Soulier syndrome (BSS) also known as giant platelet syndrome, is a rare bleeding disorder of large platelets with quantitative and qualitative defects in the platelet membrane von Willebrand receptor complex glycoprotein (GP) Ib-IX-V. This complex comprises four transmembrane polypeptide subunits – GPIb-α, GPIb-β, GPIX and GPV, the products of four distinct genes. This complex has two important functions: (i) it facilitates platelet adherence to the subendothelial matrix by binding to von Willebrand (vWf); and (ii) it promotes platelet activation by thrombin at low concentrations.

Differential diagnosis for thrombocytopenia would include: immune thrombocytopenic purpura, Wiskott–Aldrich syndrome, unlike the BSS defect (**Fig. 11.57**) is associated with very small platelets, TAR, amegakaryocytic thrombocytopenia and artefactual thrombocytopenia (**Fig. 11.58**). The artefact is usually caused by an EDTA-induced antibody and the effect can be abrogated by the use of an alternative anticoagulant such as citric acid.

TREATMENT

The only available therapy is transfusion with platelet concentrates. Affected patients usually receive this therapy only for persistent and significant haemorrhage, since the transfused patient may develop antibodies against the missing GP complex, making them permanently refractory to therapy. Antifibrinolytic agents such as tranexamic acid may be used for mucosal bleeds but is contraindicated in patients with haematuria.

VON WILLEBRAND DISEASE

CLINICAL PRESENTATION

Patients usually present with cutaneous purpura, epistaxis and mucosal bleeding, so called 'wet purpura'. Its incidence may be as high as 1% of the population. Both autosomal recessive and dominant forms are seen. There are no specific clinical features apart from bleeding.

DIAGNOSIS

Estimation of von Willebrand factor protein (vWF) along with factor VIII coagulant activity (VIII:C) are essential in making the diagnosis. Von Willebrand disease (vWD) is a heterogenous bleeding disorder with at least 20 distinct clinical subtypes. There are two main categories based on whether there is a quantitative (type I or type III) or qualitative (type II with its severe variants) defect in vWF. Type I is the commonest (70%), has an autosomal dominant inheritance and the bleeding diathesis can be mild to severe. The bleeding seen in type III is usually severe (**Fig. 11.59**) because of very low levels of VIII:C and vWF. This has recessive mode of inheritance.

Within the type II classification, type IIB needs to be distinguished from the rest, in that desmopressin (DDAVP) treatment exacerbates the bleeding tendency due to worsening of the thrombocytopenia and is, therefore contraindicated. There is increased platelet aggregation with low levels of the agonist ristocetin and intermittently low platelet counts.

TREATMENT

The majority are treated with DDAVP, which releases endogenous vWF from endothelium and megakaryocytes. Severe (type III) patients are treated with a combination of vWF and factor VIII. The prognosis is excellent and the same infective risks of blood products apply to patients with vWD as with other bleeding disorders.

SEVERE HAEMOPHILIA A AND B (CLASSIC HAEMOPHILIA AND CHRISTMAS DISEASE)

CLINICAL PRESENTATION

These disorders are related to severe deficiency of factor VIII and IX coagulation activity. Presentation is usually in early infancy with bleeding phenomena (from the umbilical cord, or recurrent bruising or haemarthrosis (**Fig. 11.60**). Classically, patients were described as bleeding following circumcision. Males are affected and females are carriers, but approximately one-third of new cases are through new mutations.

DIAGNOSIS

The diagnosis depends upon determination of levels of factor VIII or factor IX in coagulant assays. Treatment nowadays is with regular prophylactic therapy with high purity factor concentrates, preferably those produced by recombinant DNA technology. In the past, severe arthropathy (**Figs 11.60, 11.61**) was common but is rarely seen with current therapy, which aims to keep the factor level above 1% at all times. The x-ray (**Fig. 11.60**) shows severe joint damage with loss of joint space and cystic changes around the joint.

PROGNOSIS

An excellent prognosis is expected, providing factor concentrate prophylaxis is used. Patients must be regularly monitored for evidence of viral infection, especially with hepatitis viruses and for the development of inhibitors to the coagulant protein, which is a severe development that leads to an increased risk of spontaneous bleeding (**Fig. 11.62**).

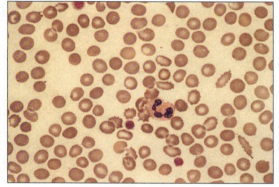

FIGURE 11.57 Bernard–Soulier syndrome: typical blood film showing macrothrombocytopenia.

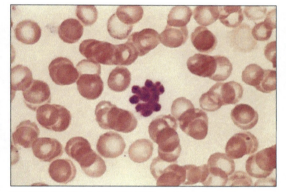

FIGURE 11.58 Artefactual thrombocytopenia, platelet clumping on blood smear.

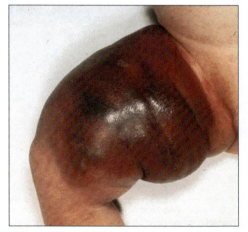

FIGURE 11.59 von Willebrand disease: effects of severe bleeding following attempted femoral cannulation.

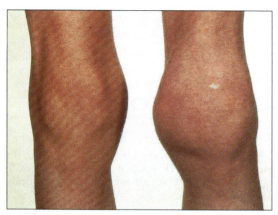

FIGURE 11.60 Severe haemophilia: marked swelling of left knee (haemarthrosis).

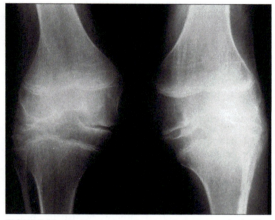

FIGURE 11.61 X-ray showing joint damage in both knees.

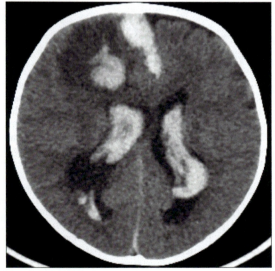

FIGURE 11.62 Large haematoma in the right frontal lobe with decompression into the ventricular system and to a lesser extent the subdural space adjacent to the falx in a 1-year-old boy with high responding FVIII inhibitors.

341

RED CELL MEMBRANE ABNORMALITIES

HEREDITARY ELLIPTOCYTOSIS

CLINICAL PRESENTATION

Hereditary elliptocytosis (HE) rarely presents in the neonatal period. HE is often asymptomatic but in approximately 10% of patients clinically significant haemolysis occurs.

DIAGNOSIS

HE comprises a heterogeneous group of red cell membrane disorders characterised by an abundance of elliptoctyes with reticulocytosis. There is a classic blood smear appearance (**Fig. 11.63B**). It is an autosomal dominant disorder with variable penetrance. Abnormalities in membrane interaction between α-spectrin, band 4.1, glycoporin C, and anion transported protein (band 3) prevent the erythrocyte biconcave shape.

TREATMENT

Most patients with HE need no therapy. As with other haemolytic anaemias, affected individuals are susceptible to hypoplastic crisis during viral infection. Human parvovirus B19, the organism responsible for erythema infectiosum, selectively invades red cell progenitors and may cause a transient arrest of red cell production. Recovery usually begins within 7–10 days after infection and is usually complete within 4–6 weeks. Those with the more severe form usually benefit from supportive transfusion therapy and splenectomy.

HEREDITARY SPHEROCYTOSIS

Hereditary spherocytosis (HS) is a primary defect in erythrocyte membranes affecting ankyrin, spectrin and other membrane proteins. It occurs worldwide, most commonly in individuals of Northern European extraction (1:2500). Inheritance can be autosomal dominant and recessive with *de novo* mutations.

DIAGNOSIS

HS is typically characterised by pallor, jaundice, splenomegaly, reticulocytosis and polymorph erythrocytes on a peripheral blood smear. Severe anaemia can be experienced by 5–10% of patients. There is a classic blood smear appearance with numerous small, dense spherocytes and bizarre erythrocyte morphology with anisocytosis (**Fig. 11.63C**).

Clinical manifestation can occur at any time, but typically in childhood with anaemia, jaundice and splenomegaly. The extent of haemolysis, jaundice, splenomegaly, and anaemia are variable. Symptoms related to cholelithiasis have to be considered.

TREATMENT

Treatment depends on the severity of haemolysis, splenomegaly and bilirubinaemia. In individuals with persistent clinical relevant symptoms, a splenectomy, which cures the intrasplenic haemolysis, needs to be considered. Individuals with HS are susceptible to hypoplastic crises (see above).

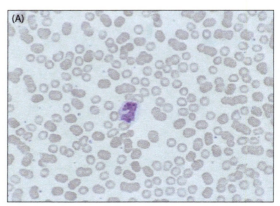
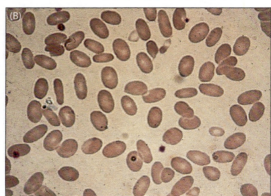
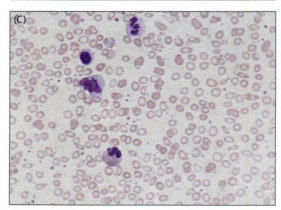

FIGURE 11.63 (A) Normal blood smear; (B) hereditary elliptocytosis showing characteristic elongated red cells; (C) hereditary spherocytosis with numerous spherocytes and bizarre erythrocyte morphology. (Courtesy of Dr. Paula Bolton-Maggs.)

BETA-THALASSAEMIA MAJOR

CLINICAL PRESENTATION

This is a severe anaemia, very often exacerbated by folic acid deficiency, which may lead to pancytopenia. At a later stage, patients who are severely affected develop overgrowth of the bones due to marrow expansion. A good example is shown in **Fig. 11.64**, where the patient on the right was not transfusion-dependent and developed narrow overgrowth because of failure of marrow suppression. The patient on the left also had beta-thalassemia major and developed hyperpigmentation of the skin, due to iron overload from blood transfusion, but the marrow was adequately suppressed and maxillary and other bony overgrowth did not occur.

If the patients are not transfused they develop massive hepatosplenomegaly and wasting (**Fig. 11.65**).

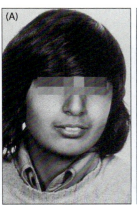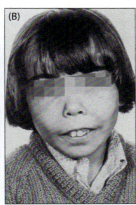
(A) (B)

FIGURE 11.64 Beta-thalassaemia major: the patient in (B) has developed bone marrow expansion of the facial bones.

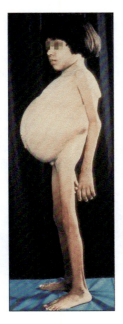

FIGURE 11.65 Beta-thalassaemia major: massive hepatosplenomegaly secondary to extramedullary haematopoiesis.

The x-rays (**Figs 11.66–11.68**) show expansion of the marrow cavity leading to a 'hair on end' appearance in the skull and expansion and thinning of the bones elsewhere.

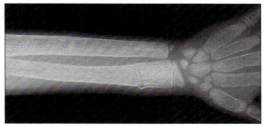

FIGURE 11.66 Beta-thalassaemia major: thinning of cortical bone results from expansion of the marrow space.

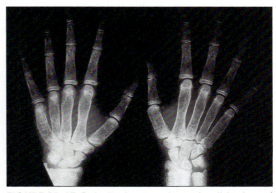

FIGURE 11.67 Beta-thalassaemia major: thinning of cortical bone results from expansion of the marrow space.

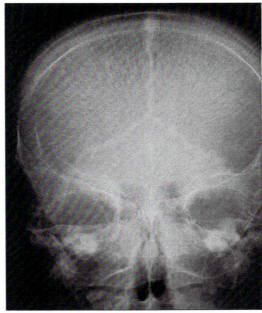

FIGURE 11.68 Beta-thalassaemia major: frontal radiograph of the skull showing the typical 'hair-on-end' appearance, with thinning of the cortical bone and widening of the marrow cavity.

343

DIAGNOSIS

The diagnosis depends on showing the presence of beta-thalassemia trait in the parents, along with either a raised haemoglobin A2 level or the existence of a coexisting haemoglobinopathy such as haemoglobin E. The blood film (**Fig. 11.69**) shows hypochromia and microcytosis, and haemoglobin electrophoresis of the patient shows mainly HbF with some haemoglobin A2. Confirmation is either with demonstration of the lack of globin chain synthesis by HPLC analysis or by molecular methods.

TREATMENT

The only curative treatment at present is with bone marrow transplantation, the outcome of which is excellent if a matched sibling donor is available and the transplant is carried out in the first few years of life. Otherwise, unrelated donor transplant could be considered, but the standard treatment at present is with regular blood transfusion, splenectomy following vaccination against *Pneumococcus*, *Haemophilus* and *Meningococcus C*, and supplementation with vitamin C, folic acid and penicillin prophylaxis (postsplenectomy). At a later stage, iron overload becomes a major problem and regular chelation with at least five times per week subcutaneous desferrioxamine is required. If iron overload ensues, multiple endocrinopathies including diabetes mellitus occur, with eventual cardiac failure.

SICKLE CELL DISEASE

CLINICAL PRESENTATION

These patients are nowadays picked up on haemoglobinopathy screening and by neonatal screening programmes. The most common problem is a painful crisis, which may involve the hand and produce dactylitis (**Fig. 11.70**), possibly leading to osteomyelitis (**Figs 11.71, 11.72**).

Sickle chest syndrome involves sequestration in the lungs (**Fig. 11.73**). The patient may also present at an early age with an aplastic crisis in which red cell production is impaired by parvovirus B19 infection. Also, an early and life-threatening problem is sickle cell sequestration in the spleen and a rapid drop in haemoglobin due to pooling of blood.

DIAGNOSIS

Diagnosis is by haemoglobin electrophoresis and family studies. The electrophoretic pattern will show haemoglobin S. In haemoglobin sickle cell disease there is an extra band on electrophoresis; in haemoglobin S beta-thalassemia one parent will have the sickle cell trait and one parent will have the beta-thalassemia trait. Blood films show the presence of sickle and target cells, the latter being more common in haemoglobin sickle cell disease (**Fig. 11.74**).

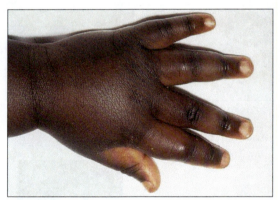

FIGURE 11.70 Sickle cell disease: swollen fingers in a 2-year-old girl (dactylitis) caused by infarction of the metacarpal bones.

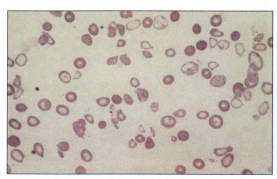

FIGURE 11.69 Beta-thalassaemia major: typical blood smear showing marked hypochromia with many different sized red cells.

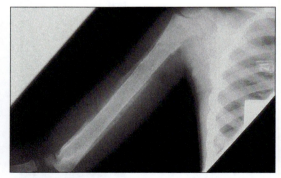

FIGURE 11.71 Sickle cell disease: periosteal elevation due to salmonellal osteomyelitis.

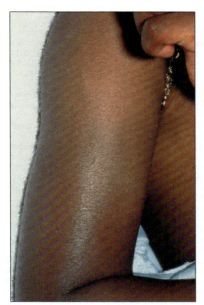

FIGURE 11.72 Sickle cell disease: salmonellal osteomyelitis.

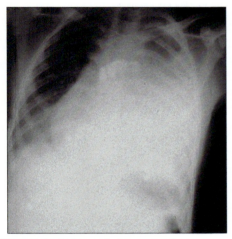

FIGURE 11.73 Sickle cell disease: pulmonary sequestration due to a combination of infection and small vessel obstruction.

TREATMENT

Early diagnosis may be picked up on neonatal screening. Early institution of penicillin prophylaxis is essential and treatment of painful crisis is with plentiful fluids and patient-controlled analgesia. For serious complications, such as chest syndrome and stroke, exchange transfusion is essential at a very early stage. Patients with recurrent severe problems may be considered for bone marrow transplantation.

GLUCOSE-6-PHOSPHATE DEHYDROGENASE DEFICIENCY

CLINICAL PRESENTATION

Most patients are asymptomatic and are picked up on screening prior to surgery or drug therapy such as antimalarial treatment. Some patients present with intravascular haemolysis and haemoglobinuria ('Coca-Cola urine'). This haemolyis is usually precipitated by the use of a drug or ingestion of broad beans (favism). Occasional patients can present with chronic haemolysis and the consequent production of gallstones.

DIAGNOSIS

The diagnosis is based on a screening test for glucose-6-phosphate dehydrogenase (G6PD). Patients with massive intravascular haemolysis often have bucket-handle forms of the red blood cells (**Fig. 11.75**). This is due to retraction of haemoglobin away from the red cell membrane.

TREATMENT

Specific treatment is not required except in the very rare case of chronic haemolysis, which may respond to splenectomy. The majority of patients should be issued with a list of drugs and foods to be avoided.

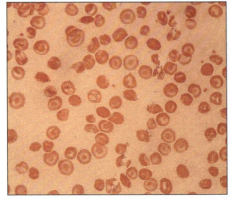

FIGURE 11.74 Sickle cell disease: blood smear showing a mixture of sickle and target cells.

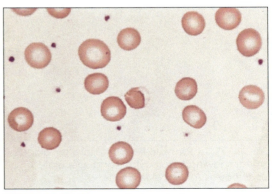

FIGURE 11.75 Glucose-6-phosphate dehydrogenase deficiency: blood smear showing 'bucket-handle' forms of red cells.

PYRUVATE KINASE DEFICIENCY

CLINICAL PRESENTATION

The child has a congenital non-spherocytic haemolytic anaemia, which may present with hyperbilirubinanaemia. Autosomal recessive inheritance is usually observed. Splenomegaly is usually present. It is found predominantly in people of Northern European descent. Erythroblastopenic crisis from parvovirus B19 infection is not uncommon.

DIAGNOSIS

Blood film shows macrocytosis and occasional shrunken, speculated erythrocytes (echinocytes, **Fig. 11.76**). Direct measurement of the pyruvate kinase (PK) enzyme shows a reduced level and there should be a concomitant high level of 2,3-diphosphoglycerate (2,3DPG). Red cell intermediates of metabolism may be helpful in those patients with a marginally low PK level, or with a dysfunctional enzyme or very high reticulocyte count.

A severe anaemia is usually present and this may be well tolerated due to a shift to the right of the oxygen dissociation curve, secondary to a raised 2,3DPG. Hyperbilirubinaemia, low haptoglobins and raised reticulocyte levels are usually found. The enzyme level may be spuriously elevated due to relatively high PK levels in the reticulocytes and the assay must be corrected for this.

TREATMENT

The patients often tolerate a low haemoglobin of around 6 g/dl very well because of the compensatory raised 2,3DPG level. Eventually the patients require splenectomy and, contrary to some previous reports, the results are usually very good. Folic acid supplementation is indicated.

FURTHER READING

Anzalone CL, Cohen PR. Acute febrile neutrophilic dermatosis (Sweet's syndrome). *Curr Opin Hematol* 2013;20(1):26–35.

Balwani M, Desnick RJ. The porphyrias: advances in diagnosis and treatment. *Hematology* Am Soc Hematol Educ Program 2012;2012:19–27.

Cairo MS, Perkins SL. *Haematological Malignancies in Children, Adolescents and Young Adults.* World Scientific Publishing, 2012.

Ching-Hon Pui. Childhood Leukaemias, 3rd edn. Cambridge: Cambridge University Press, 2012.

Gamis AS, Alonzo TA, Gerbing RB, *et al.* Natural history of transient myeloproliferative disorder clinically diagnosed in Down syndrome neonates: a report from the Children's Oncology Group Study A2971. *Blood* 2011;118(26):6752–9.

Kelly M. Kasabach-Merritt phenomenon. *Pediatr Clin North Am* 2010;57(5):1085–9.

Lo Coco F, Avvisati G, Vignetti M, *et al.* Retinoid acid and arsenic trioxide for acute promyelocytic leukaemia. *N Engl J Med* 2013;369(2):111–21.

Magrath IT (ed). *The Lymphoid Neoplasms*, 3rd edn. Hodder Arnold, 2010.

Orkin SH, Fisher DE, Ginsburg D, Look AT, Lux SE, Nathan DG. *Nathan and Oski's Hematology and Oncology of Infancy and Childhood*, 8th edn. Philadelphia: Elsevier Saunders, 2015.

Seetharam B, Yammani RR. Cobalamin transport proteins and their cell-surface receptors. *Expert Rev Mol Med* 2003;5(18):1–18.

Wanitpongpun C, Teawtrakul N, Mahakkanukrauh A, Siritunyaporn S, Sirijerachai C, Chansung K. Bone marrow abnormalities in systemic lupus erythematosus with peripheral cytopenia. *Clin Exp Rheumatol* 2012;30(6):825–9.

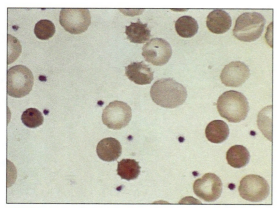

FIGURE 11.76 Pyruvate kinase deficiency: blood smear showing macrocytosis and speculated erythrocytes (echinocytes).

Haematology

12 Oncology

Gill A. Levitt, Penelope Brock, Tanzina Chowdhury,
Mark Gaze, Darren Hargrave, Judith Kingston,
Antony Michalski and Olga Slater

INTRODUCTION

Cancer affects about 1 in 600 children world-wide. Leukaemia is the commonest form (30–35% of all cancer in childhood), followed by brain tumours (20–25%), lymphomas including Hodgkin disease (10%), soft tissue sarcomas, particularly rhabdomyosarcoma (7%), neuroblastoma (7%) and Wilms tumour (5.5%)). Leukaemia and lymphoma are covered in Chapter 11 Haematology.

Survival in childhood cancer has significantly improved over the past few decades, with over 75% of all children in developed countries now being cured. This has been as a result of sequential national and international clinical trials that have optimised a multi-modality treatment approach, which, depending on the type of cancer, includes surgery, chemotherapy, radiotherapy and biological therapies. However, survival rates for many childhood cancers are now plateauing and for some aggressive malignancies, e.g. high-risk brain tumours and bone sarcomas there has been little improvement in survival over the past decade and new approaches are necessary (**Table 12.1**).

The success of multi-modality treatments (surgery, chemotherapy and radiotherapy) means that, around one in 750 young people in their twenties are long-term survivors of childhood cancer, but many will have significant long-term side-effects as a result of their primary treatment. Therefore, specialist survivorship programmes have been developed to anticipate, screen for and address these issues, but there is also a big emphasis to develop less toxic anticancer therapies to try to maintain survival rates but decrease the burden of treatment for children with cancer.

Over the past decade there has been a huge increase in the understanding of the molecular basis

TABLE 12.1 Types of childhood cancer and cure rates

Type of cancer	Percentage of childhood cancers	Average cure rate (%)
Acute lymphoblastic leukaemia	25	80–85
Brain tumours	25	Depends on the type of the brain tumour
Hodgkin disease	4	90
Non-Hodgkin lymphoma	6	80
Soft tissue sarcoma	7	70
Acute myeloid leukaemia	5	70
Neuroblastoma	7	Depends on the type and the risk category
Wilms tumour	5.5	80
Osteosarcoma	2.5	65
Ewing sarcoma	1.5	65
Malignant germ cell tumours	3.5	80–90
Retinoblastoma	3	98
Hepatoblastoma	1	90

of childhood cancer. It is being recognised that many paediatric cancers consist of a number of molecular sub-types, e.g. medulloblastoma, which are driven by abnormalities of cellular pathways that are often involved in normal development. The discovery of these abnormalities is informing new therapeutic developments, which target the underlying biology of specific cancers and subgroups of patients. New targeted therapies include small molecule and monoclonal antibodies, which block over-activated cellular pathways responsible for driving the cancer. In addition immunotherapies are being developed that harness the body's own immune system to target cancer cells. It is hoped that these new-targeted therapies will not only help to improve survival further in childhood cancer but also potentially reduce late side-effects. However, these new therapies will require rigorous clinical trial evaluation to confirm this promise and to define which patients may benefit most from their introduction to current standard therapies.

RENAL TUMOURS

Renal tumours comprise of 6–7% of childhood tumours with Wilms tumour (WT) (nephroblastoma) by far the commonest, occurring in over 90% of cases (**Table 12.2**). WT affects 1 in 10,000 children under 15 years of age, with around 80 new cases in the UK each year.

EPIDEMIOLOGY

With the exception of clear cell sarcoma of the kidney (CCSK), which is commoner in boys, the genders are almost equally affected. WT is 1.5 times more common in Afro-Caribbeans than in Caucasians and is least common in the Asian population.

GENETICS

The molecular pathology of WT is complex, with the involvement of several genes in initiation and progression, as well as disruption of normal genomic imprinting on the short arm of chromosome 11(11p). WT is usually diagnosed in healthy children. However 5% of tumours occur in children with a predisposition genetic syndrome as listed below:

- Constitutional WT1 disorders (**Fig. 12.1**):
  - 'WAGR' (**W**ilms' tumour, **A**niridia, **G**enitourinary malformations, **G**rowth **R**etardation) syndrome.
  - Denys–Drash syndrome.
  - Frasier syndrome.
- Overgrowth syndromes:
  - Beckwith–Wiedemann syndrome (associated with changes at region of chromosome 11p15.5).
  - Simpson–Golabi–Behmel syndrome (X-linked inheritance).
  - Hemihypertrophy (low risk).
  - Perlman syndrome.

Regular ultrasound surveillance to identify tumours early is recommended when the risk of developing WT is more than 5%. 1–2% of patients present with familial WT. Two WT susceptibility genes have been mapped on chromosome 17 and 19, *FWT1*/*FWT2* respectively, but in the majority of families the genetic abnormality is as yet unknown.

TABLE 12.2 Renal tumours of childhood

Tumour type	Comments
Wilms tumour	80% present <5 years 5% bilateral
Clear cell sarcoma	3–5% of renal tumours Can metastasise to bone and/or brain Overall survival 75%
Rhabdoid tumour	1% of renal tumours with 65% presenting <12 months Poor survival rates ~20% Associated with brain ATRT
Neuroblastoma	Rarely intrarenal
Soft tissue sarcoma	Desmoplastic small round cell tumours (DSRCT), rhabdomyosarcoma
Carcinoma	1.7% renal cell In adolescents, associated with Von Hippel–Lindau syndrome, medullary carcinoma
Non-Hodgkin lymphoma	Usually bilateral, diffuse involvement
Mesoblastic nephroma	Presents usually <12 months Usually benign although the cellular type can metastasise
Cystic partially differentiated nephroblastoma	Benign
Angiomyolipoma	Benign, in association with tuberous sclerosis

ATRT: atypical teratoid/rhabdoid tumour.

CLINICAL PRESENTATION

Most WTs are discovered 'incidentally' or because parents or grandparents notice abdominal enlargement (**Fig. 12.2**). They are often very large at diagnosis. Pain is uncommon and usually attributed to intratumoral bleeding, while haematuria occurs in only 10–15%. Rarely, children may present with tumour rupture, varicocoele, hypertension or symptoms of metastatic spread. Congenital anomalies are seen in 9% of patients presenting with WT.

INVESTIGATIONS

Imaging

Initial screening of abdominal masses is with ultrasound to exclude cystic lesions, although this may show the blood 'lakes' characteristic of intratumoral bleeding in WT, uncommon in other types of renal tumours. CT and MRI scanning are equally effective in demonstrating the renal origin of the primary tumours, the anatomy of the 'opposite' kidney – to exclude bilateral disease (**Fig. 12.3**) – and determining whether or not the inferior vena cava is involved (**Figs 12.4, 12.5**). MRI is preferred not just to avoid unnecessary radiation, but also because of the additional functional information it can provide.

Children with WTs should have chest x-rays and chest CT to investigate for lung metastases. Those with CCSK and rhabdoid tumour of the kidney (RTK) should have, in addition, an isotope bone scan and MRI scan of the brain.

Some patients have low haemoglobin because of intratumoral bleeding. The partial thromboplastin time (PTT) may be prolonged as some WTs make an anti-von Willebrand factor. If proteinuria is present, Denys–Drash syndrome should be suspected, and further investigated.

The histology mimics the developing kidney with triphasic components, which are namely, stromal, epithelial and blastema (**Fig. 12.6**). In the UK biopsies are performed at diagnosis above the age of 6 months to determine tumour type (WT/RKT/CCSK). The WT are classified, after a short course of preoperative chemotherapy, into low-/intermediate-/high-risk groups depending on the degree of necrosis, blastema

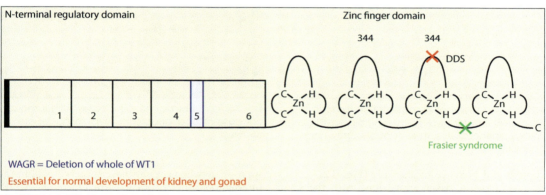

FIGURE 12.1 Effects and location of different WT1 mutations: WT1 is completely deleted in WAGR syndrome, while in Denys–Drash syndrome (DDS) WT1 mutation results in disruption of DNA binding by zinc fingers of WT1 protein. In Frasier syndrome WT1 mutation disrupts splicing.

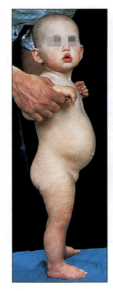

FIGURE 12.2 A 2-year-old girl on the day of diagnosis of left-sided Wilms tumour. The tumour weighed 1 kg, but was a histopathologically stage I and of favourable histology.

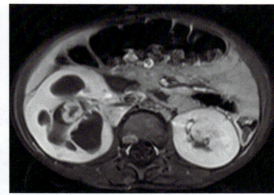

FIGURE 12.3 MRI STIR sequence of bilateral renal tumours in a child with ambiguous genitalia. Histopathology and subsequent surgery confirmed bilateral high-risk Wilms tumour.

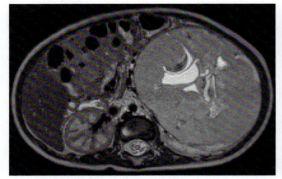

FIGURE 12.4 Large left-sided renal mass, with typical claw-like residue of normal kidney and patent left renal vein and inferior vena cava.

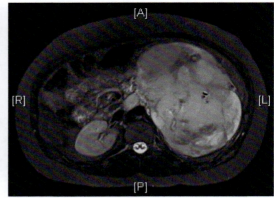

FIGURE 12.5 Large left-sided Wilms tumour with extension into the left renal vein abutting the inferior vena cava. The mass is heterogenous, suggesting internal haemorrhage.

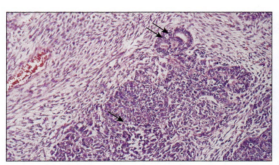

FIGURE 12.6 'Typical' triphasic Wilms tumour (favourable histology, FH) showing blastema (single arrow), epithelial structures (double arrow) and stroma.

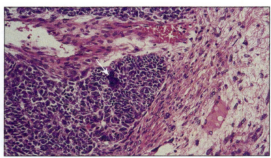

FIGURE 12.7 Unfavourable histology (UH) tumour because of focal anaplasia. Atypical nuclei are arrowed.

content and presence of anaplasia (**Fig. 12.7**). This histopathological classification along with the stage of the resected tumour determines the postoperative treatment regimen.

Nephrogenic rests are abnormal persistent embryonic tissue, found in children with multifocal or bilateral WT. These lesions are often assumed to be a precursor of WT, while multiple rests are called nephroblastomatosis.

Two staging systems are in common use. The National Wilms Tumour System (NWTS) is most

appropriate when patients have surgery first, but the International Society of Paediatric Oncology (SIOP) system is preferred for patients having preoperative chemotherapy (**Table 12.3**).

TREATMENT

There has been a divergence of opinion between Europe and North America as to the merits of preoperative chemotherapy versus immediate nephrectomy. In the UK, the UKWT3 trial randomised between

TABLE 12.3 SIOP Wilms tumour staging system

Stage I	Tumour is limited to kidney or surrounded with fibrous pseudocapsule, if outside of the normal contours of the kidney is completely resected (resection margins 'clear'); the vessels of the renal sinus are not involved
Stage II	The tumour extends beyond kidney or penetrates through the renal capsule and/or fibrous pseudocapsule into perirenal fat, renal sinus, or vena cava but is completely resected
Stage III	Incomplete excision of the tumour, which extends beyond resection margins (gross or microscopical tumour remains postoperatively), involvement of abdominal lymph nodes, tumour rupture pre/intraoperatively, tumour penetration through the peritoneal surface, tumour thrombi at resection margins of vessels or ureter, surgical wedge biopsy prior to chemotherapy
Stage IV	Hematogenous metastases (lung, liver, bone, brain, etc.) or lymph node metastases outside the abdominopelvic region
Stage V	Bilateral renal tumors at diagnosis

the two and no difference in survival was evident but less operative morbidity in the preoperative group was reported. Importantly, there was 'stage migration', with more children having lower-stage disease and less treatment, particularly radiotherapy. Treatment within Europe, including the UK, uses 4–6 weeks of preoperative chemotherapy with vincristine and actinomycin D. Postoperative treatment depends on the stage and histological subtype.

PROGNOSIS

Five year overall survival for WT is 80%, with over 90% in localised non-anaplastic disease, while with anaplastic histology overall survival is 60%. Cure is possible for WT in up to one-half of relapsing patients, especially those who have received only one or two chemotherapy drugs and no radiotherapy 'first time around'.

LIVER TUMOURS

In sharp contrast to adults, primary liver tumours in children are more common than secondary tumours. Both benign and malignant types occur (**Table 12.4**). Overall, they represent 1–2% of all children's tumours and about 1% of all children's cancers. Males are more commonly affected than females.

AETIOLOGY

Hepatoblastoma usually occurs *de novo*, but may be associated with familial adenomatous polyposis (FAP) and with Beckwith–Wiedemann syndrome. Hepatocellular carcinoma often arises in a liver previously damaged by hepatitis B or C virus, or by metabolic liver disease, especially glycogen storage disease (GSD) type I and tyrosinosis. Enormous progress has been made in reducing the incidence of hepatocellular carcinoma world-wide through perinatal hepatitis B vaccination programmes.

CLINICAL PRESENTATION

Liver tumours usually present with upper abdominal distension (**Fig. 12.8**), while pain is unusual. In very young children a differential diagnosis of stage Ms neuroblastoma with diffuse metastatic spread to the liver can usually be made by identifying an adrenal primary tumour by ultrasound. Besides increased levels of alpha-fetoprotein (AFP), which must be interpreted in the light of normal values for the patient's age, thrombocytosis (due to release of a thrombopoietin) is characteristic of hepatoblastoma and hepatocellular carcinoma.

INVESTIGATIONS

MRI alongside Doppler ultrasound is better than CT at displaying the anatomy and focality of the primary tumour, and is used to identify the pretreatment extent of disease or PRETEXT (**Fig. 12.9**). The lungs are by far the most frequent site for metastatic hepatoblastoma and hepatocellular carcinoma, so chest x-ray and CT scan of the lungs are mandatory.

TREATMENT/MONITORING/PROGNOSIS

Benign tumours are usually treated by surgery alone. Exceptions are haemangiomas (**Fig. 12.10**), especially infantile haemangioma when medical treatment (in the form of propranolol) alongside careful observation with serial imaging is preferred. Sometimes congenital haemangiomas may present with high-output cardiac failure due to the intralesional A–V shunting, in which case transarterial embolisation is preferred to surgery.

TABLE 12.4 Types of liver tumour and relationship to level* of serum alpha-fetoprotein (AFP) at diagnosis

	Undetectable	Slight elevation	Very high
Benign			
Adenoma	50%	50%	–
Haemangioma	All	–	–
Haemangioendothelioma	All	–	–
Mesenchymal hamartoma	50%	50%	–
Malignant			
Hepatoblastoma	<5%	<5%	>95%
Hepatocellular carcinoma**	25%	25%	50%
Sarcoma	All	–	–
Malignant germ cell tumour***	<5%	<5%	>95%*
Non-Hodgkin's lymphoma (NHL)****	All	–	–

*Account must be taken of the child's age in interpreting values.

**Fibrolamellar variant associated with normal serum AFP but elevated serum Vit B12 and TCII (transcobolamin II) levels.

***Can also have elevated serum β-hCG.

****In NHL, liver enlargement is usually diffuse.

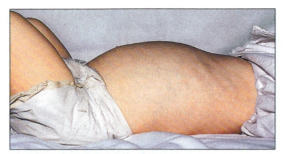

FIGURE 12.8 Distended upper abdomen in a child with hepatoblastoma. Note that there is no jaundice.

Malignant tumours are treated with chemotherapy to destroy metastases and shrink the primary tumour, followed by delayed surgical resection and then further chemotherapy. Chemotherapy is cisplatin based, including an anthracycline for high-risk hepatoblastoma and hepatocellular carcinoma. Treatment is usually dictated by international studies.

Monitoring is by serial imaging (**Fig. 12.9**) with serum AFP (**Fig. 12.11**) ultrasound, MRI and chest x-rays in the case of hepatoblastoma/hepatocellular carcinoma. It is essential to monitor serum AFP 1–2 weekly during the treatment and 3 monthly for 3 years off treatment.

PROGNOSIS

The prognosis has much improved in recent years. Overall, the cure of hepatoblastoma is now over 90% for standard risk disease and 75% for metastatic disease. Liver transplant from either living related or unknown donor is necessary for PRETEXT IV tumours responding to chemotherapy, without evidence of extrahepatic spread after completion of chemotherapy.

For hepatocellular carcinoma, prognosis is still relatively poor because tumours are often multifocal and/or metastatic at diagnosis; however, unifocal tumours are curable in at least 50% of cases.

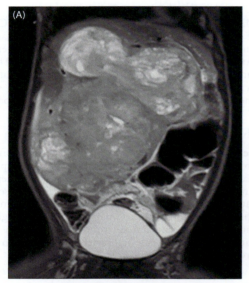

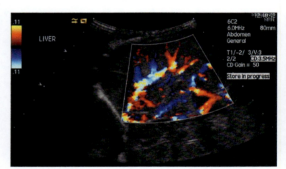

FIGURE 12.10 Ultrasound of diffuse infantile haemangioma (diffusely abnormal liver with increased vascularity).

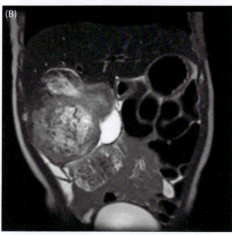

FIGURE 12.9 MRI: coronal STIR (A) and T2 (B) of a patient with hepatoblastoma at diagnosis and after 6 weeks of chemotherapy.

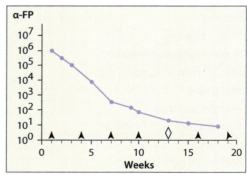

FIGURE 12.11 Serum alpha-fetoprotein response (AFP) to courses of 'PLADO' chemotherapy (solid arrows – see text) in a 1.5-year-old child with hepatoblastoma. The t1/2 is 4–5 days, indicating a major tumour response. Complete surgical resection was achieved (open lozenge). The MRI scans of this patient, who is a long-term survivor, are shown in **12.9**.

LANGERHANS CELL HISTIOCYTOSIS

Langerhans cell histiocytosis (LCH) is a rare disorder characterised by lesions with an accumulation of Langerhans cells with other immune cells, resulting in tissue damage.

EPIDEMIOLOGY

LCH occurs at all ages from the neonatal period through childhood to adulthood. The UK childhood incidence is approximately 4.1 per million children under 14 years per year with a 2:1 predominance in males. The median age at presentation is 6 years.

CLINICAL PRESENTATION

The disease may involve skeleton, skin, lymph nodes, liver, lungs, spleen, bone marrow, or CNS. Single system disease, which occurs in approximately 70% of cases, involves one organ or system, such as the skeleton (**Fig. 12.12**), skin or lymph nodes and presents with a bone or soft tissue lump or skin rash in an otherwise well child. Craniofacial involvement with proptosis or mastoiditis may result in diabetes insipidus due to involvement of the posterior pituitary and loss of hearing due to damage to the inner ear. Multi-system disease (**Figs 12.13, 12.14**) involves two or more organs or systems. Involvement of the 'risk' organs – liver, spleen and bone marrow – causes fever, failure to thrive, widespread rash, anaemia and organomegaly, with a more aggressive progression and poorer outcome.

Congenital LCH may occur at, or soon after birth, with skin nodules, diffuse rash and occasionally purpuric lesions. Isolated lesions can be treated with topical therapy but the infant must be closely monitored for symptoms of other organ involvement.

PATHOPHYSIOLOGY

LCH lesions, regardless of site and severity of disease, show the pathognomonic CD1a+ve Langerhans cell with macrophages, eosinophils, multi-nucleated giant cells and T-cells. While the Langerhans cells are clonal, this reactive background and the lack of clear malignant features have led to continuing debate whether LCH is a reactive process or a malignancy. Recently, mutations of *BRAF V600E* have been found in >50% of samples of LCH. This mutation stimulates downstream signalling via MEK and ERK, inducing proliferation and promoting transformation that has been identified in a number of malignancies. This finding in LCH may point to the underlying mechanism of disease, but ongoing studies in larger cohorts of patients are needed to validate this finding, and to understand if a correlation exists between the molecular profile and the clinical presentations to develop molecular targeted therapy for what can be a devastating disease.

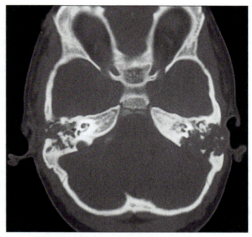

FIGURE 12.12 High-resolution CT scan of skull, showing a soft-tissue mass in the middle ear with adjacent destruction of the petrous temporal bone and invasion of the structures of the middle and inner ear. The patient, a 5-year-old female, presented with an aural polyp and deafness. Only the skeleton was involved in this patient ('single-system disease').

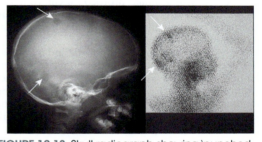

FIGURE 12.13 Skull radiograph showing 'punched-out' lytic deposits in the skull table of a 5-year-old male with 'multi-system' Langerhans cell histiocytosis. The inset shows the corresponding radionuclide scan after injection of an 111In radiolabelled mouse anti-CD1a antibody. There is increased uptake in the skull lesions and in Waldeyer's ring.

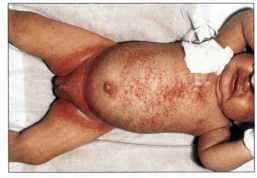

FIGURE 12.14 Widespread, confluent central truncal rash and petechiae in an infant with multi-system Langerhans cell histiocytosis (LCH) and thrombocytopenia due to 'haemopoietic failure' despite treatment. This 14-month-old male died 6 months later, from progressive LCH.

TREATMENT

Single system disease often needs minimal treatment. Isolated bone disease may respond to biopsy and curettage alone, or additional intralesional steroid, and lymph node involvement might need excision alone. Skin disease may respond to topical agents.

Multi-focal bone involvement and multi-system disease are treated with systemic therapy to induce an early response and to minimise the immediate and longer-term effects of tissue destruction by the disease, using agents that would not cause long-term morbidity.

International treatment trials for LCH are organised by the Histiocyte Society and are based on risk stratification depending on whether disease is single system or multi-system, and whether there is involvement of 'risk organs' or other sites that may predispose to the development of diabetes insipidus or long-term CNS problems (CNS risk lesions). The LCH III trial, which recently closed, recommended a 6-week induction with vinblastine and prednisolone with early reassessment and possible further 6-week reinduction, followed by 12 months of maintenance therapy with pulsed vinblastine and prednisolone and 6-mercaptopurine for multi-system disease. Multi-focal bone or CNS risk diseases were also treated with a similar protocol. 2-chlorodeoxy-adenosine (2-CdA) may be useful monotherapy in multifocal bone patients who respond poorly to first-line treatment.

Early disease response is prognostic and refractory disease requires careful discussion and planned intervention. The LCH-S-98 and LCH-S-2005 studies explored strategies for salvage in poorly responding patients who had a poor prognosis, where cytosine arabinoside combined with 2-CdA was used with success but with a significant bone marrow toxicity. Bone marrow transplantation (BMT) or reduced-intensity conditioning stem cell transplantation has also shown promise as effective salvage therapy.

The Histiocyte Society's LCH IV, seeks to refine risk stratification to allow an earlier switch to treatment intensification in refractory risk organ disease to improve outcome, and to minimise reactivation by investigating a strategy of more prolonged and intense continuation treatment. In patients with CNS risk or other special sites, the protocol seeks to minimise reactivation and long-term consequences by using prolonged maintenance therapy, while a second-line therapy for refractory or reactivating non-risk organ patients is explored.

In patients with lung LCH (**Figs 12.15–12.17**), cessation of smoking by the patient and in the household is crucially important. For patients with diabetes insipidus, DDAVP replacement is necessary together with further endocrine evaluation and hormone replacement for anterior pituitary disease (**Fig. 12.18**).

PROGNOSIS

Overall 5-year survival of patients with single system disease is close to 100%, while for those with low-risk multi-system disease; this reduces to approximately 80%. Patients with multi-system disease involving

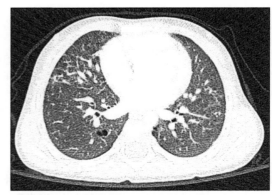

FIGURE 12.15 Langerhans cell histiocytosis pulmonary disease: CT scan demonstrating multiple lung cysts in a child with multi-system disease, whose parents were both smokers.

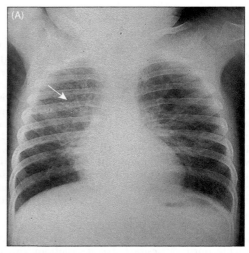

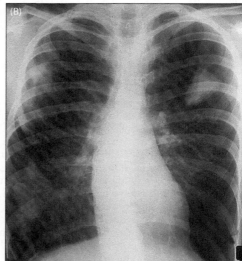

FIGURE 12.16 Langerhans cell histiocytosis pulmonary disease. X-ray showing a 4-year-old male at diagnosis (A), with interstitial infiltrate (arrow). The same patient aged 18 years had a much reduced chest volume secondary to lung fibrosis with secondary cyst formation (B).

Oncology

risk organs are less likely to respond well to initial treatment and their outcome is significantly worse.

Patients with multi-system or CNS risk disease have a higher incidence of permanent consequences including endocrine deficiency, hearing loss, chronic lung damage, learning difficulty and psychological problems that have a significant impact on quality of life (**Figs 12.19, 12.20**).

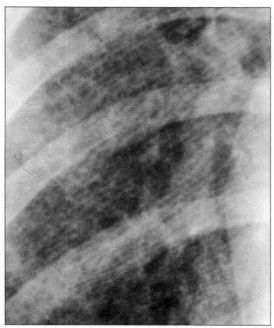

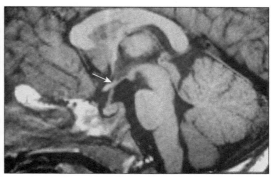

FIGURE 12.18 Pituitary stalk thickening (increased from 1 to 2–3 mm) and absence of the posterior pituitary 'bright signa;' in this T1-weighted MRI scan of a 2-year-old male with proven diabetes inspidus (DI) but normal growth. The DI was well controlled with oral desmopressin tablets. Anterior pituitary function was normal.

FIGURE 12.17 A high magnification view of the lung of another patient, who was a smoker, showing intense interstitial shadowing; biopsy confirmed 'active' Langerhans cell histiocytosis.

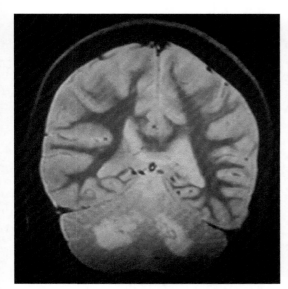

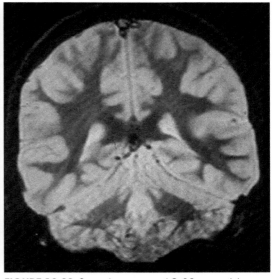

FIGURE 12.19 MRI scan (T2-weighted) of 10-year-old patient with multi-system Langerhans cell histiocytosis (LCH) since birth and cerebellar ataxia, evolving over the previous 4 years. The symmetrical changes in the white matter of both cerebellar hemispheres are characteristic of 'burnt-out' LCH.

FIGURE 12.20 Scan in a normal 9–10-year-old.

RHABDOMYOSARCOMA, OTHER SOFT TISSUE SARCOMAS AND FIBROMATOSIS

INCIDENCE

Rhabdomyosarcoma (RMS) is the commonest soft tissue sarcoma (STS) in children. 'Adult types' of sarcomas also occur, albeit rarely. STS represents 7% of all children's cancers.

RHABDOMYOSARCOMA

AETIOLOGY

More than 90% of RMS are sporadic but 5–10% can be explained by inheritance of a 'cancer predisposition gene', most often a constitutional mutation of the *TP53* gene on chromosome 17p, causing the Li–Fraumeni syndrome. *TP53* is a tumour suppressor gene, whose 'loss of function' mutations cause cells to lose regulatory control. Cell production and apoptosis become uncoupled and, if other mutations occur, clonal expansion leads to development of tumours. Brain tumours, adrenal tumours and early-developing breast cancer are also characteristic of the Li–Fraumeni syndrome and a meticulous family history is essential. Genetic and oncological counselling is available for family members with *TP53* mutations. Other genetic syndromes with predisposition to formation of RMS are neurofibromatosis type 1, Costello syndrome and Beckwith–Wiedemann syndrome.

CLINICAL PRESENTATION

Around 40% of RMS arises in the head or neck, 20–25% in the pelvis and 25–30% in the trunk and limbs. The orbit is the commonest head and neck site. Painless proptosis (**Figs 12.21, 12.22**) is usual and the differential diagnosis includes orbital cellulitis, LCH and other cancers, especially acute leukaemia, secondary neuroblastoma and optic nerve glioma. Middle ear tumours may present with aural pain or chronic discharge and delay in diagnosis is common because the problem is often first regarded as 'inflammatory'. At this and other head and neck sites, the primary tumour is often regarded as 'parameningeal' with the potential to invade directly through the meninges into the CNS.

Genitourinary and pelvic primary tumours present either as a visible mass with or without bleeding and discharge, for example at the vaginal introitus (**Fig. 12.23**) or by causing symptoms of pelvic outlet obstruction, most often retention of urine. Tumours arising under mucosa often have a tell-tale 'botryoid' appearance (**Fig. 12.23**).

Limb and trunk primaries arise as painless swellings, if they grow 'outwards' (centrifugally) or with

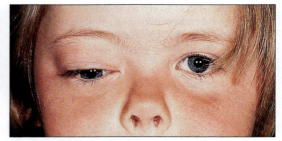

FIGURE 12.21 Orbital rhabdomyosarcoma of the right eye showing downward and outward displacement of the globe. Occasionally, the swelling looks 'inflammatory' (see text).

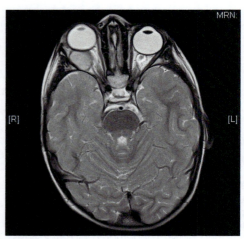

FIGURE 12.22 T2 MRI of the right orbital rhabdomyosarcoma involving lateral orbital muscles; the patient responded only partially to chemotherapy and required radiotherapy.

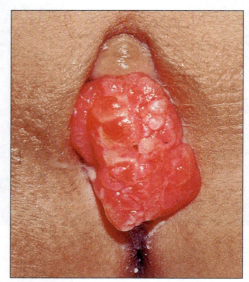

FIGURE 12.23 Vaginal submucosal embryonal rhabdomyomsarcoma with characteristic 'botryoid' appearance.

one or more of a variety of symptoms (spinal stiffness or pain, pleural effusion, intestinal obstruction) if they grow internally. Some 'primaries' can be tiny, and hard to identify, while others reach 15–20 cm or more in diameter.

DIAGNOSIS

The histology of RMS varies, with two main subtypes alveolar and embryonal found in children, while the third pleomorphic subtype is mainly diagnosed in adults (**Table 12.5**). The primary tumour is usually best imaged by MRI, including draining lymph nodes (see **Fig. 12.25**). CT of the chest, isotope bone scan and bone marrow aspirate and trephine biopsy are routine part of the staging. Biopsy, with molecular pathology studies, can be performed percutaneously or endoscopically. Immunohistochemistry for actin, myogenin and desmin are particularly useful. The alveolar subtype of RMS has pathognomonic translocation between chromosomes 1 or 2 and 13 resulting in *PAX3* or *PAX7/FOXO1* fusion gene, which enhance transcription and contribute to higher aggressiveness of this subtype. The biopsy position should be clearly marked and included in the final surgical resection. Draining lymph nodes should be biopsied if the tumour arises in the limbs, or in any location if the lymph nodes are abnormal on imaging. CSF examination is indicated if the tumour is parameningeal. The use of FDG PET/CT in paediatric sarcoma is still under scrutiny but it appears useful in evaluating nodal and metastatic disease (**Fig. 12.24**). On the both side of the Atlantic, RMS are stratified for treatment purposes according to the recognised risk factors: postsurgical stage, pathology, size, age, nodal involvement and localisation.

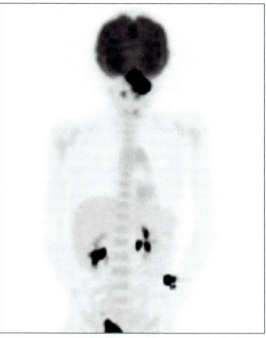

FIGURE 12.24 FDG PET/CT scan of a patient with localised embryonal rhabdomyosarcoma of the paranasal sinuses. The tumour was localised and this was confirmed by PET/CT. The patient responded well to chemotherapy and was further treated with radiotherapy. He remains well 3 years after the diagnosis.

TABLE 12.5 Subtypes of rhabdomyosarcoma (RMS)

Histological subtype/% of RMS	Age group and usual location of primary tumour	Molecular biology	Clinical behaviour	Prognosis
Embryonal 70–80	<5 years; head, neck, bladder, pelvis	Whole chromosome gains or losses, nonspecific abnormalities of 11p15	Could arise under mucosa causing botryoid appearances Lower risk of metastatic disease than alveolar tumour	Good (70%+ cure especially if in a favourable location)
Alveolar 15–20	>10 years, trunk and limb primaries	Specific translocation t(2;13)(q35q14) or t (1;13) resulting in *PAX3/FOXO1* or *PAX7/FOXO1* fusion genes; 80% of alveolar tumours harbour translocation (i.e. translocation positive)	Primary tumour has high potential to metastasise Primary tumour might be very small	Poorer than embryonal, 30–40% cure if not metastatic Translocation-positive tumours have poorer prognosis than translocation-negative tumours, which behave more like embryonal RMS

Rhabdomyosarcoma

Multi-modality treatment is required. Patients receive primary chemotherapy, either the 'IVA' (ifosfamide, vincristine and actinomycin D) favoured in Europe or VAC (vincristine, actinomycin D, cyclophosphamide) favoured in North America, without difference in efficacy between these two regimens. Other drugs, such as doxorubicin, etoposide, topotecan and irinotecan are also used. Local control may involve radiotherapy and/or surgery. Radiotherapy is effective in RMS and well tolerated by young patients but affects bony and soft tissue growth, sometimes with disastrous cosmetic results. New radiotherapy approaches as intensity modulated radiotherapy or proton beam radiotherapy have been employed recently in an attempt to minimise long-term effects. Primary surgery is only used for easily-resected 'peripheral' tumours, such as paratesticular primaries, to reduce morbidity, but less extensive surgery may be used after chemotherapy.

Response is best monitored with MRI and is usually good initially, though shrinkage is relatively slow in most cases (**Figs 12.25, 12.26**). After induction chemotherapy, depending on the response and the group stratification the patient might be treated with surgery and or RT, followed by further chemotherapy. Many children still need surgery and RT for cure, but around 50% can be spared the 'late effects' of these treatments (**Fig. 12.27**).

Embryonal tumours have significantly better prognosis than alveolar. Up to 25–30% of tumours recur, most usually locally which emphasises the value of local control. The recurrence usually happens within the first 3 years from diagnosis and is treated with second-line chemotherapy, further surgery and RT (if not given first time round). The prognosis depends on the time and type of the relapse, previous treatment given and biology of the tumour.

Metastatic disease is present in 15–20% of patients at diagnosis and has the worst outcome, which depends on the number of the involved sites and biology of the tumour.

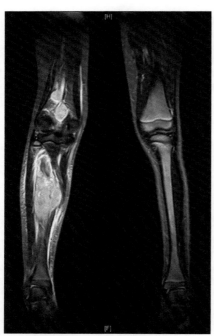

FIGURE 12.25 Alveolar rhabdomyosarcoma with primary disease in the left calf and metastatic spread in the popliteal lymph nodes.

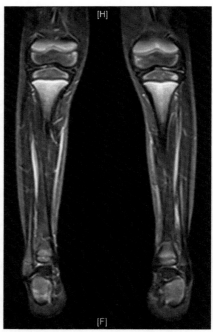

FIGURE 12.26 The same patient as in **12.25** after induction chemotherapy. He had widespread metastatic disease in the lungs, mediastinum and contralateral axillary lymph nodes. All areas showed excellent response to chemotherapy.

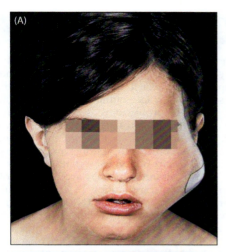

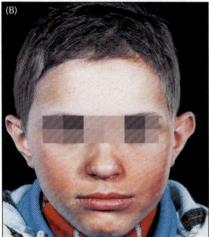

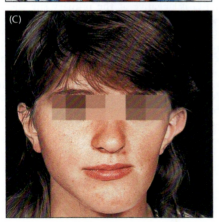

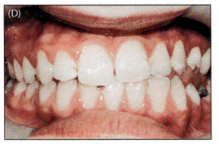

OTHER SOFT TISSUE SARCOMAS

Other STS subtypes more commonly seen in adolescents and young adults are synovial sarcoma, desmoplastic small round cell tumour and other entities, where, in general, local control of the primary tumour is the main problem and metastases are unusual. Two types of STS are seen in children.

INFANTILE FIBROSARCOMA

This entity occurs in young children affecting the limbs, especially legs, and has exceptionally low metastatic potential (**Figs 12.28, 12.29**). Almost 100% of the tumours have recurring t(12;15) translocation leading to a fusion gene *ETV6-NTRK3* abnormality not found in other STSs. Surgical resection is the mainstay of treatment, but to prevent mutilation, chemotherapy with vincristine and actinomycin D is advocated, often followed by non-morbid surgical resection.

AGGRESSIVE FIBROMATOSIS

Aggressive fibromatosis (desmoid tumour) can occur at any site. Intra-abdominal desmoids are more common in adults and could be a feature of mutation in the familial adenomatous polyposis (FAP) gene. FAP should be ruled out when desmoids are multiple or arise in young children. Aggressive fibromatosis is difficult to manage. Complete surgical excision is usually impossible and incomplete resection often provokes regrowth at a more rapid rate than that of the original tumour. Chemotherapy with vinblastine and methotrexate could produce response as well as antioestrogens (tamoxifen or toremifene). Imatinib mesylate, a selective tyrosine kinase inhibitor that targets c-kit, platelet derived growth factor receptor (PDGFR)-α and PDGFR-β has shown some activity in desmoid fibromatosis that is mediated by PDGFR kinase activity.

FIGURE 12.27 Facial appearance of girl with facial, non-parameningeal primary rhabdomyosarcoma. (A) At diagnosis, aged 7 years; (B) at the end of treatment with chemotherapy ('VAC' combination) and external beam radiotherapy; (C) showing marked facial hemiatrophy due to radiotherapy; (D) she also had severe dental caries on the side of the radiotherapy. Multiple plastic surgical and orthodontic procedures were needed, but she married and gave birth to two normal sons, despite a high cumulative dose of cyclophosphamide.

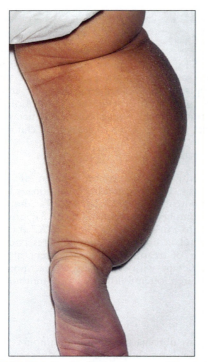

FIGURE 12.28 Infantile fibrosarcoma of the right calf at diagnosis (posterior view) in an infant. She received 6 months of chemotherapy with vincristine and actinomycin D, which initiated tumour regression.

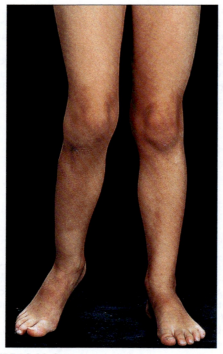

FIGURE 12.29 Spontaneous shrinkage continued in the patient in **12.28** and at the age of 5.5 years her only handicap is a shortened Achilles tendon, later successfully corrected by surgery.

NEUROBLASTOMA

Neuroblastoma arises from neural crest cells; primary tumours are located in the adrenal glands or sympathetic ganglia. It is the commonest extracranial solid tumour, accounting for 7% of all childhood malignancy. Neuroblastoma is very rarely familial. The clinical behaviour of neuroblastoma is very variable, with some tumours undergoing spontaneous regression and others progressing rapidly with a poor prognosis, in spite of aggressive multi-modality therapy. There is an internationally accepted neuroblastoma risk group classification by the International Neuroblastoma Risk Group (INRG), using criteria such as age, histology, image defined risk factors and the genomic profile, where neuroblastoma can be divided into very low risk, low risk, intermediate risk and high risk depending on outcome (**Table 12.6**). In the literature reference will also be made to an earlier surgical staging developed by the International Neuroblastoma Staging Study group (INSS).

Neuroblastoma is a disease of the very young: 40% is diagnosed in infants, 35% are patients of 1–2 years and 25% are >2 years, with the disease becoming rare after the age of 10.

INVESTIGATIONS

Urinary catecholamine metabolites are usually raised. CT or preferably MRI scans of the primary tumour will show the extent of the disease locally and allow identification of image defined risk factors L1 or L2 (**Figs 12.30, 12.31**). Tumours may be calcified. Most tumours are positive on radio-iodine labelled metaiodobenzylguanidine (MIBG) scan, which is essential to exclude distant disease (**Fig. 12.32**). If MIBG is negative at the primary site then skeletal scintigraphy or a ^{18}F-FDG PET CT will need to be done to exclude bony and soft tissue metastases. A biopsy of the primary tumour or a metastatic site is mandatory for histology, biology and the genomic profile, which also predicts outcome. Any tumour with amplification of the MycN oncongene (**MYCNA**) is high risk. Bone marrow aspirates and trephine biopsies are essential to exclude bone marrow disease. Measurement of neuron-specific enolase, ferritin and lactate dehydrogenase at diagnosis may provide further prognostic information.

TABLE 12.6 International Neuroblastoma Risk Group (INRG) Consensus Pretreatment Classification schema

INRG Stage	Age (months)	Histologic Category	Grade of Tumor Differentiation	MYCN	11q Aberration	Ploidy	Pretreatment Risk Group
L1/L2		GN maturing; GNB intermixed					A Very low
L1		Any, except GN maturing or GNB intermixed		NA			B Very low
				Amp			K High
L2	<18	Any, except GN maturing or GNB intermixed		NA	No		D Low
					Yes		G Intermediate
	≥18	GNB nodular; neuroblastoma	Differentiating	NA	No		E Low
					Yes		H Intermediate
			Poorly differenciated or undifferenciated	NA			
				Amp			N High
M	<18			NA		Hyperdiploid	F Low
	<12			NA		Diploid	I Intermediate
	12 to <18			NA		Diploid	J Intermediate
	<18			Amp			O High
	≥18			Amp			P High
MS	<18			NA	No		C Very low
					Yes		Q High
				Amp			R High

From Cohn SL, *et al.*: The International Neuroblastoma Risk Group Classification System. An INRG Task Force Report. *J Clin Oncol* 2009;27:289–97.

Neuroblastoma

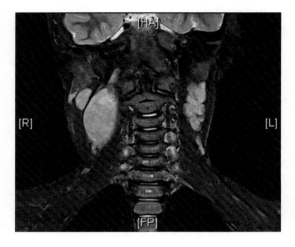

FIGURE 12.30 MRI: neuroblastoma image defined risk factors. L1, no involvement of the vital organs and structures.

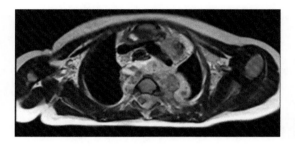

FIGURE 12.31 MRI: neuroblastoma image defined risk factors. L2, tumour compressing the trachea, extending intraspinally and encasing the aorta.

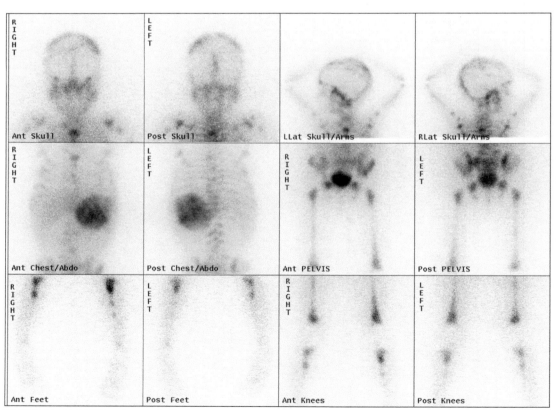

FIGURE 12.32 MIBG scan of disseminated neuroblastoma – there is avid uptake in the left abdominal tumour with diffuse metastatic disease in the bones.

VERY LOW- AND LOW-RISK NEUROBLASTOMA

INCIDENCE

The true incidence of low-risk disease is unknown. Screening all infants for urinary catecholamine metabolites detects those with low-risk disease but unfortunately not those who would go on to develop high-risk disease.

CLINICAL PRESENTATION

Congenital localised neuroblastoma, presenting within the first 3 months of life, is very low risk and can regress spontaneously. Full staging does not have to be done immediately and these infants can be monitored clinically. Infants with stage Ms (special) disease present with rapidly increasing hepatomegaly and may have skin deposits (**Fig. 12.33**). Other tumours, local groups L1 or L2 may be detected incidentally. Most children with low-risk disease are diagnosed <18 months and even if there are metastases will be treated with standard chemotherapy and surgery as long as there as there is no *MYCNA*.

HISTOLOGY/GENETICS/BIOLOGY

Low-risk tumours occur mainly in children <18 months of age, have favourable histology, may express TrkA protein and be hyperdiploid. Tumours may show segmental chromosomal abnormalities (SCAs) but no *MYCNA*.

INVESTIGATIONS

Bone marrow aspirates and trephines will be positive in metastatic disease though stage Ms disease may show <10% of nucleated non-hematopoietic cells in the bone marrow.

TREATMENT

There are different low-risk treatment groups depending on whether or not life-threatening symptoms are present or SCAs are found in the tumour. Most children will get a combination of chemotherapy and surgery. The chemotherapy mainly consists of carboplatin and etoposide. Resection of the primary tumour is often performed at diagnosis in L1 disease and after chemotherapy in L2 disease. Stage Ms can regress spontaneously but, in infants with rapid liver enlargement, chemotherapy and occasionally low-dose RT or even embolisation may be needed.

PROGNOSIS

Over 95% of patients with low-risk disease survive. Seventy percent of Ms patients survive, with uncontrolled hepatic growth accounting for the majority of the mortality.

INTERMEDIATE-RISK NEUROBLASTOMA

INCIDENCE

Approximately 30% present with intermediate-risk disease.

CLINICAL PRESENTATION

Most patients present >18 months of age and have a large primary tumour with image defined risk factors L2 and no metastases.

HISTOLOGY/GENETICS/BIOLOGY

Intermediate-risk tumours can have both favourable and unfavourable histology, often show SCAs but do not have *MYCN* amplification.

DIAGNOSIS AND GROUPING

The diagnosis is made by biopsy and grouping by full staging.

TREATMENT

Treatment includes chemotherapy and surgery. Additional RT to the site of the primary and/or 13-cis-retinoic acid therapy may be indicated. In older children and adults a more high-risk approach to treatment may be advised.

PROGNOSIS

The 5-year event free survival is >70%.

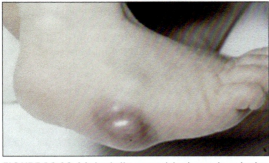

FIGURE 12.33 Metastatic neuroblastoma in a baby (Stage Ms) – deposit in the skin.

HIGH-RISK NEUROBLASTOMA

INCIDENCE

Approximately 50% of all patients present with high-risk disease.

CLINICAL PRESENTATION

The 'classic' presentation is with a hard abdominal mass in a sweaty, hypertensive, irritable child with black eyes and a limp, but many will present without all of these features, for example simply with bone pain.

HISTOLOGY/GENETICS/BIOLOGY

Histology is unfavourable, poorly differentiated neuroblastoma. No characteristic chromosomal translocations have been identified but a number of genetic changes occur in tumour cells. The following are associated with a poor prognosis: *MYCNA*, 1p or 11q deletion, 17q gain, reduced expression of the high affinity nerve growth factor receptor (TrKA) and diploid DNA index. *MYCN* amplification is used to stratify for high-risk therapy in patients with localised disease.

DIAGNOSIS AND GROUPING

Grouping should be performed according to INRG (**Table 12.6**).

TREATMENT

The majority of high-risk neuroblastoma are sensitive to both chemotherapy and radiation. Dose-intense chemotherapy aims to reduce the size of the primary tumour and clear metastatic disease. Further therapy involves resection of the primary tumour and high-dose chemotherapy with autologous peripheral blood stem cell rescue. Oral 13-cis-retinoic acid to 'differentiate' residual tumour and the addition of GD2 directed immunotherapy should further improve outcome.

PROGNOSIS

Survival is improving; however, although 50% of patients with high-risk disease survive greater than 5 years the 10-year survival rate is still only around 30%. In high-risk disease young children fare better than older patients, age being a continuous parameter.

Children can present with signs of spinal cord compression and need to be treated as a medical emergency. They should be started on oral dexamethasone, have an immediate MRI of the spine and if neuroblastoma is suspected should start chemotherapy treatment the same day. Discussion with the neurosurgeons should always take place urgently and where appropriate an intervention should be planned before the blood count drops following chemotherapy.

RETINOBLASTOMA

INCIDENCE

Retinoblastoma affects 1 in 20,000 children, which is equivalent to about 45 cases per year in the UK. More than 90% of cases are diagnosed before 5 years of age (see also Chapter 7 Ophthalmology).

CLINICAL PRESENTATION

Children with bilateral retinoblastoma present earlier (median age 8 months) than the unilateral form (median age 28 months). Presenting signs include leukocoria (**Fig. 12.34**), strabismus, red eye and reduced vision. Tumours are bilateral in 30% of cases. Five percent have deletions of chromosome 13q14 and present with dysmorphic features and failure to thrive.

GENETICS

Retinoblastoma occurs in a heritable and non-heritable form. Tumours arise following loss of function of both copies of the *RB1* tumour suppressor gene. In non-heritable cases, both copies of the gene are mutated in a single cell by random genetic events, whereas in heritable cases there is a germline mutation in one copy of the gene and then a single somatic event results in tumorigenesis (Knudson hypothesis). Patients with heritable retinoblastoma are predisposed to tumours in later life, osteosarcoma, STS and melanoma being the most prevalent.

INVESTIGATIONS

Skilled ocular examination is mandatory to define the extent of intraocular disease (**Fig. 12.35**). Eyes are classified from A–E depending on the extent of the intraocular disease. Ultrasound examination of the globe is helpful. MR head scanning is reserved for suspected extraocular disease and to exclude trilateral retinoblastoma. CSF cytology and bone marrow examinations are undertaken in patients with adverse histological features at risk of metastatic disease.

TREATMENT

Treatment of intraocular tumours is dependent on tumour size and location. Focal therapies, laser therapy and cryotherapy are used for small localised tumours. Enucleation of the eye is the treatment of choice for E eyes and the most common treatment for unilateral disease, with 80% of unilateral children undergoing primary surgery. Children with bilateral tumours usually receive primary chemotherapy with focal consolidation therapies as indicated.

Salvage therapies include intra-arterial chemotherapy for multi-focal relapses with radioactive scleral plaques for localised relapses. External beam radiation is now only rarely used, but remains an effective salvage treatment in bilateral cases where chemotherapy and focal treatments have failed.

All newly diagnosed children undergo molecular analysis of the *RB1* gene and when a germline mutation is identified, first-degree relatives are offered mutation screening. Siblings of affected individuals who cannot be excluded by molecular or linkage analysis undergo regular screening ocular examinations. Preimplantation diagnosis can be offered to parents when their mutation is known, while chorionic villus sampling is feasible for parents who desire termination of an affected pregnancy.

PROGNOSIS

Retinoblastoma has an excellent prognosis with a 98% 5-year survival rate. Deaths from second cancers are now a greater risk for patients with heritable retinoblastoma than the primary tumour itself.

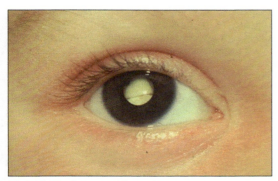

FIGURE 12.34 Lack of the red eye reflex (leucocoria) in a child with retinoblastoma.

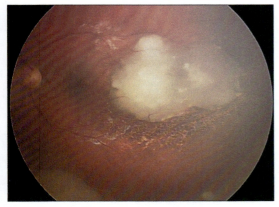

FIGURE 12.35 Retinoblastoma – fundal photograph of multi-focal tumour. (Courtesy of Dr A. Reddy, Barts and the London NHS Trust.)

FIGURE 12.36 MRI of the large mass originating in the left femoral shaft, with associated expansion of the bone, cortical irregularity and periosteal reaction and large soft tissue mass. The patient was 9 months old and had further metastatic disease in the lungs and bones.

EWING SARCOMA AND PERIPHERAL PRIMITIVE NEUROECTODERMAL TUMOUR

INCIDENCE

Ewing sarcoma classically occurs in the second decade of life, affecting fewer than three in every 1 million children under 15 years of age. Their distinction from other small round blue cell tumours of childhood could be difficult.

CLINICAL PRESENTATION

Ewing sarcoma of bone presents as pain and swelling. Pelvis, femur, tibia and fibula are most commonly affected. The soft tissue Ewing tumours or peripheral primitive neuroectodermal tumours (pPNET) present with intrathoracic disease (Askin tumour), or as paravertebral or retroperitoneal masses.

GENETICS

Both Ewing sarcoma and pPNET share the same characteristic chromosome translocation, most commonly t(11;22) with corresponding fusion genes *EWS/FLI1* or *EWS/FLI2*.

DIAGNOSIS

Plain radiographs may reveal 'moth-eaten' bone with periosteal elevation. MRI scans define the extent of soft tissue involvement (**Fig. 12.36**). Metastatic disease should be sought in the lungs (CT chest) (**Fig. 12.37**), bones (bone scan) and bone marrow (aspirate). Samples of the tumour should be analysed histopathologically (characteristically CD99 is positive on immunohistochemistry) with molecular pathology analysis for translocation.

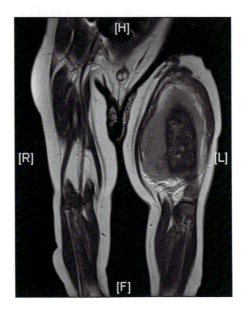

TREATMENT

Aggressive chemotherapy with alkylating agents and anthracyclines reduces disease bulk and treats micrometastatic disease. Good local control with surgery or radiotherapy is essential but difficult to achieve in pelvic sites. Intensification of chemotherapy and high-dose chemotherapy with autologous stem cell transfer could improve outcome in metastatic patients (**Fig. 12.38**).

PROGNOSIS

The tumour volume (>200 ml), poor response to chemotherapy (<90% necrosis) and the presence of metastatic disease are poor prognostic factors. With aggressive therapy, around 65% of patients with localised disease can be cured.

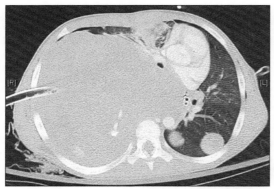

FIGURE 12.37 CT scan of a peripheral primitive neuroectodermal tumour (Askin tumour) of the right chest with pulmonary metastases and rib involvement. The patient had a long history of asthma and presented with cardiac arrest in her school.

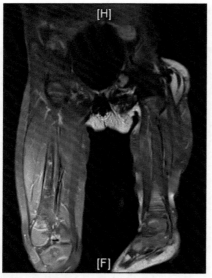

FIGURE 12.38 The same patient as in **12.36** 2 years after treatment with chemotherapy, surgery with rotationplasty and high-dose chemotherapy with autologous stem cell rescue.

OSTEOSARCOMA

INCIDENCE/AETIOLOGY

Osteosarcoma accounts for 2.5% of paediatric cancers under the age of 15 years, as the peak age coincides with a period of rapid bone growth at the time of puberty. Male to female ratio is 2:1. Several genetic conditions are associated with development of osteosarcoma: Li–Fraumeni syndrome, Rothmud–Thomson, Werner and Bloom syndromes.

CLINICAL PRESENTATION

Osteosarcoma presents with bone pain, swelling and loss of function in adjacent joints. Symptoms are often attributed to sports injuries in active adolescents. Night pain, systemic symptoms, weight loss or failure of symptoms to resolve with conservative management should alert the clinician. The presenting sites of the disease in the order of frequency are: distal femur, proximal tibia and proximal humerus. Axial tumours constitute 10% of all osteosarcomas.

DIAGNOSIS

- **Plain radiographs** show a partly lytic, partly sclerotic lesion affecting the metaphysis of a long bone, eroding the cortex, elevating the periosteum to cause a Codman's triangle, with 'sunburst' calcification extending into soft tissues.
- **MRI** of the primary site will show the extent of intramedullary tumour, and spread into surrounding soft tissues including neurovascular bundles (**Figs 12.39, 12.40**).
- **CT** of the primary site may show calcification in extraosseous tumour. CT of the lungs is mandatory to identify pulmonary metastases in 10–15% at presentation (**Fig. 12.41**).

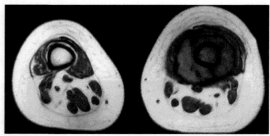

FIGURE 12.39 T1-weighted axial MRI of the distal femora, showing swelling of the left thigh caused by a tumour of the femur, which both involves the intramedullary region and extends into the soft tissues around the cortex.

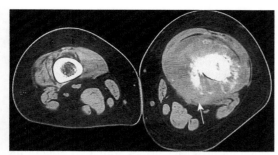

FIGURE 12.40 Axial CT of the distal femora, showing partly calcified extension of tumour into the soft tissues of the thigh around the left femur.

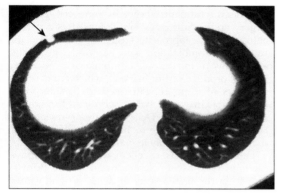

FIGURE 12.41 Thoracic CT scan showing small solitary pulmonary metastasis at the right lung base anteriorly.

- **Skeletal scintigraphy** will show the primary tumour and any bone metastases. The biopsy needle tract or incision should be placed in such a way that it can be incorporated into the final surgical excision.
- **Histologically**, there is usually osteoid with osteoblastic, chondroblastic and fibroblastic areas.

TREATMENT

Chemotherapy has improved the prognosis of operable osteosarcoma from approximately 20% to about 65%. It is given both prior (neoadjuvant) to and after definitive surgery (adjuvant). The standard chemotherapy regimen includes doxorubicin, cisplatin and high-dose methotrexate. Chemotherapy is also used for inoperable and metastatic osteosarcoma, but survival rates are poor and only 25–50% of patients survive 5 years. Prognostic factors obtained from large international multi-institutional studies are tumour site and size, presence of metastases, surgical remission and tumour necrosis after neoadjuvant chemotherapy.

Wide surgical excision remains the mainstay of surgical treatment. Advances in surgical techniques and implants have dramatically reduced the need for amputation. Most tumours arise in the metaphyseal region and abut or involve the growth plate; surgical resection will lead to limb length discrepancy. Extendible prostheses have been developed to allow *in vivo* lengthening (triggered by an external magnetic field) as the child grows (**Fig. 12.42**). The other innovative approaches use intercalary allografts and joint sparing reconstructions. In some patients

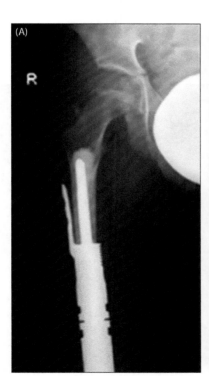
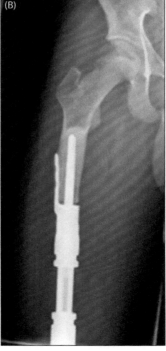

FIGURE 12.42 Radiograph of extendable growing prosthesis in a child (A) at the end of treatment and (B) several years later.

limb salvage techniques called rotationplasty can be used. This involves resection of the tumour with the amputation of the knee region, with reunion of the rotated distal limb. For responding tumours, thoracotomy and resection of pulmonary metastases is undertaken.

Radiotherapy has limited role in osteosarcoma, but it may be a useful means of achieving local control of inoperable tumours with new radiation techniques offering some further benefits.

In cases of osteosarcoma arising as a second malignancy, their prognosis may approach that of otherwise comparable patients with primary osteosarcoma if treated by an appropriate multi-modality approach.

EXTRACRANIAL MALIGNANT GERM CELL TUMOURS

INCIDENCE

Malignant germ cell tumours, derived from primordial germ cells, occur in gonadal and extragonadal sites and affect 4 children per million of the population per annum, with a childhood female to male ratio of around 3:1.

CLINICAL PRESENTATION

Sites affected include sacrococcygeal (**Fig. 12.43**), gonadal, mediastinal, vaginal, uterine and abdominal. Malignant tumours may develop in patients who have had previously 'benign' tumours resected.

DIAGNOSIS

The measurement of tumour markers AFP and beta-human choriogonadotrophin (β-hCG) helps in diagnosis and follow-up. Teratomas and germinomas secrete neither AFP nor β-hCG. Yolk-sac tumours and endodermal sinus tumours secrete AFP, choriocarcinomas secrete β-hCG, and embryonal carcinomas secrete both markers. Individual tumours may have a mixture of histopathological types within them. Accurate imaging of the primary site and evaluation for metastatic disease with a CT scan of the chest and a bone scan are important.

TREATMENT/PROGNOSIS

Chemotherapy, in particular platinum agents have revolutionised treatment efficacy in germ cell tumours. Surgery and radiotherapy are also used as a part of multi-modality approach. Cisplatin or carboplatin are used in combination with etoposide, ifosfamide or bleomycin in various combinations. Secreting tumours produce serum markers, which are excellent predictors of response, but need to be interpreted with caution in young babies whose AFP might be physiologically raised. Delayed tumour resection is the mainstay of treatment, but radiation is avoided when possible, especially in younger children.

The outcomes are excellent with overall survival reaching 80%. Most relapses occur in the primary site within the first 2 years of diagnosis and careful follow-up with serum tumour markers is mandatory as early recognition of a relapse and appropriate treatment yield good outcome. Chemotherapy, together with rigorous local control with surgery and radiotherapy are essential for cure of the relapse, which is still achievable.

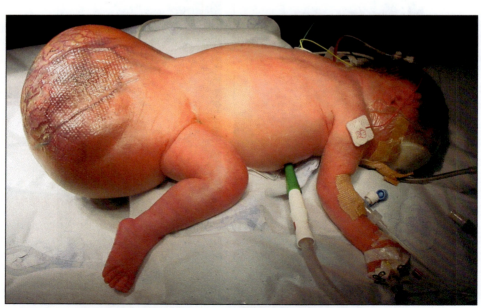

FIGURE 12.43 Sacrococcygeal teratoma in a newborn baby. Treatment is primary resection, which involves tumour mass and coccyx.

Oncology

TUMOURS OF THE CENTRAL NERVOUS SYSTEM

Primary malignancies of the CNS account for 25% of all cancers in childhood. Although there are over 120 distinct histological subtypes, the commonest tumours are low-grade gliomas, primitive neuroectodermal tumours, ependymomas, high-grade gliomas and intracranial germ cell tumours. The clinical behaviour of these tumours differs from that of their adult counterparts.

EPENDYMOMA

INCIDENCE

Ependymomas comprise 10% of all CNS tumours of childhood; 70% arise in the posterior fossa and 30% supratentorially. The mean age at diagnosis is 5 years but the peak age of incidence is 2 years. Ependymomas account for 25% of primary spinal cord tumours but present later.

CLINICAL PRESENTATION

Posterior fossa tumours present with raised intracranial pressure (ICP) and ataxia. Cranial nerve palsies and vomiting are more common than in medulloblastoma due to adherence of the tumour to the floor of the fourth ventricle. Patients with supratentorial tumours present with seizures, focal neurological deficits or raised ICP.

DIAGNOSIS

As with all CNS tumours, initial CT or MRI scans will reveal the primary tumour (**Fig. 12.44**) but full neuraxis MR imaging is required for staging. Metastases within the CNS can occur but are infrequent at diagnosis (10%). The prognostic value of histological grading is unclear.

TREATMENT/PROGNOSIS

Complete surgical resection is prognostically important but sometimes difficult to achieve due to adherence of tumour to the vital structures. Staged or second-look surgery should always be considered for residual disease. Involved field radiotherapy, rather than craniospinal radiation, is recommended, as the vast majority of relapses are at the site of the primary tumour. Modern conformal techniques (including proton radiotherapy) are allowing radiotherapy to be considered for younger patients. Chemotherapy is used in infants but its role in older children continues to be investigated. Current 5-year survival ranges from 50% to 75%.

MEDULLOBLASTOMA/ PNET

INCIDENCE

Medulloblastoma usually arises in the cerebellar vermis but, as other histopathologically similar tumours can arise elsewhere in the brain, the term primitive neuroectodermal tumour (PNET) has been used for the whole group irrespective of the site of origin (see also Chapter 8 Neurology, page 234). Classical cerebellar medulloblastoma affects 6.6 children per million per year with a median age at diagnosis of 5 years.

CLINICAL PRESENTATION

Cerebellar tumours present with ataxia and signs of raised ICP. Patients with tumours in the pineal region (pineoblastoma) may have Parinaud syndrome (failure of upward gaze, dilated pupils that react to convergence but not light, nystagmus and lid retraction).

DIAGNOSIS

MRI or CT scanning will reveal the presence of the tumour (**Fig. 12.45**). Spinal imaging (with MRI) is mandatory to exclude spinal metastases (**Fig. 12.46**). CSF should be checked for the presence of malignant cells. Histological subtypes have different outcomes: in young children extensive nodularity (desmoplastic tumours) have an excellent prognosis whereas the presence of diffuse and severe anaplasia carries a poor prognosis. Molecular genetic abnormalities are also of prognostic significance: beta catenin expression (indicative of overexpression of the Wnt pathway) carries a good prognosis whereas amplification of *MYC* genes predicts a poor outcome.

TREATMENT/PROGNOSIS

Careful risk stratification is essential in medulloblastoma as the therapy for the different risk groups differs substantially. Standard-risk disease is denoted by no evidence of metastatic disease, near total resection, age over 3 years at diagnosis and absence of worrying pathological and molecular features. In patients with standard-risk disease surgery combined with radiotherapy to the craniospinal axis at

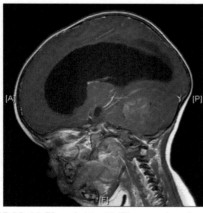

FIGURE 12.44 T1-weighted MRI scan showing a posterior fossa mass with obstructive hydrocephalus. The histopathology was in keeping with ependymoma.

a dose of 36 Gy was curative in around 60% of children. However, the addition of chemotherapy has increased survival in standard-risk disease to around 80% while allowing the dose of neuraxis radiotherapy to be reduced to 24 Gy. Various regimens are used for high-risk patients but most include neuraxis radiotherapy to a minimum dose of 36 Gy. With the use of more aggressive regimens containing chemotherapy, neuraxis irradiation and high-dose therapy with autologous stem cell rescue some groups have reported survival rates of 70% in patients with metastatic disease but the toxicity of therapy is substantial.

For children younger than 3 years, chemotherapy is used to try to delay or avoid radiotherapy, thereby decreasing the neuropsychological and endocrine sequelae. These strategies are associated with good survival in young children with tumours of desmoplastic histology but the results for children with classical medulloblastoma remain disappointing.

Relapses are local or disseminated through the craniospinal axis. Salvage therapy for children who have been irradiated as part of their primary therapy is rarely curative. Experimental therapies based on targeting the underlying biology of medulloblastoma, e.g. sonic hedgehog pathway are being explored.

HIGH-GRADE SUPRATENTORIAL GLIOMA

INCIDENCE

Malignant supratentorial gliomas comprise around 10% of childhood brain tumours and the incidence increases with age. Forty percent occur in the cerebral hemispheres and the remainder in the thalami, hypothalamic regions or basal ganglia.

CLINICAL PRESENTATION

Over one-half the patients present with signs of raised ICP. Weakness, visual disturbances, cranial nerve palsies and hemiplegia are found in around 50% of cases.

DIAGNOSIS

MRI scanning (**Fig. 12.47**) is used for diagnosis. Spread within the neuraxis is uncommon. Patients

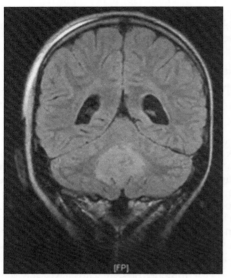

FIGURE 12.45 T2-weighted coronal MRI scan: posterior fossa mass, which proved to be medulloblastoma. This patient did not present with obstructive hydrocephalus.

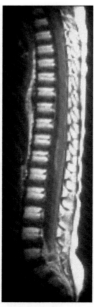

FIGURE 12.46 Sagittal MRI scan of spine showing enhancing spinal deposits.

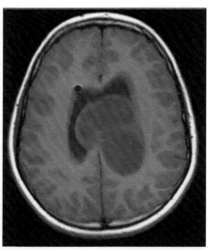

FIGURE 12.47 T1-weighted axial MRI of a large haemorrhagic tumour arising from the left thalamus and growing into the third and left lateral ventricles resulting in hydrocephalus. Right transparietal shunt is *in situ*. The histopathology confirmed high-grade glioma, in this case glioblastoma multiforme (WHO grade IV).

with glioblastoma multiforme (WHO grade IV) fare worse than those with anaplastic astrocytoma (WHO grade III).

TREATMENT/PROGNOSIS

The completeness of surgical resection is an important prognostic variable but a complete resection may be impossible due to the diffuse infiltrative nature and location of the tumour. Current standard treatment in children older than 3 years of age is combined chemo–radiotherapy with temozolomide, but the majority of patients still die from their disease, with less than 20% surviving 5 years (grade IV tumours). New insights into the molecular biology of paediatric high-grade glioma may lead to new targeted therapies.

BRAINSTEM GLIOMA

INCIDENCE

Brainstem gliomas account for 10–20% of childhood CNS tumours, with a peak incidence at 5–8 years of age. The majority (80%) are diffuse intrinsic pontine gliomas (DIPG).

CLINICAL PRESENTATION

A brief history of the classical triad of cranial nerve deficits, long tract signs and ataxia is typical for DIPG, with occasional features of raised ICP and mood disturbance.

DIAGNOSIS

Brainstem gliomas show classical appearances on MRI (**Fig. 12.48**). For DIPG, the role of biopsy remains controversial and is currently reserved for cases with an atypical history/imaging or as part of a clinical research.

TREATMENT/PROGNOSIS

Dorsally exophytic tumours or tumours of the cervicomedullary junction, which tend to be low grade, may benefit from aggressive surgical management. DIPG tumours are not amenable to surgery. Radiotherapy is useful in controlling symptoms and extends survival. Chemotherapy has currently not been shown to be of benefit. Prognosis is poor with a median survival of 9–13 months in patients with DIPG and new therapies are needed. The prognosis for localised tumours is better.

LOW-GRADE ASTROCYTOMA

INCIDENCE

Cerebellar astrocytoma accounts for 10–20% of all childhood CNS tumours and has a peak incidence in the first decade of life. Low-grade gliomas of the optic pathways comprise about 5% of CNS tumours, but patients with neurofibromatosis type 1 are predisposed to developing these tumours.

CLINICAL PRESENTATION

Cerebellar astrocytomas present with raised ICP and ataxia. Optic pathway tumours (**Fig. 12.49**) lead to squint, proptosis or visual loss. Hypothalamic involvement can produce growth disturbance, precocious or delayed puberty and changes in mood. Diabetes insipidus is rare in hypothalamic low-grade astrocytomas and its presence should raise the question of whether the tumour is a craniopharyngioma or a germ cell tumour.

DIAGNOSIS

MRI ophthalmology scan (**Fig. 12.50**) and routine spinal imaging is recommended but the incidence of neuraxis dissemination at diagnosis is under 5%. Ophthalmological and endocrine assessments are mandatory in optic pathway tumours.

TREATMENT

Over 90% of children with cerebellar astrocytoma are cured by surgery alone. Surgery has a role in unilateral optic nerve tumours with total visual loss, but the majority of optic pathway tumours can be managed with chemotherapy or radiotherapy treatment being instituted for tumour growth or an increase in symptoms. Children with NF1 have a better prognosis and sould only be treated with chemotherapy if there is 'threat' to vision or clinical/radiological evidence of tumour growth. Radiotherapy should be avoided in children with NF1 due to the increased incidence of vasculopathy in later life.

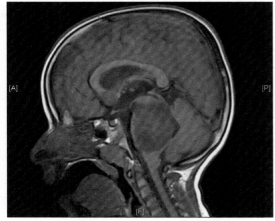

FIGURE 12.48 T1-weighted sagittal MRI showing diffuse intrinsic pontine glioma.

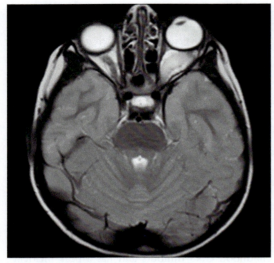

FIGURE 12.49 T2-weighted axial MRI showing left-sided optic pathway glioma with proptosis. There is no signs of neurofibromatosis-1.

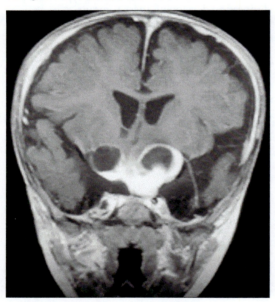

FIGURE 12.50 Coronal MRI scan showing chiasmatic glioma with cyst formation.

RARE TUMOURS

Rarer cancer types encountered in children may be truly rare paediatric cancers, or rare instances of 'adult cancers' affecting children. These tumours may pose particular problems for clinicians because there is often no standard approach to their treatment. The formation of a rare tumour group within the national (CCLG) and international (SIOP) children cancer groups aims to help alleviate this problem. Once the diagnosis is confirmed, a careful family history is mandatory, as rare tumours may be associated with an underlying genetic predisposition (**Table 12.7**). Carcinomas are epithelial malignancies, and represent only 2–3% of cancers in childhood. The sites of carcinomas also differ from those in adults.

THYROID CARCINOMA

More than 90% of childhood thyroid cancers are differentiated, with papillary carcinoma accounting for 80–90%. The major risk factor for the development of papillary carcinoma is therapeutic radiation exposure to the head and neck in children, particularly those younger than 5 years. Thyroid cancer in childhood cancer survivors is increased even in those who did not receive irradiation therapy.

CLINICAL PRESENTATION

Children usually present with a solitary, painless thyroid nodule, or diffuse or simple multinodular goiter (**Fig. 12.51**). A solitary thyroid nodule in a child should always be investigated as up to 25% may be malignant. Metastatic disease in cervical lymph nodes and the lungs is more common at presentation in children than in adults.

DIAGNOSIS

Thyroid nodules should be evaluated by thyroid function tests, thyroid and neck ultrasound scan and fine-needle aspiration cytology (FNAC). FNAC is the most efficient and accurate method of evaluating the nature of thyroid nodules in children.

TABLE 12.7 Conditions predisposing to carcinoma

Predisposing syndromes	Cancer	Molecular abnormality	
		Gene symbol	Chromosomal location
Li-Fraumeni syndrome	Adrenocortical	TP53	17p13
Beckwith-Wiedemann syndrome	carcinoma	WBS	11p15
Multiple endocrine neoplasia type 1		MEN1	11q13
Familial adenomatous polyposis	Colon carcinoma	APC	5q21
Juvenile polyposis coli			
Familial melanoma	Melanoma	MLM	9p21
Von Hippel-Lindau syndrome	Renal cell carcinoma	VHL	3p25

TREATMENT/PROGNOSIS

Treatment of differentiated thyroid cancer of follicular cell origin has three components:

1. Surgery. Total thyroidectomy, either as the first procedure when the diagnosis is clear, or as a staged procedure with an initial hemithyroidectomy and subsequent completion thyroidectomy when there is diagnostic uncertainty. Involved cervical lymph nodes should be removed surgically.
2. Radioactive iodine administration under conditions of thyroid stimulating hormone (TSH) stimulation for ablation of the thyroid remnant is usually advised. Repeated administrations may be needed if there is metastatic disease. Recent evidence suggests that radioactive iodine may not always be needed.
3. TSH suppression by overreplacement with levothyroxine sodium.

Careful monitoring with a combination of imaging and thyroglobulin measurement is necessary, and lifelong oncological follow-up is necessary as late relapses are well recognised.

The prognosis of well-differentiated thyroid cancer of follicular cell origin in children is excellent, even when there is extensive disease at presentation.

NASOPHARYNGEAL CARCINOMA

Nasopharyngeal carcinoma represents 1% of all malignant disease in children, with males being more commonly affected than females. Patients with nasopharyngeal carcinoma may have markedly elevated antibody titres to various EBV antigens, which usually correlate with the total tumour burden and decrease with successful therapy.

CLINICAL PRESENTATION

Presentation is usually with lymphadenopathy and signs of nasopharyngeal obstruction. Nasal bleeding, discharge, deafness, tinnitus or trismus may be found. Direct extension of the primary tumour into the cavernous sinus may cause multiple cranial nerve palsies. Lymph node spread is very common but metastases to other sites (bone marrow, bone, lung and CSF) occur in only 5–10% of patients.

DIAGNOSIS

Ear, nose and throat examination may reveal the diagnosis. Imaging for local and metastatic disease assessment with CT and MRI is required, and an endoscopic biopsy of the primary tumour will confirm the diagnosis.

TREATMENT/PROGNOSIS

Current chemo–radiotherapy schedules have improved survival rates, and allowed a reduction in the radiotherapy dose and consequent endocrinopathies. Use of modern radiotherapy techniques may reduce the incidence of some complications such as xerostomia. In localised disease 5-year overall survival reaches 80%.

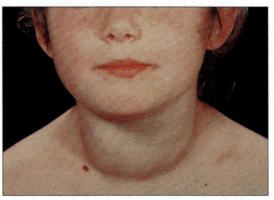

FIGURE 12.51 A discrete, painless thyroid nodule in a young girl.

ADRENOCORTICAL CARCINOMA

CLINICAL PRESENTATION

Adrenocortical carcinoma (ACC) is more common in females and presents with signs of virilisation, Cushingoid features or persistent, refractory hypertension (**Fig. 12.52**). Fifty percent of children with adrenocortical tumours (ACTs) have Li–Fraumeni syndrome and ACT might the first manifestation of the syndrome within the family. In addition 80% of sporadic childhood ACTs have atypical germline mutation of p53 associated with a lower but increased cancer risk in relatives. ACT also occurs more often in patients with hemihypertrophy and Beckwith–Wiedemann syndrome.

DIAGNOSIS

Diagnosis, treatment and follow-up of children with ACT is paradigm of multi-disciplinary approach in paediatric oncology, where endocrinologist, oncologist, surgeon, pathologist and clinical geneticist work together in management and long-term follow-up of the patients. Biochemical endocrine evaluation is invaluable in order to distinguish ACC from more common premature adrenarche or congenital adrenal hyperplasia (CAH). There is no reliable histopathological distinction between adrenal adenomas and carcinomas. Tumour size, weight and extent of surgical resection are the best available predictor of biological behaviour, and incompletely resected tumours, heavier than 100 g or greater than 200 cm^3 are associated with worse prognosis. The patients also need to be staged for possible metastatic spread, which dramatically changes the prognosis. Biopsy is contraindicated as this may cause tumour seeding.

TREATMENT/PROGNOSIS

Complete surgical resection, especially of small tumours, may be curative. In patients with incomplete resection or metastatic spread, treatment options include chemotherapy with cisplatin, etoposide, doxorubicin, 5-fluorouracil and cyclophosphamide, with or without mitotane. Radiotherapy is not advised given the high chance of a genetic cancer predisposition.

RENAL CELL CARCINOMA

CLINICAL PRESENTATION/TREATMENT

Renal cell carcinoma (RCC) presents with an abdominal mass and haematuria. The tumour may metastasise to the abdominal lymph nodes, liver, lungs and bone. The differences emerging between childhood and adulthood RCC prevent generalised application of therapies to children that are validated for adults. Forty percent of RCC in childhood are characterised by translocation involving transcription factor E3 (TFE3) family members (involving Xp11.2 or 6p21). This emphasises the importance of prospective classification of RCCs in children using molecular pathology. The treatment for RCC in children and adolescents remains radical nephrectomy, but the systemic therapy (especially in metastatic disease) is now more usually targeted therapy than conventional cytotoxic chemotherapy, which is largely ineffective, although large international studies are needed to validate this approach.

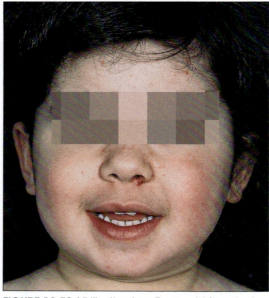

FIGURE 12.52 Virilisation in a 5-year-old female due to a functional adrenal tumour.

LATE EFFECTS OF CANCER TREATMENT

The present-day multi-modality treatment has improved overall 5-year survival, so that more than 75% of childhood cancer sufferers can expect to live to adulthood compared with only 30% 50 years ago. Unfortunately, this comes at a cost, as the treatments are not specific to tumour cells and therefore damage to normal tissue can occur. This translates into a three-fold risk of premature death after 45 years and increased morbidity compared with their peers. Long-term follow-up studies have identified that 67% of survivors suffer long-term conditions, with one-quarter of those being severe. The degree of damage depends upon the organ characteristics (cell turnover, treatment sensitivity), age and development of the patient, gender, genetic predisposition and the synergistic effects of the treatments. Furthermore, psychosocial problems can occur in both patients and their families following the cancer diagnosis and its treatment. The late sequelae can be very diverse, presenting during treatment (cisplatin-induced hearing loss, neurological deficiency after brain tumour surgery), or many decades later (second malignant neoplasms, cardiovascular disease). In certain cases the functional damage can remain static, progress or improve over time.

The most frequent fatal adverse effects are the development of second malignant neoplasms (**Fig. 12.53**) and cardiovascular disease. Important consequences that affect quality of life are endocrine dysfunction and infertility. **Table 12.8** gives examples of the consequences of treatment.

It is very important to be aware of these problems and take responsibility to provide an effective follow-up programme tailored to the needs of the survivor. Care may range from multi-disciplinary input to regular surveillance (breast cancer surveillance for survivors who received chest radiotherapy) to minimal self-care managed by the survivor. To assist this aim, all survivors and their health care providers should have treatment summaries and care plans. Effective aftercare should provide surveillance and management for late effects, support for psychosocial issues and education regarding risks of adverse effects and life style, employment and financial issues with the aim of reducing mortality, morbidity and improving quality of life.

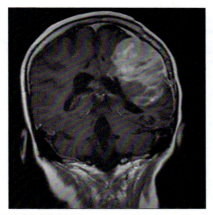

FIGURE 12.53 MRI: T1 coronal showing a large secondary tumour in the left parietal lobe – this is spindle cell sarcoma after treatment of high-grade glioma.

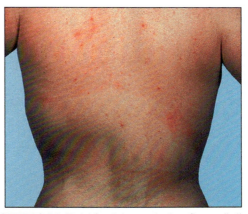

FIGURE 12.54 Right flank hypoplasia after radiation for treatment of stage III Wilms tumour.

TABLE 12.8 Consequences of childhood cancer treatment

Treatment	Organ/tissue affected	Outcome
Surgery	Brain	Neurological deficit
Radiotherapy	Organ within radiation field	Disturbance of growth and development, e.g. hypoplasia of soft tissue/bone (**Fig. 12.54**) Second malignant neoplasm presenting often many years after treatment.
	Brain	Pituitary dysfunction, degree dependant on dose
	Heart	Cardiovascular disease
Chemotherapy		
Anthracyclines	Heart	Cardiomyopathy, dose dependant
Alkylating agents	Gonadal dysfunction	Predominantly in males, dose dependant
Epidophyloxins	Bone marrow	Leukaemia
Cisplatin/carboplatin	Hearing	Hearing dysfunction occurs during treatment
	Kidney	Renal impairment occurs during treatment

FURTHER READING

Renal tumours

Szychot E, Brodkiewicz A, Pritchard-Jones K. Wilms' tumour – review of current approaches to the management. *CML-Urology* 2012;18:65–75.

Liver tumours

Maibach R, Roebuck D, Brugieres L, *et al. Prognostic stratification for children with hepatoblastoma: the SIOPEL experience. Eur J Cancer* 2012;48:1543–9.

Perilongo G, Maibach R, Shafford E, *et al.* Cisplatin versus cisplatin plus doxorubicin for standard-risk hepatoblastoma. *N Engl J Med* 2009;361:1662–70.

Zimmerman A, Perilongo G (eds). *Pediatric Liver Tumors.* Pediatric Oncology Series, 2011. Berlin: Springer-Verlag.

Zsíros J, Maibach R, Shafford E, *et al.* Successful treatment of childhood high-risk hepatoblastoma with dose-intensive multiagent chemotherapy and surgery: final results of the SIOPEL-3HR study. *J Clin Oncol* 2010;28:2584–90.

Langerhans cell histiocytosis

Badalian-Very G, Vergilio JA, Degar BA, Rodriguez-Galindo C, Rollins BJ. Recent advances in the understanding of Langerhans cell histiocytosis. *Br J Haematol* 2012;156:163–72.

Windebank K, Nanduri V. Langerhans cell histiocytosis. *Arch Dis Child* 2009;94:904–8.

Rhabdomyosarcoma and other soft tissue sarcoma

Ferrari A. Rhabdomyosarcoma – Oncopaedia, www.cure4kids.org

Oudot C, Orbach D, Minard-Colin V, *et al.* Desmoid fibromatosis in pediatric patients: management based on a retrospective analysis of 59 patients and a review of the literature. *Sarcoma* 2012;2012:475202.

Saab R, Ferrari A. Non-rhabdomyosarcoma soft tissue sarcoma – Oncopaedia, www.cure4kids.org

Neuroblastoma

Cecchetto G, Mosser V, De Bernardi B, *et al.* Surgical risk factors in primary surgery for localized neuroblastoma: the LNESG1 Study of the European International Society of Pediatric Oncology Neuroblastoma Group. *J Clin Oncol* 2005;23(33):8483–9.

Cohn SL, Pearson JAD, London WB, *et al.* The International Neuroblastoma Risk Group (INRG) Classification System: an INRG Task Force Report. *J Clin Oncol* 2009;27:289–97.

Gains J, Mandeville H, Cork N, Brock P, Gaze M. Ten challenges in the management of neuroblastoma. *Future Oncol* 2012;8(7):839–58. doi: 10.2217/fon.12.70. Review.

Maris JM, Hogarty MD, Bagatell R, Cohn SL. Neuroblastoma. *Lancet* 2007;369:2106–20. Review.

Matthay KK, Reynolds CP, Seeger RC, *et al.* Long-term results for children with high-risk neuroblastoma treated on a randomized trial of myeloablative therapy followed by 13-cis-retinoic acid: a children's oncology group study. *J Clin Oncol* 2009;27:1007–13.

Moroz V, Machin D, Faldum A, *et al.* Changes over three decades in outcome and the prognostic influence of age-at-diagnosis in young patients with neuroblastoma: a report from the International Neuroblastoma Risk Group Project. *Eur J Cancer* 2011;47:561–71.

Germ cell tumours

Gobel U, Schneider DT, Calaminus G, Haas RJ, Schmidt P, Harms D. Germ-cell tumors in childhood and adolescence. *Ann Oncology* 2000;11:263–71.

Tumours of the central nervous system

Taylor MD, Northcott PA, Korshunov A, *et al.* Molecular subgroups of medulloblastoma: the current consensus. *Acta Neuropathol* 2012;123(4):465–72.

Northcott PA, Korshunov A, Pfister SM, Taylor MD. The clinical implication of medulloblastoma subgroups. *Nat Rev Neurol* 2012;8:340–51.

Merchant TE. Ependymoma: new therapeutic approaches including radiation and chemotherapy. *J Neuroncol* 2005;75(3):287–99.

Hargrave D, Bartels U, Bouffet E. Diffuse brainstem glioma in children: critical review of clinical trials. *Lancet Oncology* 2006;7:241–9.

Late effects

Green D, Wallace H. *Late Effects of Childhood Cancer.* London: Arnold, 2004.

Skinner R, Levitt G, Wallace WHB. Therapy based long term follow up: Practice Statement. UKCCSG 2005. www.CCLG.org NHS improvement.nhs.uk/cancer/survivorship

13 Endocrinology

Mehul Dattani and Catherine Peters

THE SHORT CHILD

This is the commonest reason for referral of a child to an endocrinologist, and the algorithm (**Fig. 13.1**) gives an approach to the management of this condition.

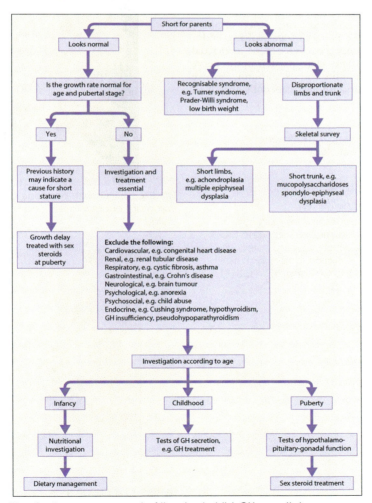

FIGURE 13.1 Algorithm for the management of the short child. GH: growth hormone.

GROWTH HORMONE DEFICIENCY/ INSUFFICIENCY

INCIDENCE/GENETICS

The incidence of growth hormone (GH) deficiency/ insufficiency (GHD/GHI) in its classical form is 1 in 3,000. Hereditary forms of GH deficiency arising as a result of a GH gene deletion or mutation or a growth hormone releasing hormone (GHRH) receptor mutation, are rare, accounting for 5–10% of cases, although Type II GHD is not an uncommon cause of GHD, and is due to a dominant negative disorder (**Table 13.1**).

DIAGNOSIS

GHD may rarely present with neonatal hypoglycaemia. Later presentation is usually with short stature (**Fig. 13.2**). The child classically looks chubby with a round immature face (**Fig. 13.3**). Micropenis may be a feature (**Fig. 13.4**). The birth weight is usually normal. However, the height velocity is slow from around the end of the first year of life. Breech delivery with obstetric trauma may be associated.

GHI may be associated with other pituitary hormone deficiencies as part of an evolving endocrinopathy. There may be evidence of associated disorders (e.g. midline cleft palate, optic nerve hypoplasia, agenesis of the corpus callosum, absence of the septum pellucidum and Fanconi's anaemia).

TABLE 13.1 GH deficiency/insufficiency pathogenesis and aetiology

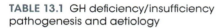

Congenital

- Hereditary – gene deletion/mutation
- Idiopathic GHRH deficiency
- Developmental abnormalities – pituitary aplasia, hypoplasia, midline brain and facial defects, many of which are associated with mutations in transcription factors such as HESX1, LHX3, LHX4, PROP1 and PIT1/POU1F1.

Acquired

- Perinatal trauma
- Hypothalamic/pituitary tumours

Secondary to

- Cranial irradiation
- Head injury
- Infection
- Sarcoidosis
- Histiocytosis

Transient due to

- Low sex hormone concentration
- Psychosocial deprivation
- Hypothyroidism

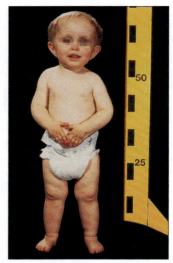

FIGURE 13.2 Growth hormone deficiency: classical appearance in a child presenting with short stature.

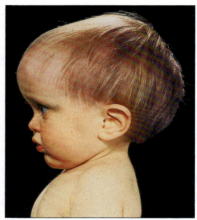

FIGURE 13.3 Growth hormone deficiency: typical immature, chubby facies and frontal bossing in a child.

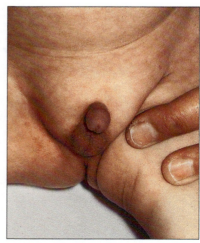

FIGURE 13.4 Growth hormone deficiency: micropenis in a child.

Endocrinology

378

The bone age is usually delayed, as is the dentition. Investigations should initially be performed to exclude non-endocrine pathology (e.g. renal and coeliac disease). The concentration of insulin-like growth factor (IGF)-I and its binding protein (IGF-BP3) may be low in GHD/GHI as these are GH-dependent factors, but the sensitivities and specificities of these tests in isolation are poor. A skeletal age may be delayed.

If the diagnosis of GHD or GHI is suspected, pharmacological or physiological tests of GH secretion may be indicated. Although physiological tests of GH secretion may be of greater relevance, they entail sampling of blood for GH concentrations at 20 minute intervals over a 12–24 hour period and are therefore expensive and time-consuming. Pharmacological testing in the form of provocative tests of GH secretion (e.g. insulin-induced hypoglycaemia, glucagon provocation, arginine provocation, clonidine stimulation and GHRH) should only be performed in children in whom a low growth velocity has been documented. Of these biochemical tests, insulin-induced hypoglycaemia and glucagon provocation are the most widely used. The results are dependent on the assay in use, and so the test results for any one centre need to be evaluated carefully. It should be noted that these tests can be dangerous if performed by inexperienced operators in units that are not tertiary referral centres.

MRI of the brain and pituitary may reveal anterior pituitary hypoplasia, often in association with an undescended/ectopic posterior pituitary and an absent infundibulum (**Figs 13.5, 13.6**).

TREATMENT

Replacement with recombinant human (rh) GH (15–20 units/m²/wk or 0.02–0.05 mg/kg/d) restores normal growth velocity after a period of catch-up growth. The smallest, most slowly growing and most severely GHI children will respond best. GH is given as a daily subcutaneous dose and is associated with minimal side-effects in replacement doses.

PROGNOSIS

The prognosis for final height in GHD/GHI is excellent, provided that treatment is begun at an early stage. If treatment is commenced late, a loss of height potential will ensue. Monitoring of IGF-1/IGF-BP3 concentrations aid in dosage optimisation.

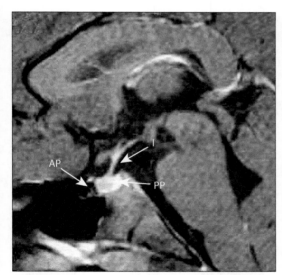

FIGURE 13.5 MRI showing a normal anterior pituitary (AP) with the posterior pituitary (PP) located normally in the sella turcica. Note the infundibulum (I) connecting the pituitary to the hypothalamus.

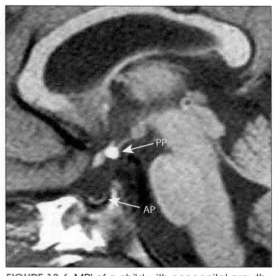

FIGURE 13.6 MRI of a child with congenital growth hormone deficiency (GHD) showing severe hypoplasia of the anterior pituitary (AP) with an undescended posterior pituitary (PP) at the level of the tuber cinereum. Note the absence of the stalk. This appearance reflects a developmental abnormality and is commonly observed in patients with isolated GHD and combined pituitary hormone deficiency.

LARON-TYPE DWARFISM

INCIDENCE/GENETICS

Classic Laron-type dwarfism is extremely rare. It is commoner in consanguineous unions as it is inherited as an autosomal recessive condition. Clusters of patients have been identified in Mediterranean countries, the Middle East and Ecuador. Molecular mutations and deletions in the gene encoding the extracellular domain of the GH receptor gene lead to GH insensitivity, although mutations in the transmembrane and intracellular domains have also been reported. Milder mutations in the GH receptor gene have been described in some cases of idiopathic short stature. Mutations in *STAT5B*, the *IGF-1* gene and the *IGFR* Type 1 have also been described in association with GH insensitivity phenotypes.

PATHOGENESIS/AETIOLOGY

The genetic lesion leads to an abnormal GH receptor. GH fails to interact appropriately with this abnormal receptor, with an inability to generate IGF-1 and ensuing growth failure. Abnormalities of the postreceptor signalling pathway including STAT5B can lead to GH insensitivity and immune deficiency, which can manifest as interstitial pneumonia. IGF-1 circulates bound to binding proteins and the acid labile subunit (ALS). Defects in the synthesis of these cotransporters also lead to IGF-1 deficiency. *IGF-1* gene deletions have been associated with deafness, microcephaly and learning difficulties.

DIAGNOSIS

It may present with hypoglycaemia in the neonatal period (with low birth weight) and, later on, with extreme short stature (**Fig. 13.7**) and an extremely poor growth rate. Clinically, they resemble GHD children, but with extreme short stature. Bone age is delayed with respect to chronological age, but advanced with respect to height age. Other features include micropenis, small hands and feet, craniofacial anomalies, such as a saddle nose (**Fig. 13.8**), excess subcutaneous fat, sparse hair growth, delayed closure of anterior fontanelles and a prominent forehead. Hip dysplasia and a chubby appearance are other associated features. Pubertal delay may be a feature. More recently, partial insensitivity to GH has been described in children who present with idiopathic short stature. Immune deficits and arthritis have been associated with *STAT5B* mutations.

Essential investigations are as for GHD/GHI (see previous pages). Unlike GHD/GHI, the basal concentration of GH in serum is elevated, with an exaggerated peak GH in response to provocation and low basal IGF-1 and IGF-BP3 concentrations. Additionally, an IGF-1 generation test fails to demonstrate an increase in the IGF-1 concentration following the administration of rhGH. GH-binding protein may be present or absent, depending on the underlying molecular lesion. In children with short stature secondary to partial GH resistance, GH-binding protein concentrations are low. GH concentrations are high, with low IGF-1 concentrations.

TREATMENT

Children with Laron-type dwarfism are now treated using recombinant IGF-1 treatment. Initial results are promising, with an initial increase in the height velocity, but close monitoring of patients is essential as the treatment is not without its side-effects (hypoglycaemia, hypokalaemia and papilloedema). In children with partial GH insensitivity, it is possible to treat with high doses of GH to improve the height velocity, but final height data are not available to date.

PROGNOSIS

The height prognosis without treatment is extremely poor. The role of recombinant IGF-1 treatment with respect to an increase in final height remains to be established.

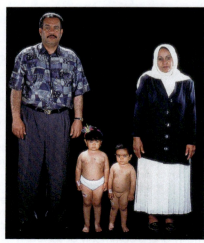

FIGURE 13.7 Laron-type dwarfism. Extreme short stature in two siblings, shown here with their parents.

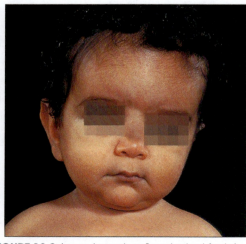

FIGURE 13.8 Laron-type dwarfism: typical facial features.

LOW BIRTH WEIGHT SYNDROME

INCIDENCE

This is common. The inheritance pattern is dependent on the underlying cause (see below). The majority are sporadic. Children with familial Russell–Silver syndrome have been described.

PATHOGENESIS/AETIOLOGY

80% of low birth weight children will catch up in the first 2 years of life. Others may have chromosomal disorders, dysmorphic syndromes such as 3M syndrome, recognised environmental insult *in utero* (e.g. rubella, CMV, alcohol, maternal smoking, anticonvulsants, placental dysfunction) and imprinting defects, as in Russell–Silver syndrome. Half of all Russell–Silver syndrome cases are found to have either hypomethylation of chromosome 11p15 or maternal uniparental disomy of chromosome 7.

DIAGNOSIS

Low birth weight syndrome may present with hypoglycaemia in the neonatal period. The majority have short stature and are usually very slim. Feeding problems in the first year of life are very common in this group of children. Birth weight is inappropriately low for gestation and in relation to the birth weight of other siblings.

The Russell–Silver syndrome shares many of these features. Children fail to demonstrate significant catch-up growth and have a very poor appetite, often requiring supplementary feeds. Additionally, clinical features include asymmetry of the face (**Fig. 13.9**) and limbs (**Fig. 13.10**), clinodactyly (**Fig. 13.11**), a small triangular facies, café-au-lait spots, genital anomalies and excessive sweating.

If hypoglycaemia is proven, investigations should be performed to exclude other pathology (e.g. congenital hyperinsulinism, β-oxidation defect). If a reduced growth velocity is documented, investigations should be carried out to exclude coincident pathology (e.g. GHI). A karyotype may be indicated if a genetic syndrome is suspected.

TREATMENT

GH treatment is approved for children who are born small for gestational age and fail to catch up. Additionally, treatment may be required for complications such as hypoglycaemia (frequent feeds).

PROGNOSIS

The prognosis for height is highly variable, and a significant proportion (~40%) will have a final height that falls considerably short of their mid-parental target height. GH treatment has been demonstrated to improve height in the short term, but effects on final height are variable. Early puberty may further limit final height. Learning difficulties may be associated.

The relationship between *in utero* growth restriction and adult cardiovascular disease risk (Barker hypothesis) suggests an increased risk of cardiovascular and metabolic disease in adulthood, particularly hypertension, diabetes mellitus and obesity.

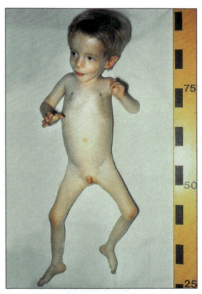

FIGURE 13.10 Russell–Silver syndrome. Full view of the child in **13.9**.

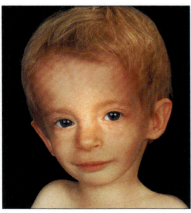

FIGURE 13.9 Russell–Silver syndrome in a child: facial asymmetry.

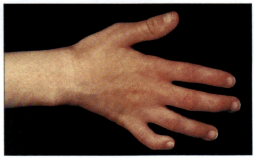

FIGURE 13.11 Russell–Silver syndrome in a child: clinodactyly.

TURNER SYNDROME

See also Chapter 15 Genetics, page 456.

INCIDENCE/GENETICS

This is the commonest abnormality of the sex chromosomes with an incidence of 1 in 2,500 live female births. Approximately 45% of cases have a 45XO karyotype in peripheral lymphocytes, with the remainder demonstrating karyotypic abnormalities or tissue mosaicism. In some cases the blood karyotype may be normal and fibroblast cell lines may need to be examined. Y chromosomal material may be present with an associated 20–30% risk of gonadoblastoma.

Short stature occurs due to loss of one copy of the *SHOX* gene located on the pseudoautosomal regions of the X and Y chromosomes. Abnormalities of this gene may also lead to short stature in children without evidence of Turner syndrome. Loss of both *SHOX* genes leads to Leri–Weill syndrome with severe skeletal abnormalities, including a Madelung deformity of the forearm (**Fig. 13.12**).

DIAGNOSIS

Turner syndrome may present in the neonatal period with lymphoedema of the hands and feet (**Fig. 13.13**) or coarctation of the aorta. Birth weight may be low (~1 standard deviation score [SDS] below the mean). Other clinical signs which may be present include widely-spaced nipples, anomalous auricles, epicanthic folds, micrognathia, low posterior hairline, webbed neck, cubitus valgus, osteoporosis, narrow hyperconvex nails (**Fig. 13.14**), excessive pigmented naevi, renal anomalies, idiopathic hypertension and aortic stenosis.

These children grow at a 25th centile height velocity during childhood, which leads to a further gradual loss of stature. Ovarian failure with streak gonads is observed in the vast majority of patients. Recurrent middle ear infections and autoimmune thyroiditis are common and sensorineural deafness, specific learning abnormalities, diabetes mellitus and coeliac disease are all associated with Turner syndrome. Renal anomalies such as horseshoe kidneys are frequently identified in these patients. Essential investigations are karyotype, ECHO, renal and pelvic ultrasound scans, gonadotrophins and thyroid function tests.

TREATMENT

Appropriate monitoring of blood pressure and treatment of cardiac and renal abnormalities, if present is instituted. Growth promotion may be achieved with the use of low-dose anabolic steroids (oxandrolone), GH and oestrogen, although the timing of these interventions remains a source of much debate. Pubertal induction with ethinyloestradiol

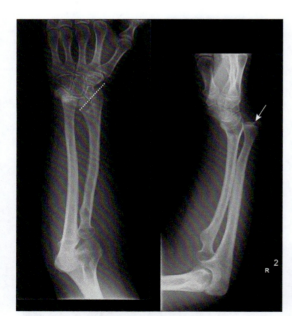

FIGURE 13.12 Leri–Weill dyschondrosteosis. AP and lateral radiographs of the right forearm in a teenage girl with heterozygous *SHOX* mutation. The radius is shortened, with a growth disturbance of the medial aspect of the distal radial physis, producing an increase tilt to the distal radius: the Madelung deformity (dotted line). In this case, the distal ulnar is dislocated due to the radial shortening.

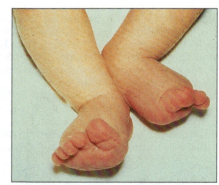

FIGURE 13.13 Turner syndrome; lymphoedema of the feet in a child.

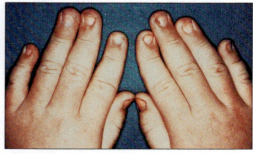

FIGURE 13.14 Turner syndrome; dysplastic nails in a child.

Endocrinology

and the later addition of progestogens is required in the majority of cases at the appropriate age. Ten percent of girls with Turner syndrome have a spontaneous onset of puberty but very few go on to achieve menarche (5–10%) and fertility (1%). Complications such as hypothyroidism are treated as they arise. If a Y chromosomal cell line has been demonstrated, the dysgenetic gonads should be removed because of the possibility of malignant change.

PROGNOSIS

The prognosis for final height is determined to a large extent by the parental heights. In the Western world, the mean final height of women with Turner syndrome is in the region of 143–146 cm, which is approximately 20 cm less than the average final height for normal adult females. The use of *in vitro* fertilisation and embryo implantation techniques have improved the prospects for childbearing.

PRADER–WILLI SYNDROME

GENETICS

Chromosomal analysis reveals a deletion in the long arm of the paternally-derived chromosome 15 (deletion of 15q11-13) or duplication of the maternal copy (uniparental disomy).

DIAGNOSIS

Prader–Willi syndrome (PWS) usually presents in the neonatal period with hypotonia and feeding difficulties. Birth weight may be low or normal. Characteristic facial features include a narrow forehead, almond-shaped eyes, strabismus and micrognathia. Small hands and feet are a feature of the condition, with tapering fingers and clinodactyly. Scoliosis, congenital dislocation of the hips, neurodevelopmental delay and hypogonadism with a micropenis, hypoplastic scrotum and bilateral cryptorchidism are other features of the condition.

Insatiable appetite from the age of 1–2 years leads to gross obesity (**Fig. 13.15**) with the ensuing complications of genu valgum, cellulitis, intertrigo, hypoventilation syndrome and diabetes mellitus. Endocrine features relate to hypothalamic defects. These include hypogonadotrophic hypogonadism, leading to poor secondary sexual development and delayed menarche and GHD. Short stature is a feature in a significant proportion of cases, with a poor pubertal growth spurt.

Essential investigations include detailed genetic analysis of chromosome 15; exclusion of other causes of obesity and hypotonia; investigation of gonadal function (luteinising hormone releasing hormone [LHRH] and human chorionic gonadotrophin [HCG] tests); and investigation of the hypothalamopituitary axis in children with a low growth velocity.

TREATMENT

The mainstay of treatment is severe dietary restriction. Energy requirements for growth are low, and these should be calculated and calorie intake appropriately restricted. Neurodevelopmental delay compounds the difficulties inherent in dietary restriction. In boys, bilateral orchidopexies may be required. Testosterone in the form of depot preparations has a role in the treatment of the hypogonadotrophic hypogonadism.

In girls, menarche may be delayed and oestrogen treatment may be required. GH treatment is licenced for use in PWS children with poor growth. It has been demonstrated to improve the hypotonia and motor development associated with PWS. However, there is a risk of lymphoid tissue overgrowth and airway obstruction necessitating Ear, Nose and Throat and sleep study assessment prior to commencing GH treatment. Central adrenal insufficiency is less common, but adrenal function should also be assessed prior to commencement of GH therapy.

PROGNOSIS

Dietary restriction and weight gain are often managed well in childhood, but become increasingly difficult in the young adult, with the consequence of gross obesity. Premature death due to bronchopneumonia or cardiorespiratory failure and Pickwickian syndrome with hypoventilation is usual. Additionally, the stress on the family is considerable.

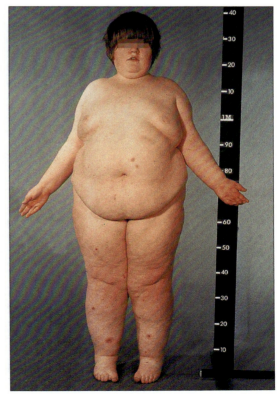

FIGURE 13.15 Prader–Willi syndrome: gross obesity in a child. Note the small hands and feet.

SKELETAL DYSPLASIAS

Several of these exist but only the commoner forms are described here – namely, achondroplasia, hypochondroplasia, spondyloepiphyseal dysplasia and multiple epiphyseal dysplasia.

INCIDENCE/GENETICS

- Achondroplasia: 1 in 10,000–15,000. It is caused by a mutation in the transmembrane domain of the fibroblast growth factor receptor-3 (FGFR3). It is inherited as an autosomal dominant condition with a fresh mutation rate of 90% and is associated with older paternal age.
- Hypochondroplasia is also inherited as an autosomal dominant trait and is due to mutations in FGFR3. In this case the defect is in the intracellular tyrosine kinase domain of the receptor.
- Spondyloepiphyseal dysplasia/multiple epiphyseal dysplasia: rare and inherited as autosomal dominant conditions.

DIAGNOSIS

Achondroplasia (**Fig. 13.16**) presents in the neonatal period with short limbs and characteristic craniofacial features. These include a large head with marked frontal bossing, a low nasal bridge and mild midfacial hypoplasia. Skeletal abnormalities include small cuboid vertebral bodies with short pedicles and progressive narrowing of lumbar interpedicular distance. Lumbar lordosis, mild thoracolumbar kyphosis, small iliac wings, short tubular bones and a short trident hand are other features of the condition (**Figs 13.17–13.19**). Mild hypotonia with some early motor delay is an occasional feature. Hydrocephalus secondary to a narrow foramen magnum is an associated feature. Spinal cord and/or root compression can occur as a consequence of kyphosis, spinal canal stenosis or disc lesions. Associated features include upper airways obstruction and recurrent otitis media. Pseudoachondroplasia resembles achondroplasia clinically.

Hypochondroplasia patients usually present with short stature in relation to mid-parental target height centile. The growth rate is initially normal, with a compromised pubertal growth spurt. Skeletal abnormalities are characteristic. Disproportion may only be apparent in puberty, although more severe cases may present earlier with disproportion (**Fig. 13.20**). Family history often reveals disproportionate short stature in one or both parents.

Spondyloepiphyseal dysplasia is characterised by prenatal onset growth deficiency, malar hypoplasia, cleft palate, severely shortened spine, lumbar lordosis, kyphoscoliosis, decreased arm span, weakness, talipes varus and developmental dysplasia of the hip.

Multiple epiphyseal dysplasia is characterised by short stature, with short metacarpals and phalanges, ovoid, flattened vertebral bodies, waddling gait, slow growth and early osteoarthritis. These features are by no means invariable.

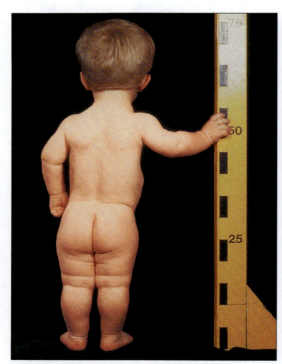

FIGURE 13.16 Achondroplasia: typical childhood appearance.

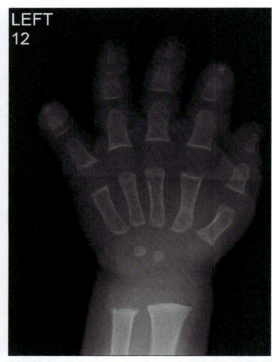

FIGURE 13.17 Left hand radiograph in a 5-month-old male with achondroplasia. There is generalised brachydactyly, with bullet shaped phalanges.

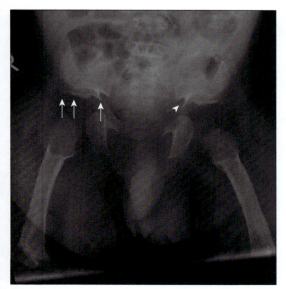

FIGURE 13.18 Pelvic radiograph in a 6-month-old male with achondroplasia. The iliac bones are small and squared off, being no wider than the acetabulum. The sacrosciatic notch (arrow head) is markedly narrowed. The acetabulum is almost horizontal and shows 'spikes' medially, centrally and laterally (white arrows): the 'trident' appearance. Note the apparent oval radiolucency in the upper femora, a typical feature at this age, due to sloping and foreshortening of the upper femoral metaphysis.

Essential investigations include a skeletal survey, especially an AP view of the spine to show diagnostic radiological features. In hypochondroplasia there is loss of the normal widening of the interpedicular distance proceeding down the lumbar spine. In achondroplasia neuroradiological imaging may be indicated if hydrocephalus is suspected.

TREATMENT

Treatment involves correction of hydrocephalus and orthopaedic abnormalities. The use of GH to treat achondroplastic children is often initially encouraging, but may increase the disproportion and has limited effect on final height. In hypochondroplasia GH treatment may enhance the pubertal growth spurt, although the effects of rhGH are variable and uncertain. GH treatment is of little use in pseudoachondroplasia, multiple epiphyseal dysplasia and spondyloepiphyseal dysplasia. Limb lengthening may be an option in achondroplasia and severe cases of hypochondroplasia. The gain in height needs to be balanced against the time and discomfort involved in these procedures.

PROGNOSIS

Without intervention, the height prognosis can be poor in achondroplasia, with a mean final height of 100–140 cm. It is more variable in hypochondroplasia.

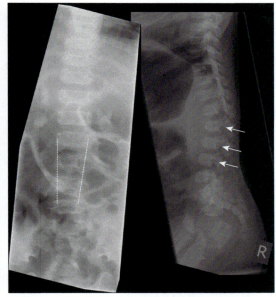

FIGURE 13.19 AP and lateral spinal radiographs in a 6-month-old male with achondroplasia. On the AP view the distance between the pedicles becomes narrower in the lower lumbar spine (dotted white lines). On the lateral view, the vertebral bodies are small, with a bullet shape and scalloping of their posterior borders (white arrows).

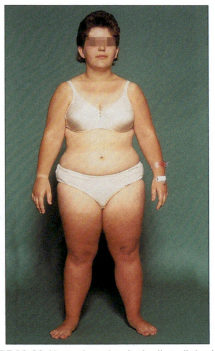

FIGURE 13.20 Hypochondroplasia: the clinical appearance shows obvious skeletal disproportion.

THE TALL CHILD

Tall children become tall adults by growing continuously at a rate greater than their smaller peers. A growth rate which is constantly around the 90th centile, a height attained that is greater than one might expect for the family and an increasing height prediction are all reasons to investigate the tall child. A plan of management for children with tall stature is presented in **Fig. 13.21**.

MARFAN SYNDROME

See also Chapter 15 Genetics, page 467.

INCIDENCE/GENETICS

Marfan syndrome is autosomal dominant, with a high *de novo* mutation rate.

PATHOGENESIS/AETIOLOGY

Heterozygous mutations in the fibrillin gene *FBN1* on chromosome 15q lead to widespread connective tissue abnormalities, and the characteristic skeletal, ocular and cardiovascular manifestations of Marfan syndrome.

DIAGNOSIS

Patients present with tall stature. Other features include arachnodactyly (**Figs 13.22, 13.23**), wide arm span, joint laxity, kyphoscoliosis, narrow face, high-arched palate, bluish sclerae, upward lenticular dislocation, aortic incompetence, dissecting aneurysm of aorta, mitral valve prolapse and inguinal or femoral herniae. The diagnosis is clinical and is often delayed until a cardiac presentation in adulthood. Investigations should include an ECHO, chromosomal analysis and measurement of urinary homocystine to exclude homocystinuria, the main differential diagnosis.

TREATMENT/PROGNOSIS

Tall stature may be limited by early induction of puberty. Cardiac lesions may need surgical intervention. Prognosis is dictated by the cardiac anomalies.

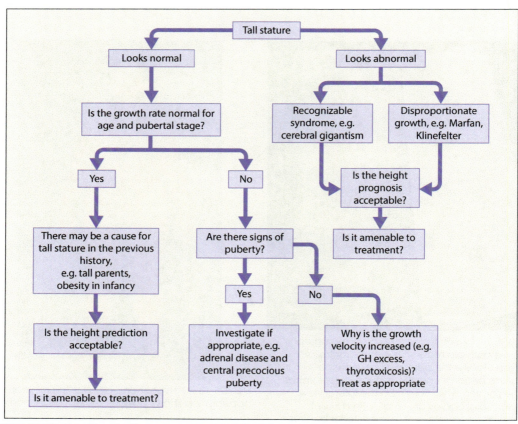

FIGURE 13.21 Algorithm for the management of the tall child. GH: growth hormone.

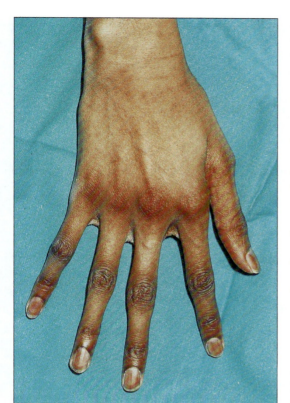

FIGURE 13.22 Marfan syndrome in a child demonstrating clinical appearance of arachnodactyly.

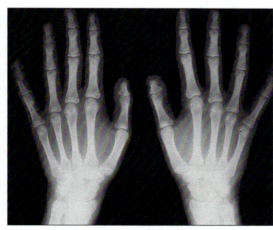

FIGURE 13.23 Radiological appearance of arachnodactyly in Marfan syndrome.

PITUITARY GIGANTISM

INCIDENCE/GENETICS

Pituitary gigantism is extremely rare. Activating Gsα mutations in signal-transducing G-proteins may account for up to 40% of adult somatotroph adenomas. Mutations in the aryl hydrocarbon interacting protein (AIP) can lead to dominantly inherited familial isolated pituitary adenomas (FIPA). The recent identification of heritable microduplications on chromosome Xq26.3 in patients with early childhood-onset pituitary gigantism, X-linked acrogigantism (X-LAG), has led to the implication of *GPR101*, encoding an orphan G-protein coupled receptor, in the aetiology of some cases of pituitary gigantism and sporadic acromegaly.

PATHOGENESIS/AETIOLOGY

The underlying lesion is usually a somatotroph adenoma. These lesions are associated with McCune–Albright syndrome (see page 393), multiple endocrine neoplasia I (MEN I), and Carney complex.

DIAGNOSIS

Children usually present with tall stature, irrespective of the mid-parental target centile (**Figs 13.24, 13.25**). The height velocity is generally greater than the 75th–97th centiles. Bone age is not advanced and precocious puberty should be excluded by clinical examination. Visual fields may reveal a deficit, although it is unlikely that a GH-secreting adenoma will be large enough to lead to such a deficit. A 24-hour GH secretory profile with measurement of serum GH concentrations at 20-minute intervals may be diagnostic. The profile is often difficult to distinguish from that of a child with constitutional tall stature. However, in gigantism, it is characterised by an inability of GH concentrations to achieve undetectable baseline concentrations (i.e. there are no troughs of GH secretion). The IGF-1 and IGF-BP3 concentrations are elevated.

Although in acromegalic adults there is a paradoxical increase in GH secretion in response to an oral glucose load or thyrotrophin releasing hormone (TRH), in childhood the situation is somewhat more complex. Paradoxical GH responses are often seen in both short and tall normal children during puberty. Imaging of the pituitary gland using MRI should be undertaken in all cases of suspected pituitary gigantism.

TREATMENT

The definitive treatment entails surgical removal of the adenoma, via the trans-sphenoidal approach. Medical treatment can be instituted using somatostatin analogues (octreotide), dopamine agonists (bromocriptine, cabergoline) or a GH receptor antagonist (pegvisomant). Pegvisomant is the most effective medical treatment and can reduce IGF-1 concentrations into the normal range, although it

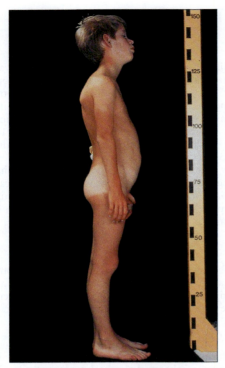

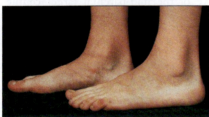

FIGURES 13.24, 13.25 Pituitary gigantism in a child. Note the large feet.

will have no effect on circulating GH concentrations or tumour size. Radiotherapy has limited effect, but may be used as second-line treatment.

PROGNOSIS

The overall prognosis in cases of isolated pituitary adenomata is generally good, once the lesion has been removed. However, there is a possibility that the lesion will recur. In the McCune–Albright syndrome and MEN I, the prognosis must be guarded, in view of the other complications associated with these conditions.

LATE PUBERTY

The algorithm in **Fig. 13.26** offers an approach to the diagnosis of conditions leading to late puberty.

KLINEFELTER SYNDROME

INCIDENCE/GENETICS

The incidence is 1 in 500 male births. Chromosomal analysis reveals at least one extra X chromosome added to the normal XY karyotype, most commonly 47 XXY.

PATHOGENESIS/AETIOLOGY

Tall stature results not only from the presence of additional chromosomal material but also from inadequate sexual development, which allows growth to continue at a normal rate far beyond its usual age of cessation.

DIAGNOSIS

This condition usually presents with tall stature and excessively long legs (**Figs 13.27, 13.28**). The patients tend to be slim initially, but can be obese as adults. Other features include hypogonadism with small testes and inadequate virilisation, infertility and gynaecomastia (**Fig. 13.28**). More severe disorders of sex development have been reported, including complete sex reversal. Children with this condition can have a low intelligence quotient (IQ) with poor school performance. Diabetes mellitus is commoner in adults with Klinefelter syndrome than in the general population. Investigations should include a karyotype and serum LH and follicle stimulating hormone (FSH), which are usually elevated (hypergonadotrophic hypogonadism). The serum testosterone is consequently low. A pelvic ultrasound scan is indicated if cryptorchidism is a feature.

TREATMENT

Some Klinefelter children enter a spontaneous puberty, but this arrests and requires testosterone treatment thereafter. In others pubertal induction and treatment with testosterone, usually in the form of depot injections administered at 2- to 4-weekly intervals may be indicated. Earlier treatment with testosterone can prevent the onset of gynaecomastia and can limit the tall stature associated with this condition.

PROGNOSIS

With the addition of testosterone therapy, pubertal development ensues. However, patients are generally infertile.

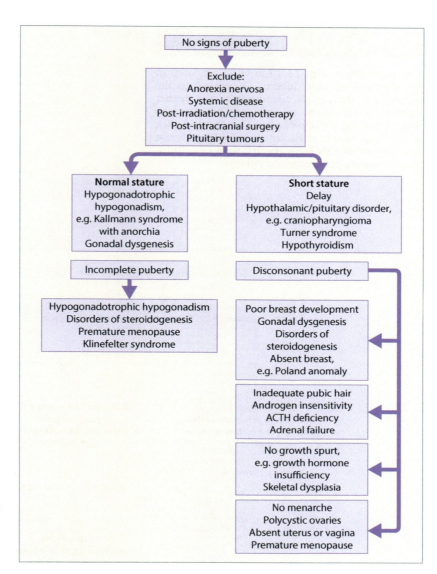

FIGURE 13.26 Algorithm for the diagnosis of late puberty. ACTH: adrenocorticotrophic hormone.

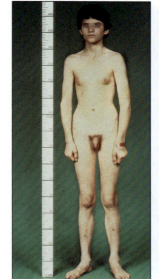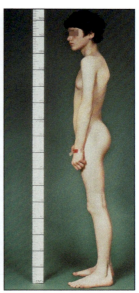

FIGURES 13.27, 13.28 Klinefelter syndrome: tall stature and slim build with eunuchoid appearances in a boy.

EARLY PUBERTY

The algorithm in **Fig. 13.29** gives an approach to the diagnosis of early puberty. Of essence to the diagnosis is the clinical assessment as to whether puberty is consonant or not (i.e. whether the sequence of pubertal development is normal or not), with enlargement of testicular size in boys and breast development in girls being the first signs of gonadotrophin-dependent precocious puberty.

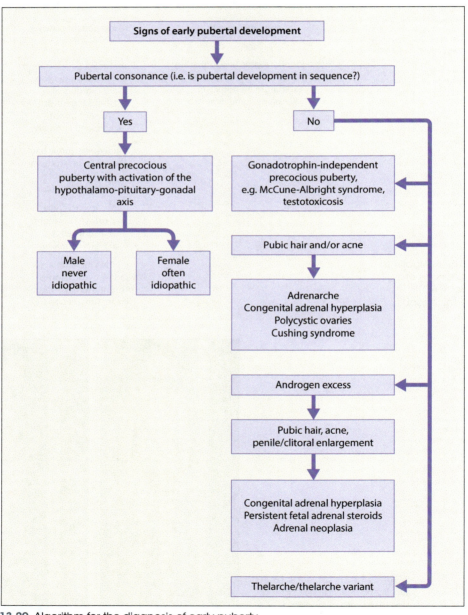

FIGURE 13.29 Algorithm for the diagnosis of early puberty.

PREMATURE THELARCHE/ THELARCHE VARIANT OR 'BENIGN' PRECOCIOUS PUBERTY

INCIDENCE/GENETICS

Premature thelarche is a sporadic condition which is commonly observed, particularly in neonates. Thelarche variant is less common and is likely to be a form of slowly progressing precocious puberty.

PATHOGENESIS/AETIOLOGY

Ovarian cyst development due to isolated pulsatile FSH secretion results in the secretion of oestrogen and isolated breast development.

DIAGNOSIS

In premature thelarche, girls usually present with isolated early breast development (**Fig. 13.30**). Over 80% of girls have cyclical breast development that waxes and wanes at intervals of 4–6 weeks. The age of onset is usually below 2 years and frequently continues as an extension of the neonatal breast enlargement, due to placental transmission of maternal oestrogens. Such development is usually associated with isolated ovarian cyst development, which is due to premature but isolated pulsatile FSH secretion. The uterus is of an appropriate size and shape for age, with no endometrial echo and only exceptionally is there a vaginal bleed. Growth is at a normal rate, and the bone age is not advanced. There are no other signs of puberty.

In thelarche variant, increased stature, advanced bone age, a small uterus, and an ovarian morphology between that for premature thelarche and precocious puberty, are characteristically associated with isolated breast development. Investigations should include a bone age in children over the age of 3 years (advanced in thelarche variant, but not in premature thelarche) and a pelvic ultrasound scan (**Fig. 13.31**). FSH concentrations are raised, with a pulsatile secretory pattern, and the response of FSH to gonadotrophin-releasing hormone (GnRH) is brisk. Thyroid function should be tested, since in primary hypothyroidism, isolated breast development may occur due to elevated FSH concentrations.

TREATMENT/PROGNOSIS

No treatment is required for these conditions. Both conditions are benign with no effect on the growth prognosis. The conditions may continue largely unchanged with waxing and waning of breast size in parallel to ovarian cyst size until puberty.

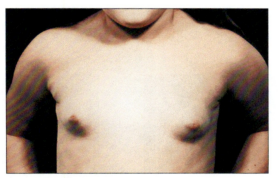

FIGURE 13.30 Thelarche in a 5-year-old girl.

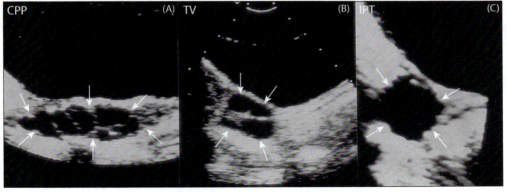

FIGURE 13.31 Pelvic ultrasound in central precocious puberty (A) compared with thelarche variant (B) and isolated premature thelarche (C).

GONADOTROPHIN-DEPENDENT (CENTRAL) PRECOCIOUS PUBERTY

INCIDENCE/GENETICS

The condition is relatively common in girls (M:F ratio of 1:10). Most cases are sporadic. In a few cases, mutations in the maternally imprinted gene *MKRN3*, encoding Makorin Ring Finger 3, have been implicated in the aetiology of central precocious puberty. The condition is inherited as an autosomal dominant and is exclusively paternally transmitted.

PATHOGENESIS/AETIOLOGY

Premature activation of the hypothalamic–pituitary gonadal axis leads to a sequence of sexual maturation that is identical to that of normal puberty. In girls, often no underlying cause can be demonstrated. In boys, pineal and other intracranial tumours and hamartomata may be present. Other causes of secondary central precocious puberty include hydrocephalus and neurofibromatosis and previous cranial irradiation.

Hypothalamic hamartomata (**Fig. 13.32**) present with early puberty in both sexes and are congenital tumours containing GnRH neurons, which secrete GnRH to induce puberty. They are otherwise benign but are associated with gelastic seizures and developmental delay in some cases.

DIAGNOSIS

Children usually present with early signs of puberty. In boys, testicular enlargement is the first sign while in girls, breast development is the first sign (**Fig. 13.33**). In boys, the aetiology is rarely idiopathic (**Fig. 13.34**), and signs of an underlying condition may be present (e.g. neurological abnormalities secondary to a brain tumour, hydrocephalus, neurofibromatosis).

Tall stature with an increased height velocity is a feature of central precocious puberty in both boys and girls. Behavioural disturbances may also be evident, with an inappropriate degree of sexualisation. A pelvic ultrasound scan in girls will reveal a multi-cystic ovarian morphology in response to pulsatile gonadotrophin secretion. The demonstration of a physiological pulsatile pattern of gonadotrophin secretion over a 24-hour period is the investigation of choice, but can be expensive and time-consuming. An LHRH test shows a brisk pubertal LH and FSH response to LHRH, with LH predominance.

The bone age will be advanced. The sex incidence of intracranial lesions is equal. However, since girls outnumber boys with precocious puberty, the majority of girls do not have an underlying lesion accounting for the precocious puberty. Neuroradiological imaging of the brain is indicated in all boys with precocious puberty, and in all girls with neurological signs and symptoms.

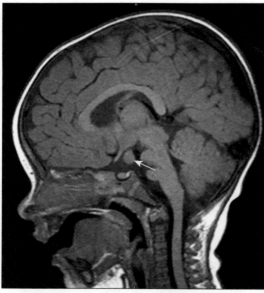

FIGURE 13.32 Hypothalamic hamartoma (arrow).

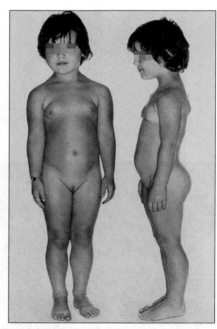

FIGURE 13.33 Idiopathic gonadotrophin-dependent precocious puberty in a 6-year-old girl.

TREATMENT

Treatment is indicated if puberty occurs at an early age with consequent psychological disturbance and implications for final height. Masturbation and other forms of inappropriate sexual behaviour can lead to major problems for the family, particularly in boys. Additionally, the onset of menarche at primary school is a cause of much distress and is also an indication for treatment. Treatment can alter the final height prognosis in the younger child; the use of GH has not been shown to improve the height prognosis. GnRH analogues are used in the treatment of this complex condition when there is likely to be compromise to final height or where there are significant psychological considerations.

PROGNOSIS

Although pubertal development can be arrested, the final height of these children may be unaffected by treatment, particularly if not started early. Early sexual maturation is associated with the early growth acceleration of puberty. In addition, rapid epiphyseal maturation occurs in response to increased sex steroid secretion, which ultimately limits growth. Although children with early puberty tend to be tall when they are young, their final height prognosis is compromised. The earlier the onset of puberty and the shorter the parental heights, the shorter the child's final height will be. Polycystic ovarian syndrome can be a late problem.

MCCUNE–ALBRIGHT SYNDROME

INCIDENCE/GENETICS

McCune–Albright syndrome is a rare condition caused by an activating mutation in the gene for the α-subunit of Gs, the G-protein that stimulates cyclic adenosine monophosphate (cAMP) formation. The mutation is found to a variable extent in different affected endocrine and non-endocrine tissues, consistent with the mosaic distribution of abnormal cells generated by a somatic cell mutation early in embryogenesis.

DIAGNOSIS

Presentation is varied, and clinical features include the presence of large irregular pigmented lesions (unilateral in 50%) (**Fig. 13.35**), polyostotic fibrous dysplasia, gonadotrophin-independent precocious puberty (**Fig. 13.36**) and other endocrinopathies (e.g. Cushing syndrome, excessive GH secretion by pituitary somatotroph adenomata and thyrotoxicosis). Patients with this condition can present at any age, including the neonatal period. Non-endocrine abnormalities include chronic hepatic disease, thymic hyperplasia and cardiopulmonary disease.

A skeletal survey and a bone scan show the characteristic bony abnormalities of polyostotic fibrous dysplasia (**Fig. 13.37**). Precocious puberty is caused by autonomously functioning follicular cysts and therefore GnRH stimulation fails to increase

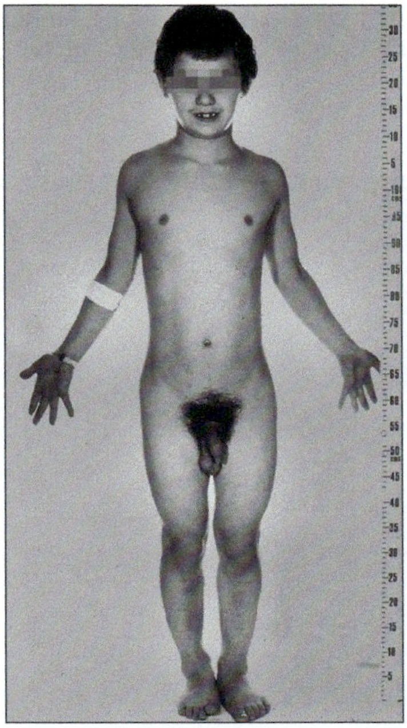

FIGURE 13.34 Gonadotrophin-dependent precocious puberty in a 7-year-old boy with a subarachnoid cyst. Note the body disproportion with the short limbs in relation to the spine.

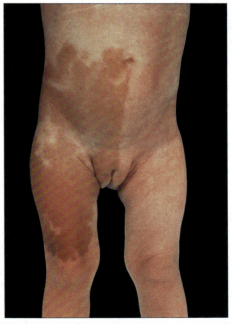

FIGURE 13.35 McCune–Albright syndrome: typical large café-au-lait pigmented area with an irregular margin in a child.

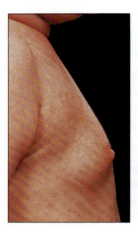

FIGURE 13.36 McCune–Albright syndrome: precocious puberty (gonadotrophin-independent) in a 2-year-old girl.

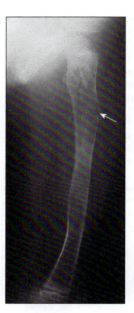

FIGURE 13.37 McCune–Albright syndrome showing polyostotic fibrous dysplasia in a child.

gonadotrophin levels. Gonadotrophin-dependent puberty occurs later. Appropriate investigations for Cushing syndrome, thyrotoxicosis and pituitary adenomata leading to GH excess are performed as and when necessary. Other investigations should include liver function tests and an ECHO.

TREATMENT/PROGNOSIS

The precocious puberty can be difficult to control. Agents used include cyproterone acetate, medroxyprogesterone and aromatase inhibitors (testolactone, letrozole, anastrozole), but they are all of limited efficacy. Abnormalities of other endocrine glands are treated as and when the problems arise (e.g. bilateral adrenalectomy for Cushing syndrome, carbimazole for thyrotoxicosis).

Prognosis is variable. It is much poorer for early-onset McCune–Albright syndrome with multi-organ involvement. Sudden death can occur due to cardiopulmonary involvement.

POLYCYSTIC OVARIAN DISEASE

INCIDENCE/GENETICS

The incidence of polycystic ovarian (PCO) disease shows a familial predisposition, although the genes implicated have not been identified to date. PCO can be found in 6% of 6-year-old girls and this increases to 25% of the female adult population on pelvic ultrasound scanning.

PATHOGENESIS/AETIOLOGY

Predisposing factors include hyperandrogenism (e.g. congenital adrenal hyperplasia), insulin insensivity, tall stature and obesity. Treatment with GH is also associated with PCO, as is diabetes mellitus.

DIAGNOSIS

This condition usually presents with late menarche and menstrual irregularities, and accounts for 87% of irregular menstrual cycles in unselected adult females. The polycystic ovarian syndrome (PCOS; Stein–Leventhal syndrome) is characterised by hyperandrogenism, oligoanovulation and evidence of PCO on ultrasound. Patients may present with oligomenorrhoea, acne, hirsutism, obesity, acanthosis nigricans or insulin insensitivity.

Pelvic ultrasound scan shows the classical appearance of large ovaries with increased stroma and a characteristic arrangement of 12 or more follicles around the periphery of the ovary (**Fig. 13.38**). Other investigations include serum LH (elevated in 70% of PCOS patients), raised concentrations of androgens, reduced sex hormone binding globulin (SHBG), an elevated fasting glucose level and

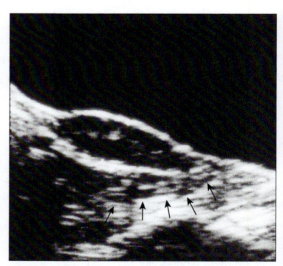

FIGURE 13.38 Polycystic ovary syndrome: classic ovarian ultrasound appearance, with a 'necklace' of cysts around the periphery of the ovary.

measurement of elevated insulin concentrations during an oral glucose tolerance test. Raised IGF-1 concentrations due to suppressed IGF binding proteins lead to further androgen stimulation. The diagnosis of late onset congenital adrenal hyperplasia (pages 403–404) and other causes of hyperandrogenism need to be excluded in children who present predominantly with hirsutism.

TREATMENT

Irregularities of the menstrual cycles can be controlled with oral contraceptive pills containing an antiandrogenic progesterone. Other antiandrogens (cyproterone acetate, spironolactone and flutamide) can also be used to alleviate the effects of hyperandrogenism. Insulin sensitisers, including metformin, and dermatological treatments may also be considered.

PROGNOSIS

Fertility can be impaired in up to 25% of women. However, in the vast majority of individuals, fertility is normal. The long-term outlook is also determined by the presence of obesity, hypertension and diabetes mellitus.

THYROID DISORDERS

CONGENITAL HYPOTHYROIDISM

INCIDENCE/GENETICS

The incidence is 1 in 4,000 newborn infants. Those cases due to an inborn error of hormonogenesis are inherited in an autosomal recessive fashion, while those due to a dysgenetic gland have a low recurrence rate (1 in 100). Mutations in several transcription factors including PAX8, TTF1 and TTF2 are associated with the latter.

PATHOGENESIS/AETIOLOGY

The thyroid gland develops from endoderm in the midline of the pharyngeal floor at the base of the developing tongue. As the thyroid descends anterior to the pharyngeal gut it remains connected to the tongue by the thyroglossal duct. This duct later obliterates, but may remain *in situ* in parts. This can predispose to the formation of a thyroglossal cyst (**Fig. 13.39**).

The primary form of the congenital hypothyroidism is due to agenesis of the thyroid gland, a dysgenetic gland or dyshormonogenesis. Failure of descent of the thyroid can lead to ectopic glands that are also usually dysgenetic (**Figure 13.40**).

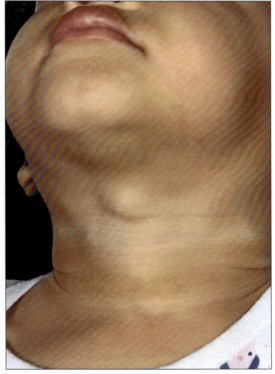

FIGURE 13.39 Thyroglossal cyst.

The much rarer secondary form of the disease is due to thyroid stimulating hormone (TSH) deficiency, either isolated or due to pituitary hypoplasia, when it may be associated with other pituitary hormone deficiencies.

DIAGNOSIS

This condition is usually detected on neonatal screening. In the UK, TSH screening occurs at 5–10 days of age; in other regions screening may be T4-based. Screening has resulted in a massive decline in cretinism, and few infants now manifest clinical evidence of severe thyroxine deficiency. Clinical features, when present, include an umbilical hernia, macroglossia, constipation, feeding problems, lethargy, respiratory distress, prolonged jaundice, hoarse cry, hypotonia, coarse facies (**Fig. 13.41**), growth failure, abundant hair, delayed closure of fontanelles, hypothermia and a dry, mottled skin. Retarded bone maturation with delayed epiphyseal ossification and epiphyseal dysgenesis are other features. These usually appear if the diagnosis has been missed for more than 6 weeks. Other congenital malformations are present in 7% of cases.

Investigations include a free thyroxine concentration (low) and serum TSH (elevated). A radioisotope scan may differentiate between thyroid dysgenesis and dyshormonogenesis, locate the thyroid gland and enable a decision to be made regarding life-long therapy. In view of the association between congenital hypothyroidism and deafness, audiological assessment should be performed in these children.

Transient hypothyroidism occurs in some children and may be due to maternal antibody transmission, drugs or iodine imbalance. In children with low thyroxine requirements, it is suggested that they have a trial off thyroxine treatment at the age of 3 years to establish if the hypothyroidism is permanent or transient.

If the hypothyroidism is secondary (due to congenital TRH or TSH deficiency), assessment of pituitary/hypothalamic function including measurement of GH, cortisol, prolactin and gonadotrophin secretion may be indicated. A TRH test may be appropriate in some instances. Isolated TSH deficiency may be due to mutations in the genes encoding TRH receptor or the TSH-β subunit. Recently, mutations in the X-linked *IGSF1* gene have been identified in some patients with central hypothyroidism and macro-orchidism.

TREATMENT

Treatment is with thyroxine at a starting dose of 8–10 μg/kg/day (maximum 50 μg once daily) with frequent initial clinical and biochemical follow-up, particularly in the first year of life. Subsequent monitoring entails careful documentation of the growth rate, which is an extremely sensitive measure of thyroid function.

PROGNOSIS

Before the introduction of screening, the major complications of late-treated congenital hypothyroidism were impaired intelligence and a range of abnormalities of neurological function, particularly with respect to co-ordination. These neuropsychological sequelae are now much less marked, following the advent of screening. Nevertheless, the IQ of these patients is closely related to the pretreatment thyroxine concentration in serum. For example, in those children with a low pretreatment thyroxine concentration (total thyroxine below 42 nmol/l or free thyroxine <5 pmol/l), a mean deficit of approximately 10 IQ points can be observed compared with controls. Subjects with pretreatment thyroxine concentrations greater than 42 nmol/l have similar IQ scores to normal children.

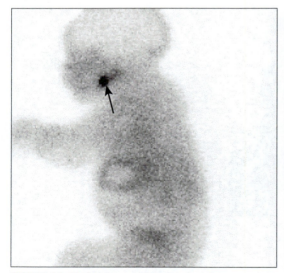

FIGURE 13.40 Sublingual thyroid gland demonstrated on technetium scan (arrow).

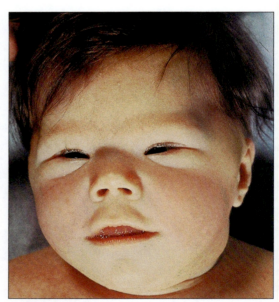

FIGURE 13.41 Congenital hypothyroidism: typical coarse facies of a child.

ACQUIRED HYPOTHYROIDISM

INCIDENCE/GENETICS

Autoimmune hypothyroidism is associated with a family history in 30–40% of cases and is one of the commonest forms of acquired hypothyroidism.

PATHOGENESIS/AETIOLOGY

World-wide, iodine deficiency is the commonest cause of hypothyroidism. Causes of acquired hypothyroidism include goitrogenic agents, thyroid dysgenesis, autoimmune thyroiditis, pituitary TSH deficiency (e.g. postcranial irradiation and craniopharyngioma), endemic iodine deficiency and cystinosis. Chromosomal disorders (i.e. Turner, Down and Klinefelter syndromes) are associated with an increased incidence of hypothyroidism, which is probably autoimmune in origin.

DIAGNOSIS

This can present at any age, usually with a gradual onset. The most important sign in childhood is growth failure. A goitre may be present. There is a modest weight gain, with disproportion between weight and height gain (**Fig. 13.42**). Isolated breast development or testicular enlargement, without other signs of puberty or an increase in height velocity, results from excessive FSH secretion. In contrast, pubertal delay or arrest can also be a feature. Other signs of classical hypothyroidism are slow to develop (e.g. mental sluggishness, cold intolerance, fatigue, constipation, bradycardia, dry skin, coarse facies, proximal myopathy). Classically, tendon reflex relaxation is slow and the bone age is delayed.

These children are usually extremely well-behaved and compliant and do well at school. There may be features of other autoimmune conditions (e.g. Addison disease, myasthenia gravis, insulin-dependent diabetes mellitus, pernicious anaemia, malabsorption and vitiligo) as thyroid disease may be a component of polyglandular autoimmune disease.

Investigations should include free thyroxine, serum TSH, thyroid peroxidase autoantibodies, thyroglobulin, FSH and prolactin (may be elevated in primary hypothyroidism). Family members are at increased risk of autoimmune hypothyroidism and should be screened where appropriate.

TREATMENT

Treatment with thyroxine should be commenced cautiously, at a dosage of 50 μg/m^2/d initially, with a subsequent increase to 100 μg/m^2/d, depending on the TSH level. Commencement of treatment can lead to severe behavioural changes, with considerable disruption to family life and the child's schooling. The model compliant child's return to a normal level of activity is often extremely traumatic. When treatment begins there is a catch-up phase of growth, followed by a subsequent return to a normal height velocity.

PROGNOSIS

The prognosis for final height, fertility and general health is excellent, provided treatment is commenced early and adherence is good.

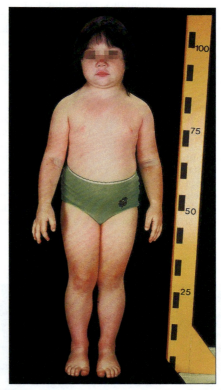

FIGURE 13.42 Acquired hypothyroidism: typical appearance of a child. Note the disproportion between height and weight.

GRAVES DISEASE

INCIDENCE/GENETICS

Autoimmune thyrotoxicosis is six to eight times more common in girls. Often, a family history of autoimmune thyroid disease can be elicited.

PATHOGENESIS/AETIOLOGY

Thyroid stimulating antibodies are present in the serum of these patients and are responsible for the clinical picture observed. Autonomous functioning thyroid nodules are rare in children, as is autonomous TSH production from the thyrotroph or pituitary tumours.

DIAGNOSIS

This can occur in preschool children, but there is a sharp increase in incidence in adolescence. The onset may be abrupt or insidious. Presenting features may include nervousness, palpitations, tremor, excessive perspiration, an increased appetite, muscle weakness, marked weight loss and behavioural abnormalities. Tachycardia, a widened pulse pressure, an overactive praecordium and heart failure may dominate the clinical picture. A goitre is the most frequent clinical sign, the size being variable (**Fig. 13.43**). A bruit and a thrill may be features of the goitre.

Eye signs of Graves disease are variable. Severe Graves ophthalmopathy is much less common in children than in adults. Malignant exophthalmos is virtually unknown. Features in childhood include lid retraction, lid lag, exophthalmos, proptosis (**Fig. 13.44**), ophthalmoplegia, chemosis of the conjunctiva, pain, swelling and irritation. Graves dermopathy, whereby there is accumulation of mucopolysaccharides in skin and subcutaneous tissues, is rare in children.

There may be evidence of other autoimmune conditions (e.g. vitiligo, Addison disease, myasthenia, pernicious anaemia and insulin-dependent diabetes mellitus). Investigations of free thyroxine, free tri-iodothyronine and TSH concentrations (suppressed) are mandatory. An autoantibody screen may show thyroid stimulating antibodies to the thyroid gland. A thyroid ultrasound scan may be required if a solitary nodule is suspected.

TREATMENT

Treatment entails reducing the secretory rate of thyroxine with the use of antithyroid medication such as carbimazole or methimazole and blunting its effects using propranolol. Carbimazole is associated with agranulocytosis and propylthiouracil is no longer recommended as a first-line treatment due to hepatotoxic side-effects. The condition may relapse once the medication is stopped; remission rates are low in children, and may be <50% after 4 years. In the long term, definitive treatment in the form of a thyroidectomy or radioactive iodine may be indicated.

Complications of surgery include hypoparathyroidism and recurrent laryngeal nerve damage. Alternatively, radioactive iodine is easy to administer and cheap. To date, concern about radiation oncogenesis and genetic damage has limited its use to adolescents, although anxieties regarding the former have largely been alleviated in adults. It is contraindicated in children with Graves eye disease. Post-treatment hypothyroidism needs to be treated with thyroxine.

PROGNOSIS

Once definitive treatment has been performed, lifelong thyroxine treatment is indicated. With this, the prognosis is good providing compliance is satisfactory. The course of the eye manifestations and the thyroid disease may differ, and exophthalmos may persist despite satisfactory treatment of the hyperthyroidism.

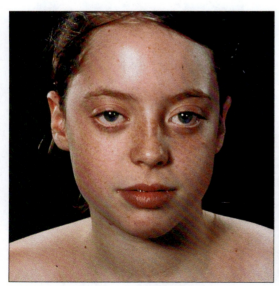

FIGURE 13.43 Graves disease; thyroid goitre.

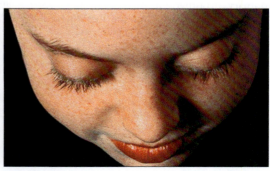

FIGURE 13.44 Graves disease: bilateral proptosis.

Endocrinology

ADRENAL DISORDERS

PRIMARY ADRENAL INSUFFICIENCY

INCIDENCE/GENETICS

The incidence of congenital adrenal hypoplasia has been reported as 1 in 12,500 births. Inheritance is either as an autosomal or X-linked recessive condition. Mutations in the *DAX1* gene are associated with the X-linked form of the disease. Autoimmune adrenal insufficiency is associated with the two types of polyglandular autoimmune syndrome (**Table 13.2**). Type I is associated with mutations in the *AIRE* (autoimmune regulator) gene on chromosome 21. Familial glucocorticoid deficiency (FGD) and triple A syndrome are characterised by an insensitivity to adrenocorticotrophic hormone (ACTH) concentrations. FGD is caused by mutations in the ACTH receptor (*MC2R*), or mutations in the MC2R accessory protein MRAP. More recently, mutations in the genes encoding nicotinamide nucleotide transhydrogenase (NNT) and minichromosome maintenance-deficient 4 (MCM4) have also been associated with FGD. Triple A syndrome is autosomal dominant and secondary to mutations in the *ALADIN* gene.

PATHOGENESIS/AETIOLOGY

Causes of primary adrenal insufficiency include congenital adrenal hypoplasia, defects of adrenal steroid biosynthesis, adrenal haemorrhage, autoimmune adrenalitis, multiple endocrinopathy, infections (e.g. tuberculosis and Waterhouse–Friederichsen syndrome), adrenoleukodystrophy (see also Chapter 14 Metabolic diseases, page 417) and iatrogenic (chemical or surgical) causes.

DIAGNOSIS

Congenital adrenal hypoplasia usually presents in the neonatal period with hypoglycaemia, salt loss, apnoeic episodes, dehydration, poor feeding, failure to thrive, vomiting and hyperpigmentation. In Addison disease, presentation is usually later and symptoms and signs include lethargy, anorexia, vomiting, weight loss, irritability, salt-losing adrenal crisis, hypoglycaemia, syncope and hyperpigmentation of the skin and mucosal surfaces (**Fig. 13.45**).

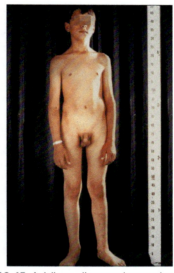

FIGURE 13.45 Addison disease: hyperpigmentation in a child.

TABLE 13.2 Polyglandular autoimmune syndrome

	Type 1	Type 2
Inheritance (autosomal)	Recessive (due to mutations in AIRE)	Dominant
Age at onset	Childhood (<12 years)	Adulthood (>30 years)
Female : male ratio	1.5:1	1.8:1
HLA association	None	B6, -Dw3, -DR3
Disease components:		
Addison disease	65%	100%
Hypoparathyroidism	80%	None
Mucocutaneous candidiasis	75%	None
Alopecia	25%	<1%
Malabsorption	22%	None
Gonadal failure	20%	20%
Pernicious anaemia	13%	<1%
Autoimmune thyroid disease	10%	70%
Chronic active hepatitis	10%	None
Diabetes mellitus	8%	5%
Vitiligo	8%	5%

In adrenoleukodystrophy, neurological symptoms and signs may develop first, with features of adrenal insufficiency developing between the ages of 4 and 8 years. In polyglandular autoimmune syndrome, features of other autoimmune conditions such as hypoparathyroidism, diabetes mellitus, vitiligo, myasthenia gravis, coeliac disease and pernicious anaemia may also be present. Mucocutaneous candidiasis is a feature of Type 1 polyglandular autoimmune syndrome.

FGD may present as acute or chronic glucocorticoid insufficiency in childhood. Production of aldosterone is generally maintained because the adrenal zona glomerulosa is regulated by the renin–angiotensin system, although rarely FGD is associated with early mineralocorticoid deficiency. Although glucocorticoid insufficiency is seen in around 80% of patients with triple A syndrome (adrenal deficiency, achalasia of the cardia and alacrima), the condition rarely presents in this manner. It is also associated with progressive neurological symptoms, sensorineural deafness, peripheral neuropathies and autonomic dysfunction.

Investigations should include plasma urea and electrolytes (hyponatraemia, hyperkalaemia), a cortisol profile (low values of cortisol), a synacthen test (no cortisol response to exogenous ACTH), a plasma ACTH level (elevated), plasma renin activity and aldosterone level (renin is raised with a low aldosterone level if mineralocorticoid deficiency is associated), an autoantibody screen, thyroid function, plasma calcium and fasting glucose (low in Addison disease, but may be elevated if associated with diabetes mellitus). Plasma very long-chain fatty acids (VLCFA) levels are useful in excluding a diagnosis of adrenoleukodystrophy.

TREATMENT

Initially, hypovolaemia should be corrected with adequate fluid and sodium replacement, followed by maintenance treatment with replacement doses of glucocorticoids in the form of hydrocortisone, with added mineralocorticoid treatment in the form of 9α-fludrocortisone if the diagnosis of mineralocorticoid deficiency is confirmed. Indication of adequate dosage is given by general well-being, normal appetite and activity, weight gain and normal growth. When hypothyroidism is present in a child with chronic adrenal insufficiency, adequate glucocorticoid therapy should be established before commencing thyroxine therapy, otherwise an adrenal crisis would be precipitated. Children with ACTH insensitivity require treatment with physiological replacement doses of glucocorticoids. The use of higher doses of glucocorticoids to suppress the ACTH concentration into the normal range should be avoided.

PROGNOSIS

Given correct treatment and adequate parental support, patients with congenital adrenal hypoplasia and Addison disease can lead a normal life with a normal life-span. However, growth and pubertal development need careful monitoring. In congenital adrenal hypoplasia, hypogonadotrophic hypogonadism is associated with the condition, and so puberty may need to be induced. The prognosis in polyglandular autoimmune disease is poor if chronic active hepatitis is also present. The prognosis in adrenoleukodystrophy is that of the underlying neurological disorder, which progresses inexorably.

CUSHING SYNDROME

INCIDENCE/GENETICS

Iatrogenic Cushing syndrome is relatively common. Endogenous Cushing syndrome is rare and the underlying lesion is usually a pituitary adenoma (Cushing disease). Adrenal tumours predominate in female infants under 2 years of age, in whom the underlying diagnosis may be that of the McCune–Albright syndrome. Ectopic ACTH production in children leading to Cushing syndrome is extremely rare. Cushing syndrome is sporadic, although very rare forms of familial hypercortisolism have been described.

PATHOGENESIS/AETIOLOGY

Cushing syndrome can be iatrogenic, due to a corticotrophin releasing hormone (CRH)- or ACTH-secreting tumour (either in the pituitary gland or due to ectopic secretion of the stimulating hormone), ACTH-independent Cushing syndrome due to adrenal neoplasms or nodular adrenal hyperplasia. This may be familial, as in the Carney complex (bilateral micronodular adrenal hyperplasia, pigmented lentigines, atrial myxomas and other tumours). Up to 50% of cases of the Carney complex are caused by mutations in the *PRKAR1A* gene. McCune–Albright syndrome (see page 393) can also lead to primary adrenal Cushing syndrome.

DIAGNOSIS

Children with this syndrome present with excessive weight gain leading to rapidly progressing obesity that is mainly truncal in nature (**Fig. 13.46**). Other features include round 'moon-like' facies (**Fig. 13.47**), a midscapular fat pad 'buffalo-hump', hypertension, purple striae (**Fig. 13.48**), hirsutism, osteoporosis, hypogonadism, proximal myopathy, susceptibility to bruising and infection, cataracts, pubertal arrest, amenorrhoea, emotional lability and growth arrest, although, initially, androgen secretion may lead to acceleration of the height velocity.

In Cushing disease (due to a pituitary adenoma), headaches and visual disturbance may be a feature, with impaired visual fields, and even papilloedema. Diagnosis can be extremely difficult, and is based upon elevated plasma cortisol concentrations with a loss of circadian rhythm and elevated 24-hour urinary free cortisol. In pituitary-dependent Cushing disease, ACTH concentrations are detectable in the face of raised cortisol concentrations. In primary adrenal Cushing syndrome, ACTH concentrations will be suppressed in the face of elevated cortisol concentrations.

In ectopic Cushing syndrome, both cortisol and ACTH concentrations are extremely high. Once the diagnosis is established, the source of the excess cortisol production needs to be established. Dexamethasone suppresses cortisol production in normal individuals. In pituitary-dependent Cushing disease, low-dose dexamethasone will not suppress cortisol secretion, but high-dose dexamethasone will suppress it in approximately 80% of cases.

Adrenal and ectopic Cushing syndrome will not suppress with any dose of dexamethasone. Administration of CRH can be helpful in differentiating an adrenal and pituitary cause of the syndrome. Imaging of the pituitary and adrenals using MRI is usually indicated in order to locate the tumour, although the sensitivity is poor (70%). Inferior petrosal sinus sampling has a similar sensitivity and can be performed to locate a pituitary lesion and to lateralise a pituitary adenoma.

TREATMENT

Pituitary-dependent Cushing disease is usually treated by trans-sphenoidal removal of the adenoma by an experienced neurosurgeon. Where an adrenal tumour is defined, surgical removal of the tumour is indicated. Medical treatment with metyrapone or ketoconazole may be required to suppress cortisol production but is not without its own problems and is generally used as a temporary measure. Adrenalectomy is usually indicated in cases of adrenal neoplasms or multi-nodular adrenal hyperplasia, although subtotal resection may be an option in certain cases.

PROGNOSIS

In untreated patients, the mortality and morbidity from this condition is high, with osteoporosis, glucose intolerance and hypertension accounting for this. Following surgical treatment of Cushing disease, there is a strong possibility that the condition either does not remit, or relapses. In this case, further exploration of the pituitary with a possible total hypophysectomy may be indicated. Radiotherapy can be used as a second-line treatment. In these situations, the child will have panhypopituitarism and therefore will need replacement hydrocortisone, thyroxine, gonadotrophins or sex steroids, growth hormone and DDAVP treatment. However, the outlook is nevertheless better than that following a bilateral adrenalectomy with consequent Nelson syndrome. If the Cushing syndrome is due to an adrenal carcinoma or an ectopic source (usually a lung carcinoid), the prognosis is much worse.

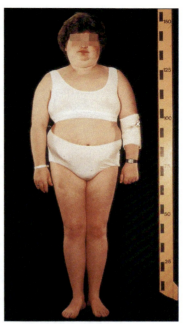

FIGURE 13.46 Cushing syndrome: central obesity.

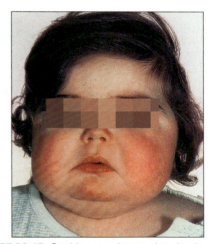

FIGURE 13.47 Cushing syndrome showing 'moonlike' facies in a child.

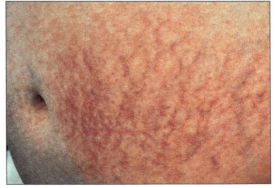

FIGURE 13.48 Cushing syndrome: purple abdominal striae in a child.

401

AMBIGUOUS GENITALIA

See also Chapter 22 Urology, page 672.

INCIDENCE/GENETICS

Congenital adrenal hyperplasia (CAH) and 5α-reductase deficiency (**Figs 13.49, 13.50**) are inherited as autosomal recessive disorders. Mutations of the genes encoding 5α-reductase, 21-hydroxylase, steroidogenic factor 1, Wilms tumour and the androgen receptor have been described. The incidence of CAH is 1 in 15,000, while 5α-reductase deficiency and androgen insensitivity are much rarer (**Table 13.3**).

DIAGNOSIS

Ambiguous genitalia are usually present at birth. The gender of the child should not be assigned without confirmation. If possible, referral to an expert Disorders of Sex Development (DSD) team should be made. Note should be made of presence or absence of palpable gonads and their position if felt. External genitalia can be described as Prader staging. The disorder may be associated with salt loss in salt-losing congenital adrenal hyperplasia (see pages 403–4). There may be associated dysmorphic features.

INVESTIGATIONS

Karyotype (or interim fluorescence *in situ* hybridisation [FISH] analysis) should be sent immediately. Further investigations should include plasma electrolytes, serum 17-hydroxyprogesterone, urinary steroid profile, plasma ACTH, testosterone, dihydro-testosterone, adrenal androgens, LH, FSH, plasma renin activity, aldosterone, HCG test and DNA analysis. Pelvic ultrasound scans may be helpful. An examination under anaesthesia by an expert DSD urologist can help to determine diagnosis and management by identification of gonads, internal anatomy and biopsy, if indicated.

TREATMENT/PROGNOSIS

- Gender assignment: aim to achieve unambiguous and functionally normal external genitalia through surgery and appropriate hormonal therapy. The decision is usually based upon the anatomy of the internal and external genitalia, although future potential for fertility must be considered.
- Psychological support is essential with medical (e.g. steroid hormone replacement in CAH, androgens for micropenis) and surgical treatments (e.g. clitoral reduction, vaginoplasty, hypospadias repair, correction of chordee) that are individualised, with gonadectomy for patients with dysgenetic or non-functional gonads, especially those with Y-bearing cell lines, which have an increased risk of malignant change in the gonad.
- Prognosis is dependent on the underlying condition and appropriateness of gender assignment.

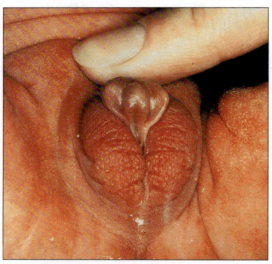

FIGURE 13.49 Virilisation in a newborn baby (karyotype 46XX) due to 21-hydroxylase deficiency.

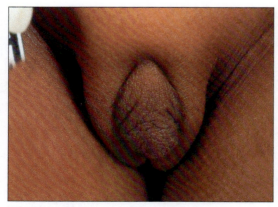

FIGURE 13.50 5α-reductase deficiency in a 9-year-old boy.

TABLE 13.3 Aetiology of ambiguous genitalia

Inadequate masculinization
Leydig cell hypoplasia
Inborn errors of testosterone biosynthesis in adrenals, testes or both
5α-reductase deficiency
Defect in target tissues, e.g. androgen insensitivity
Associated with dysmorphic syndromes –
e.g. Smith-Lemli-Opitz, Dubowitz, Aniridia-Wilms, etc.

Virilized female
Virilization by androgens of fetal origin –
e.g. congenital adrenal hyperplasia
Virilization by androgens of maternal origin –
e.g. anabolic steroids, danazol, virilizing maternal tumour
Dysmorphic syndromes – e.g. Seckel, Zellweger
Presence of testicular tissue – e.g. ovotestis

CONGENITAL ADRENAL HYPERPLASIA

INCIDENCE/GENETICS

21-hydroxylase deficiency is the commonest cause of CAH, with a frequency of 1 in 5,000–23,000 for the homozygous affected state, depending on the population studied. Simple virilising or non-classical CAH is commoner in Ashkenazi Jews. The inheritance for all forms of CAH is autosomal recessive. At the molecular level, the inheritance is best understood for 21-hydroxylase deficiency, where the gene encoding the microsomal cytochrome (CYP) P450 21-hydroxylase enzyme system (*CYP21A2*) and a pseudogene (*CYP21A* or *CYP21P*) are located in the HLA complex. Mutations and deletions in the *CYP21A2* gene are associated with the variable phenotype seen in this condition. Rarer forms include CAH due to deficiencies of 11-beta hydroxylase (CYP11B1 deficiency) or 17-alpha hydroxylase (CYP17A1 deficiency); the former can present with hypertension and virilisation, and the latter with lack of virilisation and hypertension. Some forms of CAH are due to mutations in the gene encoding P450 oxidoreductase (POR). POR is an electron donor enzyme to CYP P450 enzymes and deficiency leads to impairment of several enzymes involved in glucocorticoid and sex steroid synthesis, with a biochemical pattern indicating both CYP21A2 and CYP17A1 deficiencies.

PATHOGENESIS/AETIOLOGY

These autosomal recessive conditions result in enzyme deficiencies in the adrenal glands. These glands cannot synthesise vital steroids, with a resulting accumulation of the substrate steroid which precedes the block as a result of the excessive ACTH drive consequent upon loss of feedback. Cholesterol incorporation into the adrenal cortex is promoted by the ACTH drive, giving rise to the adrenal hyperplasia. Early genotype–phenotype studies have already shown that the correlation between clinical, biochemical and molecular genetic findings in patients with classical 21-hydroxylase deficiency is not absolute (**Table 13.4**).

DIAGNOSIS

Children with CAH may present with ambiguous genitalia at birth, a salt-losing crisis in the newborn period, hypertension, precocious puberty in males, virilisation in females and 'bilateral cryptorchidism' with breast development in puberty (i.e. females raised inappropriately as males) (**Fig. 13.51**). Hypoglycaemia is a rare feature of the condition. Clinical manifestations of POR deficiency include adrenal insufficiency without salt loss or with disorders of sex development in both sexes.

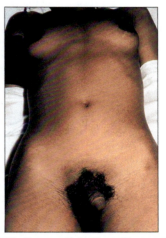

FIGURE 13.51 Congenital adrenal hyperplasia; excessive virilisation in a female raised as a male.

TABLE 13.4 Phenotypes associated with congenital adrenal hyperplasia – extra line added

Enzyme defect	Ambiguous genitalia		Salt loss	Hypertension	Puberty
	Male	Female			
CYP11A/StAR (Steroidogenic Acute Regulatory Protein)	+	–	+	–	Absent
3β-hydroxy-steroid dehydrogenase	+	+	+	–	Absent
17-hydroxylase (P450c17)	+	–	–	+	Absent
21-hydroxylase (P450c21)	–	+	+	–	Precocious
11-hydroxylase (P450c11β)	–	+	–	+	Precocious
Oxidoreductase	+/–	+	–	+/–	Normal/incomplete

In non-classical 21-hydroxylase deficiency, females are born with normal external genitalia. Subsequently, clinical manifestations from increased androgen production can occur at any time. Symptoms in female patients appearing later in childhood or adolescence include hirsutism, temporal baldness, acne, delayed menarche, menstrual irregularities, clitoromegaly and infertility. An accelerated linear growth velocity, a short final height and an advanced bone age may be other features of this condition.

In cases with genital ambiguity or virilisation, a karyotype and pelvic ultrasound scan to identify the internal organs are mandatory. A raised plasma 17-hydroxyprogesterone level (17-OHP) indicates a diagnosis of 21-hydroxylase deficiency. A urinary steroid profile may help to define the enzyme block. In cases of simple virilising CAH, a synacthen test (flat cortisol response, raised 17-OHP levels) with the collection of appropriate plasma and urine samples will assist in the diagnosis. Urea and electrolyte measurements, plasma renin activity and plasma aldosterone levels are essential in the diagnosis of salt-losing CAH. A bone age (usually advanced) may be helpful in the management of simple virilising CAH. Genetic analysis is useful, particularly if future pregnancies are being considered.

TREATMENT

In the first instance, a salt-losing crisis needs to be treated by adequate fluid and saline replacement, as well as glucocorticoid (hydrocortisone) and mineralocorticoid (9α-fludrocortisone given as crushed tablets) replacement. Subsequently, the child is maintained on these replacement hormones, the doses and timings being altered according to biochemical response and surface area (10–15 mg/m^2/d of hydrocortisone, 100 µg/m^2/d of fludrocortisone). Salt supplements should be continued until the infant is switched to normal cow's milk and diet. Girls with severe ambiguity of the genitalia may need surgical correction in the form of clitoral reduction and a genitoplasty within the first 3–12 months, although in many cases, this may be deferred until adolescence when the child can participate in decision making. Hydrocortisone clearance can be rapid in the neonate and adolescent and the hydrocortisone may need to be given more frequently than three times a day. Late-onset, simple virilising CAH is best treated with hydrocortisone in order to suppress the ACTH drive. Puberty may need to be induced in CYP11A/StAR deficiency, 3β-hydroxysteroid dehydrogenase deficiency and 17-hydroxylase deficiency.

Monitoring of the condition is by regular auxology and biochemical monitoring. Both undertreated and over-treated CAH can result in an abnormal growth pattern, with an increased or decreased growth velocity respectively. Skeletal age is advanced in under-treated CAH. Measurement of plasma renin activity and 17-OHP is useful in monitoring salt-losing CAH.

PROGNOSIS

In well-controlled CAH where compliance with medication is satisfactory, the prognosis for final height and pubertal development is good in males, while that for fertility is more guarded. Females with CAH often develop PCO disease and the prognosis for fertility may be affected by this complication. With late diagnosis and/or poor compliance, the children grow extremely rapidly with a considerable advance in bone age and early fusion of the epiphyses, leading to a compromised final height.

DISORDERS OF GLUCOSE HOMEOSTASIS

HYPERINSULINISM

INCIDENCE/GENETICS

Congenital hyperinsulinism (CHI) has an incidence of approximately 1 in 40,000 births and is the most common cause of persistent and recurrent hypoglycaemia. To date mutations in nine genes have been described, which lead to dysregulated insulin secretion from pancreatic β-cells and account for approximately 50% of cases. CHI is also associated with Beckwith–Wiedemann syndrome. Transient hyperinsulinism is most commonly seen in infants of diabetic mothers and infants with evidence of intrauterine growth restriction.

PATHOGENESIS/AETIOLOGY

Mutations in the ß-cell membrane K_{ATP} channel can lead to focal or diffuse areas of hyperinsulinism in the pancreas. This in turn leads to severe hypoglycaemia with suppression of ketones and fatty acids and failure of counter-regulatory hormone responses.

DIAGNOSIS

The majority present in the first few days after birth with symptoms of neonatal hypoglycaemia. These include tremor, jitteriness, apnoea, hypotonia, feeding difficulties, convulsions and coma. Examination may reveal macrosomia, plethora, hepatomegaly and generalised adiposity. In Beckwith–Wiedemann syndrome, characteristic abnormal somatic features may exist including exomphalos, macroglossia **Fig. 13.52**), visceromegaly, polycythaemia, hemihypertrophy and gigantism. Abnormalities of the ears are also present, and include transverse creases in the ear lobes.

Detection of insulin and C-peptide concentrations at the time of hypoglycaemia is diagnostic. Concentrations of free fatty acids, ketone bodies, glycerol and branched chain amino acids are also low. Serum GH and cortisol concentrations are generally raised, although occasionally they are suppressed. If the concentrations are low, they do not necessarily indicate GH and cortisol deficiency. An increased glucose requirement is also helpful in the diagnosis.

Other investigations including a urine organic acid screen taken at the time of hypoglycaemia and exclusion of metabolic conditions such as hyperinsulinism/hyperammonaemia (HIHA) syndrome are also helpful.

TREATMENT

The aim of treatment is to establish glucose concentrations >3.6 mmol/l. Initially glucose infusion rates of 6–20 mg/kg/min may be required. Diazoxide is first-line medical treatment and should be given in combination with chlorothiazide, to minimise fluid retention. Intravenous fluids should be restricted to 120 ml/kg/d and families counselled that diazoxide can lead to hypertrichosis lanuginosa (**Fig. 13.53**). Octreotide and glucagon may also be helpful to control hypoglycaemia.

Where possible, it is important that affected infants maintain some oral intake to minimise later feeding difficulties.

PET with fluoro-dopa is used to detect focal or diffuse disease. Surgical treatment of focal lesions is potentially curative. A 95% pancreatectomy may be required in diffuse cases that fail medical therapy.

PROGNOSIS

Impaired neurological outcome secondary to hypoglycaemic brain injury is reported in 10–40% of cases and increases with delay in diagnosis. Following a pancreatectomy, the patient is likely to later develop diabetes mellitus, characterised by an excessive sensitivity to insulin. Ketotic hyperglycaemia is very rare. Malabsorption may develop and requires treatment with exocrine pancreatic supplementation.

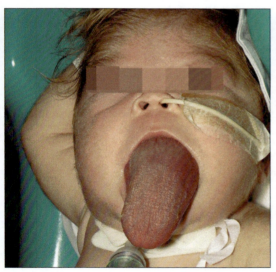

FIGURE 13.52 Massive macroglossia in a child with Beckwith–Wiedemann syndrome. Note the tracheostomy and nasogastric tube.

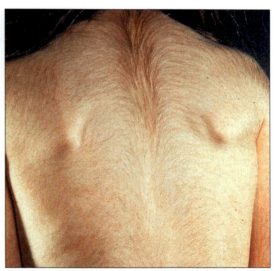

FIGURE 13.53 Hyperinsulinism; diazoxide-induced hypertrichosis lanuginosa in a child.

TYPE 1 DIABETES MELLITUS

PATHOGENESIS/AETIOLOGY

Absolute insulin deficiency results from autoimmune destruction of the beta cells in the pancreas. HLA-DR and -DQ alleles are associated with varying degrees of predisposition to, and protection against, the development of type 1 diabetes mellitus. However, 50% concordance rates for type 1 diabetes mellitus in monozygotic twins and a rapid increase in the incidence of type 1 diabetes mellitus over recent decades, suggest that as yet unidentified environmental factors modulate genetic risk.

EPIDEMIOLOGY

Type 1 diabetes mellitus is by far the commonest form of diabetes in childhood, with the highest incidence (>1 in 5,000 per year) seen in Scandinavia, Portugal, the UK, Canada and New Zealand. The lowest incidence (<1 in 100,000 per year) was found in populations from China and South America. It is estimated that the current increase in incidence is around 3%.

CLINICAL PRESENTATION

The vast majority of children with type 1 diabetes mellitus will present clinically with the classic triad of polydipsia, polyuria and weight loss. Diabetes mellitus may also present with secondary enuresis and recurrent infections. Children may present in diabetic ketoacidosis (DKA) with vomiting, dehydration, abdominal pain, hyperventilation (Kussmaul's breathing), hypovolaemia and altered consciousness.

Necrobiosis lipoidica is a rare skin condition associated with diabetes, but not the level of glycaemic control. It is most commonly found on the shins and is characterised by yellow plaques with a violaceous border, which often scale, crust or ulcerate.

DIAGNOSIS

The diagnosis can be confirmed by a random plasma glucose of >11.0 mmol/l. Rarely, a child may be found to have a high plasma glucose without having symptoms of diabetes mellitus, e.g. following the use of a family member's home blood-glucose monitoring kit. In this case diabetes should be confirmed by the presence of an HbA1c >6.5%, a fasting plasma glucose ≥7.0 mmol/l, or a 2-hour plasma glucose >11.0 mmol/l during a standard oral glucose tolerance test (OGTT). When performing these tests, results may be obtained that are outside normal limits, but do not meet the requirements for diagnosis of diabetes mellitus. In this case, the diagnosis might be impaired fasting glycaemia, or impaired glucose tolerance and follow-up is essential.

In addition to the diagnostic glucose and HbA1c concentrations, a urine dipstick test for ketonuria should also be undertaken. Absence of ketonuria might indicate type 2 diabetes or maturity onset diabetes of the young (MODY). Markers of the process of immune-mediated destruction are present in 85–98% of children with newly diagnosed type 1 diabetes. These include autoantibodies to insulin (IAA), autoantibodies to glutamic acid decarboxylase (GAD65) and autoantibodies to the tyrosine phosphatases IA-2 and IA-2β.

There is an increased risk of other autoimmune disorders, particularly coeliac disease and hypothyroidism. Screening for both of these conditions is recommended, as they can be asymptomatic with a significant morbidity if left untreated. Addison disease is a rare but recognised association.

Presymptomatic screening of at risk children, such as siblings, should not be undertaken, as it confers no benefit to the child and has the potential for psychological harm.

MANAGEMENT

Children in DKA should be treated with intravenous insulin using standardised treatment regimens such as those produced by the British Society of Paediatric Endocrinology and Diabetes (http://www.bsped.org.uk/clinical/docs/DKAGuideline.pdf).

For long-term management, only subcutaneous insulin is available, although inhaled and intranasal insulin are being studied. The injection technique should avoid intramuscular injection (with its risk of exercise-induced hypoglycaemia) or leakage of insulin from the skin. Injections should be rotated to avoid lipohypertrophy (**Fig. 13.54**), which results in variable absorption. Lipoatrophy (**Fig. 13.55**) is now rare with the available insulin analogues.

Short-acting human insulin, or insulin analogues insulin aspart and lispro, with a faster onset of action are generally given with meals and combined with intermediate-acting isophane insulin or long-acting insulin analogues, insulin glargine and detemir, for background cover. Insulin is usually delivered with a pen device, although needle and insulin syringe may be used. Four to five injections a day are commonly required. Continuous subcutaneous short-acting insulin can be administered via a pump, which provides a fixed or variable basal dose and which delivers a bolus at mealtimes.

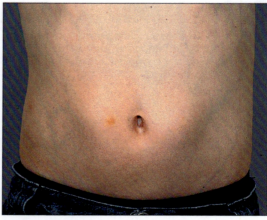

FIGURE 13.54 Lipohypertrophy in a boy who injected subcutaneously into his abdomen.

Endocrinology

The aim is to decrease the risk of microvascular complications without severe hypoglycaemia. Intensified treatment improves glycaemic control and delays the onset and slows the progression of microvascular complications, and also increases the risk of hypoglycaemia. Premixed short and intermediate insulins are available but are used less commonly as they provide little flexibility and it is harder to achieve good glucose control.

Home blood glucose monitoring is used to guide insulin dose, using meters with a memory. Continuous glucose monitoring systems allow a detailed and more visual record of patterns of glycaemic control which can be useful in guiding management. Glycated haemoglobin (HbA1c) with target <7.5% reflects medium-term glycaemic control, predicts the risk of long-term complications and should be checked 3–4 times a year.

Education is a vital part of initial management and diabetes care should be provided in a multi-disciplinary team setting, which includes nursing, medical and dietetic input by individuals with paediatric diabetes expertise. Access to psychology, podiatry and ophthalmology is also essential. Transition and transfer to adult services should be planned with the young person and occur at a time of relative stability.

Dietary advice should encourage 'healthy eating' and an active lifestyle encouraged. Carbohydrate counting is an effective way of matching the carbohydrate intake to the insulin dose administered. It requires dietetic educational input and can lead to improved blood glucose control, greater flexibility and freedom of lifestyle.

Diabetes mellitus is a chronic condition and psychological input for children with diabetes is important. Specific problems such as depression, eating and behavioural disorders, are likely to have a significant impact on diabetes control. Social work support is sometimes needed.

SHORT-TERM PROGNOSIS

The symptoms and signs of hypoglycaemia relate to autonomic activation (tremor, sweating) and neuroglycopenia (irritability, headache, confusion, convulsions, coma). Although death is an extremely rare consequence of hypoglycaemia, severe hypoglycaemia may cause long-term neuropsychological impairment. The risks of hypoglycaemia need to be balanced against the benefits of good glycaemic control. Hypoglycaemia is treated with oral glucose followed by carbohydrate-containing food or, if severe, with intramuscular glucagon or intravenous glucose.

Death from diabetes mellitus in childhood is rare (standardised mortality ratio 2.3 in the UK). DKA is the commonest cause of death (implicated in over 80% of such cases), usually as a result of cerebral oedema, which has a mortality rate of 25% and a risk of developing severe neurological sequelae in over one-third of survivors. Treatment of DKA includes rehydration with intravenous fluids, insulin and careful monitoring of fluid, electrolytes, blood glucose and neurological status.

LONGER-TERM PROGNOSIS

Diabetes mellitus is one of the most common causes of end-stage kidney disease and of blindness in people of working age. Diabetic retinopathy and nephropathy surveillance (the former using a retinal camera with pupils dilated, the latter by testing for microalbuminuria, blood pressure and renal function) should be performed annually from 12 years of age as can be modified if identified early. Microalbuminuria precedes hypertension in nephropathy. Routine screening for elevated blood lipids is not currently recommended in childhood and adolescence but may be indicated in high-risk individuals. Regular podiatry reviews are important, to emphasise preventative foot care but are not likely to identify early manifestations of diabetic foot pathology. Cataracts can occur early, unrelated to the degree of glycaemic control. Other clinical manifestations of poor diabetes control include limited finger joint mobility (**Fig. 13.56**).

Guidelines for the management of diabetes have been produced by the Scottish Intercollegiate Guidelines Network and by the National Institute for Health and Care Excellence.

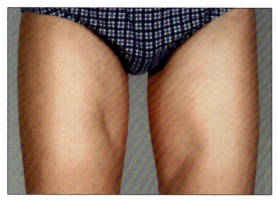

FIGURE 13.55 Lipoatrophy.

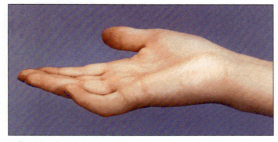

FIGURE 13.56 Limited finger joint mobility.

TYPE 2 DIABETES MELLITUS

AETIOLOGY

Type 2 diabetes mellitus occurs when insulin secretion is insufficient to compensate for insulin resistance. The prevalence is rising and it is associated with family history, obesity and certain ethnic groups, including those of African-American and South Asian origin. Risk is increased in those who were born small for gestational age or whose mothers were obese and/or diabetic. Attempts have been made to calculate the prevalence of type 2 diabetes mellitus, but these studies have mainly been in clinic populations and are therefore likely to have underestimated the prevalence, as type 2 diabetes mellitus is often asymptomatic. The prevalence increases after the onset of puberty due to the antagonistic actions of GH and sex steroids on insulin.

CLINICAL PRESENTATION

Children may have acanthosis nigricans, a velvety thickening of the skin in the neck or axillae (**Figs 13.57, 13.58**) and symptoms or signs of PCO disease (oligomenorrhoea, hirsutism), both of which are associated with insulin resistance.

Type 2 diabetes mellitus should be considered if the child is obese and particularly:

- is of non-white origin
- has a strong family history of type 2 diabetes mellitus
- has acanthosis nigricans
- has symptoms/signs of PCO disease
- has no ketones in their urine at presentation or when hyperglycaemic
- has a prolonged honeymoon phase or no insulin requirement.

Some children with type 2 diabetes can present with ketonuria.

INVESTIGATIONS

- Autoantibodies (islet cell, insulin and GAD).
- Insulin and c-peptide levels – fasting and during OGTT.
- Fasting lipid levels.

PROGNOSIS

Mortality is two to three times higher among people with type 2 diabetes mellitus than in the general population. In addition, the risk of myocardial infarction is four times greater in those diagnosed with type 2 diabetes before the age of 45 years.

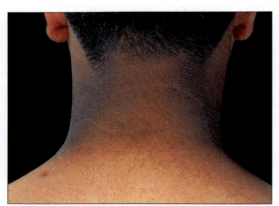

FIGURE 13.57 Insulin resistance: acanthosis nigricans in the nuchal folds of a child.

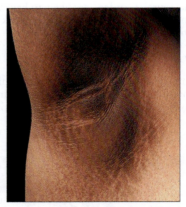

FIGURE 13.58 Insulin resistance: acanthosis nigricans in the axillary folds of a child.

MONOGENIC DIABETES

GENETICS/INCIDENCE

Monogenic diabetes results from the inheritance of a mutation or mutations in a single gene. It may be dominantly or recessively inherited or a *de novo* mutation. It includes MODY, neonatal diabetes and other genetic syndromes.

MODY affects 1–2% of people with diabetes, and is inherited in an autosomal dominant manner. Six genes have been identified to date including *HNF1A*, *Glucokinase*, *HNF1B* (including renal cysts and diabetes), *HNF4A*, *IPF1*, and *NEUROD1*.

Neonatal diabetes mellitus is usually diagnosed in the first 6 months of life and is classified as transient (TNDM) or permanent (PNDM). The majority of patients with TNDM have an abnormality of imprinting of the *ZAC* and *HYMAI* genes on chromosome 6q, while PNDM mutations include those in the *KCNJ11* gene encoding the Kir6.2 subunit of the beta cell K_{ATP} channel and homozygous or compound heterozygous mutations in glucokinase.

PATHOGENESIS/AETIOLOGY

Monogenic diabetes results from mutations in genes that regulate beta-cell function. Diabetes resulting from mutations in severe insulin resistance is discussed below.

MODY should be considered if:

- the child has no ketones in their urine at presentation or when hyperglycaemic
- or the child has a prolonged honeymoon phase, or no insulin requirement
- and there is diabetes (insulin or non-insulin dependent) in one parent
- or the child and one parent have persistent, stable, mild hyperglycaemia (fasting blood glucose 5.5–8 mmol/l), which might indicate a glucokinase mutation
- or there is glycosuria in the presence of relatively normal blood glucose levels, suggesting an HNF1 mutation.

TREATMENT OF MODY

Correct diagnosis is important. Patients with mutations in the glucokinase gene rarely require treatment and are not at increased risk of diabetic complications. Those with mutations in HNF1a and HNF4a may respond to sulphonylurea treatment.

CLINICAL PRESENTATION AND MANAGEMENT OF NEONATAL DIABETES

Diabetes associated with 6q24 is usually diagnosed in the first week of life and resolves in 3–6 months. The diabetes may recur in later childhood and adolescence. Insulin treatment is required.

Neonatal diabetes due to Kir6.2 mutations can be managed effectively with sulphonylureas and doses of up to 1 mg/kg/d may be required. Neurological features are seen in 20% of patients and severe defects can lead to developmental delay and epilepsy – developmental delay, epilepsy and neonatal diabetes (DEND) syndrome.

INSULIN RESISTANCE SYNDROMES

INCIDENCE/GENETICS

Syndromes of insulin resistance are rare. They include genetic defects in the insulin receptor (Donohue syndrome/leprechaunism; Rabson–Mendenhall syndrome; type A insulin resistance) and downstream insulin signalling defects. Acquired insulin resistance (type B) may be caused by antibodies against the insulin receptor.

Severe insulin resistance also occurs as a result of adipose tissue abnormalities. These include monogenic obesity syndromes and lipodystrophies. Congenital total lipodystrophies are usually autosomal recessive while partial lipodystrophies tend to have an autosomal dominant inheritance.

PATHOGENESIS/AETIOLOGY

There is a resistance to insulin at the receptor level, although the underlying pathogenetic mechanism is unclear. In the type A syndrome, insulin receptor mutations may cause defects in receptor expression on the cell surface, or in the signalling capacity of the receptor. Similar mutations have been described in patients with leprechaunism and lipodystrophy.

DIAGNOSIS

Abnormal glucose homeostasis with raised insulin concentrations develops in all patients although timing and severity is variable, with hypoglycaemia often preceding hyperglycaemia. Acanthosis nigricans (**Figs 13.57, 13.58**) is invariably present and is characterised by the presence of hyperkeratotic epidermal papillomatosis with increased melanocytes, leading to hyperpigmented, velvety areas of skin, predominantly in apposed and flexural regions. In girls, the condition is associated with PCO disease, where it is associated with hyperandrogenism leading to hirsutism.

Children with Donohue syndrome and Rabson–Mendenhall syndrome also have characteristic features including intrauterine growth retardation, dysmorphic facies, lipoatrophy, acanthosis nigricans and overgrowth of genitalia and viscera (**Fig. 13.59**).

Disorders of adipose tissue development or function (lipodystrophies) may lead to unusual fat distribution with areas of excessive fat distribution and areas of adipose deficiency. Hypertriglyceridaemia and hepatic steatosis are associated with these conditions. Insulin resistance leads to diabetes mellitus. Causes may be genetic, autoimmune or secondary to drugs, particularly antiretroviral therapies.

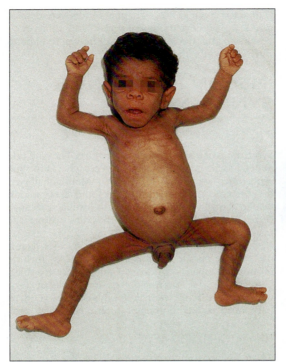

FIGURE 13.59 Donohue syndrome in a child with features of insulin resistance.

TREATMENT

At present, the main form of treatment is dietary restriction with reduced fat intake. Insulin sensitisers such as metformin and antiandrogens may have a role to play. Severe insulin receptor defects may respond to recombinant IGF-1 therapy. It is thought to act as an insulin mimetic with similar postreceptor signalling effects.

PROGNOSIS

Donohue syndrome and Rabson–Mendenhall syndrome have limited life expectancy. Other insulin resistant states lead to an increased incidence of diabetes mellitus, hypertension and coronary heart disease.

OTHER FORMS OF DIABETES

Diabetes mellitus may also be caused by diseases of the exocrine pancreas (cystic fibrosis), endocrinopathies (Cushing syndrome), drugs or chemicals (glucocorticoids, calcineurin inhibitors) and infections (congenital rubella), and may also be associated with other genetic syndromes (Wolfram syndrome).

DISORDERS OF CALCIUM METABOLISM

RICKETS

INCIDENCE/GENETICS

In the UK vitamin D deficiency is the most common cause of rickets. It is generally commoner in children in Asian communities, possibly due to a combination of genetic and dietary factors, and a lack of sunlight. Vitamin D-dependent rickets, which can be due to 1-hydroxylase deficiency (type 1) or an end-organ receptor resistance to vitamin D (type 2), is inherited as an autosomal recessive condition. Familial hypophosphataemic rickets is inherited as an X-linked, autosomal dominant or autosomal recessive condition, with a frequency of 1 in 25,000.

PATHOGENESIS/AETIOLOGY

Calciopenic causes include dietary calcium and vitamin D deficiency, malabsorption, lack of sunlight, hepatic disease, anticonvulsant treatment, renal disease, 1-α hydroxylase deficiency and end-organ resistance to vitamin D. Phosphopenic causes include Fanconi syndrome, X-linked hypophosphataemic rickets, renal tubular acidosis and oculo-cerebro-renal syndrome (Lowe syndrome).

DIAGNOSIS

This condition usually presents with bone deformity, exhibiting different patterns depending on the child's age at the onset of disease and the relative growth rate of different bones. In the first year of life, the most rapidly growing bones are the skull, the upper limbs and ribs. Rickets at this time presents with craniotabes, widening of the cranial sutures, frontal bossing, enlarged swollen epiphyses, particularly of the wrists, bulging of the costochondral joints (rachitic rosary) and a Harrison's sulcus (**Figs 13.60, 13.61**).

After the first year of life, genu varum (**Fig. 13.62**), genu valgum, abnormal dentition with enamel hypoplasia, bone pain and proximal myopathy are the dominant clinical features. In severe cases, tetany, laryngeal stridor, paraesthesiae and convulsions result from the hypocalcaemia. Growth failure is a common feature. Alopecia is a feature of vitamin D-dependent rickets type 2.

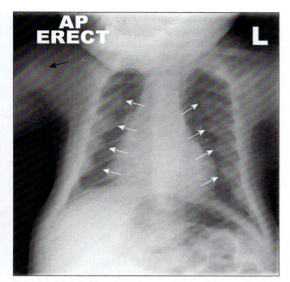

FIGURE 13.60 Chest radiograph in a 16-month-old male with severe nutritional rickets. The anterior rib ends are markedly expanded, forming an almost continuous sheet of bone around the anterior chest (white arrows), the radiological correlate of the rachitic rosary.

X-linked hypophosphataemic rickets usually presents in the male during late infancy with hypophosphataemia. Subsequently, untreated patients present with slow growth, bowing of the legs and a waddling gait. The clinical presentation is extremely variable, ranging from biochemical abnormalities to severe bony disease. Other features include poor dental development and abscesses of the teeth.

Biochemically, hypocalcaemia and hypophosphataemia may be present. The alkaline phosphatase level is high, while the 1,25-dihydroxy vitamin D concentration is low. The serum parathyroid hormone (PTH) concentration may be high. Radiologically, widening of the growth plate and fraying, cupping and widening of the metaphyses occur. Pseudofractures and signs of secondary hyperparathyroidism may also be seen (e.g. subperiosteal erosions). Other investigations may be abnormal, depending on the underlying cause (e.g. acidosis, aminoaciduria, chronic kidney disease, anaemia).

TREATMENT

Calcium, phosphate and vitamin D are used in varying combinations, in an attempt to correct the clinical, radiological and biochemical abnormalities. In vitamin D deficient states, replacement should be with preparations of cholecalciferol or ergocalciferol. Underlying abnormalities (e.g. coeliac disease) need appropriate treatment. Growth needs to be carefully monitored. In hypophosphataemic rickets, large doses of vitamin D are required. In patients with 1α-hydroxylase deficiency or end-organ resistance to vitamin D, 1,25-dihydroxy-cholecalciferol is usually required in significant doses. Regular renal ultrasound scanning is important.

PROGNOSIS

The prognosis for growth and cure of radiological and biochemical abnormalities is excellent in most children with rickets, provided that the condition is adequately treated. However, in hypophosphataemic rickets, the prognosis is less certain, and severe deformities of the limbs may result, particularly if compliance is poor.

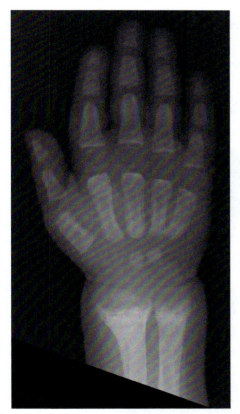

FIGURE 13.61 Radiograph of left hand and wrist in the same child as in **13.60**. There is marked fraying, cupping and splaying of the distal radial and ulnar metaphyses, with pseudowidening of the distal radial growth plate.

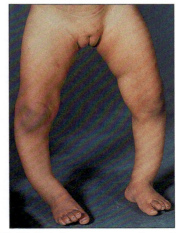

FIGURE 13.62 Rickets: genu varum in a child.

411

HYPOPARATHYROIDISM/ PSEUDOHYPO- PARATHYROIDISM

INCIDENCE/GENETICS

When due to polyglandular autoimmune syndrome type I, hypoparathyroidism is inherited as an autosomal recessive condition. DiGeorge syndrome may be due to monosomy 22q11. In pseudohypoparathyroidism, inheritance is as an autosomal dominant, and the condition is rare. Rarely, hypoparathyroidism may be associated with activating mutations in the gene encoding the calcium sensing receptor.

DIAGNOSIS

The usual presentation for both conditions is with symptomatic hypocalcaemia. Children with hypoparathyroidism may present with symptoms and signs of hypocalcaemia *per se*. These include jitteriness, apnoeas in the neonatal period, convulsions, tetany, muscle cramps, laryngospasm, carpopedal spasm, positive Chvostek and Trousseau signs, neurodevelopmental delay, basal ganglia calcification and lenticular cataracts.

In DiGeorge syndrome, hypoparathyroidism is associated with thymic aplasia and consequent T-cell defects, congenital heart disease (especially truncus arteriosus), facial anomalies such as micrognathia, cleft lip and palate and ear malformations (**Fig. 13.63**). (See also Chapter 16 Immunology, page 495.)

In pseudohypoparathyroidism, many of the children have neurodevelopmental delay and show unique somatic features, termed Albright's hereditary osteodystrophy. These include short stature, round facies (**Fig. 13.64**), a short neck, obesity and subcutaneous calcification, especially near joints. A pathognomic feature of this condition is shortening of the fourth and fifth metacarpals and metatarsals (**Fig. 13.65**). Symptoms of chronic hypocalcaemia may predominate, and include convulsions, cataracts and ectodermal changes such as dry, scaling skin and enamel hypoplasia.

Hypoparathyroidism is characterised biochemically by hypocalcaemia, hyperphosphataemia and reduced PTH concentrations. In pseudohypoparathyroidism, PTH concentrations are elevated, and the diagnosis may be confirmed genetically or clinically by an inability to increase urinary cAMP levels and phosphate excretion in response to an infusion of parathormone. In Albright syndrome, hormonal resistance may be generalised and the clinical picture includes GHD, hypogonadism and hypothyroidism.

A skeletal survey may help in the diagnosis, and reveals short metacarpals and metatarsals with ectopic subcutaneous calcification. Pseudopseudohypoparathyroidism refers to the phenotype associated with pseudohypoparathyroidism but with normal biochemistry.

PATHOGENESIS/AETIOLOGY

Hypoparathyroidism may be due to mutations in or near the PTH gene on chromosome 11, polyglandular autoimmune syndrome and post surgery. DiGeorge syndrome is due to developmental defects of the structures that derive from the third and fourth pharyngeal pouches and branchial pouches. Pseudohypoparathyroidism is due to a mutation in the α-subunit of the G-protein coupled to the PTH receptor.

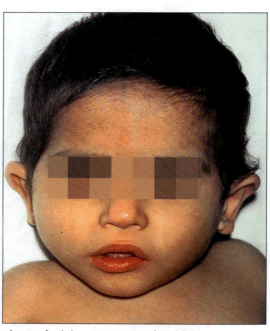

FIGURE 13.63 DiGeorge syndrome: facial appearance of a child.

TREATMENT

Treatment is with calcium supplements and vitamin D, usually in the form of 1α-calcidol, with close biochemical monitoring and regular renal ultrasound scans to detect nephrocalcinosis. In DiGeorge syndrome, recurrent infections need appropriate treatment as do cardiovascular abnormalities.

PROGNOSIS

In DiGeorge syndrome, the prognosis is dictated by the immunological and cardiovascular anomalies. In pseudohypoparathyroidism, mild to moderate neurodevelopmental delay is observed in 50–75% of cases. The prognosis in isolated hypoparathyroidism is very good, provided that the condition is not associated with chronic active hepatitis.

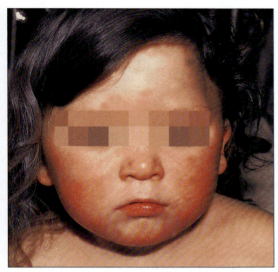

FIGURE 13.64 Pseudohypoparathyroidism: characteristic facial appearance of a child.

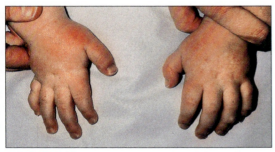

FIGURE 13.65 Pseudohypoparathyroidism: clinical appearance of the hands, with short fourth and fifth metacarpals.

HYPERCALCAEMIA

Hypercalcaemia is uncommon in paediatrics and may be attributable to genetic abnormalities of the calcium sensing receptor or mutations that are associated with parathyroid hyperplasia and/or neoplasia. Hypercalcaemia may also be attributable to disorders of bone metabolism or abnormal vitamin D metabolism, such as seen in subcutaneous fat necrosis of the newborn.

CLINICAL PRESENTATION

Symptoms may arise once the calcium concentration exceeds 3.0 mmol/l. Children may present with muscle weakness, vomiting, constipation, abdominal pain and lethargy. Nephrocalcinosis can result from long-standing hypercalcaemia. Investigations for calcium, magnesium, phosphate, alkaline phosphatase, PTH and vitamin D along with a urine calcium to creatinine ratio should be first line. Bone x-rays, renal ultrasound and DNA analysis may also be indicated.

WILLIAMS SYNDROME

See also Chapter 15 Genetics, page 457.

INCIDENCE/GENETICS

The condition is due to a deletion or mutations in the elastin gene on chromosome 7q11.

PATHOGENESIS/AETIOLOGY

A genetic defect in the elastin gene is responsible for the diverse features of the condition.

DIAGNOSIS

Infantile hypercalcaemia is associated with neurodevelopmental delay, 'cocktail party chatter', facial, cardiovascular and other features in Williams syndrome. The facial features include a broad prominent forehead, a short and turned up nose with a flat nasal bridge, full cheeks and lips with a prominent overhanging upper lip, low-set ears, stellate iris, epicanthic folds and strabismus (**Figs 13.66, 13.67**). Dental anomalies are characteristic. Cardiovascular anomalies are present in 75% and include supravalvular aortic stenosis and peripheral pulmonary artery stenosis. Low birth weight, short stature, microcephaly, hoarse voice, hyperacusis and kyphoscoliosis are other features. Infantile hypercalcaemia usually resolves spontaneously.

Investigations reveal an elevated serum calcium level, a high normal phosphate level, low normal alkaline phosphatase and PTH concentration, and hypercalciuria. Radiographic features include increased density at the metaphyseal ends of the long bones, osteosclerosis of the base of the skull, nephrocalcinosis and soft tissue calcification. The pathogenesis of the hypercalcaemia remains unclear.

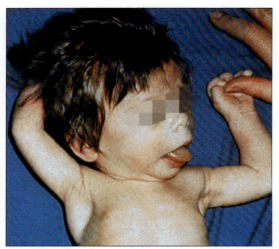

FIGURE 13.66 Williams syndrome: typical facies in a child.

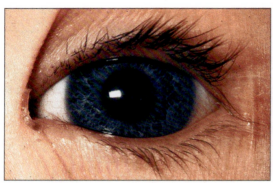

FIGURE 13.67 Williams syndrome: stellate iris in a child.

TREATMENT

The hypercalcaemia usually resolves spontaneously. A low calcium diet is indicated until the calcium level falls. If the calcium concentration is persistently elevated and leads to symptoms, treatment with bisphosphonates or prednisolone may be indicated. The cardiovascular abnormalities will also require treatment.

PROGNOSIS

The prognosis is determined by the cardiovascular anomalies and the neurodevelopmental delay. The outlook for the hypercalcaemia is good.

We acknowledge the radiology input for this chapter from Dr Alistair Calder.

FURTHER READING

Growth hormone deficiency/insufficiency

Alatzoglou KS, Webb E, LeTissier P, Dattani MT. Isolated growth hormone deficiency in childhood and adolescence: an update. *Endocrine Rev* 2014;35(3):376–432.

Kelberman D, Rizzoti K, Lovell-Badge R, Robinson ICAF, Dattani MT. Genetic regulation of pituitary gland development in human and mouse. *Endocrine Rev* 2009;30(7):790–829.

Laron-type dwarfism

David A, Hwa V, Metherell LA, *et al.* Evidence for a continuum of genetic, phenotypic, and biochemical abnormalities in children with growth hormone insensitivity. *Endocr Rev* 2011;32(4):472–97.

Wit JM. Diagnosis and management of disorders of IGF-1 synthesis and action. *Pediatr Endocrinol Rev* 2011;9(Suppl 1):538–40.

Russell–Silver syndrome

Netchine I, Rossignol S, Dufourg MN, *et al.* 11p15 imprinting center region 1 loss of methylation is a common and specific cause of typical Russell–Silver syndrome: clinical scoring system and epigenetic-phenotypic correlations. *J Clin Endocrinol Metabol* 2007;92(8):3148–54.

Turner syndrome

Gault EJ, Perry RJ, Cole TJ, *et al.* Effect of oxandrolone and timing of pubertal induction on final height in Turner's syndrome: randomised, double blind, placebo controlled trial. British Society for Paediatric Endocrinology and Diabetes. *Br Med J* 2011;342:d1980.

Prader–Willi syndrome

Siemensma EP, Tummers-de Lind van Wijngaarden RF, Festen DA, *et al.* Beneficial effects of growth hormone treatment on cognition in children with Prader–Willi syndrome: a randomized controlled trial and longitudinal study. *J Clin Endocrinol Metab* 2012;97(7):2307–14.

Pituitary gigantism

Keil MF, Stratakis CA. Pituitary tumors in childhood: update of diagnosis, treatment and molecular genetics. *Exp Rev Neurother* 2008;8(4):563–74.

Trivellin G, Daly AF, Faucz FR, *et al.* Gigantism and acromegaly due to Xq26 microduplications and GPR101 mutation. *N Engl J Med* 2014;371(25):2363–74.

Late puberty

Palmert MR, Dunkel L. Clinical practice. Delayed puberty. *N Engl J Med* 2012;366(5):443–53.

Early puberty

Carel JC, Leger J. Precocious puberty. *N Engl J Med* 2008;358(22):2366–77.

Polycystic ovarian disease

Ojaniemi M, Tapanainen P, Morin-Papunen L. Management of polycystic ovary syndrome in childhood and adolescence. *Horm Res Paediatr* 2010;74(5):372–5.

Acquired hypothyroidism

Brook, CGD and Dattani, MT. The thyroid gland. In: *Handbook of Clinical Pediatric Endocrinology*, 2nd edn. Oxford: Wiley-Blackwell, 2012, pp. 129–50.

Graves disease

Rivkees SA. Pediatric Graves' disease: controversies in management. *Horm Res Paediatr* 2010;74(5):305–11.

Ambiguous genitalia

Hughes IA, Houk C, Ahmed SF, Lee PA, and LWPES1/ ESPE2 Consensus Group. Consensus statement on management of intersex disorders. *Arch Dis Child* 2006;91(7):554–63.

Congenital adrenal hyperplasia

Khalid JM, Oerton JM, Dezateux C, *et al.* Incidence and clinical features of congenital adrenal hyperplasia in Great Britain. *Arch Dis Child* 2012;97(2):101–6.

Hyperinsulinism

Hussain, K. Congenital hyperinsulinism and neonatal diabetes mellitus. *Rev Endocr Metabol Dis* 2010;11(3):155–6.

Insulin resistance syndromes

Semple RK, Savage DB, Cochran EK, Gorden P, O'Rahilly S. Genetic syndromes of severe insulin resistance. *Endocr Rev* 2011;32(4):498–514.

Diabetes mellitus

Allgrove J, Swift P, Greene S. Evidence-based paediatric and adolescent diabetes. Br Med J books, 2007.

Ehtisham S, Hattersley AT, Dunger DB, Barrett TG. British Society for Paediatric Endocrinology and Diabetes Clinical Trials Group; First UK survey of paediatric type 2 diabetes and MODY. *Arch Dis Child* 2004;89(6):526–9.

Wolfsdorf J, Craig ME, Daneman D, *et al.* Diabetic ketoacidosis in children and adolescents with diabetes. *Pediatr Diabetes* 2009;10(Suppl 12):118–33.

Metabolic Diseases

Stephanie Grünewald, Alex Broomfield, and Callum Wilson

ADRENO-LEUKODYSTROPHY

CLINICAL PRESENTATION

Adrenoleukodystrophy (ALD) is a peroxisomal disorder with a variable phenotype. The most severe form is childhood onset cerebral ALD (COCALD). They typically present between the ages of 4 and 10 years with progressive neurological impairment. This may manifest as behavioural problems, deterioration in school performance (**Fig. 14.1**), focal neurological symptoms and/or hearing/visual impairment. Alternatively they may present with an adrenal crisis. About 8–10% may have only Addison disease; the patient is abnormally tanned and a Synacthen® test reveals the adrenal insufficiency. Approximately 30% of patients present in early adult life with evidence of spinal cord and peripheral nerve involvement; this form is known as adrenomyeloneuropathy (AMN). About one-third of these AMN patients go on to develop cerebral involvement. Adults can also develop a cerebral disease that presents, usually not as rapidly as the childhood form, with symptoms of dementia. A number of ALD patients may remain entirely asymptomatic although this number declines with age.

INVESTIGATIONS

The finding of elevated plasma very long-chain fatty acids (VLCFAs) and in particular the C26:22 and C24:22 ratios, in the presence of suggestive clinical features, is diagnostic. Once the diagnosis has been confirmed, the extent of the illness must be assessed. Neuropsychometric testing, nerve conduction studies, MRI brain (**Fig. 14.2**), visual and hearing assessment and a Synacthen® test are all required.

BIOCHEMISTRY/GENETICS

ALD is an X-linked disorder caused by a defect in a peroxisomal transmembrane transporter protein (ABCD1 gene). This leads to defective oxidation of VLCFAs, fatty acids with carbon chains lengths of 24 and 26. The cerebral forms involve a rapidly progressive inflammatory myelinopathy, that usually begins in the parieto-occipital regions and may involve autoimmune mechanisms. Degenerative

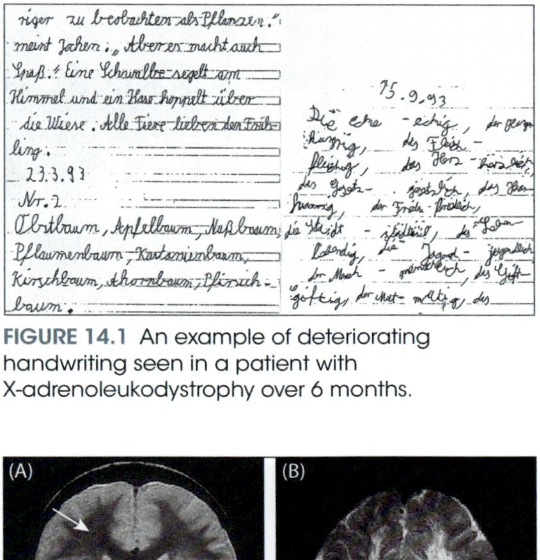

FIGURE 14.1 An example of deteriorating handwriting seen in a patient with X-adrenoleukodystrophy over 6 months.

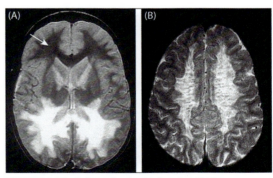

FIGURE 14.2 Adrenoleukodystrophy (ALD). (A) MRI scan showing moderately advanced leukodystrophy in a boy with COCALD. This pattern of severe temporal and parieto-occipital involvement is typical for ALD; (B) in contrast, more diffuse white matter involvement is seen in metachromatic leukodystrophy.

Adrenoleukodystrophy

417

mechanism are thought to be part of the slower onset AMN. Up to 50% of women who are heterozygous for ALD develop an AMN-like syndrome in adulthood.

TREATMENT

Cortisol and very occasionally fludrocortisone are used to manage the adrenal insufficiency. Lorenzo's oil, a 4:1 mixture of the monounsaturated fatty acids mixture of triolein and trierucin, inhibits the elongation of docosanoic acid (22:0) to 26:0 and improves/normalises the plasma VLCFA level in many patients. However, it can lead to thrombocytopenia and its impact on the neurological outcome is uncertain. Activation of peroxisomal B oxidation using peroxisome proliferator activated receptor (PPAR) alpha agonists such as fibrates has been unsuccessful, though the use of conjugated linoleic acid shows some promise. Bone marrow transplant (BMT) if performed in the early stages of COCALD does prevent the progression of the neurological disease but needs to be performed before there is significant neurological impairment and carries significant risks. Thus asymptomatic patients are monitored with regular cerebral imaging. Initial gene therapy work shown it to be effective; long-term treatment clinical trials are ongoing.

PROGNOSIS

The prognosis of COCALD without BMT is very poor. Once neurological regression has commenced there is rapid progression to a decorticate state over a period of months to years. Death usually occurs after a few years. With BMT the prognosis is much improved. The prognosis for AMN is variable; the role of gene therapy, Lorenzo's oil and BMT is unclear.

GAUCHER DISEASE

CLINICAL PRESENTATION

Gaucher disease is a heterogeneous disorder that can present at any time from birth (with hydrops fetalis +/− icthyosis) to adulthood. The severe form of the disease, the acute neuronopathic infantile (type 2) disorder, presents with a rapidly progressive neurodegeneration in the first year of life. Patients present with marked hepatosplenomegaly and go on to develop the classical signs of trismus, strabismus and opisthotonos. The most common form of the disease, the non-neuronopathic or type 1 form, can present at any age with symptoms secondary to bone marrow and visceral involvement. These include hepatosplenomegaly, anaemia and thrombocytopenia, bone pain and pathological fractures, growth failure and/or failure to thrive. Type 3 or subacute neuronopathic form has similar visceral features to type 1, but patients initially also have subtle oculomotor apraxias particularly initially with horizontal eye movements and slowly progressive neurological disease.

INVESTIGATIONS/DIAGNOSIS

The diagnosis is by enzyme analysis of glucocerebrosidase (β glucosidase) in leukocytes or fibroblasts although a strong indicator of the disease can be the presence of classical foamy 'wrinkled tissue-paper' Gaucher cell in a bone marrow aspirate (**Fig. 14.3**). The plasma levels of the enzyme chitotriosidase are markedly elevated in Gaucher disease and can be used as a screening test and to monitor treatment (caveat: 4–6 % of the population are homozygous for a common null mutation in chitotriosidase). Monitoring should include liver function test, full blood count and biomarker, such as chitotriosidase, angiotensin converting enzyme and CCL18/PARC. Abdominal ultrasound and x-rays (**Fig. 14.4**); MRI and DEXA scans are used to score severity of bone involvement. ECHO, lung function testing and eye examination may also be necessary.

BIOCHEMISTRY/GENETICS

The disease is caused by deficiency of the lysosomal enzyme glucocerebrosidase, leading to an accumulation of glucosylceramide and other sphingolipids. Prenatal diagnosis can be offered. Mutation analysis is useful as there are some limited genotype/phenotype correlations: the presence of at least one copy of the N370S mutation (found in the majority of Jewish and around half non-Jewish patients) usually results in type 1 phenotype, whereas homozygosity of the L444P mutation often results in a type 3 phenotype.

TREATMENT

Enzyme replacement therapy (usually fortnightly intravenous infusion) is the treatment of choice in type 1 and 3 disease and primarily improves the visceral and marrow symptoms. BMT has been partially effective but carries significant morbidity. Substrate reduction therapy has shown benefits and theoretically may offer better tissue penetration. Bone disease may be helped by the use of bisphosphonates. Unfortunately supportive therapy is all that is available for the acute neuronopathic form of the disease.

PROGNOSIS

The prognosis for the non-neuropathic form of the disease is generally favourable if the condition is treated early, but even in this group there is a risk of late onset neurological disease. The long-term prognosis for the subacute neurological disease in type 3 Gaucher is still unclear and therapies need to be further evaluated.

HURLER DISEASE, MPS I

CLINICAL PRESENTATION

Hurler disease is the prototype of a group of disorders collectively known as the mucopolysaccharidoses (MPS). Children with Hunter (MPS II) and Maroteaux–Lamy (MPS VI) have similar clinical features. Children with classical Hurler disease usually present in infancy with failure to attain normal developmental milestones. Affected children have hepatomegaly, thickened skin, macrocephaly and the classical 'coarse' facial features of MPS. A bone dysplasia known as 'dysostosis multiplex' is evident radiologically and later becomes obvious clinically with short stature, 'claw-like' hands (**Fig. 14.5**), a lumbar gibbus and joint contractures. Children with Hurler often have corneal clouding (**Fig. 14.6**) at presentation. Deafness, cardiac valvular disease and carpal tunnel disease are typically seen later but

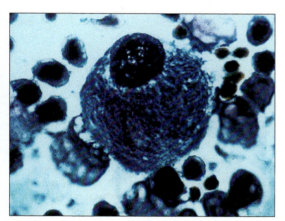

FIGURE 14.3 Typical appearance of a Gaucher cell in bone marrow.

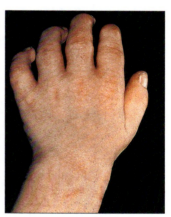

FIGURE 14.5 Typical 'claw' hand of mucopolysaccharidosis disease.

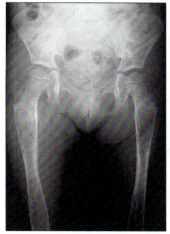

FIGURE 14.4 Severe bony involvement of the proximal femurs in a patient with Gaucher disease.

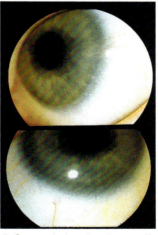

FIGURE 14.6 Corneal clouding in a patient with Hurler disease.

can occasionally be the presenting symptom. A mild variant of the disorder, Scheie disease, presents in late childhood typically with mainly bone and joint disease but without cognitive impairment. The intermediate phenotype Hurler–Scheie can display all the visceral problems of those with Hurler diseases but again with no or mild cognitive impairment.

INVESTIGATIONS/DIAGNOSIS

Measurement of urine glycosaminoglycans (GAGs) is the screening test of choice for suspected MPS disease. Children with Hurler disease have an increased secretion of dermatan sulphate and heparan sulphate. The diagnosis can then be confirmed by measurement of enzyme activity in leukocytes. Genotype phenotype correlations aid selection of patients for BMT. The extent and severity of disease needs to be established in all affected children. A skeletal survey including neck views, MRI of brain and spinal cord, neurological, visual and audiological assessment and cardiac ECHO are all required.

BIOCHEMISTRY/GENETICS

Hurler disease is caused by a defect in the gene coding for alpha-L-iduronidase, a lysosomal enzyme essential for the degradation of GAGs. They are important structurally in the extracellular matrix.

TREATMENT

Traditionally treatment has been focused on identifying and treating the various complications of the disease. This included the obstructive respiratory disease, instability of the cervical vertebrae, cardiac disease, carpal tunnel syndrome, sleep disturbances and visual and hearing impairment. BMT significantly slows the progression of the disease and although it does not reverse bone or previous neurological disease, it is the treatment of choice and should be performed early. Enzyme replacement therapy (ERT) can improve some manifestations of the disease but due to its lack of transport across the blood–brain barrier is unsuitable for those with neurological disease. The use of ERT prior to induction of BMT has improved transplant outcome.

PROGNOSIS

The prognosis for classic Hurler is poor, with progressive and severe neurodevelopmental regression. Death usually occurs before the age of 10 years from cardiac, respiratory or neurological causes. While BMT, if performed suitably early, seems to address the progressive neurological decline, it is not effective at preventing some visceral problems progressing especially the skeletal complications.

SANFILIPPO SYNDROME, MPS III

CLINCAL PRESENTATION

Sanfilippo syndrome is the most common of the MPS. Unlike the other MPS, the predominant manifestations are neurological rather than visceral, though these can also occur. The typical presentation is that of recurrent upper airway tract infections and mild speech delay in the first couple of years of life. This is followed by increasingly difficult behavioural problems that usually start around the age of 3–5 years and consist of restless, destructive, chaotic, anxious and sometimes aggressive behaviour. The aspect that most families find most difficult to deal with is the profound sleep disturbances that most patients develop. The behavioural problems do decline with age and eventually disappear due to the progressive mental retardation, finally resulting in complete loss of initiative. This decline is part of the neurological progression of the disease that ultimately results in the patient becoming fully bedridden in a vegetative state by the age of 10–30 years.

INVESTIGATIONS

Undegradated heparan sulphate will be present on testing for urinary GAGs. It can occasionally be present at low levels especially in older children and thus missed if the urine sample is overly dilute. Confirmation is by leukocyte analysis of the relevant four enzymes.

BIOCHEMISTRY

Sanfilippo syndrome is a group of four autosomal recessive lysosomal storage diseases resulting from a failure to degrade heparan sulphate. The four biochemical subtypes of MPS III (types A–D) are caused by the deficiency of one of the four enzymes required for the removal of N-acetylglucosamine at the non-reducing end of the saccharide chain. Heparan-N-sulfamidase is deficient in MPS IIIA, a-N-acetylglucosaminidase is deficient in MPS IIIB, acetylCoA:alpha-glucosaminide N-acetyl transferase is deficient in MPS IIIC and N-acetylglucosamine 6-sulfatase is deficient in MPS IIID. Type C and D are uncommon.

TREATMENT

Treatment is mainly supportive including the use of antipsychotics, melatonin and gastrostomies. Genistein, an isoflavone, has been trialed for substrate reduction therapy, though the clinical results thus far are disappointing. There are trials in progress for intrathecal and/or intravenous ERT for MPS IIIA and B.

MORQUIO SYNDROME, MPS IV

CLINICAL PRESENTATION

Patients with MPS IVA appear healthy at birth. The initial signs and symptoms are usually identifiable by the age of 3 years, with unusual skeletal features including striking short trunk, odontoid hypoplasia, pectus carinatum, kyphosis, scoliosis, genu valgum, coxa valga, hypermobile joints and abnormal gait. Patients with MPS IVA have normal intelligence and also, unlike most other MPS, have a degree of ligamentous laxity. The odontoid hypoplasia is the most critical skeletal feature, which in combination with the ligamentous laxity and extradural muco-polysaccharide deposition, can result in atlantoaxial subluxation, cervical myelopathy or even death (**Fig. 14.7**). Other potential complications include pulmonary compromise, valvular heart disease, hearing loss, hepatomegaly, corneal clouding, coarse facial features and abnormal dentition.

INVESTIGATIONS

Urinary GAG profiling will reveal an excess of keratan sulphate. However, this can be falsely negative and enzymatic analysis of leukocytes should be considered if a strong clinical suspicion is present.

BIOCHEMISTRY

Two enzyme of keratan suphate metabolism can be deficient: either N-acetylgalactosamine-6 sulfatase (frequent type A) or beta-galactosidase, also mutated in GM1-gangliosidosis.

TREATMENT

Supportive measures include NSAIDs for joint pain, antibiotics for pulmonary infections and respiratory support for the pulmonary compromise and obstruction. Orthopedic and spinal interventions are commonly required with cervical spinal fusion being performed in most patients. ERT for MPS IVA is currently being trialed.

PROGNOSIS

Patients with a severe phenotype often do not survive beyond the second or third decade of life, primarily related to cervical instability and pulmonary compromise. Patients with mild manifestations of MPS IVA have been reported to survive into the seventh decade of life.

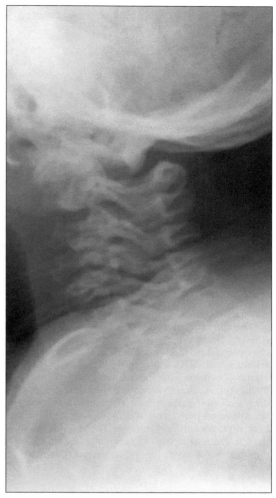

FIGURE 14.7 Cervical x-ray showing atlantoaxial subluxation in a patient with Morquio syndrome.

HOMOCYSTINURIA – CLASSICAL AND SECONDARY TO REMETHYLATION DISORDERS

CLINICAL PRESENTATION

Classical homocystinuria (HCU) typically presents with mental retardation, ectopia lentis and/or thromboembolic episodes. The optic lens dislocation occurs by age 6 years in 50% of those with untreated vitamin B6 (pyridoxine) non-responsive disease and by age 10 years in 50% of untreated B6-responsive individuals. As patients get older there is increasing skeletal involvement with many patients developing a marfanoid body habitus though with restriction rather than joint laxity. Mental retardation, is moderate with the historical mean IQ of 58 for untreated adults with pyridoxine-unresponsive HCU compared with IQ of 72 for pyridoxine-responsive individuals.

The remethylation disorders have a more heterogeneous phenotype, with the severest presenting in the neonatal period with failure to thrive, hypotonia, seizures and MRI changes that can include white matter changes and occasionally communicating hydocephalus that may require shunting. Older children are often globally developmentally delayed and later develop peripheral neuropathies and are at risk of respiratory failure. However, at the mildest end of the spectrum, patients can be asymptomatic and may only present in adult life, often with cerebrovascular thrombosis.

BIOCHEMISTRY/GENETICS

Classical HCU is due to cystathionine b-synthase (CBS) deficiency, an enzyme that utilises pyridoxine as a cofactor. Enzyme deficiency results in elevated total homocysteine and methionine with the latter being used in a number of newborn screening programs around the world. Approximately one-half of individuals with HCU are pyridoxine responsive. There are some genotype/phenotype correlations: the common c.833T>C (p.I278T) mutation that may account, world-wide, for some 21% of all CBS-inactivating alleles, being B6 responsive. However, in Ireland, 71% of the defective CBS alleles are G307S, resulting in pyridoxine non-responsiveness.

In contrast, in remethylation disorders high homocysteine but low methionine levels are seen. Remethylation is the process by which methionine is reformed from homocysteine and requires the enzymes methionine synthase and methionine synthase reductase methyltetrahydrofolate and cobalamin (vitamin B12). They should be considered when a high level of homocysteine is not accompanied with a proportional rise in methionine.

TREATMENT

The treatment of classical HCU is firstly adding pyridoxine and assessing response. In those patients that do not or only partial respond, a diet low in methionine and homocysteine is recommended. This may require the use of homocysteine-free essential amino acids preparations. No dietary treatment will help the remethylation disorders though the block can be bypassed by using betaine (utilising the alternative betaine:homocysteine methyltransferase system) while remnant activity may be stimulated by vitamin B_{12} addition.

PROGNOSIS

In those children picked up with classical HCU by newborn screening, that are able to comply with diet, the long-term neurological outcome is favourable. Some improvement is noted in behaviour even in those diagnosed late. At any age a reduction in total homocysteine levels reduces the thomboembolic risk and thus long-term treatment is essential. The prognosis of the remethylation disorders is much more guarded with the severity at presentation often determining the long-term outcome.

WOLMAN/CHOLESTEROL ESTER DISEASE

CLINICAL PRESENTATION

Wolman disease is the term for the most severe clinical variant of acid lipase deficiency. Patients are symptomatic at birth and develop progressive feeding intolerance, diarrhoea, massive hepatosplenomegaly, liver cirrhosis and pulmonary infiltrates/inflammation secondary to lipid deposition. Death usually occurs during infancy. Patients frequently have enlarged adrenal glands with calcifications. The less severe phenotype, which often presents much later in childhood, is known as cholesterol ester disease.

BIOCHEMISTRY/GENETICS

Lysosomal acid lipase (LAL) hydrolyzes cholesteryl esters and triglycerides taken up via receptor-mediated endocytosis of plasma lipoprotein particles. Normally LAL-mediated release of free cholesterol intracellularly causes down-regulation of HMG-CoA reductase and LDL receptor genes and up-regulation of cholesterol esterification by the activation of ACAT enzyme. However, in LAL deficiency the intralysosomal accumulation of fats is accompanied by a combined hyperlipidaemia plasma lipid profile.

TREATMENT

A number of case reports documented successful BMT for Wolman disease, though success was mainly seen in early diagnosed and siblings of families with a previous index case. The early results from ERT trials have also been impressive but these need to be further evaluated.

PROGNOSIS

With just supportive treatment Wolman patients die before 1 year of age usually from a combination of liver, adrenal and pulmonary disease.

FRUCTOSE 1, 6-BISPHOSPHATASE DEFICIENCY

CLINICAL PRESENTATION

50% of patients present in the first days of life with metabolic acidosis, marked hypoglycaemia, raised lactate and often a degree of hepatomegaly. Decompensation is triggered by catabolism that often accompanies a febrile illness and/or refusal to eat. Episodes may also be triggered by large fructose loads (>1 g/kg/dose). Between attacks, patients are usually well though mild, intermittent or chronic acidosis can persist. The frequency of attacks decreases with age.

DIAGNOSIS/INVESTIGATIONS

Hypoglycaemia, high lactate and a variable degree of ketosis are seen during periods of decompensation. Increased levels of glycerol and lactate excretion may be found on urinary organic acids analysis. Measurement of low fructose 1, 6-bisphosphatase (FB) activity in a mixed leucocyte preparation or, more reliably, in isolated monocyte cultures is diagnostic. This can be confirmed by mutation analysis. Liver biopsies for enzymatic activity are now rarely performed.

BIOCHEMISTRY

Fructose 1, 6 bisphosphatase is a key enzyme in the gluconeogenic pathway, with deficiency impairing the production of glucose from all gluconeogenic precursors including fructose. Children with fructose 1, 6-bisphosphatase deficiency have a greater tolerance to fructose than those with hereditary fructose intolerance as they can still metabolise fructose 1-P to lactate.

TREATMENT

Emergency management is the provision of adequate glucose during decompensations. Additional supplementation of bicarbonate is only occasionally necessary. The cornerstone of therapy is the avoidance of fasting and the restriction of fructose, sucrose and sorbitol, particularly during unwell episodes.

PROGNOSIS

The prognosis is favourable and fasting tolerance improves with age.

NEURONAL CEROID LIPOFUSINOSES

CLINICAL PRESENTATION

These are a group of inherited progressive neurodegenerative diseases. They are grouped together due to the accumulation of autofluorescent lipopigments in the lysosomes. They typically present with psychomotor retardation, seizures, visual loss and early death. They are subclassified by their age of onset into infantile, late infantile, juvenile and adult. The late infantile is the most common and in this form children, typically between the ages of 2 and 4 years, present with delayed speech and seizures. They then develop ataxia and developmental regression. Vision is usually lost by the age of 6 years with death typically following a period of being bedridden.

BIOCHEMISTRY/GENETICS

Three genes encoding lysosomal enzymes and five encoding lysosomal transporters have been delineated. *CLN1* and *CLN2* encode palmitoyl protein thioesterase and tripeptidyl peptidase type 1, respectively and their activity can be measured on white cell assay. However, if the history is strongly suggestive but enzymology is negative, electron microscopy of leukocytes/fibroblasts may be performed, searching for the presence of characteristic inclusions. Gene sequencing is needed for subtyping. While there is generally good genotype–phenotype correlation there is also genetic heterogeneity whereby, for instance, different mutations in *CLN1* can cause infantile or adult onset disease.

DIAGNOSIS

Electron microscopy on whole blood or fibroblasts is complemented by white cell assay of palmitoyl protein thioesterase and tripeptidyl peptidase type 1. Direct sequencing for other variants should be undertaken if these are non-informative.

TREATMENT

Symptomatic management adjusted to the individual's needs and disease progression are the cornerstone of treatment. Carbazepine and phenytoin can worsen symptoms and the recommended antiepileptic medication of choice is lamotrigine. ERT and gene therapy trials are ongoing.

UREA CYCLE DISORDERS

CLINICAL PRESENTATION

Patients usually present in the neonatal period with lethargy, poor feeding, apnoea and encephalopathy. These symptoms reflect the toxic effects of ammonia on the brain and may be initially mistaken for signs of sepsis. Ammonia, the key diagnostic metabolite in the acute setting, is a respiratory stimulant and a respiratory alkalosis may be found early in the illness. Early treatment of hyperammonaemia determines the long-term outcome for the patients (**Fig. 14.8**).

Older children with milder disease present with variable symptoms. These can range from episodic nausea, vomiting and behavioural changes to encephalopathy. There may be a history of protein intolerance. Clinical examination is often without diagnostic clues other than possible hepatomegaly. The most common urea cycle disorder (UCD) is ornithine transcarbamylase deficiency (OTC). This is the only x-linked inherited UCD. Affected males often die with overwhelming hyperammonaemia in the newborn period. Female carriers, although usually much less severely affected, can also present with life-threatening hyperammonaemic episodes.

DIAGNOSIS/INVESTIGATIONS

The key investigation is the plasma ammonia. Obtaining a reliable ammonia level can be challenging, particularly in the sick patient. Ideally it should

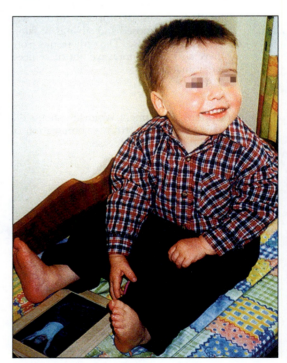

FIGURE 14.8 A 3-year-old boy with the urea cycle disorder citrullinaemia. He has short stature and had failure to thrive secondary to his restrictive diet and recurrent episodes of illness. He is of normal intelligence.

be from a free flowing sample, sent to the laboratory, on ice, and analysed immediately. A concentration greater than 200 μmol/l in neonates and 100 μmol/l in older children is highly suspicious of a metabolic condition – a repeat sample should be obtained for confirmation. Plasma amino acids and urine organic acids are urgently required to establish the exact diagnosis. Molecular analysis of the suspected gene is needed for confirmation.

BIOCHEMISTRY/GENETICS

The urea cycle converts toxic ammonia to urea. Deficiencies in the enzymes and transporters of this cycle result in hyperammonaemia.

TREATMENT

Any new hyperammonaemic patient should be transferred to a metabolic centre. Ammonia is neurotoxic and lowering the plasma concentration immediately is essential. In general, stopping normal feeds and commencing intravenous 10% dextrose at high infusion rates is recommended to avoid catabolism. The sick neonate will frequently require haemofiltration. Sodium benzoate and sodium phenylbutyrate lower the ammonia by conjugating with amino acids and reducing the nitrogen load.

Depending on the location of the urea cycle defect, arginine or citrulline can be used in very high treatment doses to remove nitrogen, or are semi-essential and only need to be supplemented in more modest doses. Once the situation has stabilised, protein is gradually reintroduced. The long-term management of these patients includes a low protein diet, the use of ammonia scavenger drugs above and the use of an emergency regime whenever the child is unwell. Diet and medication need to be adjusted to the patient's needs regularly.

PROGNOSIS

The outcome depends on the diagnosis, severity and duration of the initial hyperammonaemic crisis. Children who present in the neonatal period with severe encephalopathy will frequently die and those that survive will invariably have some degree of neurodevelopmental delay. Once treated, children often have further episodes of metabolic decompensation, especially during periods of intercurrent illness. Children with milder disease who present later may do remarkably well, with the outcome dependent on the severity of hyperammonaemic events prior to diagnosis and the implementation of emergency treatments, when unwell, after diagnosis. Prenatal testing should be offered to families.

GALACTOSAEMIA

CLINICAL PRESENTATION

Affected neonates classically present in the early neonatal period with jaundice, vomiting and lethargy. They are often initially thought to have sepsis. Once the lactose (galactose)-containing feeds are stopped the children improve. The frequent finding of an *Escherichia coli*-positive blood culture may confuse the diagnosis. Less commonly, children may also present in infancy with failure to thrive and vomiting (**Fig. 14.9**). Hepatomegaly and jaundice often present on examination and there is usually biochemical evidence of liver dysfunction. Cataracts are characteristically present (**Fig. 14.10**). In many countries galactosaemia is part of the newborn screening panel and affected children are diagnosed, ideally, prior to becoming significantly unwell.

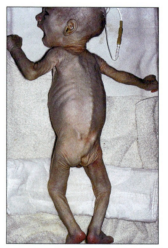

FIGURE 14.9 Severe failure to thrive seen in a late-diagnosed patient with galactosaemia.

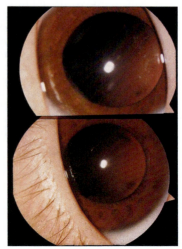

FIGURE 14.10 'Oil-drop' cataracts seen in the condition.

DIAGNOSIS/INVESTIGATIONS

Positive urine reducing substances can suggest the diagnosis but the sensitivity of the test is limited and would be negative in a galactosaemia child that has not yet been exposed to galactose. Direct measurement of the enzyme galactose-1-phosphate uridyltransferase (Gal-1-PUT) in red blood cells is diagnostic. The parents of affected children will have Gal-1-PUT levels in the heterozygotes range and this is useful in diagnosing the infant who has received a recent blood transfusion. Affected children should have their eyes examined and their liver function should be assessed.

BIOCHEMISTRY/GENETICS

The disease is autosomal recessive and is caused by a deficiency in the enzyme Gal-1-PUT. Lactose, the disaccharide in breast, formula and cow's milk, consists of galactose and glucose. It is the metabolites of galactose that are toxic to the liver and eyes. The cause of the neurological problems seen in later life is largely unknown with a variety of mechanisms suggested.

TREATMENT

Galactose (i.e. lactose) should be eliminated from the diet. Essentially this means switching to a soya-based formula and later a dairy products-free and 'minimal galactose foods' diet. Galactose is present in many processed foods and in general these should also be avoided. In later life, a very strict galacotose-free diet is probably not required and adults appear to be able to tolerate moderate amounts without apparent clinical problems. Bone health should be monitored and calcium and vitamin D supplements are usually recommended.

PROGNOSIS

Death from liver failure or sepsis is seen if the patient remains on a lactose diet. The cataracts are reversible if treatment is started early.

With treatment, however, the immediate prognosis is generally good, although early feeding problems and speech delay due to an oral motor dyspraxia are common. Older children and adults might have problems with verbal planning and 'concepts' in mathematics and science. Motor function, co-ordination and balance may also be affected. The majority of women develop hypergonadotrophic hypogonadism and there is a high risk for ovarian failure. Individually, females need to be assessed to start hormone replacement therapy as indicated.

FATTY ACID OXIDATION DEFECTS

CLINICAL PRESENTATION

Prior to expanded newborn screening, children with fatty acid oxidation defects (FAODs) frequently presented with encephalopathy due to severe hypoketotic hypoglycaemia. Often there was evidence of hepatic dysfunction. Usually there was a history of a preceding viral-like illness and a period of catabolic stress such as a missed meal(s). There was often little to find on examination apart from some hepatomegaly. 'Found dead in bed' during an intercurrent illness was unfortunately also a relatively common presentation. By far the most common FAOD is medium-chain acyl Co-A dehydrogenase (MCAD) deficiency and this is now screened for in most Western countries in the newborn period. Thus while MCAD should be suspected in the above clinical scenario the most common presentation is with a positive screening test. Babies can however, become unwell prior to screening and older children born prior to the commencement of expanded newborn screening might present symptomatically in later life.

Muscle preferentially oxidises fat as an energy source, so alternative presentations for the FAODs, especially the so-called long-chain disorders, are with cardiomyopathy, especially in infancy, and/or rhabdomyolysis, potentially occurring after significant exercise, as an older child or adult.

DIAGNOSIS/INVESTIGATIONS

The finding of hypoglycaemia with inappropriately low ketones (urine or blood) is suggestive of a FAOD. There may be acidosis, hepatic dysfunction, an elevated creatine kinase and/or hyperammonaemia. The specific disorder can usually be diagnosed on the acylcarnitine profile (**Fig. 14.11**). Cardiological assessment is essential in any suspected cases. Confirmation of the diagnosis is by fatty acid oxidation flux studies of fibroblasts (skin biopsy and culture) and/or on molecular genetic testing.

BIOCHEMISTRY/GENETICS

There are a series of enzymes necessary for the oxidation of fat to ketones and energy. The FAODs are inherited in an autosomal recessive fashion.

TREATMENT

Catabolism should be avoided. The child must not be subjected to significant catabolic stress such as fasting, especially during periods of intercurrent illness. If the child is unwell, they should take a high calorie carbohydrate drink frequently until well (the 'emergency regime'). If they are not tolerating this, or if there are any other concerns, then they should be admitted to their local hospital.

Regular feeds, in some FAOD even overnight feeds and the avoidance of long-chain fats are recommended, particularly necessary in long-chain disorders (long-chain L-3 hydroxyacyl-CoA dehydrogenase deficiency [LCHAD] and very long-chain L-3 hydroxyacyl-CoA dehydrogenase deficiency [VLCAD]).

PROGNOSIS

Once diagnosed and treated, the prognosis for MCAD is generally favourable. Prior to screening many children, however, did die or suffered significant morbidity. The long-term outcome for some of the long-chain disorders is less favourable even on treatment, as the children may develop peripheral neuropathy, retinopathy and cardiomyopathy.

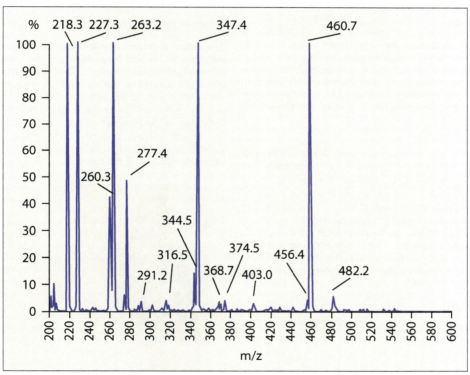

FIGURE 14.11 Acylcarnitine profile of a patient with medium-chain acyl co-A dehydrogenase (MCAD) deficiency showing the characteristic peak of octanycarnitine at 344.5.

DISORDERS OF KETONE BODY METABOLISM

CLINICAL PRESENTATION

The initial presentation is that of profound hypoglycaemia, with possible seizures, triggered by a catabolic stresses such as infection or decreased oral intake. Acidosis is a common co-presenting feature and in the ketone body utilisation defects, massive ketosis may be present.

INVESTIGATIONS

Any patient with hypoglycaemia should be tested for ketones. Excessive ketones and/or very high unexplained anion gap is suspicious of a ketone disorder, although a exaggerated normal physiological response is a much more common explanation. The urine organic acids may show a non-specific dicarboxylic aciduria (as seen in 3-hydroxy-3-methylglutaryl-coenzyme A synthase [HMG CoA synthase]) or the presence of diagnostic leucine metabolites (3-hydroxy-3-methylglutary-coenzyme A lyase, HMG CoA lyase) or isoleucine metabolites (beta-ketothiolase deficiency). The latter diseases also results in an increased hydroxy C5 levels on carnitine profiling, thus making it possible to diagnose these conditions on newborn screening. A clue to the presence of the ketone body utilisation defects can be the persistence of ketones after a meal in an otherwise well child. Definitive functional enzymatic testing can be performed on leukocytes and fibroblasts.

BIOCHEMISTRY

Ketone bodies acetoacetate and 3-hydroxybutyric acid are metabolites derived from fatty acids and ketogenic amino acids, such as leucine. They are mainly produced in the liver, via reactions catalysed by the ketogenic enzymes HMG CoA synthase and HMG CoA lyase. After prolonged starvation, ketone bodies can provide up to two-thirds of the brain's energy requirements. The rate-limiting enzyme of ketone body utilisation (ketolysis) is succinyl-coenzyme A: 3-oxoacid coenzyme A transferase. The subsequent step of ketolysis is catalysed by 2-methyl-lactoacetyl-coenzyme A thiolase (beta-ketothiolase), which is also involved in isoleucine catabolism.

TREATMENT

The avoidance of fasting and the use of a high energy carbohydrate emergency regime at times of catabolic stress, e.g. infections, is the cornerstone of management. A low leucine diet has been recommended in HMG CoA lyase patients but the need for this has been questioned. HMG CoA lyase and beta-ketothiolase patients may be given carnitine to avoid secondary deficiencies in carnitine.

PROGNOSIS

The prognosis is determined by the severity of the first presentation. Overall the prognosis tends to be excellent although individual HMG CoA lyase patients have developed white matter lesions and cardiomyopathies.

TYROSINAEMIA

CLINICAL PRESENTATION

Tyrosinaemia (tyrosinaemia type 1), usually presents as 'acute' neonatal liver failure with jaundice, coagulopathy, failure to thrive and often sepsis. These children can be very sick and prior to nitisinone (NTBC) treatment the mortality was high.

Alternatively, the 'chronic' presentation in later infancy is of failure to thrive, rickets (due to renal tubular dysfunction) (**Fig. 14.12**) and liver dysfunction. Other problems include neurological crises with porphyria-like pain and paraesthesia, renal failure and hepatocarcinoma (**Figs 14.13, 14.14**). It is possible to diagnose tyrosinaemia on expanded newborn screening although the diagnostic metabolite tyrosine is often elevated in non-tyrosinaemia liver disease and thus a second-line test is required.

DIAGNOSIS/INVESTIGATIONS

The presence of elevated levels of succinylacetone in the urine organic acids is diagnostic.

BIOCHEMISTRY/GENETICS

The defect is in the enzyme fumarylacetoacetase, the last enzyme in the breakdown of the amino acids phenylalanine and tyrosine. The 'upstream' metabolites are alkylating agents and are thought to be responsible for the hepatorenal damage. Decreased activity of fumarylacetoacetase in fibroblasts or lymphocytes, in the presence of the classical biochemical and clinical features, confirms the diagnosis although the diagnosis is usually confirmed on mutation analysis. The disorder is recessive.

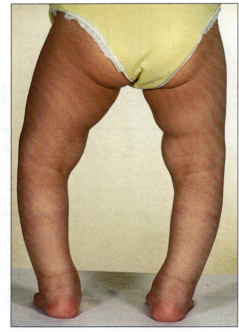

FIGURE 14.12 Tyrosinaemia: involvement of the bones (rickets) is seen in untreated tyrosinaemia.

TREATMENT

Normal feeds should be stopped and the hepatorenal dysfunction and rickets treated as indicated. Prior to 1991, the only successful long-term treatment of tyrosinaemia type I was liver transplantation but, with the advent of NTBC (2-(2-nitro-4-trifluoromethyl-benzoyl)-1, 3-cyclohexanedione) – a potent inhibitor of the up-stream enzyme 4-hydroxyphenylpyruvate dioxygenase – effective treatment is now available. NTBC prevents the toxic metabolites forming and is effective in both the acute and chronic forms of the disease. A dose of 1 mg/kg/d is recommended. Because the children still have a 'metabolic block', they require a low phenylalanine and tyrosine diet with a supplementary phenylalanine-/tyrosine-free amino acid formula. Growth, tyrosine levels and residual liver damage all need to be monitored, including regular liver imaging for hepatoma.

PROGNOSIS

Provided there is no substantial liver damage or malignant transformation, the long-term prognosis is likely to be excellent.

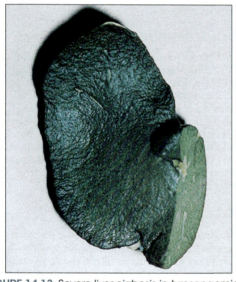

FIGURE 14.13 Severe liver cirrhosis in tyrosenaemia.

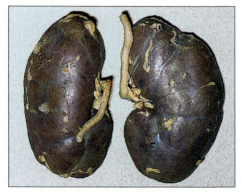

FIGURE 14.14 Tyrosinaemia: involvement of the kidneys.

GLYCOGEN STORAGE DISEASE TYPE I

CLINICAL PRESENTATION

Children with glycogen storage disease type I (GSDI) usually present in infancy with failure to thrive, abdominal distension secondary to hepatomegaly and/or symptoms of hypoglycaemia. The latter can occur after a short fast, yet the child, especially in early infancy, may surprisingly be asymptomatic. On examination there is often massive hepatomegaly (**Fig. 14.15**), truncal obesity, short stature, mild hypotonia and a 'doll-like' face.

DIAGNOSIS/INVESTIGATIONS

There is often a significant lactic acidosis that decreases with feeding. Hypertriglyceridaemia and hyperuricaemia are also characteristically present. These findings, along with the typical clinical appearance, are highly suggestive of GSDI and subsequent diagnostic investigations should be based on molecular testing rather than a liver biopsy for enzymology.

BIOCHEMISTRY/GENETICS

GSDIa is caused by a deficiency of glucose-6-phosphatase. A transport protein, responsible for the transport of glucose-6-phosphate, is defective in GSDIb. This disorder is additionally associated with neutropenia and immune deficiency. Molecular analysis is available for both GSDIa and Ib.

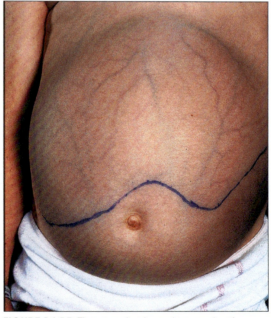

FIGURE 14.15 The massive hepatomegaly of glycogen storage disease type I.

TREATMENT

Maintaining normal glucose homeostasis is the key and is likely to reduce the long-term complications greatly. This is achieved by frequent daytime feeds and a continuous overnight feed via a naso-gastric tube or gastrostomy. Specialist dietary input is essential. After the age of 2 years, uncooked cornstarch may be used to improve fast tolerance. Individual fasting tolerance needs to be assessed. Allopurinol lowers uric acid levels while granulo-cyte colony stimulating factor (G-CSF) can improve the neutropenia seen in GSDIb. Long-term management also includes regular monitoring of the biochemistry (lactate, triglycerides and glucose profiles), growth, renal function, liver (ultrasound for adenomas) and bone mineralisation status. Liver transplantation may be an option in some patients.

PROGNOSIS

Adults who have had relatively poorly controlled disease frequently have the complications of short stature, renal disease, osteoporosis and liver adenomas. The latter may become malignant. It is hoped the current treatment guidelines will greatly reduce the frequency and severity of these complications. It is likely that there is a good correlation between metabolic control (i.e. normoglycaemia) and outcome.

PEROXISOMAL BIOGENESIS DISORDERS

CLINICAL PRESENTATION

Peroxisomal biogenesis disorders (PBD) are a group of disorders that include the phenotypes Zellweger, neonatal ADL and infantile Refsum disease. The most severe form, Zellweger presents at birth with severe hypotonia, hepatomegaly and the characteristic features of a prominent forehead, large anterior fontanelle, mild dysmorphic features (**Fig. 14.16**) and stippled epiphyseal calcification (**Fig. 14.17**). The much milder infantile Refsum disease presents with subtle facial features and developmental delay in early childhood. Patients may have autistic features and/or seizures.

INVESTIGATIONS/DIAGNOSIS

Elevation of VLCFAs is the key diagnostic finding. Measurement of plasma bile acids, red cell plasmalogens and fibroblast enzyme analysis is needed to elucidate the aetiology further. Liver and renal function are often impaired in these patients and need to be assessed.

BIOCHEMISTRY/GENETICS

Peroxisomal functions include the beta-oxidation of VLCFAs, pristanic acid and bile acid synthesis and others. PBDs are caused by a failure of protein (enzyme) import into the peroxisome, encoded by various *PEX* genes. A variety of gene defects can result in the same phenotype (locus heterogeneity) and yet the various phenotypes can also be allelic. In addition there are single enzyme peroxisomal disorders that can give rise to an infantile Refsum-like phenotype. All the conditions are inherited in an autosomal recessive manner.

TREATMENT/PROGNOSIS

There is no specific treatment for these disorders. The prognosis for the severe Zellweger form of the disease is very poor, with death usually in the first year of life. Children with infantile Refsum disease can live much longer with very little disease progression.

Metabolic diseases

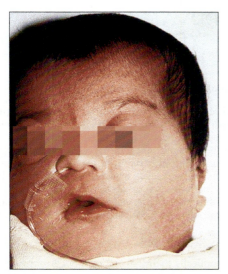

FIGURE 14.16 Typical facial appearances of Zellweger syndrome.

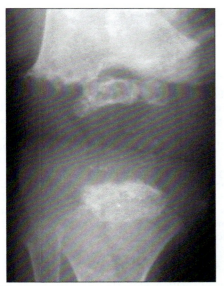

FIGURE 14.17 Radiograph showing the punctate calcification seen in peroxisomal disorders.

LEIGH SYNDROME

CLINICAL PRESENTATION

Leigh syndrome (LS), also called subacute, necrotising encephalopathy, is a devastating neurodegenerative disorder, characterised by defined changes on CNS imaging, i.e. focal, bilaterally symmetric lesions, particularly in the basal ganglia, thalamus and brainstem (**Fig. 14.18**). Patients can however, exhibit considerable clinical and genetic heterogeneity. The course of the illness is unpredictable, although the onset is frequently in infancy often coinciding with an intercurrent illness. The child may present acutely with encephalopathy, respiratory abnormalities or a stroke-like illness. Alternatively, there may be no clear onset of symptoms or there are non-specific symptoms such as failure to thrive, generalised myopathy or polyneuropathy and only occasionally developmental delay. The children may have evidence of basal ganglia dysfunction on examination, with variable combinations of abnormal eye movements, dysarthria, dystonia, ataxia, autonomic dysfunction and cognitive delay present. They are not typically dysmorphic though midline defects such as cleft palate and long thin philtrum have been described and there is normally no significant hepatomegaly.

INVESTIGATIONS/DIAGNOSIS

While LS remains a neuropathological/neuroimaging-based diagnosis, the characteristic clinical features, typical radiological findings and the frequent finding of an elevated blood and/or CSF lactate, allow a diagnosis to be made ante-mortem in most patients. If a lumbar puncture is being performed diagnostically then an assessment of CSF methylentetrahydrofolate should be considered as folate levels in brain

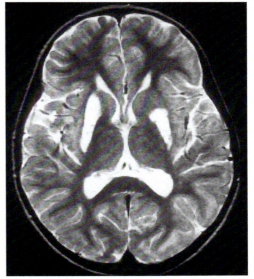

FIGURE 14.18 MRI showing changes typical of Leigh syndrome, with involvement of the lentiform nuclei bilaterally.

can be low. A muscle biopsy for histology, histochemistry, respiratory chain enzymology and coenzyme Q levels is essential to help to genetically define the diagnosis. Fibroblasts studies for pyruvate dehydrogenase defects and mitochondrial DNA analysis should also be performed.

BIOCHEMISTRY/GENETICS

Recent studies have demonstrated various molecular or biochemical defects of the pyruvate dehydrogenase complex (PDHC) and the mitochondrial respiratory chain complexes I and IV in particular and to a lesser extent complex II/III, ubiquinone and complex V can result in LS. While many of the defects are likely to be inherited in an autosomal recessive manner, some forms of LS are caused by mutations in the mitochondrial genome and thus genetic counselling can be difficult. Now that sequencing of the mitochondrial DNA is commonly available, many of the nuclear genes for mitochondrial disease are being identified.

TREATMENT

There is no curative therapy so treatment is generally supportive. A variety of vitamins and other medications have been tried with anecdotal reports of their benefit. These include thiamine, riboflavin, coenzyme Q, carnitine, biotin and folinic acid. Ketogenic diet has been used in pyruvate dehydrogenase defects.

PROGNOSIS

The long-term prognosis is generally poor although there may be long periods (i.e. many years) of stability. Children who present in early infancy can be expected to have a very poor prognosis.

PYRUVATE DEHYDROGENASE DEFICIENCY

CLINICAL PRESENTATION

Typically children with deficiency of the pyruvate dehydrogenase complex (PDHC) present with global developmental delay, hypotonia, epilepsy, ataxia (that may be intermittent), progressive encephalopathy and/or Leigh-like symptoms (LS) and peripheral neuropathy, which can be acute. They may have brain malformations such as agenesis of the corpus callosum, dilatation of the ventricles or abnormalities of the midbrain and basal ganglia (**Figs 14.19, 14.20**).

INVESTIGATIONS

Biochemically their hall mark is a persistent lactic acidosis (and correspondingly high alanine in plasma amino acids) with a normal/low lactate to pyruvate ratio. Occasionally, in the E3 defects elevated leucine, isoleucine and valine can be seen. Enzymatic activity can be assayed in fibroblasts. Immunoblotting is used to define which subunit is affected before genetic investigations are initiated.

BIOCHEMISTRY/GENETICS

PDHC is a multi-subunit enzyme complex, governing the conversion of pyruvate into acetyl CoA. Its four main subunits are E1 – the decarboxylase that is a heterodimer of an α (PDHA1) and β (PDHB) subunit; E2 – the dihydrolipoamide acetyltransferase (DLAT); E3 – dihydroliopamide dehydrogenase(DLD), which is also a component of branched chain α-ketoacid dehydrogenase complex; and E3BP – the E3 binding protein. PDHC uses thiamine as a cofactor. Only the E1 α subunit is encoded on the X chromosome, but defects are typically the result of new mutations.

TREATMENT

Supplementation with thiamine has been tried at doses up to 2 g/d. The early institution of a ketogenic diet may lead to improved overall survival and neurological outcome. In acute increased lactic acidosis, dichloroacetate has been used in doses up to 50 mg/kg/d, though prolonged use may cause polyneuropathy.

PROGNOSIS

The prognosis is often poor but depends on the severity of the defect and its response to therapy.

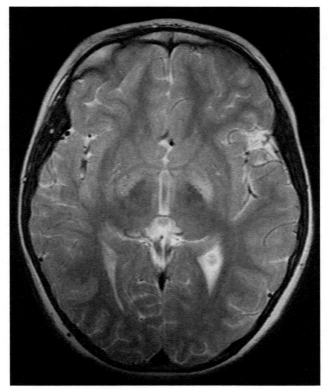

FIGURE 14.19 Bilateral globus pallidus involvement in pyruvate dehydrogenase deficiency.

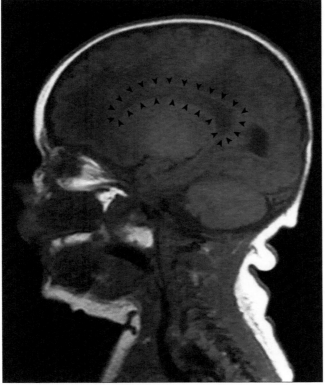

FIGURE 14.20 Absent corpus callosum (arrow heads) in pyruvate dehydrogenase deficiency.

PYRUVATE CARBOXYLASE DEFICIENCY

CLINICAL PRESENTATION

There are three distinct types of presentation of pyruvate carboxylase deficiency: type A patients typically become severely ill between 2 and 5 months of age with progressive hypotonia, recurrent episodes of vomiting and dehydration and metabolic acidosis typically precipitated by catabolic stress, before developing pyramidal tract signs. Hepatomegaly and renal dysfunction may also be present. Central imaging might show subepidymal cysts and delayed myelination; type B, the so-called French phenotype, presents shortly after birth with severe neurological dysfunction with rigidity and Parkinson-like features. Most of these patients die in the neonatal period. The third form is the most benign and uncommon, with patients presenting with episodes of lactic acidosis and ketoacidosis, though recovering well from these and being asymptomatic inbetween.

INVESTIGATIONS/DIAGNOSIS

PC should be considered in any child with hypoglycaemia and lactic acidosis with neurological abnormalities. In neonates a high lactate/pyruvate ratio with a low hydroxybutyrate/acetoacetate ratio is suggestive, while high plasma citrulline and low glutamine/glutamate is almost pathognomic. Enzymatic assay to confirm the diagnosis can be performed on fibroblasts (**Fig. 14.21**).

BIOCHEMISTRY/GENETICS

Pyruvate carboxylase is a tetramere of four identical subunits and uses biotin as a cofactor. The most severe phenotypes have been linked to null mutations. Mosaicism has been reported in several patients having a milder phenotype.

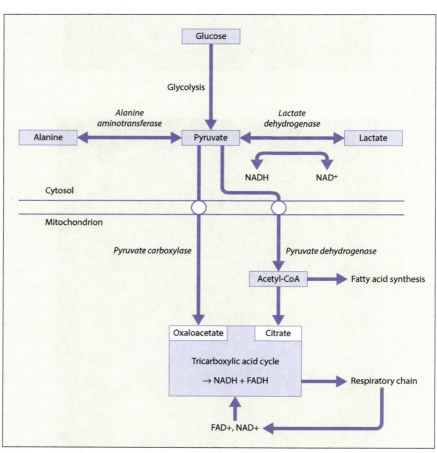

FIGURE 14.21 Pyruvate metabolism.

Metabolic diseases

TREATMENT

Type A and B should be treated acutely with bicarbonate and 10% dextrose on acute presentation. Overall the results of treatment with biotin, thiamine, dichloroacetate and ketogenic diets have been poor.

PROGNOSIS

Prognosis is determined by the severity of the defect, though some patients with very limited enzyme activity have lived beyond 5 years. Those milder phenotypes may survive longer with differing degrees of impairment.

MENKE DISEASE

CLINICAL PRESENTATION

Menke disease is a disorder of copper transport which, in the classic form, causes severe neurological disease. Apart from neonatal jaundice, children are usually relatively normal during early infancy but develop symptoms of poor feeding, vomiting and failure to thrive at 2–4 months (**Fig. 14.22**). Seizures and developmental delay are often the presenting features. Neurological regression is rapid, with a wide range of symptoms reported. Seizures are often difficult to control. Death is usually within the first 2 years of life.

The facial appearance is highly characteristic, with a pale complexion, sagging jowls, wide nasal bridge and abnormal hair. The hair is striking; it is lustreless, brittle and has an unkempt appearance (**Figs 14.23, 14.24**). Microscopically it shows pili torti. Menke patients, because of the role of copper in elastin and

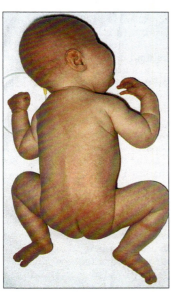

FIGURE 14.22 Infant with Menke disease who presented with failure to thrive and seizures.

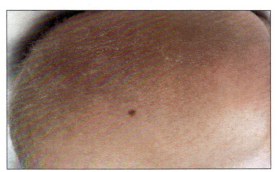

FIGURE 14.23 The short, brittle hair of Menke disease.

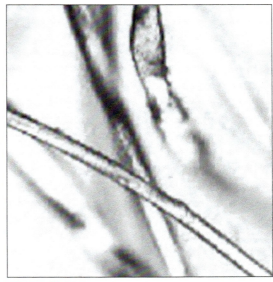

FIGURE 14.24 Pili torti and trichorrhexis nodosa seen in Menke disease.

collagen synthesis, can also have problems with joint laxity, bladder diverticulum and rupture, arterial bleeds and bony abnormalities. These features are also seen in the milder forms of the disease such as the occipital horn syndrome.

INVESTIGATIONS/DIAGNOSIS

The clinical features are usually highly suggestive, and the subsequent finding of low serum copper and caeruloplasmin establishes the diagnosis. Copper levels can be (very) low in the normal neonate and thus biochemical diagnosis at this age can be difficult. Measurement of neurotransmitters can be a useful adjunct to diagnosis at this age. Copper uptake and release studies in fibroblasts can be performed to confirm the diagnosis, although mutational analysis is the gold standard confirmatory test and is important for future prenatal testing.

BIOCHEMISTRY/GENETICS

Menke disease is caused by a defect in copper transmembrane transporter that results in enhanced uptake but decreased efflux in intestinal and renal tubular cells. This results in an increased concentration of copper in these areas but a deficiency elsewhere. This deficiency affects copper-containing enzymes such as cytochrome oxidase and lysyl oxidase, essential in cellular energy production and collagen/elastin synthesis, respectively. The disease is inherited as an X-linked recessive trait.

TREATMENT/PROGNOSIS

Treatment is palliative. Intravenous or subcutaneous copper histidinate therapy may be partially successful if started very early (in patients less than 1 month old) although these children still have a significant morbidity, with a severe connective tissue disorder and developmental delay.

PHENYLKETONURIA

CLINICAL PRESENTATION

The classical childhood features of phenylketonuria (PKU) are now rarely seen, as a result of the highly effective neonatal screening programmes. This is based on the detection of elevated phenylalanine concentrations measured in the neonatal Guthrie card blood spot, taken when the child is 2–10 days old. Untreated, PKU leads to progressive mental retardation. Patients may also develop spasticity and an abnormal gait, while a minority have focal neurological signs and seizures. The severe neurodevelopmental delay may be partially reversible if treatment is started in early childhood. If treatment is not started until late childhood, an improvement in behaviour is the best one can expect. Children with untreated PKU may have blond hair, blue eyes and fair skin due to metabolic defect restricting melanin production.

INVESTIGATIONS/DIAGNOSIS

PKU is easily diagnosed by measuring the concentration of phenylalanine in blood (Guthrie card blood spot or plasma). In classical severe PKU, the levels are above 1200 µmol/l (normal 40–100 µmol/l) whereas in mild PKU, which still requires treatment, levels on a normal diet are above 400 µmol/l. Molecular testing is not essential for diagnosis but is increasingly being performed. A rare but important group of disorders are pterin defects, also presenting with elevated levels of phenylalanine on the neonatal blood spot. Tests for defects in the 'pterin' pathway must be done in all patients with raised blood phenylalanine, as the treatment and prognosis are different from that for PKU.

BIOCHEMISTRY/GENETICS

PKU is caused by a defect in the gene for phenylalanine hydroxylase, the enzyme responsible for the conversion of phenylalanine to tyrosine. It is the high concentrations of phenylalanine that cause the cognitive damage. The disease is inherited in an autosomal recessive manner.

TREATMENT

The aim of treatment is to maintain the phenylalanine concentrations in the range 100–350 µmol/l in the first 5 years of life and less than 600 µmol/l throughout childhood. The immature brain is much more susceptible to hyperphenylalaninaemia and thus good control is essential in early childhood (**Fig. 14.25**). The diet can be relaxed in adulthood, except for women contemplating pregnancy (see below), although the long-term consequences of this are unknown and 'diet for life' is probably ideal but not achieved in many. Treatment consists of a very restricted natural protein (phenylalanine) intake and a supplementary phenylalanine-free formula. This diet can be difficult and compliance is often a problem.

Metabolic diseases

Recently the use of the natural cofactor tetrahydrobiopterin in pharmacological doses has shown to increase significantly the residual enzyme activity in some patients with PKU and thus allows for a liberalisation of the diet.

PROGNOSIS

With early treatment, the prognosis is excellent, although there is probably a mild deficit in IQ in some. Women with PKU are at risk of having children with severe complications due to intrauterine exposure of high concentrations of phenylalanine and thus must be on a very strict diet prior to and throughout the pregnancy.

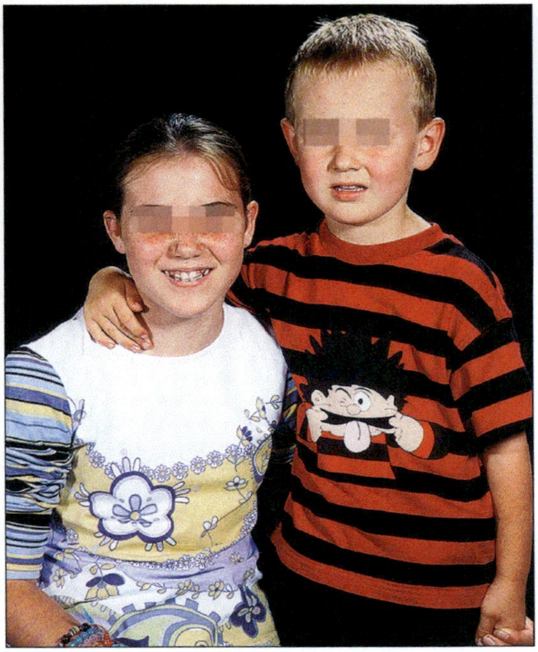

BIOTIN DISORDERS

CLINICAL PRESENTATION

There are two main forms of biotin disorders: holocarboxylase synthetase and biotinidase deficiency. The former tends to present in the neonatal period while the latter usually presents in infancy. The presentation is variable and ranges from acute metabolic decompensation with ketosis, lactic acidosis and a 'septic'-like picture, to failure to thrive and developmental delay. Frequently, children present with neurological complaints such as ataxia, hypotonia and especially seizures. There may be a characteristic erythematous rash, which may be generalised or confined to the perioral regions (**Figs 14.26, 14.27**). There may be blepharoconjunctivitis and a glossitis. Both conditions can be diagnosed by newborn screening, so ideally patients will be treated prior to symptoms developing.

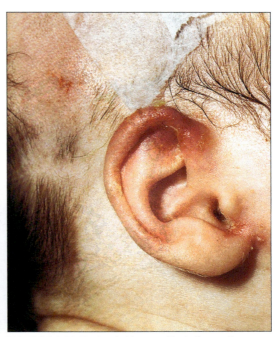

FIGURE 14.26 Typical skin manifestations of biotinidase deficiency.

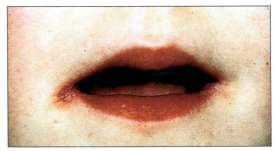

FIGURE 14.27 Typical skin manifestations of biotinidase deficiency.

FIGURE 14.25 Brother and sister seen with early diagnosed and treated phenylketonuria. They are healthy and of normal intelligence.

437

INVESTIGATIONS/DIAGNOSIS

Acutely unwell children have lactic acidaemia with the typical urinary organic acid picture of 3-methylcrotonylglycine and methylcitrate – highly suggestive of a biotin pathway defect. The child with the chronic form of the conditions may not always have the typical organic acids, although lactic acidaemia is often present. Biotinidase activity can be directly measured in blood, while holocarboxylase synthetase enzymology requires fibroblasts.

BIOCHEMISTRY/GENETICS

The carboxylase enzymes require the attachment of biotin to their apocarboxylase precursors to be active. Biotinidase recycles biocytin to supply biotin while holocarboxylase synthetase is involved in catalysing the attachment of biotin to the apoenzyme. Both conditions are autosomal recessive.

TREATMENT/PROGNOSIS

Treatment is with 5–20 mg of biotin daily. This dramatically improves the biochemical abnormality, the skin rash and general wellbeing. Seizures tend to improve but significant neurological impairments to hearing, vision and cognition may remain.

GLUTARIC ACIDAEMIA TYPE I

CLINICAL PRESENTATION

Patients with glutaric acidaemia type 1 (GA1) are typically well, although they may be macrocephalic, and are often only diagnosed after suffering an acute metabolic encephalopathy that is usually precipitated by an intercurrent illness. This can result in severe neurological sequelae secondary to destruction of the striatum and these children commonly are left with a severe dystonic–dyskinetic movement disorder.

INVESTIGATIONS

The characteristic MRI changes are predominately in the striatum and prominent sylvian fissues and fronto-occipital enlargement of the CSF spaces are observed (**Fig. 14.28**). The finding of elevated 3-hydroxyglutarate and glutaric acid in the urine organic acids and/or elevation of C5DC in plasma or blood spot acylcarnitine profile are diagnostic for GA1. The latter is very useful as it allows for the diagnosis of the condition by newborn screening. Confirmation of the diagnosis can be made molecularly.

BIOCHEMISTRY/GENETICS

GA1 is an autosomal recessive organic academia caused by the deficiency of the enzyme glutaryl-CoA dehydrogenase. The enzyme is involved in the catabolism of the amino acid lysine and it is thought that the protein catabolism that can occur during an undercurrent illness releases large amounts of lysine, which leads to the accumulation of the neurotoxic compound glutaric acid and related metabolites.

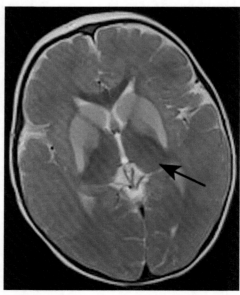

FIGURE 14.28 Bilateral symmetrical abnormalities of the basal ganglia (arrow) with sparing of the thalamus in a patient with glutaric aciduria type 1.

This can result in an acute severe permanent neurological insult. Less frequently a high protein intake may result in a similar but typically more gradual onset neurological disease.

TREATMENT

The key to treatment is early diagnosis, ideally by newborn screening and then aggressive treatment of periods of catabolic stress with high carbohydrate intake, either orally or intravenously, and supplementation with L-carnitine. When well, a low lysine diet achieved by the use of a special low lysine milk formula and/or a low protein product, is advised. This is complemented by oral L-carnitine. The latter helps remove glutaric acid through renal excretion and prevents carnitine depletion.

PROGNOSIS

With presymptomatic diagnosis through newborn screening and aggressive management of catabolic crisis throughout early childhood, the prognosis is excellent and severe neurological sequelae can be prevented. If diagnosis is late and once brain damage has occurred however, the typical severe dystonia and movement disorder is resistant to satisfactory management.

GLUT 1 TRANSPORTER DEFICIENCY

CLINICAL PRESENTATION

Children with GLUT 1 transport deficiency (GLUT 1) typically present with developmental delay and/or seizures. There may be a history of developmental regression or more commonly failure of developmental progression. There is often a degree of microcephaly. The phenotype is wide with some patients having severe disability and others relatively mild symptoms. Especially in the more mildly affected cases there is often a history of symptoms being better after eating and worsening after a short fast. Paradoxically there may be a history of the children being more alert or having fewer seizures during a period of significant sickness, reflecting the positive effect of a ketogenic state at the time.

INVESTIGATIONS

The critical and relatively easy investigation is the plasma/CSF glucose ratio. This is normally greater than 0.6. If it is less than 0.4, and if there is no other cause of hypoglycorrachia (low CSF glucose), for instance infection, then the diagnosis is highly likely, especially if the result is repeatable. If the ratio is between 0.4 and 0.6, then the diagnosis should still be considered. A repeat sample should be obtained on a fasted sample, e.g. in the morning. An elevated plasma glucose due to stress can lead to a falsely reduced ratio. The MRI brain may reveal mild generalised atrophy but is not diagnostic. Erythrocyte glucose uptake can be measured, but usually the diagnosis is confirmed molecularly.

BIOCHEMISTRY/GENETICS

GLUT 1 is caused by an autosomal dominant, usually *de novo*, molecular defect of the glucose transporter across the blood–brain barrier. This results in inadequate glucose being delivered to the brain despite a normal blood sugar level.

TREATMENT

The mainstay of treatment is ketogenic diet. This often results in a dramatic decrease of seizures and increase in cognitive function. The diet is particularly burdensome however, and some children struggle to tolerate it. The ratio of calories deriving from fat to other sources needed is individually different and ranges from 4:1 to a 3 or even a 2.5:1 ratio. In mild cases maintaining a high blood glucose level with regular high carbohydrate meals, including cornstarch supplements, can result in improved neurological function without having to implement a ketogenic diet.

PROGNOSIS

The earlier the diagnosis and thus the earlier treatment is commenced, the better the prognosis. Early treatment reduces the severity of intellectual disability. While the ketogenic diet results in a significant improvement in symptomatic patients it is not a cure and thus has to be continued long term.

FABRY DISEASE

CLINICAL PRESENTATION

Fabry disease is a multi-system disease that is extremely heterogeneous. Presentations include painful burning extremities in late childhood that are typically exacerbated by exercise or extremes of temperature. Gastrointestinal complaints, e.g. diarrhoea and abdominal pain, as well as signs of vestibular dysfunction and tinnitus are also common. Presentation with severe renal impairment, heart failure, stroke and/or psychiatric disease in adulthood is also well recognised and make up the classical, severe, life-threatening pathology of the disease. Many patients are asymptomatic with the diagnosis following family screening. Physical findings include angiokeratoma and cornea verticillata on slit-lamp examination.

INVESTIGATIONS

The presence of classical features of the disease (cardiomyopathy, renal disease, etc.) in a patient who has a relative with confirmed Fabry disease and in whom an X-linked inheritance pattern is possible (e.g. son of a known affected female as opposed to the son of a known affected male) is highly suggestive of the diagnosis. The condition can be confirmed by measuring the activity of the enzyme alpha-galactosidase in white cells. Females can sometimes have false negative enzymology and a molecular or biochemical test may be required.

BIOCHEMISTRY/GENETICS

Fabry disease is a lysosomal storage disease and accumulation of α-D-galactosyl moieties, particularly of globotriaosylceramide (Gb3) appears to be the initiation factor of the pathological cascades. While these include features suggestive of a classic vasculopathy, the overall pathological process is still poorly understood. Once significant end-organ damage has occurred, it is largely irreversible. The gene for Fabry disease, *GLA*, is on the X chromosome. Males tend to have more severe and earlier disease many females are also affected. There is a degree of genotype–phenotype correlation but no particular common mutation.

TREATMENT

A key to the treatment is the early diagnosis of potential affected family members. Genetic counselling and family cascade testing is thus important. Patients with the condition should be regularly screened for any manifestations of the disease. Medications such as ACE inhibitors are useful in the treatment of renal and cardiac disease. Carbamazepine and gabapentin can decrease pain. Specific treatment of the condition is available with ERT. This is most beneficial when started prior to significant end-organ damage occurring. Gb3 has been shown to fall on commence of enzyme replacement and even to rise on establishment of antibodies (a common occurrence in Fabry), but it has never been correlated to overall outcome.

POMPE DISEASE

CLINICAL PRESENTATION

Patients affected by Pompe disease (glycogen storage disease type II) classically present either as the 'floppy neonate' with skeletal myopathy and severe hypertrophic cardiomyopathy (**Fig. 14.29**) or as the adult with a slowly, but relentlessly, progressive myopathy with no cardiac disease. The infantile presentation may include failure to thrive, symptoms of heart failure, and respiratory distress and increasingly hearing and visual defects are being recognised. The natural history of the early presentation is death in the first year of life. The adult or late onset form typically presents with a history of gross motor dysfunction such as weakness going up stairs and climbing or exercise intolerance. The condition progresses to the point whereby the patient is wheel chair and later ventilator dependent. This tends to occur over a decade or two. There is also a less common juvenile presentation of progressive skeletal myopathy.

INVESTIGATIONS

All patients with signs and symptoms of Pompe disease should be tested for the condition. This can be done on enzyme testing of the specific lysosomal enzyme involved, a-1, 4-glucosidase (GAA). This can be performed on blood spots or on leukocytes, muscle or cultured fibroblasts. Measurement of a patients cross-reactive immunological material (CRIM) status is important in predicating which infantile patients might develop neutralising antibodies to ERT.

BIOCHEMISTRY/GENETICS

The condition is autosomal recessively inherited. Pompe disease results in the accumulation of intra-lysosomal glycogen, which itself results in myo- and cardiocyte hypertrophy, dysfunction and cell death, due to both dysfunction of the lysosomal and autophagocytic pathways.

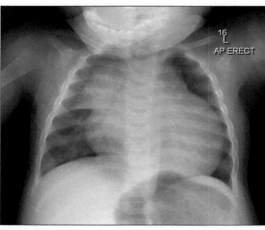

FIGURE 14.29 Cardiomegaly seen in a patient with infantile Pompe disease.

TREATMENT

Infantile patients normally require significant assistance feeding, respiratory and cardiac support. Pompe disease is associated with hearing loss and this should be assessed and treated as appropriate. Arrhythmias are common and continuous Holter monitoring may be appropriate. The decision to commence ERT is based on age of diagnosis, CRIM status and disease severity. CRIM negative patients are likely to produce antibodies and therefore are given immunomodulation prior to the start of ERT to decrease potential antibody formation. In general the earlier treatment is commenced the better. A clear plan of when to discontinue ERT should be in place and discussed early, as the response to therapy might be disappointing.

Adults with late onset disease require regular review by a multi-disciplinary team experienced in the needs of the progressively myopathic patient. The benefits of ERT are not yet fully explored although it appears that many patients can expect disease stabilisation if not a degree of improvement.

PROGNOSIS

The prognosis for early onset Pompe disease is variable and very dependent on age of onset of ERT. In many affected adults a reasonable quality of life is possible for many years. ERT has significantly improved the prognosis in many patients, although long-term observations are still outstanding.

CREATINE DEFICIENCY DISORDERS

CLINICAL PRESENTATION

These conditions present with intellectual disability and speech delay, autistic features and epilepsy. The conditions are variable and can cause mild or severe neurological disease. The more severe end of the clinical spectrum tends to present in the first few years of life. Severely affected patients may have microcephaly. Patients with guanidinoacetate methyltransferase (GAMT) deficiency in addition may have muscular hypotonia, weakness, progressive extrapyramidal signs and autistic and/or self-aggressive behaviour.

INVESTIGATIONS

Patients will have low creatine peaks on magnetic resonance spectroscopy (MRS) of their brains. Thus in any patient having MRI for the investigation of developmental delay or seizures, additional MRS should be performed. Urine guanidinoacetate levels are high in GAMT deficiency, while in the more common creatine transporter disorder the urine creatine/creatinine ratio is elevated; thus measuring these compounds in urine and blood, is usually the diagnostic test of choice. The diagnosis should be confirmed molecularly.

BIOCHEMISTRY/GENETICS

Creatine is required for the formation of creatine phosphate, an important short-term source for cellular energy. There are three known defects of creatine metabolism, arginine glycine amidinotransferase (AGAT), GAMT and creatine transporter defect. The latter is responsible for the transport of creatine across the blood–brain barrier. All three diseases result in decreased cerebral creatine. However, the additional peripheral symptoms seen in GAMT deficiency are thought to arise from the toxicity of accumulating guanidinoacetate. AGAT and GAMT deficiencies are inherited in an autosomal recessive manner, whereas defects in the creatine transporter are due to a defect in the X-linked gene *SLC6A8*. Several female carriers of *SCL6A8* mutation have been recorded having a phenotype of mild learning problems.

TREATMENT

Oral creatine supplementation can be effective, especially if commenced early, in GAMT and AGAT deficient patients. Doses of 300–500 mg/kg/d of creatine are used. This improves the creatine levels but does not reduce the toxic elevated guanidinoacetate in GAMT. This is achieved by reducing the arginine content in the diet (the amino acid required for the synthesis of guanidinoacetate); this improved clinical outcome has been reported in isolated cases. Arginine restriction is often complemented by ornithine supplementation. The creatine transporter defects unfortunately do not respond to oral creatine or other dietary manipulations, as while these increase blood creatine levels, brain levels remain unchanged. Thus conventional treatment of the epilepsy and educational support are primarily what can be offered. Genetic counselling is important in all conditions.

PROGNOSIS

Providing the diagnosis is made early, the prognosis for AGAT is favourable while in GAMT a degree of developmental delay, even with treatment, is to be expected. The outcome for the severe, classical creatine transporter is generally poor and more specific effective treatments are required.

METHYLMALONIC AND PROPIONIC ACIDAEMIA (MMA, PA)

CLINICAL PRESENTATION

These variable conditions classically present in the neonatal period during episodes of catabolism. Presentation is with unspecific clinical signs, i.e. lethargy, vomiting, irritability and eventually encephalopathy. Investigations reveal a severe metabolic acidosis, and often hyperammonaemia. Although the initial presentation is often in the first few days of life, milder affected patients may not become clinically unwell until their first significant intercurrent illness. Sometimes the history is more subacute, with failure to thrive, recurrent unwellness, developmental delay or occasionally a later onset with cardiomyopathy or hepatomegaly.

INVESTIGATIONS

Routine investigations, especially when unwell, usually reveal a metabolic ketoacidosis. Urine organic acids show grossly elevated methylmalonic acid or propionic acid. An acylcarnitine profile reveals an elevated propionylcarnitine (C3). Vitamin B_{12} and total homocysteine level should be measured in methylmalonic acidaemia (MMA) to rule out the associated disorders of cobalamin metabolism.

Diagnosis can be confirmed by enzymology and/or molecular genetics.

BIOCHEMISTRY/GENETICS

MMA and PA are autosomal recessive disorders in the catabolism of odd chain fats and some amino acids. These come from, respectively, bacterial gut metabolism and mainly from protein in the diet; toxic metabolites can cause slowly progressive end-organ disease. However, the cause of most episodes of acute severe classical decompensation is from body protein catabolism and secondary accumulation of toxic metabolites that occurs during an intercurrent illness.

TREATMENT

The key to treatment is early diagnosis, ideally prior to the first episode of metabolic decompensation. Aggressive treatment during periods of intercurrent illness with high-dose calories stopping catabolism, either orally or intravenously, is essential. Some patients with MMA may respond to regular vitamin B_{12} injections. In the acute setting patients with severe disease may require haemofiltration until metabolically stable. The long-term prognosis is generally guarded, with both diseases prone to episodes of recurrent decompensation. MMA patients frequently suffer chronic renal impairment; cardiomyopathy is more often seen in PA. Liver transplantation, replacing the defective enzyme, has a role in PA and possibly in MMA, although some patients have still decompensated post-transplant and long-term neurological complications have still occurred. Renal transplantation might be needed in chronic renal failure in MMA and also results in partial enzyme recovery. Various forms of gene therapy offer hope for future treatment.

PROGNOSIS

The prognosis often depends on the severity of decompensation at the first admission. Traditionally these patients have done poorly with few living to adulthood and those that did often having significant learning problems and renal disease (in MMA). It is hoped early diagnosis, improved management and the use of organ transplantation may improve the prognosis.

NEUROTRANSMITTER DISORDERS (L-DOPAMINE-RESPONSIVE DYSTONIA, TYROSINE HYDROXYLASE DEFICIENCY, PTERIN DISORDERS)

CLINICAL PRESENTATION

This group of conditions present with a variety of neurological signs and symptoms. These can include combinations of hypotonia, dystonia, ataxia, dysarthria, drooling, seizures, tremor, ptosis, oculogyric crisis, hypokinesia and developmental delay. Symptoms can be variable and patients' symptoms may display diurnal variation and periods of exacerbation with intercurrent illness.

INVESTIGATIONS

The group of disorders known as the pterin (or more correctly tetrahydrobiopterin disorders) are usually diagnosed following the routine measurement of urine 'pterins' that is required in every child who has an elevated phenylalanine level (as seen in PKU) on newborn screening. The key investigation of the other disorders is the measurement of neurotransmitters in the CSF following a set protocol. These conditions can be suspected in patients showing a favourable response to a trial of L-dopa.

BIOCHEMISTRY/GENETICS

The conditions result in a deficiency of the cerebral neurotransmitters dopamine and/or serotonin. These rare conditions are generally autosomal recessively inherited. However the condition GTP cyclohydrolase deficiency (also called L-dopa-responsive dystonia) is not that uncommon and inherited in a dominant manner. Thus a number of family members can be affected and they can be surprisingly variable in their symptoms, with one member having perhaps simple intermittent cramping whereas another may have more severe generalised neurological dysfunction.

TREATMENT

The conditions usually respond to a combination of L-dopa (combined with carbidopa) and 5-(OH) tryptophan, the latter being the precursor to serotonin. Tetrahydrobiopterin may be needed in the hyperphenylalaninaemia pterin disorders. Their precise dosing requires regular lumbar punctures for accurate assessment.

PROGNOSIS

On individually adjusted treatment, the prognosis is generally favourable in most of the conditions although some degree of developmental delay can be expected in the severe or late diagnosed patients.

SPHINGOLIPIDOSIS DISORDERS (TAY SACHS/SANDHOFF/GM1/NIEMANN–PICK/METACHROMATIC DYSTROPHY/KRABBE)

CLINICAL PRESENTATION

The sphingolipidosis disorders refer to a group of lysosomal storage disorders that in their classical form are notable for progressive and relentless neurological decline with relatively few other organ manifestations. In the severe forms of the conditions, onset is in infancy and is rapidly progressive over months leading to severe encephalopathy and death. These children usually have, albeit sometimes brief, a period of normal development followed by a plateauing of developmental progress and then actual regression. This may be exacerbated by intercurrent illness. Features such as epilepsy, macrocephaly, hyperacusis, visual impairment and spasticity are seen. The degree of irritability especially in Krabbe is extremely distressing to the family. There are no skeletal manifestations, usually minimal hepatomegaly (except in Niemann-Pick disease) and unlike in MPS disorders, coarse facial features are not seen. Retinal cherry red spots can sometimes be observed and loss of vision is common. The late infantile onset metachromatic leukodystrophy (MLD) has a very classical presentation whereby the previously near normal development plateaus at between 12 months to 2 years with subsequent aggressive regression and loss of any skills.

In the mild forms onset may not be until late childhood or even adulthood and early symptoms can include mild motor dysfunction such as difficulties climbing stairs or psychiatric manifestations. Progression of the late onset forms can be very slow and patients can survive for decades.

INVESTIGATIONS

Any child who presents with developmental regression should be investigated for these lysosomal storage disorders. The key investigation is the measurement of white cell enzymes in white blood cells. This test is essentially diagnostic although this should be confirmed molecularly. Patients may have characteristic MRI brain scans changes. Krabbe and MLD in particular often have very suggestive imaging.

BIOCHEMISTRY/GENETICS

The lysosome is a cell organelle that is often described as the recycling centre of the cells. It is responsible for the degradation of large complex molecules. This occurs in a stepwise manner and the deficiency of any enzyme results in the accumulation of a specific compound. This eventually results in cell – and in these conditions particularly neuronal, cell death. These conditions are inherited in an autosomal recessive manner.

TREATMENT

Due to the very limited curative treatment options the cornerstone of management is to provide individually adjusted palliative care. Seizures, manifesting especially early on, can usually be controlled with conventional anticonvulsants. Problems such as spasticity, drooling, feeding difficulties, constipation and visual impairment should be anticipated and managed accordingly. Support for the family and genetic counselling are always necessary.

BMT in the very early stages of some of the conditions may ameliorate and slow down the progression of the disease but the exact role of BMT is still to be evaluated. ERT is not effective as the large enzyme molecules do not cross the blood–brain barrier. Giving the medication intrathecally may be an option in the future.

PROGNOSIS

In general the prognosis for these conditions is poor and new treatments are required. Gene therapy probably offers the best hope for a cure.

CONGENITAL DISORDERS OF GLYCOSYLATION

CLINICAL PRESENTATION

Congenital disorders of glycosylation (CDG) are a group of inherited conditions, usually presenting as multi-organ disease, and often affecting the CNS. The most frequently diagnosed deficiency of phosphomannomutase deficiency, PMM-CDG, presents with the diagnostic triad of cerebellar hypoplasia, abnormal fat pads and inverted nipples (**Figs 14.30–14.32**). Very few CDG disorders (over 50 genetic disorders are known) present with normal neurological development. In PMI-CDG, due to phosphoisomerase deficiency, patients primarily present with gastrointestinal symptoms (failure to thrive, protein-losing enteropathy and liver fibrosis). Other CDG diseases, belonging to the group of muscular dystroglycanopathies, affect primarily the muscle, brain and eye.

DIAGNOSIS/INVESTIGATIONS

The most commonly used screening test for N-glycosylation defects is transferrin isoelectric focusing (IEF, **Fig. 14.33**); the majority of O-glycosylation defect can be detected by IEF of ApoCIII. However, only specific enzyme and/or molecular genetic testing can identify the precise CDG subtype of the patient.

BIOCHEMISTRY/GENETICS

CDGs affect the glycosylation of glycoproteins and glycolidids. They are usually inherited in an autosomal recessive matter. Defects can be localised to the cytoplasma, endoplasmatic reticulum or Golgi network. Depending on the defects, disorders are grouped as N-glycosylation defects, O-glycosylation defects, combined defects or others.

TREATMENT

There is no curative treatment available for any CDG disorder. However, supplementation of several different carbohydrates, such as mannose in PMI-CDG or galactose in galactose transporter deficiency, has been reported to be of some benefit.

PROGNOSIS

The prognosis of CDG patients depends on the subtype of the disease. Around 30% of PMM-CDG patients die in early infancy secondary to complications such as liver failure, cardiomyopathy and severe seizures. Regression of skills is rarely seen in patients with CDG.

Metabolic diseases

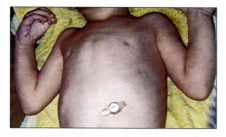

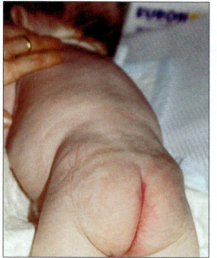

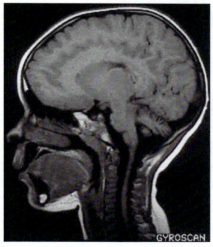

FIGURES 14.30–14.32 Features suggestive of congenital disorders of glycosylation 1A: **14.30**: inverted nipples; **14.31**: abnormal fat pads; **14.32**: cerebellar hypoplasia.

NON-KETOTIC HYPERGLYCINAEMIA (GLYCINE ENCEPHALOPATHY)

CLINICAL PRESENTATION

The clinical manifestation of non-ketotic hyperglycinaemia (NKH) is one of increasingly encephalopathy and hypotonia associated with a resistant seizure disorder. Presentation is typically towards the end of the first week of life.

DIAGNOSIS/INVESTIGATIONS

General bloods are normal. Urine and blood reveal significantly elevated glycine but this can be seen in other metabolic disorders (the term non-ketotic hyperglycinaemia was used to distinguish this from the organic acidaemias, which are typically ketotic hyperglycinaemia) and sometimes can be physiological. The diagnosis of NKH is made by the finding of an elevated CSF to plasma glycine ratio. Care must be taken for the CSF not to be blood stained as this can significantly elevate the CSF glycine level and thus the ratio.

BIOCHEMISTRY/GENETICS

Enzyme activity can be measured on liver biopsy; however, the interpretation of results can be challenging. Glycine is degradated by the glycine cleavage system that is encoded by three different large genes (P, T and H protein). Hence mutation analysis can be laborious.

TREATMENT

Primarily, seizure control is needed in NKH patients. Additionally to conventional anticonvulsants, sodium benzoate is used, as it binds glycine and therefore can lower glycine levels. Dextromethorphan is an inhibitor of the neuroexcitatory effect of glycine on the brain and can be used as an add-on therapy for NKH patients.

PROGNOSIS

Prognosis of NKH is poor and little developmental progress is seen in patients affected. There is a rare presentation of transient hyperglycinaemia that can complicate counselling in the neonatal period.

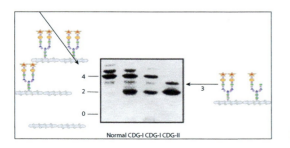

FIGURE 14.33 Transferrin isoelectric focusing.

445

SMITH–LEMLI–OPITZ SYNDROME

CLINICAL PRESENTATION

Smith–Lemli–Opitz syndrome (SLO) patients usually display characteristic dysmorphic features (**Figs 14.34, 14.35**) including syndactyly of the 2nd and 3rd toe, hypospadia and structural visceral and neurological abnormalities. There is usually global developmental delay with very slow progression of development. Challenging behaviour and sleeping difficulties can be a major task for families looking after these patients.

DIAGNOSIS/INVESTIGATIONS

The classical clinical features often raises suspicion for SLO alongside the observation of low total cholesterol levels. Patients need to be carefully clinically assessed as manifestation of SLO can be on any organ system. Structural abnormalities of brain, heart and gastrointestinal systems have been reported. Any patient with SLO needs a detailed abdominal ultrasound, brain imaging and cardiac assessment.

BIOCHEMISTRY/GENETICS

Low cholesterol levels might be seen on baseline testing. The characteristic biochemist results are elevation of 7- and 8-dihydrocholesterol. The diagnosis is usually confirmed on molecular genetic testing.

TREATMENT/PROGNOSIS

There is no curative treatment. Supplementation of cholesterol (cholesterol powder) has been reported to improve the behavioural challenges of some patients. Melatonin might be useful in some patients to improve their sleep quality. Statins have been used in some patients with few proven benefits.

Life expectancy in SLO is probably decreased. General health of the patient is usually satisfactory.

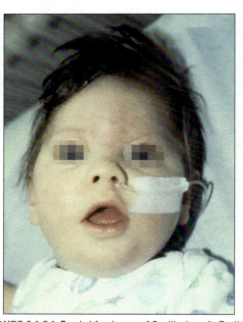

FIGURE 14.34 Facial features of Smith–Lemli–Opitz syndrome.

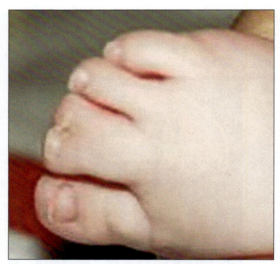

FIGURE 14.35 Smith–Lemli–Opitz syndrome: an example of the 2–3 syndactyly seen.

HYPER-CHOLESTEROLAEMIA

CLINICAL PRESENTATION

Clinically familial hypercholesterolaemia (FH) presents with premature atherosclerosis and myocardial infarction. On clinical examination xanthomas, xanthelasma and thickened tendons and arcus corneae can sometimes be seen. Homozygeous FH results in severe artherosclerosis and the onset of symptoms can be in early childhood.

DIAGNOSIS/INVESTIGATIONS

Lipid profile should be determined on a fasted blood sample. In FH, LDL cholesterol levels above 160 mg/dl (4.0 mmol/l) should be treated with a low-fat healthy diet and particularly if there is a positive family history of early cardiac manifestations, with additional drug therapy in patients >10 years.

BIOCHEMISTRY/GENETICS

FH is multigenetic with mutations mainly found in the low-density lipoprotein (LDL) receptor or Apo-B gene. The inheritance is autosomal dominant. Incidence is as high as 1:500.

TREATMENT/PROGNOSIS

Initially healthy life style and low-fat diet is promoted, followed by additional drug therapy usually started around the age of 10 years. Drugs used are cholestyramine and statins mainly. In homozygeous FH removal via LDL apheresis is recommended and liver transplantation could be considered.

Early initiation of treatment should prevent/postpone lipid deposition and secondary early cardiac manifestation.

FURTHER READING

Aggarwal A, Puri K, Thangada S, Zein N, Alkhouri N. Nonalcoholic fatty liver disease in children: recent practice guidelines, where do they take us? *Curr Pediatr Rev* 2014:10(2):151–61.

Blau N, Duran M, Gibson KM, Dionisi-Vici C. *Physician's Guide to the Diagnosis, Treatment, and Follow-Up of Inherited Metabolic Diseases.* Berlin: Springer, 2014.

Coutinho MF, Matos L, Alves S. From bedside to cell biology: a century of history on lysosomal dysfunction. *Gene* 2015;555(1):50–8.

Hoffmann GF, Nyhan WL, Zschocke J, Kahler SG. *Inherited Metabolic Disorders.* Berlin: Springer, 2010.

Kaler SG. Inborn errors of copper metabolism. *Handb Clin Neurol* 2013;113:1745–54.

Ng V, Nicholas D, Dhawan A, Yazigi N, *et al.* PeLTQL Study Group. Development and validation of the pediatric liver transplantation quality of life: a disease-specific quality of life measure for pediatric liver transplant recipients. *J Pediatr* 2014;165(3):547–55.e7.

Ruegger CM, Lindner M, Ballhausen D, *et al.* Cross-sectional observational study of 208 patients with non-classical urea cycle disorders. *J Inherit Metab Dis* 2014;37:21–30.

Rahman S. Gastrointestinal and hepatic manifestations of mitochondrial disorders. *J Inherit Metab Dis* 2013;36:659–73.

Saudubray JM, van der Berghe G, Walter JH. *Inborn Errors of Metabolic Diseases,* 5th edn. Berlin: Springer, 2011.

Turmnacioglu S, Gropman AL. Developmental and psychiatric presentations of inherited metabolic disorders. *Pediatr Neurol* 2013;48:179–87.

Walterfang M, Bonnot O, Mocellin R, Velakoulis D. The neuropsychiatry of inborn errors of metabolism. *J Inherit Metab Dis* 2013;36(4):687–702.

15 Genetics

Jane A. Hurst and Richard H. Scott

INTRODUCTION

The management of genetic disorders is a major part of the role of a paediatrician in developed countries. Approximately 50–60% of admissions and deaths in paediatric hospitals are due to malformations or genetic disorders including many of the conditions discussed elsewhere in this book.

The correct diagnosis of genetic disorders, and their differentiation from sporadic or environmentally-caused malformations is important in the proper care of children and their families. It allows the institution of optimal management and surveillance programmes for the affected individuals, guides advice regarding natural history and prognosis, as well as risk of recurrence of the disorder in further pregnancies.

COMMON CONGENITAL MALFORMATIONS

About 2–3% of newborns have a major congenital anomaly (**Table 15.1**). This rate doubles with follow-up throughout childhood. Monozygous twins have double the rate of malformations. Infants of diabetic mothers and mothers on some antiepileptic medications have about double the risk of congenital malformation. Alcohol and other drugs also increase the risk.

- **Genetic aetiology/Pathogenesis**: most isolated malformations are described as having a multifactorial aetiology caused by a combination of environmental and genetic effects. It is important to assess if the malformation is an isolated anomaly or part of a syndrome where the prognosis and inheritance pattern are specific to that syndrome.
- **Natural history**: dependent on the specific condition.
- **Differential diagnosis**: see **Table 15.1**. If the malformation is not isolated, consider syndromes where the specific malformation is a frequently found feature.
- **Treatment/Management/Surveillance**: good control of diabetes in mothers in a subsequent pregnancy and folic acid to prevent recurrence of neural tube defects. Prenatal diagnosis may be possible in future pregnancies by ultrasound scan.

TABLE 15.1 Incidence of congenital malformations

Malformation	Livebirth incidence	Syndromes to consider
Congenital heart disease	7 in 1,000	Chromosomal trisomy (page 452), del 22q11 (page 258), Noonan syndrome (page 464), CHARGE syndrome (page 464)
Hypospadias	6.4 in 1,000 males	*WT1*-associated syndromes, Smith–Lemli–Opitz syndrome
Neural tube defects	2 in 1,000	Occipital encephalocoele: Meckel syndrome, muscle–eye–brain disease
Talipes (club foot)	1.6 in 1000	Congenital myotonic dystrophy (page 466)
Cleft lip and palate	1 in 700–1,000	Van der Woude syndrome
Cleft palate	0.4 in 1000	Stickler syndrome (page 467)
Diaphragmatic hernia	0.3 in 1000	30% have chromosomal abnormality

CHROMOSOME DISORDERS

CHROMOSOMES – STRUCTURAL ABNORMALITIES AND IMBALANCE

Until 2010 the majority of cytogenetic reports from a routine laboratory were based on analysis of G-banded chromosomes under light microscopy (**Table 15.2**). This allowed a visual representation of structural anomalies visible at that level of magnification. In order to diagnose submicroscopic abnormalities of less than 5 Mb, laboratories first used specific fluorescence *in situ* hybridisation (FISH) testing and now array comparative genomic hybridisation (CGH). Array CGH has the advantage that it detects abnormalities genome wide (i.e. at any location in the genome) in a single test.

GENETIC AETIOLOGY/PATHOGENESIS

Loss or gain of the DNA content of the chromosome is known as an unbalanced rearrangement. Array CGH is a molecular technique and does not detect structural chromosome abnormality where there is no gain or loss of the DNA content of the chromosome – a balanced chromosome abnormality.

The chromosome structure can be altered by:

- deletion of part of a chromosome
- duplication of part of a chromosome
- inversion of part of a chromosome – two breaks form on a single chromosome and the middle section rotates through 180° (**Fig. 15.1**)
- translocation of part of a chromosome to another chromosome. This can either result in a *balanced translocation* if there is no overall gain or loss of chromosome material (**Fig. 15.2**), or an *unbalanced translocation* if there is a net loss or gain of chromosomal material. Translocations are also classified as either *reciprocal*, where there is an exchange between two chromosomes, or *Robertsonian* (page 452) where two acrocentric chromosomes are joined.

TABLE 15.2 Incidence of structural chromosome abnormalities

Deletion	8% of abnormal results based on G-banded analysis
Duplication	2% of abnormal results based on G-banded analysis
Inversion	Many are normal variants; 1 in 100 population
Balanced reciprocal translocation	1 in 1,000 population

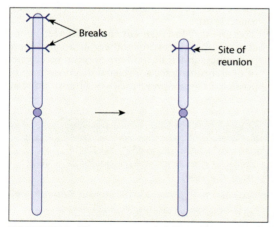 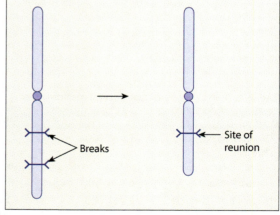

FIGURE 15.1 Chromosome deletion. (With permission from Oxford University Press, Firth, Hurst and Hall, *Oxford Desk Reference – Clinical Genetics*, 2005.)

Genetics

450

- **Clinical presentation**: a child with congenital malformations and/or developmental delay.
- **Diagnosis**: cytogenetic analysis (now usually by array CGH) (**Fig. 15.3**); if there is a family history of an inversion, translocation or recurrent miscarriage, G-banded analysis is required.
- **Inheritance**: deletions and duplications usually follow a dominant pattern of inheritance. The inheritance of inversions and translocations is more complex and requires referral to clinical genetics. They may be associated with a high miscarriage rate or risk of a child with severe developmental delay and malformation caused by chromosome imbalance.

- **Natural history**: although the natural history of the common deletion syndromes is well delineated, the majority of chromosome abnormalities are unique to a family. Databases such as DECIPHER can give guidance about the phenotype and prognosis.
- **Differential diagnosis**: single gene and environmental causes of syndromes and malformations.
- **Treatment/Management/Surveillance**: refer to clinical genetics; family follow-up and chromosome testing are necessary. Prenatal diagnosis by chorionic villus sampling or amniocentesis can be offered.

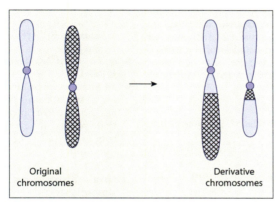

FIGURE 15.2 Balanced reciprocal chromosome translocation.

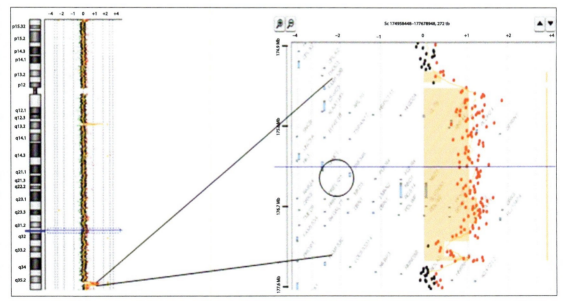

FIGURE 15.3 Ideogram of chromosome 5 and array CGH data, showing a 1.91 Mb deletion at 5q35.2, including *NSD1*, identified using an Oxford custom 4 × 180 K array; deletion of *NSD1* causes Sotos syndrome.

Chromosomes – structural abnormalities and imbalance

451

ROBERTSONIAN TRANSLOCATION

GENETIC AETIOLOGY/PATHOGENESIS/INCIDENCE

In a Robertsonian translocation there is fusion of the long arms (q) of two chromosomes (**Fig. 15.4**). This can occur only with chromosomes known as acrocentric chromosomes, where the short arms contain only repetitive DNA sequences. In humans these are chromosomes 13, 14, 15, 21 and 22.

Incidence is 1 in 1,000. The most common is the rob(13q14q) translocation found in 1 in 1,300.

A balanced carrier of a Robertsonian translocation has 45 chromosomes. A baby with Down syndrome due to an unbalanced Robertsonian translocation has 46 chromosomes due to a fused 21 with another acrocentric chromosome and an additional chromosome 21. Similar situations can arise with the others, notably including 13, with a risk of Patau syndrome.

CLINICAL PRESENTATION

- Fetal loss or syndrome related to **aneuploidy** (chromosome imbalance).
- Abnormal phenotypes in babies with apparently balanced translocations involving chromosomes 14 or 15 associated with **uniparental disomy** (UPD).

DIAGNOSIS

Conventional G-band karyotype is used to distinguish between simple trisomy 21 or trisomy 13 and their Robertsonian counterparts, as the children with Robertsonian translocations are phenotypically indistinguishable.

INHERITANCE

An unbalanced Roberstonian translocation may have arisen *de novo* or have been inherited from a parent who is a carrier of a balanced Roberstonian translocation. If it has arisen *de novo* then risk in another pregnancy is <1%. If one parent is a carrier of a balanced translocation, there will be increased risk in another pregnancy of aneuploidy. This may result in pregnancy loss/miscarriage or in some cases a liveborn child with aneuploidy. The level of risk depends on the chromosomes involved and sex of the carrier parent. With Roberstonian translocations involving chromosomes 14 or 15 there is a risk of UPD in future pregnancies due to trisomy rescue.

For instance, the fetus of a parent with a balanced Roberstonian (14;21) translocation may have:

- a *normal* karyotype
- a *balanced* Roberstonian translocation (as in the parent)
- a *balanced* Roberstonian translocation with UPD 14
- an *unbalanced* product of the translocation resulting in spontaneous pregnancy loss
- an *unbalanced* product of the translocation that results in Down syndrome, e.g. 46,XY rob(14;21)+21 (**Fig. 15.5**); this risk is 10–15% if the mother carries the translocation.

Natural history: as for specific chromosome abnormality.

Differential diagnosis: other chromosomal mechanisms can cause the same phenotype.

Treatment/Management/Surveillance: carrier testing of parents and extended family; prenatal chromosome and UPD testing as appropriate.

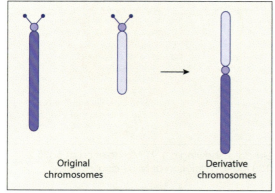

FIGURE 15.4 Balanced Robertsonian translocation. (With permission from Oxford University Press, Firth, Hurst and Hall, *Oxford Desk Reference – Clinical Genetics*, 2005.)

Original chromosomes

Derivative chromosomes

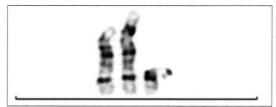

FIGURE 15.5 A Robertsonian translocation rob(14:21), the cause of 2% of Down syndrome. A normal chromosome 14 is pictured on the left, a normal chromosome 21 on the right and a derivative rob(14:21) between the two.

CHROMOSOME MOSAICISM

INCIDENCE

- 1 in 50 chorionic villous samples.
- 1 in 200 amniocentesis samples.

GENETIC AETIOLOGY/PATHOGENESIS

Chromosome mosaicism is the presence of two or more cell lines with different chromosomal complements (**Table 15.3**). Mosaicism can also occur for point mutations in single gene disorders (e.g. neurofibromatosis type 1).

CLINICAL PRESENTATION

- Hypomelanosis of Ito.
- Trisomy 8.
- Tetrasomy 12p (Pallister–Killian syndrome).
- Mosaic UPD 11p15 (Beckwith–Wiedemann syndrome, page 482).

DIAGNOSIS

Extended count of G-banded chromosomes, array CGH or testing of another tissue (buccal swab or skin biopsy) is required.

TRISOMY 13 (PATAU SYNDROME)

INCIDENCE

1 in 12,000 livebirths (increases with maternal age).

GENETIC AETIOLOGY/PATHOGENESIS

- Trisomy 13 – 90% of cases and associated with increased maternal age. Low recurrence risk in future pregnancies, although risk is dependent on maternal age and if prenatal diagnosis is offered.
- Translocation – 5–10% of cases: Robertsonian translocation (see page 452).
- Mosaic trisomy 13 – up to 5% of cases. The phenotype is milder and babies live longer but the developmental outcome is poor.

CLINICAL PRESENTATION

Children present with low birth weight, major facial malformations (holoprosencephaly sequence, clefts, microphthalmia) (**Fig. 15.6**), postaxial polydactyly, cardiac defects and exomphalos.

DIAGNOSIS

A rapid result is obtained by FISH or PCR; confirmation by G-banded karyotype can be sought to exclude Robertsonian translocation.

TABLE 15.3 Mechanisms and outcomes of chromosome mosaicism

Mechanism leading to mosaicism	Karyotype at conception	Karyotype in fetus/baby
Mitotic non-disjunction	Normal	47N+abn/46N
Trisomy rescue	Trisomy	47N+abn/46N Consider if UPD features contributing to phenotype
Somatic recombination	Normal	46N/46 with structural chromosome abnormality or UPD, for example causing syndromes such as Beckwith–Wiedemann syndrome (page 482)

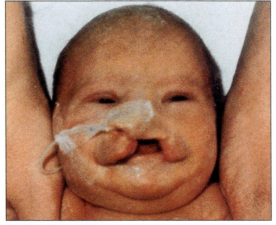

FIGURE 15.6 A child with trisomy 13 (Patau syndrome).

INHERITANCE

- Trisomy 13: sporadic, maternal age-related.
- Robertsonian translocation: see page 452. Refer to clinical genetics for advice regarding risks in future pregnancies.
- Mosaic: refer to clinical genetics.
- **Natural history**: median survival 7–10 days, 5–10% survive after the 1st birthday.
- **Differential diagnosis**: autosomal recessive disorders such as ciliopathies (e.g. Meckel syndrome) and severe Smith–Lemli–Opitz syndrome; other unbalanced chromosome abnormalities.
- **Treatment/Management/Surveillance**: after confirmation of the diagnosis, supportive treatment only is indicated.

TRISOMY 18 (EDWARDS SYNDROME)

INCIDENCE

1 in 7,900 livebirths (increases with maternal age).

GENETIC AETIOLOGY/PATHOGENESIS

47XXorXY+18. Most are due to an error during meiosis and 85% are of maternal origin. The aetiology is associated with increased maternal age.

CLINICAL PRESENTATION

Prematurity is common and many trisomy 18 fetuses are lost spontaneously during pregnancy. The birth weight is low (mean 2240 g) and the head shape is abnormal with a prominent occiput. Limb abnormalities are found with contractures of the fingers, short hallux, prominent heels and sometime a radial deficiency of the forearms. 90% have a congenital heart defect and the sternum is short. Cleft lip and palate, exomphalos and diaphragmatic hernia are common additional malformations (**Fig. 15.7**).

DIAGNOSIS

A rapid result is obtained by FISH or PCR, with confirmation by G-banded karyotype. The phenotype is not as distinctive as trisomy 21 or 13 so it is wise to wait for the rapid FISH result before discussing the diagnosis with the parents.

INHERITANCE

There is a low recurrence risk in future pregnancies, though risk is dependent on maternal age and if prenatal diagnosis is offered.

- **Natural history**: mean survival after birth is 4 days with failure to establish respiration probably secondary to CNS malformation with contribution from chest and heart malformations.
- **Differential diagnosis**: other chromosome abnormalities; syndromic causes of distal arthrogryposis.
- **Treatment/Management/Surveillance**: sadly once the diagnosis is confirmed supportive treatment only is indicated.

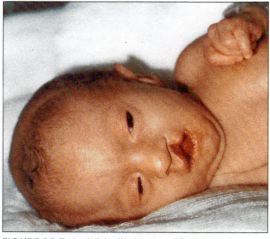

FIGURE 15.7 A child with trisomy 18 (Edwards syndrome).

TRISOMY 21 (DOWN SYNDROME)

INCIDENCE

The incidence is 1 in 600, but the livebirth rate is influenced by the uptake and availability of prenatal screening and is about 1 in 1100 in the UK. There is an increase with maternal age from 1 in 1500 at 17 years to 1 in 100 at 40 years.

GENETIC AETIOLOGY/PATHOGENESIS

- Trisomy 21 – 95% of cases (**Fig. 15.8**). Risk is associated with increased maternal age. There is a low recurrence risk in future pregnancies, although risk is dependent on maternal age and if prenatal diagnosis is offered.
- Translocation Down syndrome – 2% of cases: Robertsonian translocation (see page 452).
- Mosaic Down syndrome – 2% of cases: phenotype may be milder but the ratio of normal to Down syndrome cells in bloodprenatal testing is not a reliable indicator of the ratio in other tissues.

CLINICAL PRESENTATION

Paediatricians are familiar with the clinical features (**Fig. 15.9**). Enquire about serum screening in pregnancy. The child typically present as a floppy neonate with upslanting palpebral fissures, flat facial profile, large fontanelle(s), poor suck and cardiac murmur. 50% have congenital heart disease and there is a two-fold increase for all congenital anomalies.

DIAGNOSIS

A rapid result is obtained by FISH, with confirmation by G-banded karyotype to exclude Robertsonian translocation.

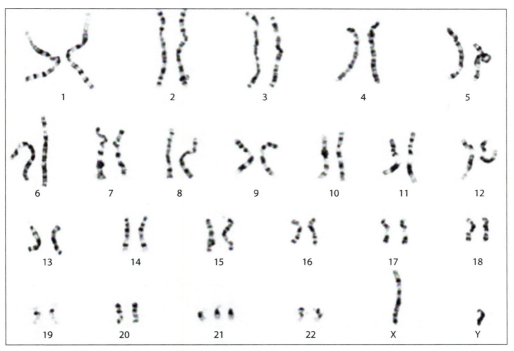

FIGURE 15.8 G-banded karyotype showing trisomy 21.

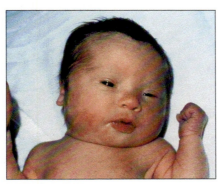

FIGURE 15.9 Down syndrome.

INHERITANCE

- Trisomy 21 – sporadic, maternal age-related.
- Robertsonian translocation: see page 452. Refer to clinical genetics.
- Mosaic: Refer to clinical genetics. An individual with mosaic Down may have a child with complete trisomy 21.

NATURAL HISTORY

Median survival is close to 50 years unless there is a significant cardiac or other malformation. Mean IQ for young adults is 45–50 but this declines later due to early onset dementia.

DIFFERENTIAL DIAGNOSIS

Usually no diagnostic difficulty but:

- mosaic trisomy 21 may not be detected with basic genetic testing.
- deletion of chromosome 9q34.3 has a similar facial profile.
- Zellweger syndrome – extremely floppy with large fontanelle.

TREATMENT/MANAGEMENT/ SURVEILLANCE

ECHO for cardiac disease. Referral to a community paediatrician for surveillance of medical (thyroid function, visual and hearing checks, increased risk for coeliac disease, increased risk of leukaemia) and developmental issues is necessary.

TURNER SYNDROME, 45,X AND VARIANTS

INCIDENCE

1 in 2,500 female livebirths.

GENETIC AETIOLOGY/PATHOGENESIS

The clinical features are due to monosomy (one copy) of all or part of the second X chromosome in females. About 50% of females with Turner have 'pure' monosomy X, whereas the other 50% shows mosaicism for a second cell line (**Table 15.4**). There is a high rate of loss during pregnancy of about 65% between 12 and 40 weeks.

CLINICAL PRESENTATION

- Neonate: a history of increased nuchal measurement, cystic hygroma or hydrops in pregnancy is almost always found and prenatal karyotype may have been performed. Peripheral oedema, excess skin around the neck. coarctation of the aorta and renal anomalies may be present.
- Childhood: short stature, neck webbing, ptosis (**Fig. 15.10**).

TABLE 15.4 X chromosome abnormalities found in Turner syndrome

X chromosome abnormality	Frequency
45,X	50%
45,X/structural abnormality of other X	20%
45,X/46,XX	20%
46,XX with structural abnormality of second X	10%

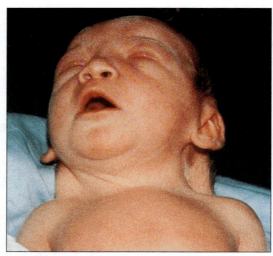

FIGURE 15.10 A child with Turner syndrome with neck webbing.

- Adolescent: primary ovarian failure with scant of or pubertal development and amenorrhoea.
- **Diagnosis**: karyotype with 30 cell count to investigate possible mosaicism.
- **Inheritance**: this is sporadic. The majority of women with Turner are infertile. *In vitro* fertilisation (IVF) with donor oocytes has resulted in successful pregnancy for some women with Turner syndrome.
- **Natural history**: although there are some well-documented behavioural and developmental difficulties, the majority of girls attend mainstream school and have a normal independent adult life. The average adult height is 147 cm.
- **Differential diagnosis**:
  - other causes of primary ovarian failure.
  - syndromes with overlapping features (e.g. Noonan syndrome).
- **Treatment/Management/Surveillance**:
  - Neonate: ECHO, renal ultrasound, audiogram.
  - Childhood: paediatric endocrinology review. Short stature can be partially corrected by administration of growth hormone in childhood.
  - Adolescents/adults: in addition to primary ovarian failure, adults with Turner syndrome are also susceptible to a range of disorders, including osteoporosis, hypothyroidism and renal and gastrointestinal disease. They have a particularly high cardiovascular risk and it is imperative that patients are screened by ECHO, assessed by a cardiologist and advised of the potential risks before attempting to become pregnant by IVF – there is a 2% risk of rupture or dissection of the aorta.

WILLIAMS SYNDROME

INCIDENCE

1 in 20,000.

GENETIC AETIOLOGY/PATHOGENESIS

Williams syndrome is due to a monoallelic deletion of chromosome 7q11.23 encompassing the elastin *ELN* gene. This microdeletion is not detectable by G-banded karyotype but identified by specific FISH and array CGH analysis.

CLINICAL PRESENTATION

The typical cardiac defects are supravalvular aortic stenosis and supravalvular pulmonary stenosis. There is a history of poor feeding and developmental delay. Facial features include periorbital oedema, small nose with upturned nasal tip, wide mouth with full lips and sagging cheeks due to elastin deficiency (**Figs 15.11, 15.12**). The facial features coarsen with age.

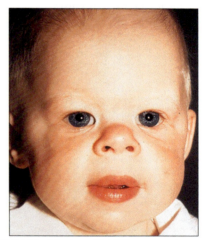

FIGURE 15.11 A baby with Williams syndrome.

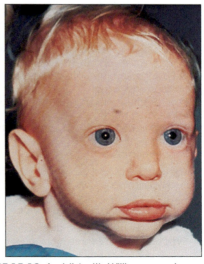

FIGURE 15.12 A child with Williams syndrome.

There is a typical behavioural phenotype that has been well delineated. There are visual–spatial deficits but strengths in communication. Hyperacusis is a problem to some. Adults are not usually able to live an independent life.

- **Diagnosis**: by specific FISH or array CGH analysis.
- **Inheritance**: the vast majority arise *de novo*, the remainder have a parent with the deletion. The deletion is inherited as an autosomal dominant. There is full penetrance. Parents are offered the availability of prenatal diagnosis in a subsequent pregnancy but the risk is low when parents do not have Williams syndrome.
- **Differential diagnosis**:
  ○ elastin mutation.
  ○ Noonan syndrome.
- **Treatment/Management/Surveillance**:
  ○ screening for hypercalcaemia and nephrocalcinosis.
  ○ surveillance for later onset arterial hypertension and renal artery stenosis.
  ○ referral to clinical genetics to discuss parental testing and prenatal diagnosis.

22Q11 DELETION SYNDROME (DIGEORGE SYNDROME)

INCIDENCE

1 in 2,000–4,000.

GENETIC AETIOLOGY/PATHOGENESIS

DiGeorge syndrome is due to a monoallelic deletion of chromosome 22q11 (del22q11.2) (**Fig. 15.13**). These microdeletions are typically ~3 Mb of genomic DNA and are not detectable by G-banded karyotype. The *TBX1* gene within the area of deletion is of particular importance in the phenotype.

CLINICAL PRESENTATION

In the neonate, cardiac defects and cleft palate lead to identification of the deletion. In older children speech delay, velopharyngeal insufficiency and the facial features are more common reasons for testing. The facial features are not distinctive but there are subtle changes to the shape of the nose and ears. The ear abnormalities include overfolded or squared off helices. A prominent nasal root and bulbous nasal tip is sometimes observed in older children. (See other features in **Table 15.5**.)

- **Diagnosis**: specific FISH analysis or array CGH.
- **Inheritance**: approximately 90% arise as new mutations, the remainder have a parent with the deletion.

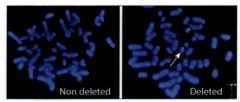

FIGURE 15.13 FISH using specific 22q11 probe (red) and control chromosome 22 probe (green) showing 22q11 deletion (absent red signal on the deleted chromosome).

TABLE 15.5 Features of 22q11 deletion (DiGeorge) syndrome

Age	Feature	Frequency
Infant	Congenital heart disease (all types but particularly associated are tetralogy of Fallot, pulmonary atresia–ventricular septal defect, interrupted aortic arch, truncus arteriosus)	75%
	Cleft palate, including submucous cleft)	15%
	Hypocalcaemia	Up to 60%
	Defects in cell-mediated immunity (hypoplasia of the thymus) and recurrent infections	1% have a major immune defect
	Renal anomalies	30–40%
Child	Speech delay and velopharyngeal insufficiency	30%
	Pachygyria/polymicrogyria	
	Craniosynostosis	1%
	Hypocalcaemia/hypoparathyroidism	30%
Older child	Schooling and learning difficulties	60–70%
	Hypocalcaemic seizures	
Adult	Psychiatric problems	15–20%

Genetics

The deletion is inherited as an autosomal dominant. There is full penetrance but huge variability of expression. Parents are offered the availability of prenatal diagnosis in a subsequent pregnancy. If parents do not have the deletion, risk to a subsequent pregnancy is about 2% due to gonadal mosaicism.

- **Differential diagnosis**:
  - CHARGE syndrome.
  - VATER/VACTERL (see page 480).
  - Goldenhar/oculo-auricular-vertebral syndrome (see page 479).
- **Treatment/Management/Surveillance**: immune function should be checked prior to vaccination with live vaccines and whole blood transfusion; referral to clinical genetics should be offered to discuss family testing and prenatal diagnosis.

SINGLE GENE DISORDERS

The human genome contains approximately 20,000 genes and many disorders are caused by mutations affecting just one gene. Often referred to as single gene disorders, they can follow a number of different patterns of inheritance depending on whether they reside on an autosome or sex chromosome and whether disease is caused by mutations affecting one or two alleles (copies) of the gene.

Mutations in single gene disorders can be single nucleotide alterations, for example inserting a premature 'stop' codon to cause the production of a non-functional, truncated protein. They can also be larger scale, for example deletions affecting a several exons of the gene or even the whole gene. Testing for single gene disorders can be performed by DNA sequencing (searching for single nucleotide and other small-scale sequence alterations) and copy number testing (looking for deletions or duplications).

CLINICAL PEDIGREES

Drawing and interpretation of clinical pedigrees are important skills and aid the recognition of the likely underlying pattern of inheritance (**Fig. 15.14**). A pedigree is usually started from the presenting individual (the consultand), who is marked with an arrow. The pedigree should encompass three generations, usually the consultand's generation, their parents' generation and their grandparents. If there is relevant history in the wider family, the pedigree may need to be extended more widely. The person through whom the family was first brought to medical attention is referred to as the proband.

When constructing pedigree, the clinician should specifically but tactfully ask about consanguinity, miscarriages and still births.

'FIRST GENERATION' GENETIC TESTING TECHNIQUES

Since the 1980s, the mainstay of DNA sequencing has been Sanger sequencing, a technique which requires PCR amplification of the target gene in small fragments followed by sequencing of the amplified fragment. This is a highly accurate but labour intensive and therefore expensive technique. Sanger sequencing does not usually detect larger-scale copy number alterations. For many genes, comprehensive mutation testing therefore also requires the use of a copy number analysis technique such as multiplex ligation-dependent probe amplification (MLPA).

NEXT GENERATION SEQUENCING

In the 2000s, a number of 'next generation' sequencing technologies have been developed. Unlike Sanger sequencing where single fragments must be sequenced individually, these techniques allow 'massively parallel' sequencing of millions of fragments simultaneously. This allows larger scale genetic testing with consequent lower cost per gene.

While it is possible to use next generation sequencing to sequence the whole genome of an individual, the cost of this remains high and the time and cost of searching for a single disease causing mutation amongst many thousands of innocent genetic variants have favoured more targeted approaches when testing for single gene disorders. Targeting of next generation sequencing has been developed using a

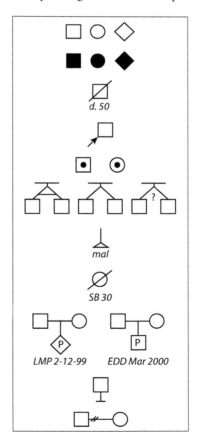

FIGURE 15.14 Standard symbols for pedigree drawing. (See further Bennett RL, *et al.* Recommendations for standardized human pedigree nomenclature. Pedigree Standardization Task Force of the National Society of Genetic Counselors. *Am J Hum Genet* 1995;56:745–52.)

number of different sequence capture techniques prior to the sequencing stage.

Examples of clinical use of next generation sequencing include:

- **Single gene sequencing**: sequencing of large numbers of samples through a single gene in conditions with a readily recognisable clinical phenotype, for example the cystic fibrosis gene *CFTR*.
- **Gene panel sequencing**: sequencing of panels of genes with overlapping phenotypes, for example a panel of 50 genes that can cause severe developmental delay disorders (page 468).
- **Whole exome sequencing**: sequencing the coding sequencing of all ~20,000 known genes. This is 1% of the whole genome. It can be employed in malformation syndromes where the phenotype does not allow sequencing to be targeted to a single gene or gene panel.
- **Whole genome sequencing**: sequencing of the entire genomic sequence. As discussed above, the diagnostic utility is limited by the large number of innocent sequence variants it detects and the fact that the large majority of known disease causing variants are located in the exome.

At the time of writing, many clinical diagnostic laboratories are transferring some of their high throughput single gene tests to next generation technologies and developing gene panel sequencing tests. Clinical whole exome and/or whole genome testing is still in its infancy but is expanding through projects such as the DDD study and the UK government funded 100,000 Genome Project.

Next generation sequencing is capable of detecting copy number alterations but this remains technically difficult. Therefore, currently, conventional copy number testing techniques are used where a copy number abnormality is likely.

AUTOSOMAL DOMINANT INHERITANCE

Autosomal dominant (AD) disorders are caused by mutations in genes on the autosomes (i.e. not the X or Y chromosome) (**Table 15.6**).

GENETIC AETIOLOGY/PATHOGENESIS

Children (and adults) with AD conditions have a mutation on one the two alleles of the gene ('monoallelic' or heterozygous mutation). Aspects of inheritance in AD disorders include:

- Differences in expression with inter- and intrafamilial variability.
- Penetrance: the percentage of individuals who have any features of the disorder. This may be age-dependent penetrance or incomplete penetrance (not all mutation carriers will develop the condition).
- Somatic mosaicism: a new mutation arising at an early stage in embryogenesis may result in a partial or modified phenotype.
- Germline/gonadal mosaicism: a new mutation arising during oogenesis or spermatogenesis may cause no phenotype in the parent but can be transmitted to the offspring.
- Paternal age effect: for some AD disorders the chance of a new mutation from the father increases with his age. However, the absolute risk of recurrence following a new mutation remains low.
- Anticipation: worsening of disease severity in successive generations.

TABLE 15.6 Common autosomal dominant conditions

Disease	Incidence	Gene	Particular features
Osteogenesis imperfecta	1 in 500 incidence 1 in 1,000 prevalence	COL1A1/A2	Severe types lethal Gonadal and somatic mosaicism
Neurofibromatosis	1 in 5,000	NF1	Variable expression, age-dependent expression, somatic mosaicism
Myotonic dystrophy	1 in 8,000	DMPK	Anticipation
Tuberous sclerosis	1 in 10,000	TSC1/2	Variable expression, age-dependent expression, somatic and gonadal mosaicism
Craniosynostosis (Apert/Crouzon/Pfeiffer)	Apert: 1 in 100,000 Crouzon: 1 in 50,000	FGFR2	Paternal age effect
Achondroplasia	1 in 27,000	FGFR3	Paternal age effect

FIGURE 15.15 A typical family tree showing AD inheritance. An affected parent has a 50% risk of transmitting the condition to each child whether they are male or female. (With permission from Oxford University Press, Firth, Hurst and Hall, *Oxford Desk Reference – Clinical Genetics*, 2005.)

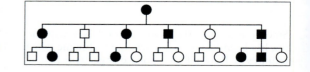

Genetics

CLINICAL PRESENTATION

Many AD conditions are more commonly encountered in adults (due to age-dependent penetrance). Others are more frequently considered in children (see **Table 15.6**), particularly those severe dominantly inherited conditions that have arisen as the result of a new mutation (e.g. osteogenesis imperfecta, Apert syndrome), or where anticipation is a feature of the condition (e.g. congenital muscular dystrophy).

- **Diagnosis**: confirmatory genetic testing is available for some but not all AD conditions.
- **Inheritance**: see **Fig. 15.15**.
- **Natural history**: dependent on the specific condition.
- **Differential diagnosis**: dependent on the specific condition.

TREATMENT/MANAGEMENT/ SURVEILLANCE

Carrier and predictive testing should be considered for the wider family. However, there are ethical considerations in the testing of children with adult onset conditions and this is usually only performed when the diagnosis will lead to better treatment and/or surveillance. Surveillance for age-dependent features that require treatment (e.g aortic dilation in Marfan syndrome) should be carried out. Prenatal diagnosis is often possible in future pregnancies.

AUTOSOMAL RECESSIVE INHERITANCE

Autosomal recessive (AR) disorders are caused by mutations affecting both of the two alleles of genes on the autosomes (i.e. not the X or Y chromosome). **Table 15.7** presents common AR conditions.

GENETIC AETIOLOGY/PATHOGENESIS

Affected children have mutations in both of the two alleles of the gene ('biallelic' mutation). They are either homozygotes (two identical mutations) or compound heterozygotes (two different mutations). Individuals with a mutation in one allele are known as carriers. They either do not have features of the condition (e.g. cystic fibrosis), or if they do this is very mild in comparison with the disease state (e.g. sickle cell trait vs. sickle cell disease). Many of the more common AR conditions have higher frequencies in certain populations.

Rare AR conditions are more common in the children of consanguineous parents.

INHERITANCE

Autosomal recessive inheritance is depicted in **Fig. 15.16**. There is a 25% risk of an affected child in any pregnancy, independent of gender. The diagram in (**B**) illustrates a consanguineous relationship between first cousins. A common ancestor is a carrier for a recessive mutation that may occur in homozygous form in a descendent as a consequence of consanguinity.

- **Natural history**: dependent on the specific condition.
- **Differential diagnosis**: dependent on the specific condition.
- **Treatment/Management/Surveillance**:
  - carrier testing for the wider family.
  - prenatal diagnosis is often possible in future pregnancies.

TABLE 15.7 Incidence of some of the common autosomal recessive conditions

Disease	Carrier frequency in general population	Gene
α1-antitrypsin deficiency	1 in 25 for Z allele and 1 in 17 for S allele in Northern European populations	SERPINA1
Congenital adrenal hyperplasia	1 in 50 for CYP21	CYP21
Cystic fibrosis	1 in 23 in North European populations	CFTR
Gaucher	1 in 25 in Ashkenazi Jewish population	GBA
Haemochromatosis	1 in 10 in North European populations	HFE
Phenylketonuria	1 in 50	PAH
Sickle cell disease	>1 in 10 in equatorial Africa	HBB
Spinal muscular atrophy	1 in 50	SMN1
Tay Sachs disease	1 in 30 in Ashkenazi Jewish population	HEXA
Beta-thalassaemia	1 in 30 in Greek/Italian population	HBB

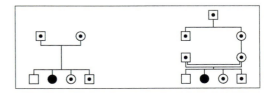

FIGURE 15.16 Family trees to illustrate autosomal recessive inheritance. (With permission from Oxford University Press, Firth, Hurst and Hall, *Oxford Desk Reference – Clinical Genetics*, 2005.)

X-LINKED INHERITANCE

X-linked (XL) disorders are due to mutation in genes on the X chromosome.

- X-linked recessive (XLR) – males are hemizygous and affected; females are heterozygous carriers.
- X-linked dominant (XLD) conditions are lethal to males and the affected individuals are heterozygous females.

INCIDENCE

The incidence of common X-linked conditions is shown in **Table 15.8**.

GENETIC AETIOLOGY/PATHOGENESIS

In XLR conditions males are hemizygotes and manifest the condition. Carrier females have one normal and one mutated X-chromosome. In some disorders females have symptoms due to non-random X-inactivation and age-dependent penetrance.

In Duchenne or Becker muscular dystrophy, there is a significantly high gonadal mosaic risk.

CLINICAL PRESENTATION

XL conditions should be considered where a genetic condition affects males more severely and there is no male to male transmission of the condition.

DIAGNOSIS

Confirmation is by mutation analysis if possible.

INHERITANCE

Inheritance of X-linked conditions is shown in **Fig. 15.17**.

- **Natural history**: dependent on the specific condition.
- **Differential diagnosis**: dependent on the specific condition.
- **Treatment/Management/Surveillance**:
    - referral to clinical genetics to evaluate the family history.
    - carrier testing for females in the wider family.
    - prenatal diagnosis is often possible in future pregnancies.

TABLE 15.8 Common X-linked conditions

Disease	Frequency in males	Gene	Particular features
Duchenne muscular dystrophy	1 in 3,000–4,000	*DMD*	High new mutation and gonadal mosaic risk
Haemophilia A	1 in 5,000	*F8*	Most mothers are carriers
Fragile X syndrome	1 in 5,500	*FMR1*	Anticipation, normal transmitting males, permutations, premature ovarian failure in carrier females

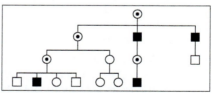

FIGURE 15.17 A typical family tree showing X-linked recessive inheritance. The condition is expressed in males, but not in females. For a carrier female, on average, 50% of her sons will be affected and 50% of her daughters will be carriers. All daughters of an affected male are obligate carriers and none of his sons inherit the condition. (With permission from Oxford University Press, Firth, Hurst and Hall, *Oxford Desk Reference – Clinical Genetics*, 2005.)

MITOCHONDRIAL CONDITIONS AND INHERITANCE

INCIDENCE

Under 6 years 1 in 11,000. These occur in older children and adults in 1 in 8,500.

GENETIC AETIOLOGY/PATHOGENESIS

Table 15.9 presents common mitochondrial (mt) conditions.

CLINICAL PRESENTATION

These conditions present insidiously and diagnosis is often delayed. Key clinical features are myoclonus, external ophthalmoplegia, ptosis, sensorineural deafness, cardiac conduction defects and diabetes mellitus.

DIAGNOSIS

Diagnosis is based on a combination of biochemical abnormalities (raised lactate in blood/CSF), characteristic muscle biopsy 'ragged red fibres', brain MRI and genetic testing.

INHERITANCE

Mitochondrial DNA (mtDNA) is exclusively maternally inherited (**Fig. 15.18**) and for the purposes of genetic counselling the risk of paternal inheritance of a mitochondrial mutation is zero. The severity in children is difficult to predict.

TABLE 15.9 Common mitochondrial (mt) conditions

Disease	Features	Mechanism	Inheritance
Kearns Sayre	CPEO, ataxia, cardiac conduction defect	mt DNA deletion	Sporadic or rarely maternally inherited
Leber's hereditary optic neuropathy	Loss of vision	mt DNA mutation	Maternal
Leigh syndrome	Developmental delay/regression, seizures, raised lactate, abnormal brain MRI	Both mt DNA mutations (*NARP* mutations) and nuclear encoded gene mutation	Maternal and autosomal recessive
Aminoglycoside deafness	Progressive sensorineural deafness	mtDNA mutation, usually mt.A1555G	Maternal
Pearson syndrome	Transfusion dependent anaemia, exocrine pancreatic failure	mtDNA deletion	Usually sporadic

CPEO: chronic progressive external ophthalmoplegia.

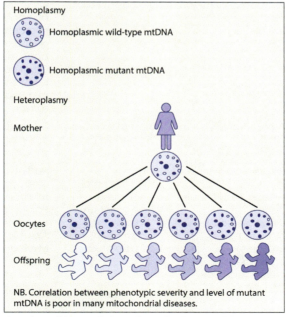

FIGURE 15.18 Illustration of maternal transmission of a mitochondrial (mt) mutation. (With permission from Oxford University Press, Firth, Hurst and Hall, *Oxford Desk Reference – Clinical Genetics*, 2005.)

Important note: many disorders of mitochondrial function are caused by mutations in nuclear genes and show AR inheritance.

- **Natural history**: progressive conditions. Prognosis depends on the diagnosis and age of presentation.
- **Differential diagnosis**: clinical overlap with inborn errors of metabolism.
- **Treatment/Management/Surveillance**: management and care should be provided by a neurologist or a metabolic physician. Family members require specialist genetic counselling because of the complexities of estimating risks to another pregnancy, and prenatal testing.

GENETIC SYNDROMES WITH CARDIAC MALFORMATION AS A MAJOR FEATURE

INCIDENCE

While most congenital heart disease is sporadic and isolated, cardiac malformation is a frequent and diagnostically discriminating feature of some inherited genetic syndromes caused by mutation with a specific gene. Those most commonly encountered in paediatric practice are listed in **Table 15.10**, along with the inheritance and cardiac malformation(s) most typical of the syndrome to use a guide to the diagnosis.

DIFFERENTIAL DIAGNOSIS OF CARDIAC MALFORMATIONS

- Environmental/maternal factors: maternal diabetes, fetal alcohol, thalidomide.
- Chromosomal conditions (trisomy and microdeletion or microduplication and syndromes).
- VATER/VACTERL association (page 480).

TABLE 15.10 Genetic syndromes with cardiac malformation as a major feature

Syndrome	Inheritance and gene	Typical cardiac malformation	Non-cardiac features
Noonan syndrome and related phenotypes of RAS-MAPK pathway: 1 in 1,000–2,000 **(Fig. 15.19)**	Autosomal dominant *PTPN11*	Pulmonary stenosis and hypertrophic cardiomyopathy	Prenatal nuchal oedema/hydrops and polyhydramnios, neck webbing, wide-spaced nipples, feeding difficulties, increased risk of bleeding problems Developmental delay in some
CHARGE syndrome: 1 in 10,000	Autosomal dominant Most are *de novo* mutations *CHD7*	Tetralogy of Fallot	**C**oloboma of the eye; **h**eart anomaly; **a**tresia choanae; **r**etardation of development; **g**enital anomalies; **e**ar abnormalities and/or deafness Other common features are facial palsy, tracheo-oesophageal atresia and hypoplasia of the semicircular canal
Holt–Oram syndrome: 1 in 100,000	Autosomal dominant *TBX5*	Atrioseptal defect, right bundle branch block	Radial ray/thumb hypoplasia, triphalageal thumb, sloping shoulders
Fanconi anaemia: 1 in 130,000 Rate increased in consanguineous families and with Ashkenazi heritage	98% are autosomal recessive At least 15 different genes Diagnosed clinically by increased chromosome breakage in presence by DEB and mitomycin C	Mostly ventriculoseptal defect, but a whole spectrum of cardiac malformations have been reported	Radial ray/thumb hypoplasia, renal agenesis, short stature and microcephaly Patchy increased skin pigmentation Aplastic anaemia in childhood Myelodysplasia and acute myeloid leukaemia Head and neck tumours in adulthood

Genetics

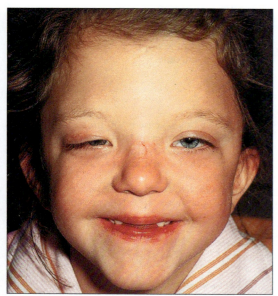

FIGURE 15.19 Noonan syndrome.

THE FLOPPY BABY

Babies with congenital hypotonia are often referred to as floppy infants. After excluding sepsis and other acute problems, the differential diagnosis is wide but with a careful pregnancy and neonatal history and examination it is possible to reduce the list and to assess the likelihood of a primarily CNS aetiology (e.g. brain malformations, complex chromosomal syndromes, metabolic disorders) versus a PNS abnormality of the nerves, neuromuscular junction and muscle.

Many paediatricians request the triad of tests for Prader–Willi syndrome, myotonic dystrophy and spinal muscular atrophy but these are clinically distinguishable with different modes of presentation and inheritance.

PRADER–WILLI SYNDROME

INCIDENCE

1 in 10,000–25,000.

GENETIC AETIOLOGY/PATHOGENESIS

Disruption of the imprinted domain at 15q11.2-13 with loss of the paternal allele in >95% of cases and include:

- microdeletions deleting the paternally inherited 15q11.2-13 (approximately 70% of cases)
- maternal UPD of chromosome 15 (25%)
- methylation defects at 15q13 (<1%) and paternally inherited unbalanced chromosome
- translocations with deletion of 15q11.2-13 (<1%).

These changes are reciprocal to those seen in Angelman syndrome (see page 470).

CLINICAL PRESENTATION/NATURAL HISTORY

Hypotonia and poor feeding arise from the neonatal period and improve during infancy. Developmental milestones are delayed with a mean age of walking approximately 2 years. Learning difficulties fall in the mild to moderate range. Hyperphagia and obesity are present from 12–18 months. Hypogonadotrophic hypogonadism is common and cryptorchidism is present in >80% of males.

DIAGNOSIS

Molecular testing is used to confirm the diagnosis and is carried out by methylation and copy number analysis at 15q11.2-13.

INHERITANCE

The majority of causes are *de novo* molecular events, with a low risk of familial recurrence. However, unbalanced translocations and some methylation defects and microdeletions can be inherited and have recurrence risks of up to 50%.

DIFFERENTIAL DIAGNOSIS

- Other causes of neonatal hypotonia.
- Other causes of obesity and learning difficulties including Albright hereditary osteodystrophy (page 484), Bardet–Biedl syndrome (page 481) and Alstrom syndrome.
- Other chromosomal abnormalities that can mimic either presentation.

TREATMENT/MANAGEMENT/ SURVEILLANCE

Developmental evaluation and support should be provided as appropriate, including, for example speech therapy and physiotherapy. Dietetic support is important for early feeding problems/failure to thrive and later for hyperphagia and obesity. Endocrine and, where appropriate, surgical referral should be provided for assessment and management of hypogonadism/cryptorchidism, with monitoring and interventions for secondary complications of obesity (e.g. type 2 diabetes mellitus).

MYOTONIC DYSTROPHY (MYOTONIC DYSTROPHY TYPE 1)

INCIDENCE

1 in 8,000.

GENETIC AETIOLOGY/PATHOGENESIS

Myotonic dystrophy is caused by CTG triplet repeat expansion in the 3' non-coding region of the *DMPK* gene. Repeat lengths of >34 are pathogenic.

CLINICAL PRESENTATION

Congenital muscular dystrophy manifests with respiratory insufficiency, hypotonia and talipes. Babies often require ventilation and the neonatal mortality is 20%. There is subsequent developmental delay. It is almost always inherited from the mother who may be only minimally affected. Traditional teaching is to shake hands with the mother to try and detect her inability to relax her grip but a genetic test has higher diagnostic sensitivity.

Later onset disease presents with progressive muscular weakness and myotonia (sustained muscle contraction) with variable age of onset. Systemic features can include cataracts, type 2 diabetes mellitus and cardiac rhythm disturbance including heart block.

DIAGNOSIS

EMG shows myotonia. Creatine kinase (CK) may be mildly elevated. Muscle biopsy is rarely used now as molecular testing is easily available and accurate. Southern blotting and/or PCR analysis is used to identify the causative expansion mutation in the *DMPK* gene.

INHERITANCE

Inheritance is AD with anticipation. The risk of expansion of the mutated allele (and therefore risk of earlier/congenital disease) is increased when passed on by females.

NATURAL HISTORY

The natural history depends on the severity of disease and there is a continuum of age of presentation. This is broadly dependent on the size of the expanded allele. Congenital muscular dystrophy can be fatal in infancy. Classical disease typically presents in the 20s or 30s. Mildly affected individuals may remain symptom free into old age or have minimal symptoms.

DIFFERENTIAL DIAGNOSIS

- Congenital muscular dystrophy.
- Other causes of a 'floppy baby'.
- Moebius syndrome.

TREATMENT/MANAGEMENT/ SURVEILLANCE

- Supportive management of muscular weakness including physiotherapy and orthoses.
- Medicalert and/or documentation in health records to alert anaesthetists to avoid agents such as vecuronium.
- Offer predictive testing to the wider family.
- Prenatal diagnosis is often possible in future pregnancies.

SYNDROMES ASSOCIATED WITH FEATURES OF A CONNECTIVE TISSUE DISORDER

The structural support proteins collagen and along with other proteins such as the fibrillins, elastin and components of the transforming growth factor-beta (TGFB) pathway maintain the strength and integrity of the connective tissue. **Table 15.11** shows how there are overlapping features but some features are more diagnostically discriminating for a particular syndrome.

TREATMENT/MANAGEMENT/ SURVEILLANCE

These conditions are all associated with serious and often progressive medical problems, the most acute of which are vascular dissection/rupture and rupture of the bowel and uterus. Referral for confirmation of the diagnosis and the appropriate surveillance by an experienced team is necessary.

TABLE 15.11 Syndromes associated with features of a connective tissue disorder

Syndrome	Inheritance and gene	Joint laxity	CVS	Eye	Palate	Skin	Bone fracture	Deaf	Other
Marfan syndrome	AD *FBN1*	++	Aortic root dilation and dissection	Myopia, lens dislocation, Cataract	High	Striae			Arachnodactyly Pneumothorax
Loeys Dietz syndrome	AD *TGFBR1* and *TGFBR2*	+++	Aortic root dilation Rupture, aneurysm, and/or dissection of major or minor arteries	Myopia, blue sclerae	Cleft palate/uvula	Thin, 'velvety', translucent, easy bruising, poor wound healing with scarring			Arachnodactyly Congenital joint contractures e.g talipes, craniosynostosis Aortic dissection/rupture Uterine rupture during pregnancy
Ehlers–Danlos I, II (Hypermobility types)	AD *COL5A1* and *COL5A2*	+++ Disloc	Mild mitral valve prolapse and aortic dilatation			Thin, 'velvety', hyperelastic skin. Poor wound healing with scarring			Inguinal hernia PROM in pregnancy
Ehlers–Danlos IV (Vascular type)	AD *COL3A1*	+ Disloc	Rupture, aneurysm, and/or dissection of major or minor arteries			Thin, translucent, easy bruising			Congenital joint contractures e.g talipes Spontaneous rupture of bowel Pneumothorax Inguinal herniae
COL2A1 spectrum (Stickler syndrome, Kneist, spondyloepiphyseal dysplasia)	AD *COL2A1* (Fig. 15.20)	++	Mild mitral valve prolapse	Myopia, retinal detachment cataract	Cleft palate/uvula			+	Short stature Early onset arthritis due to epiphyseal dysplasia
Osteogenesis imperfecta (Fig. 15.21)	Most are AD and due to mutation in *COL1A1* and *COL1A2*	++	Mild mitral valve prolapse	Blue sclerae			Yes	+	Short stature and bony deformity Type II is lethal

AD: autosomal dominant; PROM: premature rupture of membranes.

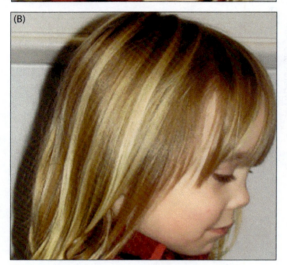

(A)

(B)

FIGURE 15.20 Facial features associated with *COL2A1* mutation.

A number of disorders present with marked developmental delay, often with absent or little speech. Common features seen in association with this include microcephaly and seizures.

The differential diagnosis includes Angelman syndrome, Rett syndrome, metabolic disorders, and an increasing number of other single gene disorders are recognised to cause this presentation and they can be difficult to distinguish clinically. Antenatal and perinatal insults are also a cause, but before this diagnosis is made other causes should be ruled out and a strongly suggestive history and supportive brain scan findings should be present.

A careful pregnancy, birth, developmental and medical history should be obtained. Routine assessment of these children should usually include chromosome testing, plasma amino acid, urine amino acid and organic acid analysis. MRI scan and EEG are often also indicated.

A number of features can help guide further specific gene testing (**Table 15.12**). Note a number of the disorders are X-linked.

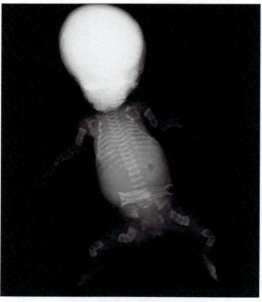

FIGURE 15.21 Radiograph showing lethal osteogenesis imperfecta type II.

Genetics

468

TABLE 15.12 Recognisable syndromes associated with severe developmental delay

Syndrome	Inheritance and gene	Developmental delay	Seizures	Other features
Angelman syndrome	Epigenetic (see text); usually sporadic) *UBE3A*	Severe Speech usually absent	80%; usually by 3 y Characteristic EEG (see text)	Jerky movements, ataxic gait, fair complexion in some, wide mouth, microcephaly, frequent laughter
Rett syndrome	X-linked dominant i.e. females *MECP2*	Severe Usually with normal early development followed by regression at 6–18 months	80% Early seizures are sometimes seen in 'variant' Rett syndrome, e.g. as part of a severe infantile epileptic encephalopathy	Stereotypic midline hand movements and loss of purposeful hand movements, microcephaly
FOXG1-related disorders	Autosomal dominant Mutations *de novo*	Severe-profound; often without a period of apparently normal development	+	Abnormal midline movements; dyskinesia/ abnormal movements; microcephaly; MRI: absent or hypoplastic corpus callosum
CDKL5-related disorders	X-linked dominant, i.e. females Mutations *de novo*	Severe-profound often without a period of apparently normal development Often 'early infantile epileptic encephalopathy'	~100% Often initially with infantile spasms	Stereoptypic hand movements; microcephaly
ARX-related disorders	X-linked recessive, i.e. males *ARX*	Mild-severe Variable; some with early infantile epileptic encephalopathy	Yes Infantile spasms in some	Dystonic hand movements; dysarthria; microcephaly; abnormal/ambiguous male genitalia; MRI: absent or hypoplastic corpus callosum; lissencephaly
ATRX-related disorders	X-linked recessive, i.e. males *ATRX*	Mild-severe Absent speech in some	~30%	Flat face; depressed nasal bridge; tented upper lip; coarse facial features; abnormal/ambiguous male genitalia Mild anaemia and HbH bodies on blood film (as seen in alpha-thalassaemia)
Mowat–Wilson syndrome	Autosomal dominant Mutations *de novo* *ZEB2*	Moderate-severe Speech usually absent	70%; usually by 2 y	Prominent chin; uplifted earlobes; Hirschprung disease (50%); constipation; genitourinary abnormalities; cardiac malformations; microcephaly MRI: absent or hypoplastic corpus callosum (40%)
Pitt–Hopkins syndrome	Autosomal dominant Mutations *de novo* *TCF4*	Severe	Yes	Coarse facial features; wide mouth; bow-shaped upper lip; episodes of hyperventilation and hypoventilation; microcephaly

ANGELMAN SYNDROME

INCIDENCE

1 in 20,000.

GENETIC AETIOLOGY/PATHOGENESIS

Disruption of the imprinted domain at 15q11.2-13 results in loss of the maternally expressed *UBE3A* gene in approximately 90% of cases, and includes microdeletions deleting the maternally inherited 15q11.2-13 (approximately 70% of cases), paternal UPD of chromosome 15 (10%), maternally inherited *UBE3A* mutations (10%), methylation defects at 15q13 (5%) and maternally inherited unbalanced chromosome translocations with deletion of 15q11.2-13 (<1%). These changes are reciprocal to those seen in Prader–Willi syndrome (see page 465).

CLINICAL PRESENTATION/NATURAL HISTORY

Severe developmental delay occurs, particularly speech delay. Motor delay and characteristic jerky movements are often noticed from around 1 year. Seizures occur in >80% from 1–3 years. The child presents with frequent laughter, often inappropriate to the situation and a dysmorphic appearance, including a wide mouth (**Figs 15.22, 15.23**). One-half of patients develop microcephaly by 1 year. Patients have good physical health in the teenage and adult years with the exception of seizures. Fair colouration may be seen in those caused by 15q11.2-13 deletions if they encompass the nearby *P* gene.

DIAGNOSIS

EEG may also be useful, showing runs of high-amplitude delta activity with intermittent spike and slow-wave discharges. Molecular testing is by methylation and copy number analysis at 15q11.2-13 together with *UBE3A* mutation analysis.

INHERITANCE

The majority of these are *de novo* events, with a low risk of familial recurrence. However, unbalanced translocations, *UBE3A* mutations and some methylation defects can be inherited and have recurrence risks of up to 50%.

DIFFERENTIAL DIAGNOSIS

See Table 15.12. X-linked recessive Angelman syndrome-like disorder caused by *SCL9A6* mutations.

TREATMENT/MANAGEMENT/SURVEILLANCE

Developmental evaluation and support should be provided as appropriate including, for example, speech therapy and physiotherapy. Seizures, if present, should be monitored and treated. Sleep disturbance should be managed, including behavioural measures and use of melatonin considered.

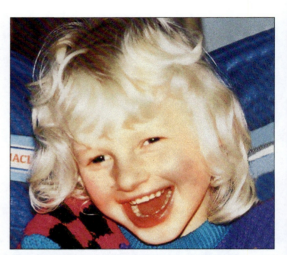

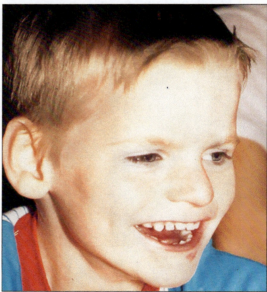

FIGURES 15.22, 15.23 Facial features of Angelman syndrome.

Genetics

RETT SYNDROME

INCIDENCE

1 in 10,000–20,000 females.

GENETIC AETIOLOGY/PATHOGENESIS

Heterozygous loss of function mutations in the *MECP2* gene at Xq28 in females.

CLINICAL PRESENTATION

Classical Rett syndrome affects females. There is apparent normal early development followed by a period of developmental regression in terms of language and motor skills at between 6 and 18 months of age. Subsequently, speech is typically absent and development remains severely delayed in all areas (**Fig. 15.24**). Stereotypic midline hand movements are common, replacing purposeful hand movements. Head growth decelerates. Occasionally males are observed with *MECP2* mutations. They manifest with a severe neonatal encephalopathy.

- **Diagnosis**: mutation analysis of the *MECP2* gene.
- **Inheritance**: X-linked dominant with almost all mutations occurring *de novo*.
- **Differential diagnosis**: see Table 12; metabolic disorders.

TREATMENT/MANAGEMENT/ SURVEILLANCE

Developmental evaluation and support should be provided as appropriate including, for example, speech therapy and physiotherapy. Seizures, if present, should be monitored and treated. Melatonin can be useful in the treatment of sleep disturbance.

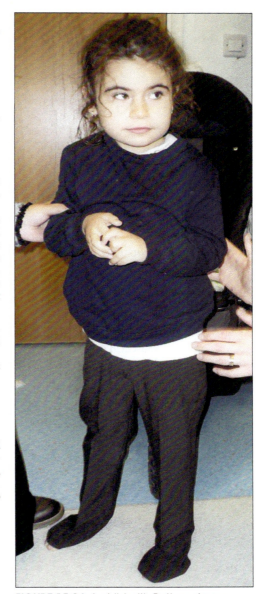

FIGURE 15.24 A child with Rett syndrome.

OTHER COMMON SINGLE GENE DISORDERS

DUCHENNE MUSCULAR DYSTROPHY

INCIDENCE

1 in 3,600 males.

GENETIC AETIOLOGY/PATHOGENESIS

Hemizygous Duchenne muscular dystrophy (DMD) (i.e. affecting the single X chromosome of a male) invloves loss of function mutations in the *Dystrophin* gene. These can be point mutations or larger structural abnormalities (e.g. multi-exon deletions).

CLINICAL PRESENTATION

Delayed motor milestones are apparent in a boy, particularly walking. There is a waddling gait as a result of the proximal muscular weakness and calf 'pseudohypertrophy'. A positive Gowers sign is found, where the arms are used to rise from a seated position on the floor. About 30% have a mild non-progressive learning disability.

DIAGNOSIS

Neonatal screening is performed in some parts of the UK/USA. Measurement of CK, muscle biopsy with dystrophin studies and *Dystrophin* mutation analysis (positive in approximately 90% with current techiniques) can help in diagnosis of DMD.

INHERITANCE

DMD is X-linked recessive. One-third are *de novo* mutations, i.e. in two-thirds the mother is a carrier and at risk of having a further affected boy.

NATURAL HISTORY

Weakness is progressive. Most affected boys are wheelchair bound by the teenage years. Dilated cardiomyophathy is usually present by 18 years of age and this with scolioisis and respiratory failure is the typical cause of death; few survive beyond the age of 30 years. The milder *Dystrophin*-related disorder Becker muscular dystrophy presents with later onset muscular weakness and patients remain ambulant into their 20s.

DIFFERENTIAL DIAGNOSIS

- Emery–Dreyfuss muscular dystrophy.
- Limb girdle muscular dystrophy.

TREATMENT/MANAGEMENT/SURVEILLANCE

Supportive management of muscular weakness and prevention of contractures should be provided, including physiotherapy and nocturnal respiratory support. Children should be under surveillance for, and management of, cardiac failure using standard therapies. Gene therapy and upregulation of the dystrophin-related protein utrophin are therapeutic hopes for the future.

Carrier testing should be offered for the wider family; prenatal diagnosis is often possible in future pregnancies.

FRAGILE X SYNDROME

INCIDENCE

1 in 2,000 males.

GENETIC AETIOLOGY/PATHOGENESIS

Fragile X is caused by a triplet repeat expansion within the *FMR1* gene. Repeat lengths of >200 are referred to as 'full mutations' and cause fragile X syndrome. Alleles with 55–200 repeats are referred to as 'premutations' and are associated with an increased risk of expansion to >200 repeats when transmitted.

CLINICAL PRESENTATION

Males with fragile X typically have moderate learning difficulties. Behavioural difficulties, often leading to a diagnosis of autism, are common. Physical features present in some include relative macrocephaly, a long face, prominent ears, squint, joint laxity, mitral valve prolapse and large testes (**Fig. 15.25**). Affected females typically have mild learning difficulties.

- **Diagnosis**: Southern blotting and/or PCR analysis to identify the causative expansion mutation in the *FMR1* gene.
- **Inheritance**: X-linked recessive.

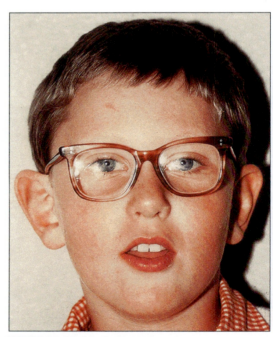

FIGURE 15.25 Fragile X syndrome.

- **Natural history**: the features of the fragile X syndrome are largely static.
- **Differential diagnosis**:
  - chromosome abnormalities.
  - Sotos syndrome.
  - Non-syndromic autism of unknown cause.

TREATMENT/MANAGEMENT/SURVEILLANCE

Developmental evaluation and support should be provided as appropriate, including speech therapy and behavioural management. Children should receive routine medical management of concomitant problems such as squint or mitral valve prolapse.

Carrier testing should be offered for the wider family; prenatal diagnosis is often possible in future pregnancies.

NEUROFIBROMATOSIS TYPE 1

INCIDENCE

1 in 5,000.

GENETIC AETIOLOGY/PATHOGENESIS

90% of neurofibromatosis type 1 (NF1) patients have monoallelic (dominant) loss of function mutations in the *NF1* gene; 10% have a microdeletion of 17q11.2 encompassing *NF1*.

CLINICAL PRESENTATION

Patients with NF1 shows considerable variability between affected individuals. Diagnostic features include multiple café-au-lait (hyperpigmented) patches, axillary and inguinal freckling, Lisch nodules (iris hamartomas), cutaneous neurofibromas, plexiform neurofibromas, relative macrocephaly, osseous dysplasia such as tibial pseudarthrosis or sphenoid wing dysplasia, scoliosis and renal artery stenosis (leading to hypertension) (**Figs 15.26–15.29**). Optic nerve and other CNS gliomas are seen, as are malignant peripheral nerve sheath tumours, but the excess cancer risk of the condition is only approximately 5%. Mild learning difficulties occur in up to 50%.

DIAGNOSIS

Clinical assessment remains the main means of diagnosis in the majority. To reach a clinical diagnosis, an individual must have two or more of the following: a) six or more café-au-lait patches (>0.5 mm before puberty of >15 mm after); b) two or more cutaneous neurofibromas or one plexiform neurofibroma; c) two or more Lisch nodules (on slit-lamp examination); d) optic glioma; e) pseudarthrosis or sphenoid wing dysplasia; f) first-degree relative with NF1 as defined above.

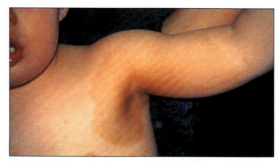

FIGURE 15.26 Café-au-lait patches/macules in neurofibromatosis type 1.

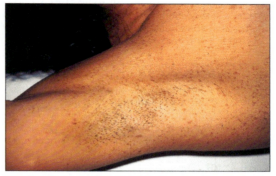

FIGURE 15.27 Axillary freckles in neurofibromatosis type 1.

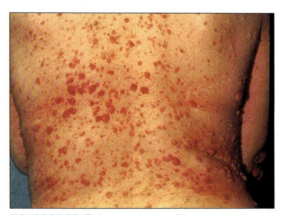

FIGURE 15.28 Cutaneous neurofibromas in neurofibromatosis type 1.

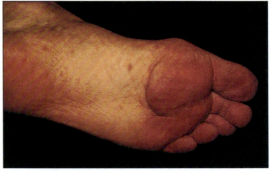

FIGURE 15.29 Plexiform neurofibroma on the sole of the foot in neurofribromatosis type 1.

Mutation analysis of the *NF1* gene is an expensive test and it is currently reserved for individuals who cannot be managed by clinical assessment alone or where prenatal diagnosis is planned.

INHERITANCE

Autosomal dominant.

NATURAL HISTORY

Café-au-lait patches are usually the first feature and can be seen from birth. Bony manifestations are also usually congenital. Optic gliomas rarely develop after 6 years of life, whereas Lisch nodules are rarely found before 6 years of age. In some cases, scoliosis develops in the first decade but it is more common in the teenage years. Cutaneous neurofibromas usually develop in the teenage years.

DIFFERENTIAL DIAGNOSIS

- Legius syndrome. Cafe-au-lait macules, axillary freckles, macrocephaly but no neurofibromas. *SPRED1* mutations.
- Mismatch repair deficiency syndrome (caused by biallelic – recessive – mutations in hereditary non-polyposis colon cancer genes).
- NF2: the typical multiple café-au-lait skin macules of NF1 are not seen in NF2 but NF1-like neurofibromas can lead to diagnostic uncertainty.
- LEOPARD and Noonan syndrome (see page 464).

TREATMENT/MANAGEMENT/ SURVEILLANCE

Annual assessment by a paediatrician should be undertaken in childhood. This should include assessment of developmental needs, blood pressure, scoliosis, growth, skin lesions and any other new features. Children should also have annual slit-lamp examination by an ophthalmologist. The annual review should continue in adulthood but can be performed in primary care.

TUBEROUS SCLEROSIS

INCIDENCE

1 in 10,000.

GENETIC AETIOLOGY/PATHOGENESIS

Tuberous sclerosis is caused by monoallelic (dominant) mutations in the *TSC1* or *TSC2* genes. Mutations are found in approximately 85% of cases. *TSC1* mutations account for approximately 25% and *TSC2* mutations in approximately 60%.

CLINICAL PRESENTATION

Tuberous sclerosis shows considerable variability with some individuals showing only very subtle features. Others are severely affected, for example manifesting initially with infantile spasms and going on to have severe developmental delay and intractable seizures. Overall, seizures occur in up to 80% of individuals and developmental delay/learning difficulties in 50%. In general, more severely neurologically impaired individuals have more florid CNS involvement including with corticle tubers and subependymal nodules (**Fig. 15.30**). Supepdendymal giant cell astrocytomas can also occur.

A number of other systems can also be involved. Cutaneous manifestations are present in almost 100% of individuals and include hypopigmented ('ash leaf') skin macules, adenoma sebaceum, Shagreen patches and ungal fibromas. Renal features include angiomyolipomas and renal cell carcinoma. Cardiac rhabdomyomas and pulmonary lymphangiomyomatosis are also seen.

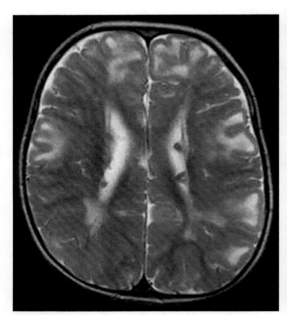

FIGURE 15.30 T2-weighted MRI brain image showing multiple parenchymal tubers and subependymal nodules in tuberous sclerosis.

DIAGNOSIS

A definite clinical diagnosis of tuberous sclerosis can be made in the presence of two major features (listed above) and one minor feature such as multiple renal cysts, hamartomatous rectal polyps, gingival fibromas and retinal achromic patches. Increasingly, molecular diagnosis is used. This is by mutation analysis of the *TSC1* and *TSC2* genes.

INHERITANCE

Autosomal dominant.

NATURAL HISTORY

Presentation can be from the prenatal period with cardiac rhabdomyomas. These can cause dysrhythmia and occasionally outflow tract obstruction in the neonatal period but typically resolve during infancy. Seizures are the leading cause of death and can occur initially as infantile spasms or develop later. Renal disease is also an important cause of mortality, and 80% of cases have an identifiable renal lesion by 10 years. Progressive pulmonary lymphangiomyomatosis is principally a disease of women with tuberous sclerosis in adulthood and can be life threatening.

DIFFERENTIAL DIAGNOSIS

- Subependymal nodules need to be distinguished from periventricular nodular heterotopia.
- Many of the other features can occur sporadically (i.e. in isolation and not as part of tuberous sclerosis), for example, cardiac rhabdomyomas, renal angiomyolipomas, pulmonary lymphangiomatosis.
- Vitiligo and other skin lesions mimicking those seen in tuberous sclerosis.

TREATMENT/MANAGEMENT/SURVEILLANCE

Seizures should be managed with antiepileptic drugs and occasionally surgery. mTOR inhibitors have been used for enlarging tuberous sclerosis-related lesions including astrocytomas, angiomyolipomas and lymangiomatosis in adults. Surgical management can also be used. MRI brain scan is suggested at 2 and 8 years of age. Annual reviews should be conducted by a paediatrician, to include: history and examination (including cardiac, respiratory, abdominal ocular and skin examination), blood pressure measurement and urine dipstick testing. Renal ultrasound scan is recommended every 2 years after the age of 8 years. CT chest is recommended in females at 16 years.

OTHER RARE RECOGNISABLE SYNDROMES

KABUKI SYNDROME

INCIDENCE

Approximately 1 in 30,000.

GENETIC AETIOLOGY/PATHOGENESIS

There is heterozygous (dominant) loss of function mutations in the *MLL2* gene in approximately 60% of cases. The cause in the remainder is unknown.

CLINICAL PRESENTATION

The facial appearance is characteristic but may be difficult to recognise in early infancy. Features include arched eyebrows with lateral sparseness, long palpebral fissures with eversion of the lateral portion of the lower lid and prominent cupped ears (**Figs 15.31, 15.32**). Growth retardation including

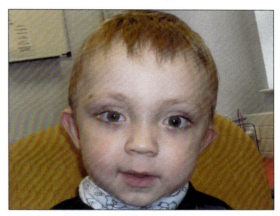

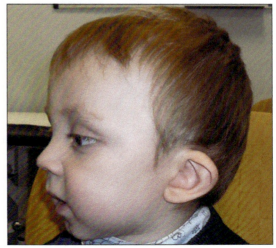

FIGURES 15.31, 15.32 Facial features of Kabuki syndrome.

microcephaly occurs, often with other congenital anomalies including congenital heart disease, cleft palate and structural renal abnormalities. Immune dysfunction is often present. Hypotonia is common in infancy and development is delayed. Learning difficulties are typically moderate.

DIAGNOSIS

Diagnosis is clinical, with recognition of the characteristic facial appearance in the context of other supportive features. *MLL2* mutation analysis is particularly useful in cases where the diagnosis is uncertain.

INHERITANCE

Autosomal dominant. However, the large majority of cases arise as a result of *de novo* mutations, meaning that the parents of an affected child are usually at low risk of having a further affected child.

TREATMENT/MANAGEMENT/ SURVEILLANCE

Initial work-up should include ECHO, renal ultrasound scan, hearing assessment, T-cell subsets and immunoglobulins, and formal palatal assessment. Subsequently management focuses on monitoring and support of development, growth and specific abnormalities identified in initial work-up.

RUBINSTEIN–TAYBI SYNDROME

INCIDENCE

1 in 125,000–300,000.

GENETIC AETIOLOGY/PATHOGENESIS

This syndrome is caused by heterozygous (dominant) deletions or loss of function mutations affecting the *CREBBP* gene in 50–70% of cases. Heterozygous loss of function mutations in the *EP300* gene have been found in a small number of cases (approximately 3%). The cause in the remainder is unknown.

CLINICAL PRESENTATION

Children present with microcephaly with short stature and developmental delay. Learning difficulties are moderate to severe. The facial appearance is often recognisable with downslanting palpebral fissures, prominent columella and a grimacing smile (**Fig. 15.33**). Thumbs and great toes are often broad and medially deviated (**Figs 15.34, 15.35**). Structural cardiac and renal tract abnormalities are common and cryptorchidism is almost invariably present in males. The phenotype may be more subtle in individuals with *EP300* mutations.

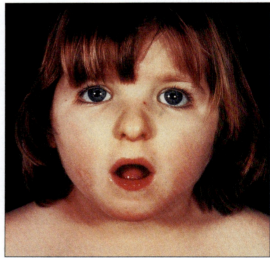

FIGURE 15.33 Facial features in Rubinstein–Taybi syndrome.

DIAGNOSIS

Diagnosis is by recognition of the characteristic facial and other physical features in the context of other supportive features. *CREBBP* copy number and mutation analysis and *EP300* mutation analysis can provide molecular confirmation.

INHERITANCE

Rubinstein–Taybi syndrome is autosomal dominant; the large majority of cases arise as a result of *de novo* mutations, meaning that the parents of an affected child are usually at low risk of having a further affected child.

DIFFERENTIAL DIAGNOSIS

Floating–Harbour syndrome (caused by a gene in same pathway as *CREBBP*).

TREATMENT/MANAGEMENT/SURVEILLANCE

Initial evaluation should include ECHO and renal ultrasound scan. Subsequent management focuses on monitoring and support of development, growth and other specific abnormalities.

de LANGE SYNDROME

INCIDENCE

1 in 10,000–30,000.

GENETIC AETIOLOGY/PATHOGENESIS

Heterozygous (dominant) deletions and loss of function mutations of the *NIBPL* gene cause typical de Lange. Mutations in other genes occur in a small percentage of cases (usually with atypical features).

CLINICAL PRESENTATION

The facial appearance is characteristic including synophrys, long thick eyelashes, upturned nasal tip, long smooth philtrum and thin upper lip (**Figs 15.36, 15.37**). Additional features are pre- and postnatal growth retardation with microcephaly, limb abnormalities (**Figs 15.38, 15.39**), hirsuitism and learning difficulties. Limb defects range from phocomelia or ectrodactyly to more subtle hand abnormalities such as proximally placed thumbs or fifth finger clinodactyly. Most children with typical de Lange have severe learning difficulties.

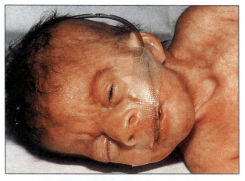

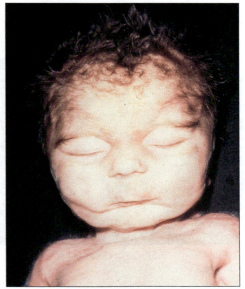

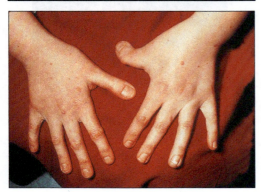

FIGURES 15.34, 15.35 Features of digits in Rubinstein–Taybi syndrome.

FIGURES 15.36, 15.37 Facial features of De Lange syndrome.

DIAGNOSIS

Characteristic facial and other physical features in the context of other supportive features diagnose De Lange. *NIBPL* copy number and mutation analysis and *SMC/SMC1A* mutation analysis can provide molecular confirmation.

INHERITANCE

NIBPL mutations are autosomal dominant. However, the large majority of cases arise as a result of *de novo* mutations, meaning that the parents of an affected child are usually at low risk of having a further affected child. *SMC1A* mutations are X-linked recessive.

TREATMENT/MANAGEMENT/ SURVEILLANCE

Children are monitored and given support for development, growth and other specific abnormalities including limb defects. Management of gastroesophageal reflux is often required.

SOTOS SYNDROME

INCIDENCE

1 in 10,000–20,000.

GENETIC AETIOLOGY/PATHOGENESIS

Heterozygous (autosomal dominant) loss of function mutations and deletions in the *NSD1* gene occur in 90% of cases.

CLINICAL PRESENTATION

Sotos syndrome is an overgrowth disorder, which often initially presents with pre- and postnatal macrosomia including macrocephaly. Bone age is advanced in the majority of cases. The facial appearance is characteristic with a tall forehead, high frontal hairline, downslanting palpebral fissures and a prominent chin (**Figs 15.40, 15.41**). Developmental delay is very common and learning difficulties are usually present, but to a variable degree.

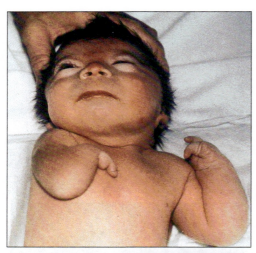

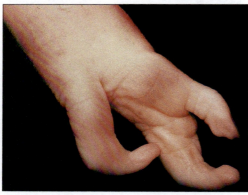

FIGURES 15.38, 15.39 Limb defects in De Lange syndrome.

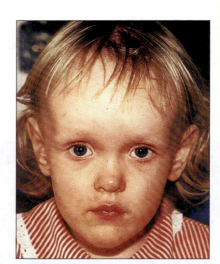

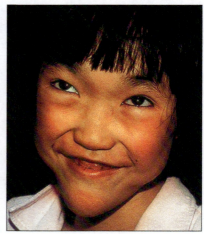

FIGURES 15.40, 15.41 Facial features of Sotos syndrome.

Genetics

DIAGNOSIS

Diagnosis is on characteristic facial appearance in the context of overgrowth and developmental delay/learning difficulties. *NSD1* mutation and copy number analysis provides molecular confirmation.

INHERITANCE

Inheritance is autosomal dominant; the large majority of *NSD1* mutations arise as *de novo* mutations meaning that the parents of an affected child are usually at low risk of having a further affected child.

DIFFERENTIAL DIAGNOSIS

Other overgrowth syndromes and fragile X.

TREATMENT/MANAGEMENT/SURVEILLANCE

Children are monitored and given support for development, growth and other specific abnormalities. Annual surveillance should include assessment for scoliosis and blood pressure measurement. Unlike some overgrowth syndromes, additional cancer screening is not recommended.

GOLDENHAR SYNDROME (HEMIFACIAL MICROSOMIA)

INCIDENCE

1 in 5,000.

GENETIC AETIOLOGY/PATHOGENESIS

Goldenhar is considered to be a non-genetic disorder that results from a vascular insult early in development.

CLINICAL PRESENTATION

This is a disorder principally affecting the derivatives of the first and second branchial arches. Its features include facial asymmetry, macrostomia with lateral oral clefting, cleft palate and microtia (**Figs 15.42, 15.43**). Preauricular ear tags and epibulbar dermoids of the eye are key features (**Fig. 15.44**). Microphthalmia and coloboma also occur. Common extracranial features include hemivertrebrae, fused

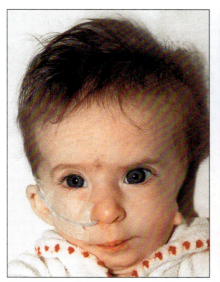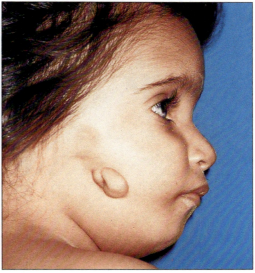

FIGURES 15.42, 15.43 Facial features in Goldenhar syndrome.

vertebrae and structural cardiac and renal abnormalities. Hearing is often affected.

- **Diagnosis**: is based on clinical findings and eliminating other diagnoses.
- **Inheritance**: sporadic.
- **Differential diagnosis**: chromosome 22 abnormalities, particularly duplication and additional marker 22.
- **Treatment/Management/Surveillance**: management is best co-ordinated by a multidisciplinary craniofacial team including craniofacial surgeons, speech therapists, audiologists and ophthalmologists.

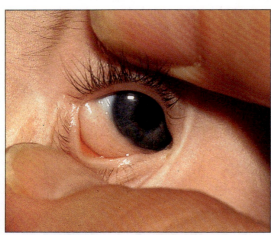

FIGURE 15.44 An epibulbar dermoid in a child with Goldenhar syndrome.

VATER/VACTERL ASSOCIATION

INCIDENCE

1 in 5,000.

GENETIC AETIOLOGY/PATHOGENESIS

The cause of VATER /VACTERL association is unknown. It is speculated to be a non-genetic disorder that results from a vascular insult early in development.

CLINICAL PRESENTATION

VATER or VACTERL are acronyms referring to the principal features of the condition: **v**ertebral defects (usually hemivertebrae or hypoplastic vertebrae), **a**nal anomalies (anal atresia or stenosis), structural **c**ardiac defects, oesophageal abnormalities (typically oesophageal atresia with **t**racheo-oesophageal fistula with **o**esophageal atresia), **r**enal defects (including renal agenesis and other structural abnormalities) and **l**imb defects (typically radial ray abnormalities ranging from radial aplasia with severe forearm shortening to hypoplastic or proximally placed thumbs).

DIAGNOSIS

Diagnosis is by presence of the above features and differentiation from related, genetic disorders that affect the radius and thumb. In VATER the radial abnormalities are typically unilateral.

- **Inheritance**: sporadic.
- **Differential diagnosis**:
  - Fanconi anaemia.
  - thrombocytopenia absent radius (TAR) syndrome.
  - chromosome abnormalities.
- **Treatment/Management/Surveillance**: management is dependent on the individual features present and typically involves early surgical intervention for tracheo-oesophageal fistula and gastrointestinal abnormalities.

Genetics

480

BARDET–BIEDL SYNDROME

INCIDENCE

1 in 150,000.

GENETIC AETIOLOGY/PATHOGENESIS

Biallelic (recessive) loss of function mutations occurs in one of the more than 14 currently known Bardet–Biedl syndrome (BBS) genes. In some cases there is evidence of modification of the phenotype by the presence of an additional mutation in a second BBS gene. BBS is a 'ciliopathy' and BBS genes are important in the function of cilia.

CLINICAL PRESENTATION

BBS causes truncal obesity (in 70%) and mild to moderate learning difficulties. Postaxial polydactyly (that may affect all four limbs) is often also present and the major other features include progressive rod–cone dystrophy and renal disease with cystic kidneys and chronic kidney disease. Other features include male hypogonadotrophic hypogonadism and complex female genital abnormalities (e.g. hydrometrocolpos).

DIAGNOSIS

Until recent technological and service developments, molecular diagnosis has been difficult and costly due to the large number of different genes. Prior to this, diagnosis was often solely clinical and based on the presence of four major features (above) or three major features and one or more minor features such as brachy/syndactyly, ataxia/poor co-ordination or diabetes mellitus. Renal ultrasound scan, renal function testing and ophthalmological assessment including electrodiagnostic testing are useful in detecting occult renal and ophthalmological disease.

INHERITANCE

BBS is autosomal recessive.

NATURAL HISTORY

Initial presentation is with pre- or early postnatal detection of structural physical abnormalities such as postaxial polydactyly (**Fig. 15.45**) or cystic kidney disease. Truncal obesity is present in approximately 70% and usually develops during the first year (**Fig. 15.46**). Progressive rod–cone dystrophy causes night blindness by 8 years. The mean age of registered visual loss is 15–16 years. Renal disease is also progressive and end-stage kidney disease is present in 10% of patients. Diabetes mellitus and abnormal lipid profiles are also features.

DIFFERENTIAL DIAGNOSIS

- Other causes of childhood obesity/marcrosomia.
- Other disorders caused by mutations in ciliary genes (e.g. AR polycystic kidney disease, Joubert syndrome).

- Alstrøm syndrome (retinal dystrophy, obesity, sensorineural deafness, cardiomyopathy).
- AD HNF1β mutations (isolated renal disease).

TREATMENT/MANAGEMENT/ SURVEILLANCE

Regular ophthalmologic evaluation should be performed with monitoring of renal function, blood pressure, blood lipids and screening for diabetes mellitus and annual blood pressure measurement. In the UK, this is usually co-ordinated through the National Specialist Bardet–Biedl service http://www.specialisedservices.nhs.uk/serv/bardet-biedl-syndrome. Prenatal diagnosis may be available in future pregnancies.

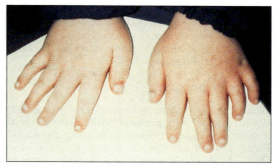

FIGURES 15.45 Postaxial polydactyly in Bardet–Biedl syndrome.

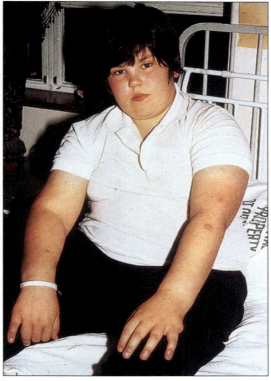

FIGURE 15.46 Truncal obesity in Bardet–Biedl syndrome.

BECKWITH–WIEDEMANN SYNDROME

INCIDENCE

1 in 10,000.

GENETIC AETIOLOGY/PATHOGENESIS

Disruption of the imprinted domain at 11p15 result in increased expression of growth promoting genes such as *IGF2* and/or decreased expression of growth suppressing genes such as *CDKN1C*. Abnormalities at 11p15 are identifiable in approximately 80% of cases and include loss of methylation at KvDMR1 (approximately 50% of cases), paternal UPD 11p15 (20%), hyperrmethylation at *H19* DMR (5%), maternally inherited mutations in *CDKN1C* (<5%) and duplications of the paternal 11p15 allele, including those occurring as part of unbalanced translocations (<1%). These abnormalities are reciprocal to those seen in Silver–Russell syndrome.

CLINICAL PRESENTATION

Beckwith–Wiedemann syndrome is an overgrowth disorder and often presents with increased birth weight and increased growth in early childhood. Facial appearance may be coarse in some cases (**Fig. 15.47**). Other features include neonatal hypoglycaemia, macroglossia, exomphalos, growth asymmetry (hemihypertrophy), earlobe creases and posterior helical pits and predisposition to embryonal tumours, particularly Wilms tumour. It should be noted that there is no evidence of increased Wilms risk in cases with loss of methylation at KvDMR1 (the largest molecular group).

DIAGNOSIS

The condition is variable and clinical features may be subtle. Diagnosis is by characteristic clinical features (above) and/or confirmatory molecular genetic testing. Molecular testing is carried out by methylation and copy number analysis at 11p15 and (in selected cases) mutation analysis of *CDKN1C*.

INHERITANCE

The majority of causes are *de novo* molecular events, with a low risk of familial recurrence. However, unbalanced translocations, copy number defects and *CDKN1C* mutations can be inherited and have recurrence risks of up to 50%.

DIFFERENTIAL DIAGNOSIS

- Isolated hemihypertrophy (that can also be caused by 11p15 defects).
- Simpson–Golabi–Behmel syndrome.
- Sotos syndrome (page 478).
- *WT1*-related Wilms predisposition disorders.

TREATMENT/MANAGEMENT/SURVEILLANCE

Monitoring of prefeed glucose is performed for the first 48 hours. Three to 4-monthly renal ultrasound scans for Wilms tumour surveillance are carried out for those at risk (i.e. not those with isolated loss of methylation at KvDMR1). Referral to a clinical geneticist is advised to guide this.

Children should be referred to a speech therapist in cases with macroglossia and have orthopaedic referral in cases with marked leg length discrepancy.

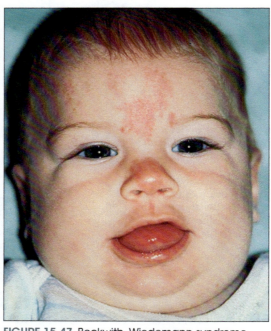

FIGURE 15.47 Beckwith–Wiedemann syndrome.

SILVER–RUSSELL SYNDROME

INCIDENCE

1 in 20,000.

GENETIC AETIOLOGY/PATHOGENESIS

Disruption of the imprinted domains at 11p15 or on chromosome 7 occurs. Abnormalities at 11p15 are found in approximately 60% of cases and include loss of methylation at *H19* DMR (60%) and duplications of the maternal 11p15 allele (<1%). These abnormalities are reciprocal to those seen in Beckwith–Wiedemann syndrome. Approximately 10% have maternal UPD for chromosome 7.

CLINICAL PRESENTATION

Growth retardation is present, characterised by pre- and postnatal growth retardation and relative macrocephaly. Children have a recognisable facies with a triangular configuration (small chin with frontal prominence), thin lips and down-turned corners of the mouth (**Fig. 15.48**). Other features include fifth finger clinodactyly, growth asymmetry and hyperpigmented skin patches. Some individuals have developmental delay/learning difficulties. Average adult height is approximately 150 cm for males and 140 cm for females.

DIAGNOSIS

Molecular testing is by methylation and copy number analysis at 11p15 and microsatellite testing for maternal UPD7.

INHERITANCE

The majority of causes are *de novo* molecular events, with a low risk of familial recurrence. However, duplications at 11p15 can be inherited and have recurrence risks of up to 50%.

DIFFERENTIAL DIAGNOSIS

- Placental insufficiency, other maternal and environmental causes of prenatal growth retardation, other causes of failure to thrive.
- Chromosome disorders causing overlapping phenotypes, e.g. 15q26.6 deletions.
- 3M syndrome.
- DNA repair disorders associated with poor growth, e.g. Fanconi anaemia.
- Isolated hemihypertrophy (which can also be cause by 11p15 defects).

TREATMENT/MANAGEMENT/SURVEILLANCE

Monitoring and supportive management of development, growth and feeding is provided and endocrinology referral for management of growth retardation. Growth hormone therapy is beneficial in some cases, even in the absence of deficiency. Orthopaedic referral is provided in cases with marked leg length discrepancy.

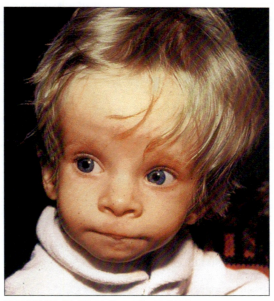

FIGURE 15.48 Silver–Russell syndrome.

ALBRIGHT HEREDITARY OSTEODYSTROPHY (PSEUDOHYPOPARA-THYROIDISM TYPE 1A)

INCIDENCE

1 in 300,000.

GENETIC AETIOLOGY/PATHOGENESIS

This is caused by maternally inherited mutations in the imprinted *GNAS1* gene that encodes Gs-α G protein subunit.

CLINICAL PRESENTATION

Children present with short stature, stocky build, round face and brachydactyly and short metacarpals (especially the 4th and 5th). There is peripheral resistance to parathyroid hormone (PTH), resulting in pseudohypoparathyroidism including hypocalcaemia and hyperphosphataemia. Subcutaneous calcification is seen in some individuals. Resistance to other hormones including thyroid stimulating hormone and gonadotrophins also occur. Learning difficulties are present in some individuals.

DIAGNOSIS

Diagnosis is by presence of the characteristic physical and biochemical features. Radiographs of the hands can provide further supportive evidence, including the presence of cone-shaped epiphyses. Genetic confirmation can be provided by mutation analysis of *GNAS1*.

INHERITANCE

Autosomal dominant inheritance when inherited from a female.

DIFFERENTIAL DIAGNOSIS

- Pseudohypoparathyroidism type 1b (peripheral resistance to PTH and other hormones in the absence of the physical features of Albright hereditary osteodystrophy).
- Chromosome abnormalities, including 2q37 deletions and 17p11 deletions (Smith–Magenis syndrome).
- *HDAC1* mutations.
- *RAI1* mutations.

TREATMENT/MANAGEMENT/SURVEILLANCE

Children are referred to an endocrinologist for management of endocrine disturbance including calcium and vitamin D supplementation, thyroxine and other endocrine therapies as appropriate. Support of developmental and learning needs is provided.

FURTHER READING

Web resources

Dyscerne http://www.dyscerne.org/dysc/Guidelines; this included management guidelines for Angelman syndrome, Kabuki syndrome, Noonan syndrome and Williams syndrome.

Gene Clinics http://www.geneclinics.org; this includes reviews of the majority of the single gene and epigenetic disorders covered in this text.

OMIM – Online Mendelian Inheritance in Man www.ncbi.nlm.nih.gov/omim/

General genetics texts

Firth HV, Hurst JA. *Oxford Desk Reference – Clinical Genetics*, 1st edn. Oxford: Oxford University Press, 2005. ISBN 9780192628961.

Gardner RJM, SutherlandGR. *Chromosome Abnormalities and Genetic Counseling*, 3rd edn. Oxford Monographs on Medical Genetics no 31, 2004.

Turnpenny P, Ellard S. *Emery's Elements of Medical Genetics*, 13th edn. Churchill Livingstone, 2007. ISBN 9780702029172.

Young ID. *Medical Genetics*. Oxford: Oxford University Press, 2005. ISBN 0198564945.

Dysmorphology texts

Jones KL, Jones MC, Del Campo Casanelles M (eds). *Smith's Recognisable Patterns of Human Malfomations*, 7th edn. Philadelphia: WB Saunders, 2013.

Hennekam RCM, Krantz ID, Allanson JE (eds). *Gorlin's Syndromes of the Head and Neck*, 5th edn. Oxford: Oxford University Press, 2010.

Databases

Baraitser M, Winter R. Baraitser–Winter Dysmorphology Database. www.lmdatabases.com

DECIPHER database of chromosomal imbalance and phenotype http://decipher.sanger.ac.uk/

Other key references

British Society for Human Genetics Report on testing in children 2010. http://www.bshg.org.uk/GTOC_Booklet_Final_new.pdf

Ferner RE, Huson SM, Thomas N, *et al*. Guidelines for the diagnosis and management of individuals with neurofibromatosis 1 (NF1). *J Med Genet* 2007;44:81–8.

O'Malley M, Hutcheon RG. Genetic disorders and congenital malformations in pediatric long-term care. *J Am Med Dir Assoc* 2007;8(5):332–4.

Stevenson DA, Carey JC. Contribution of malformations and genetic disorders to mortality in a children's hospital. *Am J Med Genet A* 2004;126A(4):393–7.

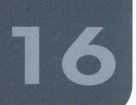

16 Immunology (Primary Immunodeficiency Syndromes)

Stephan Strobel and Alison M. Jones

BACKGROUND

Primary immunodeficiency syndromes (PIDs) are rare disorders caused by genetic defects affecting development and function of adaptive and/or innate immunity. More than 250 single gene defects have been defined, with many more emerging. Most are extremely rare, but collectively they form a significant group of childhood diseases. The overall incidence of PID is thought to be about 1 in 5000.

Secondary immunodeficiencies, which are not discussed in this chapter, are more common than PIDs. Causes include HIV/AIDS, malignancy and immunosuppressive drugs.

PRESENTING FEATURES OF PID

The most frequent presenting feature of PID in children is infection. However, only approximately 10% of children referred with recurrent infections have a demonstrable immunodeficiency. Other causes include atopy (which may co-exist with PID) and other chronic disorders, and in many children with recurrent infection no underlying cause can be defined. These children usually have normal growth and development, respond quickly to appropriate treatment, recover completely, and are healthy between infections.

With regard to infection the acronym 'SPUR' can be useful:

- **S**evere.
- **P**ersistent.
- **U**nusual.
- **R**ecurrent.

In the following scenarios investigation for possible PID should be considered:

- Need for intravenous antibiotics to clear infections on more than one occasion.
- Six or more new infections per year.
- Two or more episodes of sepsis or meningitis.
- Recurrent or resistant candidiasis (**Fig. 16.1**).
- Deep-seated or recurrent abscesses.
- Infection with an opportunistic organism.
- Complications after live vaccines (e.g. bacillus Calmette–Guérin [BCG]).

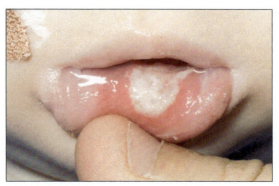

FIGURE 16.1 Persistent oral candidiasis in an 8-month-old male; X-linked immunodeficiency before bone marrow transplantation.

Background

485

Other clinical features that may suggest PID include:

- Chronic diarrhoea.
- Autoimmune phenomena.
- Poor wound healing.
- Persistent lymphopenia (<1500 cells/µl in patients >5 years and <2500 cells/µl in younger children).
- Granulomatous disease – any organ.
- Haemophagocytic lymphohistiocytosis (HLH).
- Lymphoma in infancy.
- Other features typical of syndromic primary immunodeficiencies – see **Table 16.1**.

CLASSIFICATION OF PIDs

A broad classification of PIDs is shown in **Table 16.2**. In practice the most frequently encountered disorders are those affecting antibody production. Isolated T-cell defects are very rare. Severe combined immunodeficiency (SCID) is a paediatric emergency; urgent referral to a specialist centre is required if SCID is suspected.

TREATMENT

Management of children affected by PIDs includes supportive and corrective treatment. Supportive measures focus on prevention and treatment of infection; non-infective complications may require anti-inflammatory and/or immunosuppressive treatment. For severe life-threatening or life-limiting PIDs, corrective treatment by stem cell transplantation is required; in highly selected cases gene therapy and thymus transplant trials are in progress.

Combined immunodeficiencies/T cell defects:

- Protective isolation.
- Antipneumocystis prophylaxis: cotrimoxazole (dapsone or pentamidine if intolerant).
- Antifungals: fluconazole (itraconazole if neutropenic).
- Antivirals may be required in specific situations.
- Immunoglobulin replacement (see below).
- Stem cell transplantation (or gene therapy in specific situations).
- Thymus transplantation is being developed for 'complete DiGeorge syndrome'.

Antibody deficiencies

- Lifelong immunoglobulin replacement is the mainstay of treatment for significant antibody deficiency. Immunoglobulin can be given intravenously (IVIg) or subcutaneously (SCIg). IVIg is usually given 3-weekly in hospital, and SCIg requires weekly infusion but in almost all cases is given at home (**Fig. 16.2**).

TABLE 16.1 Patterns suggestive of specific immunodeficiency syndromes

Symptom/sign	Syndrome
Petechiae/bruising/bleeding, eczema, recurrent infection	Wiskott–Aldrich syndrome
Coarse facial features, chronic infected eczema, deep-seated abscesses	Hyper-IgE syndrome
Short stature, chondrodystrophy, fine hair, recurrent infection	Cartilage hair hypoplasia
Congenital heart disease, facial dysmorphism, hypocalcaemia, absent thymus	DiGeorge syndrome
Severe erythrodermic dermatitis, hepatosplenomegaly, lymphadenopathy, eosinophilia, severe infections	Omenn syndrome
Recurrent lymphadenitis, deep-seated abscesses, oral gingivitis and ulceration	Chronic granulomatous disease
Delayed separation of the umbilical cord, omphalitis, severe soft tissue infection without pus formation, high circulating neutrophil count	Leukocyte adhesion deficiency
Oculocutaneous albinism, recurrent infections; giant granules in neutrophils	Chediak–Higashi syndrome
Abnormal dentition, reduced sweating, sparse hair	Ectodermal dysplasia with immunodeficiency (NEMO)
Extensive warts/molluscum contagiosum	T-cell defects, especially DOCK-8 deficiency WHIM (warts, hypogammaglobulinemia, infections, myelokathexis) syndrome
Lupus-like rash	Early complement component defects

(Adapted from: Approach to the child with recurrent infections, Stiehm ER. Up-to-date 2014, accessed 01/09/2014; http://www.uptodate.com/contents/approach-to-the-child-with-recurrent-infections.)

TABLE 16.2 Classification of PIDs (Adapted from Al-Herz W, *et al*. Primary immunodeficiency diseases: an update on the classification from the International Union of Immunological Societies Expert Committee for Primary Immunodeficiency. *Front Immun* 2011;2:54.)

	Broad category	Example
I Combined immunodeficiencies	Severe combined immunodeficiency (SCID)	Adenosine deaminase deficiency X-linked SCID Omenn syndrome
	Other combined immune deficiencies	X-linked hyper-IgM syndrome (CD40 ligand deficiency syndrome)
II Other well-defined syndromes		Wiskott–Aldrich syndrome Cartilage hair hypoplasia Ataxia telangiectasia
III Thymic defects		DiGeorge syndrome (22q11 microdeletion syndrome) CHARGE syndrome
IV Antibody deficiency syndromes		X-linked agammaglobulinaemia Common variable immunodeficiency
IV Hyper-IgE syndromes		Job syndrome
VI Defects of immune regulation	With hypopigmentation	Chediak–Higashi syndrome
	FHL syndromes (HLH)	
	Lymphoproliferative syndromes	X-linked lymphoproliferative syndrome
VII Phagocytic defects		Chronic granulomatous disease Leukocyte adhesion defects
VIII Innate immune defects		Interferon gamma/IL12 pathway defects

FHL: familial haemophagocytic lymphohistiocytosis; HLH: haemophagocytic lymphohistiocytosis; IL: interleukin.

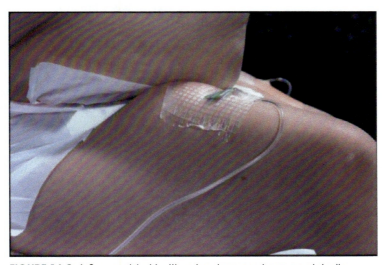

FIGURE 16.2 A 3-year-old girl with subcutaneous immunoglobulin infusion (markedly swollen thigh during infusion: normal finding).

- Antibiotics: for mild antibody deficiencies antibiotic prophylaxis (or early recourse to antibiotics) can be highly effective. Azithromycin is a frequent first choice. Early treatment of breakthrough infection, guided by microbiology where possible.
- Monitoring for evidence of organ damage includes chest CT scanning and regular lung function tests.
- Autoimmune complications may require immunosuppression or monoclonal antibody treatment – e.g. rituximab (anti-CD20) for autoimmune haematological complications.

Phagocytic disorders and innate immune defects

- Antibiotics/antifungals: antibiotic prophylaxis is chosen according to likely infections; e.g. for chronic granulomatous disease (CGD) cotrimoxazole is first choice as effective prophylaxis against intracellular bacterial infection. Aggressive treatment of infection may be needed: e.g. mycobacterial infection in defects of the interferon gamma/IL12 pathway, or aspergillus infection in CGD.
- Stem cell transplantation is indicated in some of these disorders depending on availability of donors and severity of phenotype.

All children affected by primary immunodeficiency should be monitored regularly in a specialist paediatric immunology centre.

SEVERE COMBINED IMMUNODEFICIENCY

Severe combined immunodeficiency (SCID) encompasses a group of inherited rare disorders characterised by the absence of functional T- and B-lymphocytes. SCID is clinically, immunologically and genetically heterogeneous. If untreated, these disorders are usually fatal within the first 12–24 months of life. In all subtypes of SCID lymphocyte development and function are severely impaired, as a result of absence or defective function of essential membrane, cytoplasmic or nuclear proteins, or in some cases presence of toxic metabolites that affect lymphocyte development. Many genetic defects underlying SCID have been identified (**Table 16.3**).

INCIDENCE

Rare, approximately 1 in 75,000 live births.

PRESENTATION

Infants usually present within the first year of life with failure to thrive, diarrhoea, recurrent/severe respiratory viral infections and opportunistic infections. There may be a family history of unexplained early infant death, or parental consanguinity. In some infants an exanthematous skin rash due to maternal graft-versus-host disease (**Figs 16.3, 16.4**) may be present. There is a risk of transfusional graft-versus-host disease (usually fatal) with transfusion of non-irradiated blood products.

DIAGNOSIS

Infants are usually **lymphopenic** (although a normal absolute lymphocyte count does not exclude a diagnosis of SCID). Chest x-ray may show absence of the thymus gland. Lymphocyte phenotyping and T-cell proliferation responses demonstrate abnormalities of T-, B- and natural killer (NK)-cell numbers and poor T-cell function. The immunophenotype can predict the likely underlying molecular defect. (see **Table 16.3**). Serum immunoglobulin levels may be helpful although they are variable in young infants and confounded by the presence of maternal IgG in infants less than 6 months of age. Further molecular and genetic investigations allow specific diagnosis in approximately 80% of cases.

TREATMENT

First-line treatment includes protective isolation, immunoglobulin replacement and antimicrobial prophylaxis to prevent infection. Any existing infections require aggressive treatment. All blood products must be CMV-negative and irradiated. Definitive treatment with allogeneic stem cell transplantation (SCT), or, in selected cases, gene therapy, should be performed as soon as possible.

TABLE 16.3 Severe combined immunodeficiency – molecular defects

	Inheritance	Defect	Other features
T- B+ NK-			
Common γ chain deficiency	X-linked	Defect in γ chain of receptors for IL-2,-4,-7,-9,-15,-21	
Jak-3 deficiency	AR	Abnormal Janus-associated kinase-3	
T- B+ NK+			
IL-7R α deficiency	AR	Defect of IL-7 receptor α chain	
CD3 deficiencies	AR	Defects of CD3δ/ CD3ε/CD3ζ	Absent γ/δ T-cells
Coronin 1A deficiency	AR	Defect of thymic egress	Thymus present
T- B- NK+			
RAG1 and RAG2 defects	AR	Defective VDJ recombination	Leaky variants may present with Omenn syndrome
Artemis deficiency	AR	Defective VDJ recombination	Leaky variants may present with Omenn syndrome
T- B- NK-			
ADA and PNP def	AR	Defect of purine metabolism	

ADA: adenosine deaminase; B: B-lymphocyte; IL: interleukin; NK: natural killer-cell; PNP: purine nucleoside phosphorylase; RAG: recombination activating gene; T: T-lymphocyte.

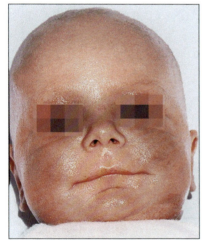

FIGURE 16.3 Severe combined immunodeficiency (SCID): face of a boy aged 4 months with X-linked SCID (common gamma chain deficiency).

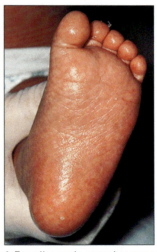

FIGURE 16.4 Exanthematous rash caused by graft-versus-host disease mediated by maternally-acquired T-cells in X-linked SCID.

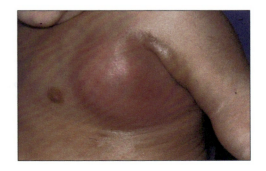

FIGURE 16.5 BCG abscess in a child with severe combined immunodeficiency (SCID).

PROGNOSIS

Without treatment SCID is fatal in infancy or early childhood. After SCT or gene therapy 70–95% disease-free survival can be achieved, depending on donor tissue type matching and clinical condition at the time of treatment (**Fig. 16.6**).

Notes

- BCG immunisation is contraindicated in infants at risk of SCID (i.e. in families with previous affected infants) until immunity has been confirmed as normal (see **Fig. 16.5**).
- Infants with SCID and other severe immune deficiencies requiring SCT or gene therapy should be referred urgently to a specialist centre (see **Fig. 16.6**).

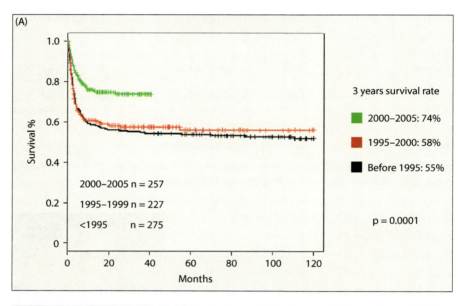

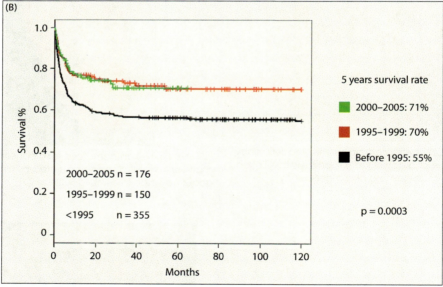

FIGURE 16.6 (A) European analysis after haematopoetic stem cell transplantation (HSCT) in severe combined immunodeficiency (SCID patients); (B) survival analysis in non-SCID primary immunodeficiency after HSCT.

SPECIFIC SCID SUB-TYPES

OMENN SYNDROME (SCID VARIANT)

Omenn syndrome is a variant of SCID associated with the presence of oligoclonal autoreactive T-cells, associated with a generalised erythrodermic dermatitis (**Figs 16.7, 16.8**) and other inflammatory changes. Expanded oligoclonal populations of activated and antigen-stimulated T-cells generate inflammatory changes, eosinophilia and elevated IgE levels. Mutations that causes a partial loss of function (hypomorphic mutations) in the recombinase-activating genes (*RAG-1* and *RAG-2*) are the most frequent underlying genetic defects in infants with Omenn syndrome. However, mutations in a number of other SCID-causing genes have also been associated with Omenn syndrome, including adenosine deaminase, common gamma chain, IL-7 receptor alpha, Artemis and DNA ligase 4 genes.

INCIDENCE

Very rare; unknown.

PRESENTATION

Affected infants present as for other SCIDs, but, in addition, have prominent generalised erythrodermic dermatitis; lymphadenopathy and hepatosplenomegaly may also be present.

DIAGNOSIS

A suggestive phenotype (see above) with elevated total lymphocyte numbers, eosinophilia and raised IgE are clinical indicators. Lymphocyte immunophenotyping will show activated T-cells, abnormal T-cell proliferative responses and an abnormal V-beta repertoire with oligoclonal expansions. IgG, IgA and IgM levels are usually decreased. Initial genetic analysis should focus on mutations in *RAG* genes.

TREATMENT

Inflammatory skin disease may require immunosuppression with steroids and/or ciclosporin. Prophylactic measures are required as described above, and SCT should be performed as soon as possible as for other forms of SCID, although the mortality rate is higher in Omenn syndrome.

PROGNOSIS

Outlook is very poor without corrective treatment.

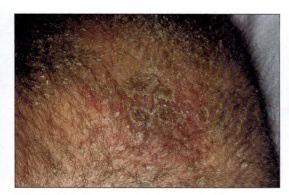

FIGURE 16.7 Omenn syndrome: scalp of a 2-month-old girl, showing erythrosquamous exanthema and hair loss.

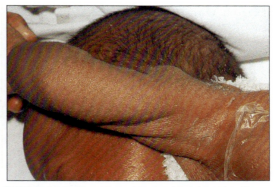

FIGURE 16.8 Omenn syndrome: head and axilla of the same girl as in **16.7**, showing erythrodermic rash and lymphadenopathy.

ADENOSINE DEAMINASE (ADA) DEFICIENCY

INCIDENCE/AETIOLOGY

Adenosine deaminase (ADA) is involved in the purine metabolism pathway; absence of ADA results in accumulation of toxic metabolites, which interfere with lymphocyte survival. ADA is variably expressed in all body tissues and ADA deficiency frequently causes extralymphoid manifestations. These often include neurological, neurodevelopmental (especially deafness) and skeletal abnormalities. ADA deficiency is responsible for approximately 15% of cases of SCID. Most infants present as typical SCID (T-, B-, NK-). Milder variants may present in later childhood. The accurate incidence is unknown, but is approximately 1 in 50,000 live births.

CLINICAL PRESENTATION

Clinical presentation is as for SCID. Chest x-ray may show splayed anterior rib ends. Developmental and behavioural abnormalities are common. Milder variants presenting later in childhood or even early adulthood have been recognised.

DIAGNOSIS

Immunological diagnosis as for SCID (**Fig. 16.9**). Reduced ADA levels in red and/or white blood cells, in combination with raised levels of metabolites in plasma and urine, confirm the metabolic defect and diagnosis. Carriers have intermediate levels of ADA.

TREATMENT

Treatment is as for SCID. Bovine polyethylene gly-cosylated (PEG)-ADA (intramuscular) improves immune function in a subgroup of patients. SCT (or gene therapy in a selected subgroup) restores immune function but does not correct non-immunological manifestations.

PROGNOSIS

Cure of immune deficiency can be achieved by SCT or gene therapy, but many patients have significant long-term developmental and behavioural problems.

II OTHER WELL-DEFINED SYNDROMES

WISKOTT–ALDRICH SYNDROME

Wiskott–Aldrich syndrome typically consists of the triad of thrombocytopenia, atypical eczema and immunological abnormalities. It is inherited as an X-linked recessive disorder, and is caused by mutations in the '*WASP*' (Wiskott–Aldrich syndrome protein) gene, located at Xp11.

INCIDENCE

Wiskott–Aldrich syndrome is rare, probably approximately 1 in 50,000–100,000 live births.

PRESENTATION

Affected male infants usually present with bruising and bleeding and severe eczema, in combination with recurrent upper and lower respiratory tract infections including otitis media (**Fig. 16.10**). A clinical variant, termed 'X-linked thrombocytopenia' (XLT) represents a milder form, also caused by mutations in the *WASP* gene. There is a positive family history with a typical 'X-linked pedigree' in only approximately 30% of cases.

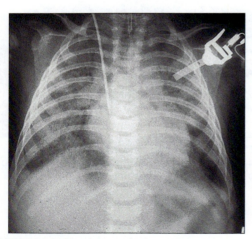

FIGURE 16.9 Chest x-ray of a boy with severe combined immunodeficiency due to adenosine deaminase deficiency who presented with tachypnoea, hypoxia, and interstitial pneumonitis caused by *Pneumocystis jirovecii* (previously known as *Pneumocystis carinii*). Note the interstitial infiltration predominantly in the left upper lobe and absence of retrosternally located thymus shadow.

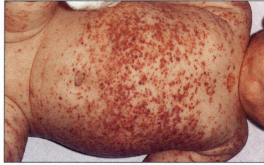

FIGURE 16.10 Wiskott–Aldrich syndrome: extensive eczema and purpuric skin rash.

DIAGNOSIS

Laboratory investigations reveal thrombocytopenia, with small volume platelets. Immunoglobulin levels often reveal low IgM, normal IgG and raised IgA. Lymphocyte subpopulations and T-cell function are usually normal in the first few years of life, but there is usually progressive reduction in T-cell numbers. Most affected boys have absent WASp expression in peripheral blood mononuclear cells. All have mutations in the *WASP* gene.

COMPLICATIONS

There is a high risk of autoimmune disease, including autoimmune haematological complications including vasculitis and lymphoma.

TREATMENT

Supportive treatment with immunoglobulin replacement and antibiotic prophylaxis is required, as well as appropriate treatment of eczema. Autoimmune complications may require immuno-suppression and/or monoclonal antibodies. For most affected boys SCT is indicated if there is a matched donor available. Gene therapy trials are in progress.

PROGNOSIS

The prognosis is variable and the phenotype can vary even within families. Some boys survive to adulthood with few complications. Overall outlook is poor in the absence of SCT because of the above risks. Successful transplant cures the underlying syndrome, but the effect on the risk of later malignancy is unknown.

CARTILAGE HAIR HYPOPLASIA

Cartilage hair hypoplasia (CHH) is an autosomal recessive disorder that usually results in short-limb skeletal dysplasia, sometimes associated with T-cell and B-cell deficiencies. It is caused by mutations of the *RMRP* gene (RNA component of mitochondrial RNA processing endoribonuclease) on chromosome 9p12.

INCIDENCE

The frequency of CHH varies in different populations. There is a high incidence in the Amish population, and in Finns. The overall frequency is around 1 in 25000 live births. The frequency of an associated immunodeficiency varies (~50% in small series) and CHH as a cause of SCID is rare.

PRESENTATION

The dominant clinical feature of CHH is short-limbed skeletal dysplasia, which is evident at birth and can also be detected *in utero* through shortening and bowing of the femur. Additional features include fine, sparse hair, nail dysplasia, skin hypopigmentation, microdontia and gastrointestinal malformation and/or diseases. Individuals with severe immunodeficiency present in early infancy and have increased susceptibility to (opportunistic) infections as in other infants with SCID. Recently infants with a SCID phenotype cause by *RMRP* mutations, but who have little evidence of skeletal dysplasia have been recognised.

DIAGNOSIS

The extent of T-cell or B-cell immunodeficiency varies. Individuals with reduced T-cell immunity show lymphopenia, decreased percentages and numbers of CD3+ and CD4+ T-cells, and usually normal percentages and numbers of B-cells and NK-cells. T-cell function is decreased. The diagnosis is confirmed by demonstration of a disease-causing mutation in *RMRP*.

COMPLICATIONS

There is a risk of gastrointestinal obstruction. Individuals with impaired cellular immunity are more susceptible to malignancies, especially leukaemia and lymphoma.

TREATMENT

Affected children without associated immunodeficiency do not require prophylactic intervention. Those with immunodeficiency need immunoglobulin replacement and prophylactic antibiotics. Live vaccines must be avoided until the extent of the immunodeficiency has been evaluated. SCT is required for those with severe immunodeficiency. This will restore immunity but does not affect the altered bone growth.

PROGNOSIS

The outlook depends on the extent of the underlying immunodeficiency and the occurrence of autoimmune phenomena and lymphomas.

ATAXIA TELANGIECTASIA

See also Chapter 8 Neurology, page 214.

Ataxia telangiectasia (AT) is characterised clinically by cerebellar ataxia, oculocutaneous telangiectases, immunodeficiency, sensitivity to radiomimetic agents and cancer predisposition. AT is inherited as an autosomal recessive disorder, caused by mutations in the *ATM* (ataxia telangiectasia mutated) gene, (chromosome 11q22-23). The ATM protein is a member of a novel family of large proteins implicated in the regulation of the cell cycle and response to DNA damage.

INCIDENCE

Incidence of AT is unknown (very rare).

PRESENTATION

There is great variability in the onset of symptoms. Slurred speech, strabismus, cerebellar and extrapyramidal signs, and muscle weakness usually develop during progression of the disease (**Fig. 16.11**). Neurodevelopmental delay is present in some patients. There may be bronchiectasis if infections are a prominent feature. Ocular telangiectases appear later in childhood. The frequency of recurrent infections depends on the extent of any associated immunodeficiency, which is very variable, as well as other neuromuscular factors (**Fig. 16.12**).

DIAGNOSIS

Serum alpha-fetoprotein levels are increased. There is abnormal DNA irradiation sensitivity. Lymphopenia and IgA deficiency are present in 60–70% of patients. T- and B-cell numbers may be low, and T-cell proliferative responses to mitogens may be impaired. The diagnosis is confirmed by demonstration of a mutation in the *ATM* gene.

TREATMENT

Depending on the degree of immunological abnormality, supportive treatment with prophylactic antibiotics and in some cases immunoglobulin replacement may be required. There is no cure for the disease. SCT would only correct the immune defect, and is not indicated because of the progressive nature of the neurological disorder.

PROGNOSIS

There is great variability in outlook, but most patients are wheelchair-bound by the second decade of life. Survival into the early adult life has been reported.

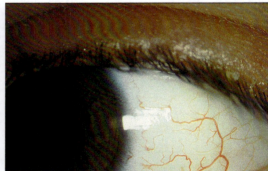

FIGURE 16.12 Ataxia telangiectasia: appearance of the eye.

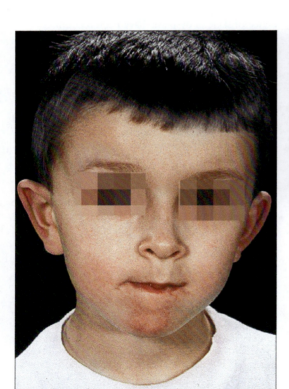

FIGURE 16.11 Ataxia telangiectasia: typical facial appearance.

Immunology (primary immunodeficiency syndromes)

III THYMIC DEFECTS

DIGEORGE SYNDROME

DiGeorge syndrome refers to the complex of hypoparathyroidism, congenital heart disease, cleft lip/palate and absent thymus, and represents the severe end of the spectrum of disorders caused by chromosome 22q11 microdeletion syndrome. The 'complete' form with absent T-cells is very rare, while there is a wide spectrum of less severe immunodeficiencies in other affected children. It is caused by a hemizygous microdeletion of chromosome 22q11, inherited as an autosomal dominant trait, but many cases arise as new mutations. A similar thymic defect is associated with various other complex syndromes, the most common being CHARGE syndrome, caused by mutations in CHD7 (chromodomain helicase DNA binding protein 7).

INCIDENCE

The incidence of 22q11 microdeletion is of the order of 1 in 4000.

PRESENTATION

There is a wide variation in clinical presentation and severity. The classical combination includes hypocalcaemia, congenital heart disease (conotruncal abnormalities), characteristic facies, cleft lip/palate, and absent thymus. Later manifestations include speech problems, neurodevelopmental delay and growth retardation. Susceptibility to infection may be increased, depending of the degree of immune deficiency.

- Facial appearance (**Figs 16.13, 16.14**): low set, posteriorly rotated ears, hypertelorism, short philtrum and a small mandible.
- Congenital heart disease: most frequently interrupted aortic arch (type B), also truncus arteriosus and tetralogy of Fallot.

- Hypocalcaemia: tetany or convulsions; onset usually within 24–48 hours of birth and persists after 14 days; usually associated with low levels of parathyoid hormone (PTH).
- Thymus: absent thymus may be evident on chest x-ray or may be noted at cardiac surgery. Absent or very low total and naïve T-cells in complete DiGeorge syndrome.

DIAGNOSIS

DiGeorge is confirmed by demonstration of a chromosome 22q11 microdeletion – usually by microarray analysis. Immunological finding are very variable: Patients with the 'complete' form show absent total and naïve T-cells, and absent T-cell receptor excision circles, with normal B- and NK-cells, normal total immunoglobulin levels but poor specific antibody production. Incomplete forms may have low T-cells and varying degrees of antibody deficiency. T-cells may increase spontaneously during the first few years of life.

TREATMENT

Infants affected by 22q11 microdeletion syndrome often require complex cardiac surgery, and may require calcium supplements and vitamin D. For complete DiGeorge syndrome survival is very unlikely without corrective therapy for the thymic defect. SCT may be successful if there is an HLA-identical sibling. Thymic transplantation is becoming increasingly successful. Patients with less severe T-cell defects may benefit from antibiotic prophylaxis, and, rarely, immunoglobulin replacement. Most patients can receive all routine immunisations safely although T-cell function should be evaluated carefully if BCG is required.

PROGNOSIS

The long-term outlook is very variable depending on individual clinical characteristics.

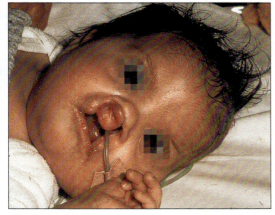

FIGURE 16.13 DiGeorge syndrome: characteristic facies.

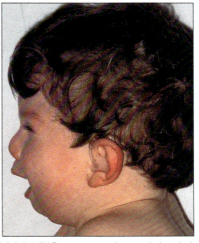

FIGURE 16.14 DiGeorge syndrome: lateral view of face showing small jaws and low ears.

IV ANTIBODY DEFICIENCY SYNDROMES

COMMON VARIABLE IMMUNODEFICIENCY

Common variable immunodeficiency (CVID) is the most frequent PID encountered in later childhood and adult life. It is a heterogeneous disorder of unknown aetiology in most cases. Several genes have been identified recently in consanguineous families, which underly a very small minority of cases, but most cases are likely to have polygenic basis with multiple environmental triggers. There is usually no clear pattern of inheritance, but there is an increased familial incidence, and in some families a suggestion of autosomal dominant inheritance with variable penetrance. Coinheritance with certain HLA haplotypes (HLA-A1, HLA-B8, HLA-DR3 and HLA-DQB1*0201) has been found in some families. Other family members may have selective IgA deficiency, and minor immunoglobulin abnormalities in infancy or early childhood may evolve to become CVID.

INCIDENCE

Incidence of CVID is probably approximately 1 in 20,000 live births.

PRESENTATION

The most frequent age of diagnosis is early adulthood, but CVID can present at any age. Most patients have a history of recurrent sinopulmonary bacterial and viral infections, or unusually severe episodes of common infections (**Figs 16.15, 16.16**). Non-specific symptoms such as fatigue, general malaise and poor growth are often associated. Chronic diarrhoea is common, and caused by various underlying gastrointestinal pathologies; autoimmune manifestations such as autoimmune haemolytic anaemia or thrombocytopenia also occur frequently, and may be the presenting problem.

DIAGNOSIS

International criteria for diagnosis of CVID include:

- Patient over the age of 2 years (to distinguish from transient hypogammaglobulinemia of infancy).
- Hypogammaglobulinaemia – low levels of at least two of three major immunoglobulin isotypes.
- Poor specific antibody responses to vaccine antigens.
- Exclusion of other defined genetic defects, e.g. X-linked agammaglobulinaemia (BTK deficiency) or hyper-IgM syndrome (CD40 ligand deficiency).
- Lymphocyte subpopulations are frequently normal, but there may be low T-cells and/or low B-cells. There may also be abnormalities of memory B-cell populations.
- Causes of secondary hypogammaglobulinaemia must be excluded (e.g. drugs and protein-losing states).

COMPLICATIONS

Repeated or chronic infections may lead to permanent organ damage, particularly bronchiectasis. Autoimmune and inflammatory complications include haematological autoimmunity (which may be the presenting feature), inflammatory bowel disease, lymphoid hyperplasia, splenomegaly, and lymphoproliferative or granulomatous disease affecting any organ. There is an increased incidence of malignancy, especially lymphoma.

TREATMENT

Lifelong immunoglobulin replacement is required. Antibiotic prophylaxis may be required, particularly if there is established lung damage, as well as early recourse to antibiotics for breakthrough infections. Inflammatory and autoimmune complications may require immunosuppression and/or monoclonal antibody treatment (e.g. rituximab (anti-CD20), infliximab [anti-TNF-alpha]).

PROGNOSIS

The outlook is good in most patients provided that the diagnosis is made early, before organ damage occurs, and that treatment is optimised. However, this is influenced by the occurrence of inflammatory and/or autoimmune complications. Occasional patients with a very severe phenotype may justify SCT.

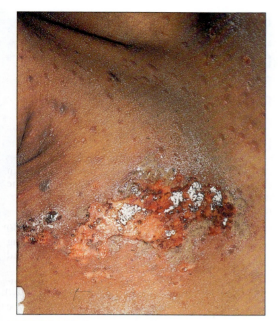

FIGURE 16.15 Herpes zoster becoming generalised in a child with common variable immunodeficiency.

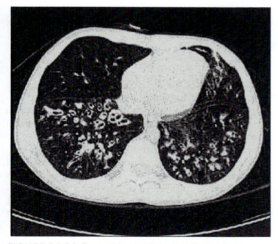

FIGURE 16.16 Bronchiectasis in inadequately treated common variable immunodeficiency.

X-LINKED AGAMMA-GLOBULINAEMIA (BRUTON DISEASE)

X-linked agammaglobulinaemia (XLA) was described in 1952 by Bruton. It is caused by mutations in the *BTK* (Bruton tyrosine kinase) gene, located at Xq22. *BTK* is essential for B-cell development and is involved in signalling.

INCIDENCE

The accurate incidence unknown – probably approximately 1 in 50,000–100,000 live births.

CLINICAL PRESENTATION

Affected boys usually present with recurrent bacterial infections, which are often severe (e.g. pneumonia, osteomyelitis, bacterial meningitis), with onset between 6 months (after maternal IgG has declined) and 2 years. Occasionally the history may be of less severe infections and/or later presentation (**Fig. 16.17**).

DIAGNOSIS

There may be a positive family history with a typical X-linked pedigree, but only in approximately 30% of cases. The remaining 70% arise as new mutations. Typical laboratory findings include:

- Absent or very low circulating mature B-cells.
- Absent or very low immunoglobulins of all isotypes.
- Absent specific antibody response to vaccines.
- Absence of BTK protein by Western blotting or FACS analysis.
- Disease-causing mutation in *BTK* gene.

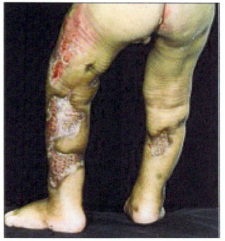

FIGURE 16.17 Severe pseudomonas fasciitis in XLA requiring skin grafting.

Attenuated variants of XLA are now recognised, with some detectable immunoglobulin and some circulating mature B-cells. The severity of the clinical phenotype may vary within families.

COMPLICATIONS

The most frequent complication, particularly if diagnosis is delayed or treatment is inadequate, is bronchiectasis. Historically there has been an increased incidence of enteroviral meningoencephalitis, but this occurs less frequently since improvements in diagnosis and management have become established. Neutropenia may be present at diagnosis, and usually responds to immunoglobulin therapy.

TREATMENT

Lifelong regular immunoglobulin replacement is required, either intravenously or subcutaneously. IgG levels should be maintained >8 g/l). Intercurrent infections require prompt antibiotics, ideally guided by microbiology; antibiotic prophylaxis may be required, especially if there is established chronic lung disease. Clinical and CT scan surveillance for 'silent' lung damage is important.

PROGNOSIS

The outlook should be excellent with early diagnosis, optimal immunoglobulin replacement, prompt treatment of infection and monitoring for complications.

HYPOGAMMAGLOBULINAEMIA WITH HYPERIGM (CLASS-SWITCH RECOMBINATION [CSR] DEFECTS) (INCLUDING CD40 LIGAND DEFICIENCY)

A group of disorders affecting immunoglobulin class-switch recombination. All are rare, but the most frequent is the X-linked form; several autosomal recessive genes cause a similar syndrome.

- **X-linked**: caused by mutations in the CD40 ligand (CD154) gene, located at Xq26, causing defective expression of CD40 ligand on activated T-cells and endothelial cells.
- **Autosomal recessive**: mutations in (i) activation-induced cytidine deaminase (*AID*) gene; (ii) *CD40* gene; (iii) *UNG* gene. All result in defective isotype switching.

A similar syndrome may be triggered by congenital rubella infection, drugs (e.g. phenytoin), pulmonary disease, tumours and haemolytic anaemia.

INCIDENCE

CSR defects are rare, probably approximately 1 in 50,000–100,000 live births.

PRESENTATION

Manifestations of the X-linked form reflect functional defects of both humoral and cell-mediated immunity, with recurrent bacterial infections, *Pneumocystis jirovecii* (previously known as *Pneumocystis carinii*) pneumonia, and susceptibility to liver disease (especially sclerosing cholangitis) (**Fig. 16.18**). Neutropenia is also common and may cause oral ulceration and gingival hypertrophy. Presentation is usually after 6 months of age, when maternal IgG has declined. Autosomal recessive forms present with recurrent infections, but do not carry risks of opportunistic infection or liver disease.

DIAGNOSIS

All forms are characterised by very low levels of IgG and IgA, with normal or high IgM. Lymphocyte subpopulations and T-cell proliferative responses to mitogens are usually normal.

The X-linked form:

- Absence of CD40 ligand expression on activated T-cells.
- May have abnormal antigen-induced T-cell proliferation.
- Positive family history in approximately 30% of cases.
- Disease-causing mutation in the CD154 gene.

TREATMENT

All types require immunoglobulin replacement. Boys affected by X-linked hyper-IgM syndrome require prophylaxis against *Pneumocystis jirovecii* with cotrimoxazole, and anticryptosporidial precautions (boil drinking water). SCT is recommended if a suitable donor is available.

COMPLICATIONS

There is a risk of end-organ damage as a result of repeated infections, especially bronchiectasis, in all forms. In the X-linked variety autoimmune manifestations include haemolytic anaemia, thrombocytopenia and neutropenia, and there is a high risk of liver disease, particularly sclerosing cholangitis and liver tumours.

PROGNOSIS

- Autosomal recessive varieties: good with early diagnosis and adequate immunoglobulin replacement and monitoring.
- X-linked: high risk of liver disease/autoimmune complications. The outlook is good with successful SCT.

V HYPER-IGE SYNDROMES

Hyper-IgE syndromes (HIES) are a heterogeneous group of disorders, all characterised by extremely high levels of IgE and severe infections.

AUTOSOMAL DOMINANT HYPER-IGE SYNDROME

This disorder (previously known as Job syndrome) is caused by mutations in Stat-3 (signal transducer and activator of transcription 3), which mediates cellular responses to interleukins and other growth factors.

INCIDENCE

AD-HIES is rare; accurate incidence unknown.

PRESENTATION

Affected patients suffer recurrent staphylococcal infections, particularly of skin and lungs, on a background of severe atypical eczema and other atopic symptoms. Facial features may be coarse (**Fig. 16.19**). Other systemic features include delayed loss of primary dentition, skeletal abnormalities (particularly scoliosis) and increased risk of fractures. Severe staphylococcal lung infections lead to pneumatocoele formation. There is a risk of vascular complications in older individuals.

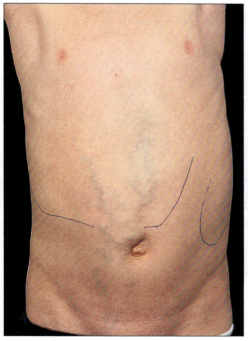

FIGURE 16.18 Caput medusae and hepatosplenomegaly (outlined) in a boy with CD40 ligand deficiency complicated by sclerosing cholangitis.

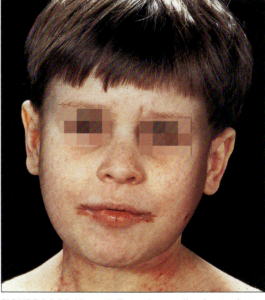

FIGURE 16.19 Hyper-IgE syndrome: the face of an affected child showing coarse, pitted skin.

DIAGNOSIS

All patients have extremely high IgE levels, varying with age at presentation. Under 1 year IgE may be >1000 IU/ml, but in older patients may be 10,000–20,000 IU/ml or higher. Patients with severe atopic disease alone may also have very high IgE levels but usually do not exhibit other clinical features of HIES. Other immunology investigations are usually normal, although defects in neutrophil function have been described. The diagnosis is confirmed by demonstration of a mutation in *Stat-3*.

TREATMENT

The mainstay of therapy is antibiotic prophylaxis with an antistaphylococcal agent. Immunoglobulin treatment is rarely indicated. SCT has been successful in a small number of cases. Immunosuppressive therapy has been used to control inflammatory complications.

PROGNOSIS

Prognosis is variable depending on the severity of phenotype.

AUTOSOMAL RECESSIVE HYPER-IGE SYNDROME

This is caused by mutations in DOCK-8 (dedicator of cytokinesis-8) or, very rarely, Tyk-2 (tyrosine kinase-2).

DOCK-8 DEFICIENCY

Presentation

Patients usually have severe eczema and recurrent superficial staphylococcal skin infections, and recurrent respiratory infections. Severe skin viral infections, particularly molluscum contagiosum, viral warts and herpes simplex infections, occur frequently. There is also an increased risk of malignancy. DOCK-8 deficiency is distinguished from autosomal dominant hyper-IgE syndrome by lack of pneumatocoele formation, absence of systemic features, and the excess of skin viral infections (**Figs 16.20, 16.21**).

Diagnosis

Patients usually have high IgE levels as in autosomal dominant HIES. There are usually progressive abnormalities of immunology, including low T-cells and poor T-cell proliferative responses to mitogens. Immunoglobulin levels may be low. The diagnosis is confirmed by demonstration of a mutation in DOCK-8.

Treatment

Antibiotic prophylaxis and immunoglobulin replacement help to control infections and minimise risk of organ damage; SCT is indicated.

Prognosis

The long-term outlook is poor without corrective treatment.

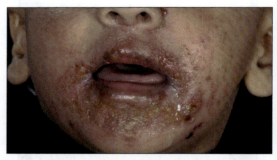

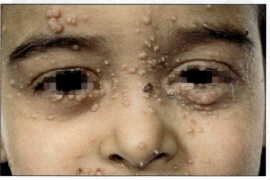

FIGURES 16.20, 16.21 DOCK-8 deficiency. Extensive perioral herpes simplex (**16.20**) and facial viral warts (**16.21**) in a 5-year-old boy.

VI DEFECTS OF IMMUNE REGULATION

X-LINKED LYMPHOPROLIFERATIVE DISEASE (DUNCAN SYNDROME)

X-linked lymphoproliferative disease (XLP) type 1, also known as Duncan syndrome or Purtilo syndrome, is characterised by inability to mount an appropriate immune response to EBV infection (infectious mononucleosis) and sometimes other viruses. XLP-1 is caused by mutations in a gene known as *SH2D1A*, which encodes SLAM-associated protein (SAP). A similar syndrome, XLP type 2, is caused by mutations in XIAP (X-linked inhibitor of apoptosis protein), and is associated with a high incidence of inflammatory bowel disease.

INCIDENCE

XLP is very rare; exact incidence is unknown.

PRESENTATION

There are several presenting syndromes, including:

- Fulminant (sometimes fatal) infectious mononucleosis, with secondary haemophagocytic lymphohistiocytosis (HLH) (**Fig. 16.22**).
- Progressive hypogammaglobulinaemia.
- Aplastic anaemia.
- B-cell lymphoma/lymphoproliferative disease (**Figs 16.23, 16.24**).
- Inflammatory bowel disease (in XIAP).

DIAGNOSIS

The diagnosis is usually suggested by a typical clinical presentation. A positive family history is only found in approximately 30% of cases. Immunological abnormalities, such as a markedly reversed CD4/CD8 ratio and panhypogammaglobulinaemia may be present. Absence of SAP expression, and demonstration of a mutation in the *SH2D1A* gene confirms XLP-1, and mutations in XIAP confirm XLP-2.

TREATMENT

Patients presenting with fulminant EBV disease require aggressive anti-EBV therapy with anti-CD20 monoclonals and antivirals, as well as specific anti-HLH chemotherapy, followed by SCT as soon as possible after remission is achieved. Boys presenting with hypogammaglobulinaemia require immunoglobulin replacement, and those presenting with HLH or lymphoproliferative disease/lymphoma without EBV require immunosuppression and chemotherapy followed by SCT. Gene therapy is currently in development.

Apparently healthy male siblings should be screened for the genetic defect.

PROGNOSIS

XLP has a high mortality rate without SCT.

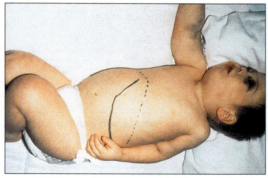

FIGURE 16.22 Patient with Duncan syndrome, bruises and oedema in intensive care unit.

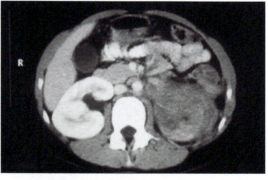

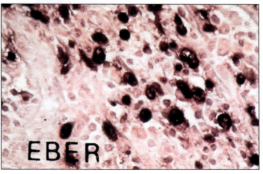

FIGURES 16.23, 16.24 Example of EBV lymphoproliferative disease. An 11-year-old female developed progressive combined immunodeficiency and presented with renal mass on CT (**16.23**) while histology (**16.24**) showed xanthogranulomatous pyelonephritis. Retrospective confirmation of EBV in liver and kidney was obtained.

CHEDIAK–HIGASHI SYNDROME

Chediak–Higashi syndrome (CHS) is an autosomal recessive disorder that causes oculocutaneous albinism, associated with varying degrees of immune deficiency and a risk of progression to an 'accelerated' haemophagocytic lymphohistiocytosis phase. It is caused by mutations in the '*LYST*' (lysosomal trafficking regulator) gene, which is involved in lysosomal function. Giant granules fail to discharge during phagocytosis (**Fig. 16.25**).

INCIDENCE

The incidence of CHS is unknown (very rare).

PRESENTATION

Affected children demonstrate partial oculocutaneous albinism, usually associated with recurrent infections. Occasionally the first clinical presentation is in 'accelerated phase' with haemophagocytic lymphohistiocytosis.

DIAGNOSIS

The diagnosis is usually suggested by typical clinical findings (**Figs 16.26–16.28**). There may be neutropenia and large cytoplasmic inclusions in neutrophils are seen on peripheral blood film. Demonstration of a mutation in the *LYST* gene confirms the diagnosis.

TREATMENT

Recurrent bacterial infections require prophylaxis and early treatment with antibiotics. Treatment of the accelerated phase includes steroids, cytotoxic and immunosuppressive agents, followed by early SCT. SCT may be considered before progression to the accelerated phase in selected children depending on phenotype and family history.

PROGNOSIS

The prognosis is poor without successful transplantation if the patient presents in the accelerated phase. However, some patients remain free of complications well into adult life. In long-term survivors post-transplantation there is an increased incidence of neurological and behavioural problems.

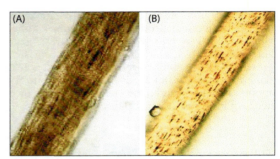

FIGURE 16.26 Chediak–Higashi syndrome. (A) Appearance of normal hair under the microscope; (B) patient with Chediak–Higashi syndrome.

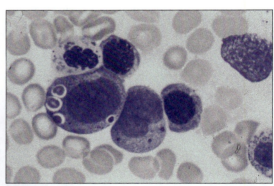

FIGURE 16.27 Bone marrow with giant inclusions in Chediak–Higashi syndrome.

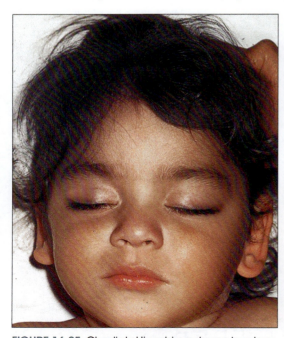

FIGURE 16.25 Chediak–Higashi syndrome in a boy, showing greyish appearance of the hair.

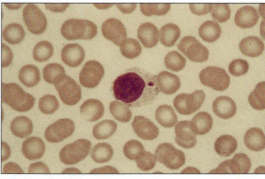

FIGURE 16.28 Normal marrow.

AUTOIMMUNE LYMPHOPROLIFERATIVE SYNDROME

Autoimmune lymphoproliferative syndrome (ALPS) is a dysregulatory disorder of the immune system, characterised by impaired regulation of lymphocyte homeostasis by apoptosis. It is most frequently caused by mutations in the *Fas* gene (autosomal dominant); other causes include defects in *Fas-ligand* and *caspase 10*, and in some cases no genetic cause can be defined.

INCIDENCE

ALPS is rare; incidence is unknown.

PRESENTATION

ALPS usually presents during childhood with persistent widespread non-malignant lymphadenopathy, frequently a history of autoimmune cytopenias, splenomegaly and sometimes hepatomegaly. There may be a family history of similarly affected individuals. There is an increased risk of lymphoma. Malignancy must be excluded by lymph node biopsy. There are overlaps with CVID.

DIAGNOSIS

The clinical history is usually suggestive, and there may be a positive family history. Laboratory abnormalities include elevated 'double negative' (CD4+/CD8+) T-cells, defective *in vitro* Fas-mediated apoptosis, and elevated 'biomarkers' (soluble Fas-ligand, plasma IL-10, plasma or serum Vitamin B_{12}, plasma IL-18). Definitive diagnosis is confirmed by demonstration of mutation in *Fas, Fas-L* or *caspase 10*.

TREATMENT/PROGNOSIS

Treatment depends on the clinical manifestations. Chronic lymphadenopathy may not require active intervention. Autoimmune manifestations may require immunosuppression or treatment with monoclonal antibodies (e.g. rituximab for autoimmune cytopenias). Monitoring for progression to lymphoma is necessary. Successful SCT has been reported in patients with severe refractory disease. Prognosis depends on the severity of disease.

CHRONIC MUCOCUTANEOUS CANDIDIASIS

CMC is a heterogeneous group of disorders, causing increased susceptibility to superficial *Candida* infection. In a subgroup of patients there is a high incidence of organ-specific autoimmunity in older children; this syndrome is known as autoimmune polyendocrinopathy ectodermal dysplasia (APECED). APECED is inherited as an autosomal recessive disorder, and is caused by mutations in the *AIRE* (autoimmune regulator) gene. AIRE is involved in generation of self-tolerance in the thymus by elimination of autoreactive T-cells. Patients affected clinically by CMC without autoimmunity form a heterogeneous group, and in most cases the underlying genetic defect is not known. In some families there is an autosomal dominant pattern of inheritance. Deficiencies of IL-17 and IL-17 receptor, STAT-1 gain of function and CARD 9 mutations have been described.

INCIDENCE

The incidence of CMC is unknown (rare).

PRESENTATION

Patients present during infancy with persistent, often treatment-resistant oral and perineal thrush. There may be secondary bacterial infection. Increased mucosal spread of *Candida* leads to extensive involvement of buccal mucosa, lips, and finger or toe nails. Systemic *Candida* infections are not a feature. Autoimmunity particularly affecting parathyroid, adrenal and thyroid glands occurs in older children. Pancreatic islet cell and gastric parietal cell antibodies are also common, although the presence of autoantibodies is not always associated with organ dysfunction. Vitiligo, alopecia and oral aphthous ulceration are also common (**Figs 16.29–16.31**).

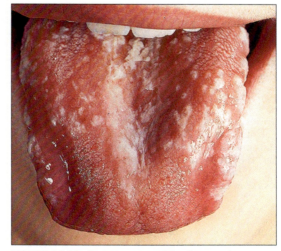

FIGURE 16.29 Appearance of the tongue in chronic mucocutaneous candidiasis.

503

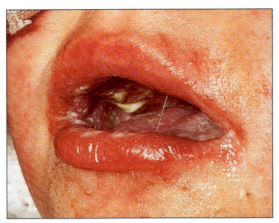

FIGURE 16.30 Mouth of a toddler with chronic mucocutaneous candidiasis.

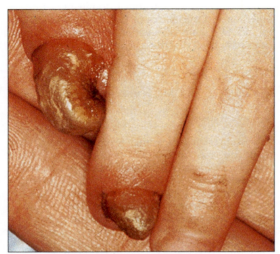

FIGURE 16.31 Nail infection in chronic mucocutaneous candidiasis.

DIAGNOSIS

In patients without autoimmunity the diagnosis is made clinically, with a suggestive clinical picture with excess *Candida* infections. There are no specific laboratory immunological abnormalities. For those affected by APECED the diagnosis is confirmed by demonstration of a mutation in the *AIRE* gene.

TREATMENT

In most cases treatment is symptomatic, with topical and/or systemic antifungals. In patients with autoimmunity hormone replacement therapy may be required for restoration of endocrine function. Immunosuppressive therapy is of no value. In extreme cases, SCT can be considered.

PROGNOSIS

The outlook is usually satisfactory (no robust data are available) with good long-term surveillance and early treatment of infections and underlying endocrinopathies.

VII PHAGOCYTIC DEFECTS

CHRONIC GRANULOMATOUS DISEASE

Chronic granulomatous disease (CGD) is a disorder of neutrophil function, characterised by recurrent bacterial infection of the skin, lungs and lymph nodes and other deep sites, with formation of widespread granulomata. CGD is caused by mutations in components of the phagocyte NADPH oxidase, which result in failure of phagocyte respiratory burst and defective killing of pathogens. Two-thirds of cases are X-linked and are due to mutations in the gene encoding the 91 kDa component of the membrane-bound NADPH oxidase (*gp91phox*). One-third of patients have autosomal recessively inherited mutations in the genes encoding cytosolic proteins, the most common being the *p47phox* and *p67phox*.

PRESENTATION

Most cases present in early childhood but CGD can present at any age. There is particular susceptibility to staphylococcal and other catalase positive bacteria, and fungi, especially *Aspergillus*. Frequent manifestations include suppurative lymphadenitis, recurrent staphylococcal skin infections, perianal abscesses, deep-seated abscesses and pneumonia. Inflammatory (granulomatous) lesions can cause gastric outlet and bladder neck obstruction. Occasionally the presenting syndrome is inflammatory bowel disease, which can be mistaken for Crohn disease (**Figs 16.32–16.35**).

DIAGNOSIS

The diagnosis can be established by the nitro-blue tetrazolium test. This test depends on the conversion of the yellow dye (NBT) to dark blue formazan by superoxides generated by normal phagocytes. In affected individuals, >90% of phagocytes fail to

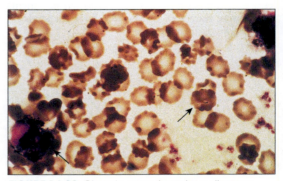

FIGURE 16.32 Chronic granulomatous disease: nitro-blue tetrazolium test of a carrier showing normal (blue-stained, left) and abnormal phagocytes.

reduce the dye. Carriers of the X-linked form of the disease demonstrate intermediate (10–90%) NBT dye reduction. The respiratory burst can also be evaluated using the dihydrorhodamine (DHR) test. The genetic subtype can be confirmed by Western blotting, followed by mutation analysis.

TREATMENT

Initial management includes aggressive treatment of infection, followed by antibiotic and antifungal prophylaxis. Cotrimoxazole is the usual antibiotic of choice because of its antibacterial spectrum and concentration in the phagocyte. Itraconazole prophylaxis is usually used for *Aspergillus* prophylaxis (**Fig. 16.36**). Interferon-gamma may have a role as an adjunct to the treatment of deep-seated infections. The long-term outlook is poor without corrective therapy and SCT is recommended if there is a suitable donor. Gene therapy trials for the X-linked form are currently in progress.

PROGNOSIS

Prognosis for CGD is usually poor in the long-term without corrective therapy, although there is considerable phenotypic variation.

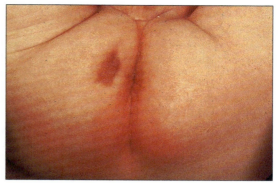

FIGURE 16.33 Chronic granulomatous disease: buttock abscess.

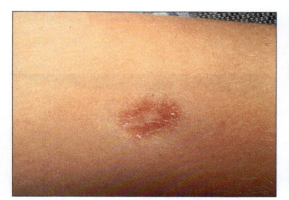

FIGURE 16.34 Chronic granulomatous disease: granulomatous healing of a forearm.

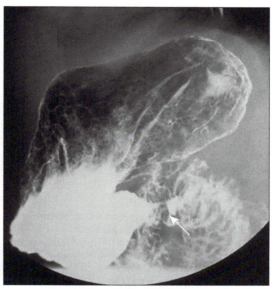

FIGURE 16.35 Chronic granulomatous disease: gastric outlet obstruction.

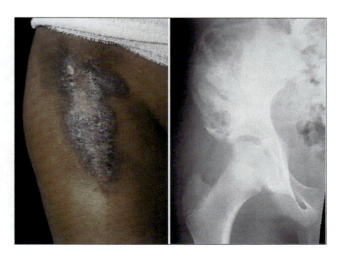

FIGURE 16.36 *Aspergillus* osteomyelitis and skin infection in a 6-year-old boy with X-linked chronic granulomatous disease before subsequent successful gene therapy.

LEUKOCYTE ADHESION DEFICIENCIES

Leukocyte adhesion deficiencies (LAD) are a group of defects of neutrophil adhesion, causing recurrent soft tissue and skin infections. Several subtypes have been defined, all of which are autosomal recessive disorders. The most frequent is LAD type 1, caused by mutations in the common beta subunit (CD18) gene of the lymphocyte function-associated antigen 1 (LFA-1, CD 11a) located on chromosome 21. Defective neutrophil adhesion leads to diminished margination with an increased neutrophil pool in the circulation.

INCIDENCE

The incidence of LAD is unknown (very rare).

PRESENTATION

Severe forms of the disease can present with omphalitis, neonatal septicaemia and delayed cord separation (>3 weeks), where the umbilical cord remains 'fleshy' and may need to be manually separated. Superficial skin lesions begin as small non-purulent nodules that fail to heal and progress to form large ulcers and surrounding cellulitis. Hallmarks of LAD are absence of pus formation, and a high baseline circulating neutrophil count. Healing of wounds is delayed leaving dysplastic scars. Gingivitis and peridontitis are common features in older children (**Figs 16.37–16.39**).

DIAGNOSIS

Recurrent infections and poor wound healing, associated with neutrophil counts persistently >15,000 µl even when well, usually rising to over 40,000 µl during infections, are highly suggestive. The absence of neutrophilia makes LAD very unlikely. In LAD-1 CD18 is absent from lymphocytes and neutrophils. Reduced expression may be found in a subgroup of patients with an attenuated clinical phenotype. Functional assays show severely impaired adhesion, migration and complement receptor 3 binding. Adhesion-independent functions (microbicidal activity and the oxidative burst) are unaffected.

TREATMENT

Early and aggressive treatment of bacterial infections and prophylactic antibiotic therapy are essential. Dental hygiene with antiseptic mouthwashes reduces the painful gingivitis in some patients. Anti-inflammatory agents and steroids may be of benefit. SCT is indicated.

PROGNOSIS

The prognosis is poor without corrective treatment in the complete form of LAD. Patients with attenuated phenotypes can live into the second or third decade of life without transplantation.

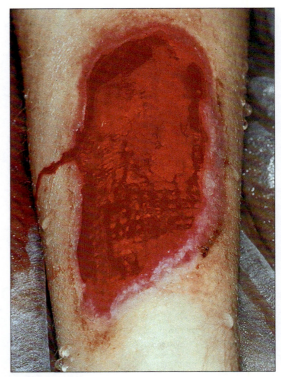

FIGURE 16.37 Large clean ulcer in leukocyte adhesion defects.

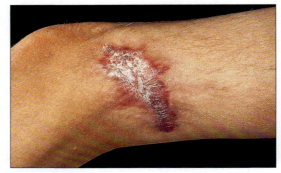

FIGURE 16.38 Dysplastic scar in leukocyte adhesion defects.

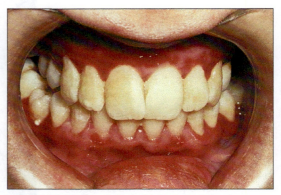

FIGURE 16.39 Gingivitis in leukocyte adhesion defects.

X-LINKED IMMUNODEFICIENCY ASSOCIATED WITH ECTODERMAL DYSPLASIA

Hypohidrotic ectodermal dysplasia associated with varying degrees of immunodeficiency is caused by mutations in the NFkappaB essential modulator (*NEMO*) gene, on chromosome Xq28.

INCIDENCE

This defect is very rare; incidence is approximately 1:250,000.

PRESENTATION

Affected children have absent sweat glands, hypo/oligodontia with abnormal peg-shaped teeth, sparse hair, eczema and typical facial features with frontal bossing and a depressed nasal bridge. There is increased susceptibility to pyogenic infections, mycobacterial infection and herpes viruses. Diarrhoea and failure to thrive are common. Autoimmunity also occurs frequently. There may be a family history of incontinentia pigmenti.

DIAGNOSIS

Immunology investigations show variable abnormalities. There may be leukocytosis with eosinophilia and immunoglobulins may be low. T- and NK-cell numbers and function are also variable. The diagnosis is confirmed by demonstration of a mutation in the *IKBKG* (inhibitory kappa B kinase gamma) gene, which encodes for *NEMO*.

TREATMENT/PROGNOSIS

Early treatment and prophylaxis of bacterial, viral, mycobacterial and fungal infections are required. SCT may be indicated.

The long-term outcome is variable depending on clinical phenotype. Curative treatment with SCT has been reported

INTERFERON-GAMMA/ IL-12 PATHWAY DEFECTS

Defects in the interferon-gamma (IFNγ)/IL-12 pathway result in increased susceptibility to intracellular pathogens, especially non-tuberculous mycobacterial infection and *Salmonella* species. Mutations in several genes can be responsible, including IFNγ receptor, IL-12 receptor beta1 (IL-12Rbeta1) and IL-12 p40 genes.

INCIDENCE

The incidence is very rare.

PRESENTATION

Clinical suspicion is raised by a narrow spectrum of persistent infections caused by weakly virulent non-tuberculous environmental mycobacterial, BCG and non-typhoidal *Salmonella* species. Non-invasive mucocutaneous candidiasis may be an additional feature.

DIAGNOSIS

Peripheral blood mononuclear cells show impaired production of IFNγ in response to IL-12. In patients affected by IL-12R beta1 deficiency surface expression of this molecule is absent. Other immunological parameters are usually normal. The diagnosis is confirmed by demonstration of a mutation in one of the above genes.

TREATMENT

Supportive treatment focuses on management and prevention of the most common severe infections with *Mycobacteria* and non-typhoidal *Salmonella* species. INFγ is indicated in some patients. Trials with exogenous administration of recombinant IL-12 have been reported. Outcomes following SCT have not been favourable.

PROGNOSIS

The outlook varies depending on the underlying molecular defect. In patients with IL-12R defects the overall mortality rate is about 30% and penetrance of disease about 40–60%. However, in those with IFNγR defects the outlook is poor. The only potentially curative treatment is bone marrow transplantation, for which there is limited experience world-wide, and results are poor.

FURTHER READING

Abolhassani H, Sagvand BT, Shokuhfar T, *et al*. A review on guidelines for management and treatment of common variable immunodeficiency. *Exp Rev Clin Immunol* 2013;9(6):561–74; quiz 75.

Aiuti A, Bacchetta R, Seger R, Villa A, Cavazzana-Calvo M. Gene therapy for primary immunodeficiencies: Part 2. *Curr Opin Immunol* 2012;24(5):585–91.

Al-Herz W, Bousfiha A, Casanova JL, *et al*. Primary immunodeficiency diseases: an update on the classification from the International Union of Immunological Societies Expert Committee for Primary Immunodeficiency. *Front Immunol* 2014;5:162.

Battersby AC, Cale AM, Goldblatt D, Gennery AR. Clinical manifestations of disease in X-linked carriers of chronic granulomatous disease. *J Clin Immunol* 2013;33(8):1276–84.

Cavazzana-Calvo M, Fischer A, Hacein-Bey-Abina S, Aiuti A. Gene therapy for primary immunodeficiencies: Part 1. *Curr Opin Immunol* 2012;24(5):580–4.

Chan WY, Roberts RL, Moore TB, Stiehm ER. Cord blood transplants for SCID: better B-cell engraftment? *J Pediatr Hematol Oncol* 2013;35(1):e14–8.

De la Morena MT, Nelson RP, Jr. Recent advances in transplantation for primary immune deficiency diseases: a comprehensive review. *Clin Rev Allergy Immunol* 2014;46(2):131–44.

Dvorak CC, Cowan MJ, Logan BR, *et al*. The natural history of children with severe combined immunodeficiency: baseline features of the first fifty patients of the Primary Immune Deficiency Treatment Consortium prospective study 6901. *J Clin Immunol* 2013;33(7):1156–64.

Gaspar HB, Aiuti A, Porta F, *et al*. How I treat ADA deficiency. *Blood* 2009;114(17):3524–32.

Gelfand EW, Ochs HD, Shearer WT. Controversies in IgG replacement therapy in patients with antibody deficiency diseases. *J Allergy Clin Immunol* 2013;131(4):1001–5.

Hernandez-Trujillo V. New genetic discoveries and primary immune deficiencies. *Clin Rev Allergy Immunol* 2014;46(2):145–53.

Lee PP, Woodbine L, Gilmour KC, *et al*. The many faces of Artemis-deficient combined immunodeficiency: Two patients with DCLRE1C mutations and a systematic literature review of genotype-phenotype correlation. *Clin Immunol* 2013;149(3):464–74.

Massaad MJ, Ramesh N, Geha RS. Wiskott–Aldrich syndrome: a comprehensive review. *Ann NY Acad Sci* 2013;1285:26–43.

Mogensen TH. STAT3 and the Hyper-IgE syndrome: clinical presentation, genetic origin, pathogenesis, novel findings and remaining uncertainties. JAK-STAT 2013;2(2):e23435.

Mukherjee S, Thrasher AJ. Gene therapy for PIDs: progress, pitfalls and prospects. *Gene* 2013;525(2):174–81.

Notarangelo LD. Primary immunodeficiencies. *J Allergy Clin Immunol* 2010;125(2Suppl 2):S182–94.

Notarangelo LD. Functional T-cell immunodeficiencies (with T-cells present). *Ann Rev Immunol* 2013;31:195–225.

Notarangelo LD. Combined immunodeficiencies with non-functional T-lymphocytes. *Adv Immunol* 2014;121:121–90.

Ocampo CJ, Peters AT. Antibody deficiency in chronic rhinosinusitis: epidemiology and burden of illness. *Am J Rhinol Allergy* 2013;27(1):34–8.

Prasse A, Kayser G, Warnatz K. Common variable immunodeficiency-associated granulomatous and interstitial lung disease. *Curr Opin Pulmon Med* 2013;19(5):503–9.

Shearer WT, Dunn E, Notarangelo LD, *et al*. Establishing diagnostic criteria for severe combined immunodeficiency disease (SCID), leaky SCID, and Omenn syndrome: The Primary Immune Deficiency Treatment Consortium experience. *J Allergy Clin Immunol* 2014;133(4):1092–8.

Sillevis Smitt JH, Kuijpers TW. Cutaneous manifestations of primary immunodeficiency. *Curr Opin Pediatr* 2013;25(4):492–7.

Sokolic R. Neutropenia in primary immunodeficiency. *Curr Opin Hematol* 2013;20(1):55–65.

Immunology (primary immunodeficiency syndromes)

17 Rheumatology

Clarissa Pilkington, Kiran Nistala, Helen Lachman and Paul Brogan

INTRODUCTION

Over the last 10 years, there have been many advances in paediatric rheumatology. New biological therapies have improved the treatment of the inflammatory disorders resulting in better disease control. International collaboration has led to pooling of rare disorders to enhance diagnostic and classification criteria, disease assessments and clinical trials. Genetic breakthroughs in the periodic fever syndromes have led to a better understanding of these autoinflammatory disorders, with improved treatment.

JUVENILE IDIOPATHIC ARTHRITIS

Juvenile idiopathic arthritis (JIA) is a heterogenous group of clinically and genetically distinct forms of chronic arthritis. The incidence is approximately 1 in 10,000 and prevalence is 1 in 1,000 (15–20,000 children have JIA in the UK).

SYSTEMIC JIA

- Incidence: 1 in 100,000.
- Onset: 1–5 years old; SJIA can occur throughout childhood and into adult years (adult onset Still disease).
- Pathogenesis: dysfunction of the innate immune system, in particular elevation of interleukin (IL)-1 and IL-6, is important.

DIAGNOSIS

- Arthritis (**Fig. 17.1**).
- Rash: salmon pink, macular and evanescent (not fixed), but can be erythematous, urticarial, or pruritic (**Fig. 17.2**).

- Spiking fevers (**Fig. 17.3**) lasting for 2 weeks with a quotidian (once a day) pattern for at least 3 days.
- Pericarditis, peritonitis (mimicking acute abdomen) and pleuritis can occur.
- Growth failure is common, secondary to disease or high-dose corticosteroids.

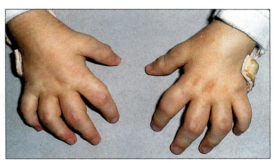

FIGURE 17.1 Symmetrical polyarthritis and tenosynovitis in a young child with systemic onset juvenile idiopathic arthritis.

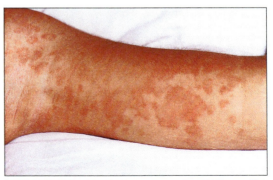

FIGURE 17.2 Typical 'salmon-pink' rash in the axilla and upper arm of a child with systemic onset juvenile idiopathic arthritis.

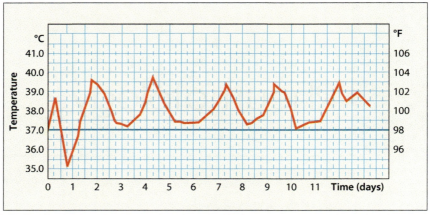

FIGURE 17.3 Typical swinging high fever chart in a child with systemic onset juvenile idiopathic arthritis.

TREATMENT

NSAIDs in high doses are used to control fever, pain and stiffness (e.g. ibuprofen, naproxen, diclofenac). Corticosteroids are required by most patients. Methotrexate is used as a second-line agent when arthritis is the predominant clinical feature. Newer biological agents, such as anakinra (IL-1 receptor antagonist) or tocilizumab (anti IL-6) are used if systemic features (fever and rash) continue. Rehabilitation, including physiotherapy and occupational therapy, are essential.

PROGNOSIS

Prior to the availability of biologic drugs, <50% of SJIA patients went into long-term remission. However, biologics targeting IL-1 and IL-6 have improved outcomes significantly.

POLYARTICULAR ONSET: RHEUMATOID FACTOR (RF)-NEGATIVE JIA

INCIDENCE

RF-negative JIA occurs in 1 in 25,000 children. The commonest onset is under 6 years of age, but it is seen throughout childhood.

DIAGNOSIS

- Five or more joints are involved at onset.
- Affects both large and small joints (symmetrical or asymmetrical).
- Early predilection for cervical spine and tempero-mandibular joint (TMJ) involvement (with resultant micrognathia) is common (**Figs 17.4, 17.5**).
- Knee, ankle, wrist, hip and elbow are frequently involved.
- Contractures of joints or cervical vertebra fusion (**Fig. 17.6**) can occur if untreated.
- Up to 50% of patients are antinuclear antibody (ANA) positive, with increased risk of chronic anterior uveitis (**Fig. 17.7**).

TREATMENT

- NSAIDs.
- Corticosteroids (either as intra-articular injection or systemically).
- Methotrexate.
- Biological agents targeting the tumour necrosis factor (TNF)-alpha pathway (etanercept and adalimumab) are second-line treatments for resistant disease.
- Physiotherapy and occupational therapy are mandatory, podiatry may be required.

PROGNOSIS

Approximately 50% go into remission (2–10 years after onset). The remainder continue with disease activity into adult years, with variable severity.

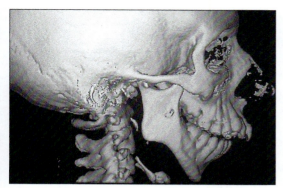

FIGURE 17.4 3D CT scan reconstruction, showing severe micrognathia in a 12-year-old boy with juvenile idiopathic arthritis.

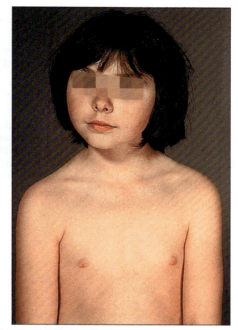

FIGURE 17.5 Torticollis due to cervical spine involvement in an 8-year-old girl with juvenile idiopathic arthritis.

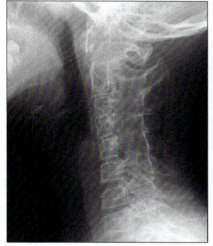

FIGURE 17.6 Cervical spine fusion and osteoporosis in a child with severe progressive juvenile idiopathic arthritis.

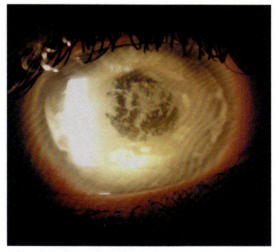

FIGURE 17.7 Uveitis: end-stage chronic anterior uveitis with visible calcium deposits of band keratopathy.

POLYARTICULAR ONSET: RF-POSITIVE JIA

The incidence of RF-positive JIA is <1 in 100,000 in childhood.

DIAGNOSIS

The disease is the equivalent of adult onset 'seropositive', i.e. RF-positive rheumatoid arthritis. Onset is usually over 8 years, most commonly in females. Children present with symmetrical polyarthritis (**Fig. 17.8**), involving proximal interphalangeal joints (PIPs), metacarpophalangeal joints (MCPs), wrists, knees and feet. There is a high risk of erosion if not treated aggressively.

TREATMENT/PROGNOSIS

Treatment is as for RF-negative polyarthritis, with a rapid escalation of therapy in patients failing to respond to methotrexate. Physiotherapy is mandatory to maintain joint function.

The disease is destructive unless treated early and has a worse long-term remission rate compared with RF-negative polyarthritis.

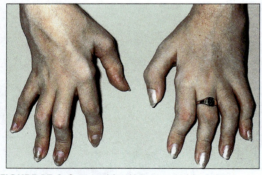

FIGURE 17.8 Symmetrical 'swan-neck' and 'boutonnière' deformities in a 15-year-old girl.

OLIGOARTICULAR ARTHRITIS

INCIDENCE

Oligoarticular arthritis is the most common type of JIA (60% of cases), occurring in 1 in 15,000 children. It is commonest in young females, with onset typically between 1 and 5 years of age, peak age of onset at 3 years.

DIAGNOSIS

- Four or fewer joints are involved.
- ANA positive (>75%).
- Significant risk of anterior uveitis (approximately 25%):
  - clinically silent, diagnosed on slit-lamp examination.
  - usually occurs in the first 5 years after onset of arthritis.
  - slit-lamp examinations are recommended every 3 months.
  - untreated uveitis can lead to visual impairment or blindness.
- Arthritis is usually asymmetric, involving large joints and the lower limbs (knees and ankles).
- Extends to multiple joints in up to 25% of cases (after the first 6 months); in this case, called extended oligoarticular JIA, the course is identical to polyarticular JIA.

TREATMENT

- NSAIDs.
- Intermittent intra-articular corticosteroid injections.
- Uveitis: topical steroids and mydriatics.
- Methotrexate is used if eye or joint disease remains active.

PROGNOSIS

Significant bony overgrowth may occur in affected joints, which leads to leg-length discrepancies and angular deformity (**Figs 17.9, 17.10**). The extended form affects 10–20%, with greater risk for joint destruction and loss of function. 75% or more of patients tend to go into remission in late childhood, but the disease can persist or recur in adult years.

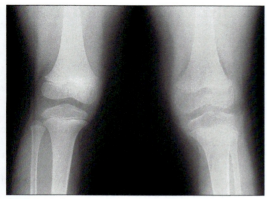

FIGURE 17.9 X-ray of a 6-year-old boy with oligoarticular arthritis of the left knee, showing medial overgrowth of the femoral and tibial condyles, osteoporosis and early valgus deformity.

ENTHESITIS-RELATED ARTHRITIS

Formerly known as juvenile onset spondyloarthropathy or juvenile ankylosing spondylitis.

INCIDENCE

1 in 100,000 children are affected per year, usually in males >8 years of age.

DIAGNOSIS

The pattern is of a lower limb, large joint, asymmetric arthritis (**Fig. 17.11**). Acute, painful, anterior uveitis occurs, but rarely causes permanent visual loss if treated. Enthesitis (inflammation of ligament and tendon insertions) is typical, often very painful (**Fig. 17.12**). It affects the Achilles tendon insertion and proximal plantar fascial insertion into the calcaneum; inflammation of patella tendon (quadriceps) insertion also occurs.

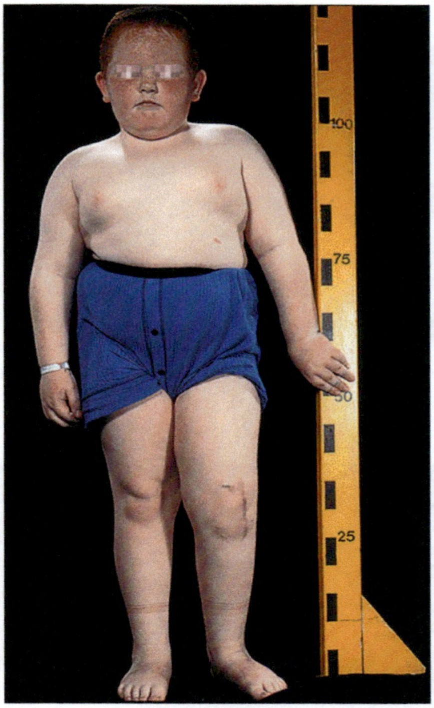

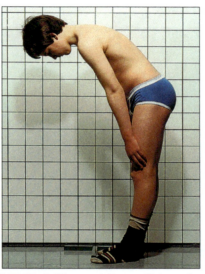

FIGURE 17.11 A 12-year-old boy with juvenile ankylosing spondylitis showing limited flexion of the lumbar spine and loss of lumbar lordosis.

FIGURE 17.10 The child in **17.9**, showing swelling and fixed flexion deformity of the left knee.

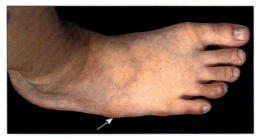

FIGURE 17.12 Enthesitis at the base of the right 5th metatarsal (arrow) in an 8-year-old girl with enthesitis-related arthritis.

Spinal and sacroiliac involvement (ankylosing spondylitis) is uncommon in childhood but may occur in later life (**Fig. 17.13**). Arthritis may progress to involve hip joints in adolescence and be very destructive. A family history of HLA-B27 associated disorders is common.

TREATMENT

- NSAIDs.
- Corticosteroid joint injections.
- Disease-modifying agents: sulphasalazine, methotrexate.
- Anti-TNF therapy is highly effective at controlling spinal and sacroiliac inflammation.
- Physiotherapy and occupational therapy input are critical.

PROGNOSIS

Enthesitis-related arthritis persists or recurs intermittently into adult years in many patients. In some, remission occurs in late childhood.

PSORIATIC ARTHRITIS

- Incidence: fewer than 1 in 100,000 children.
- Diagnosis:
  - arthritis associated with psoriasis (**Fig. 17.14**).
  - may closely mimic oligo- or polyarticular JIA.
  - characteristic dactylitis or swelling of toes/fingers (**Fig. 17.15**) (sausage-shaped).
  - nail pitting and a psoriatic rash (or a first-degree relative with psoriasis) are part of the diagnostic criteria.
  - psoriasis may occur many years after the onset of arthritis.
  - ANA positive in 50% of patients, with increased risk of chronic anterior uveitis.
- Treatment: as for oligo/polyarticular JIA; skin disease may respond to corticosteroids or methotrexate.
- Prognosis: remission may occur in late childhood, but can persist in a number of patients.

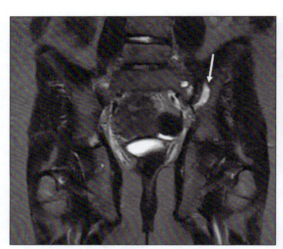

FIGURE 17.13 Sacroiliitis: short T1 inversion recovery MRI left sacroiliac joint showing bone marrow oedema (arrow).

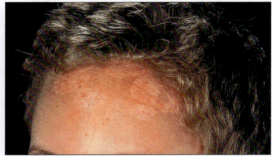

FIGURE 17.14 Psoriasis on the forehead of a child with psoriatic arthritis.

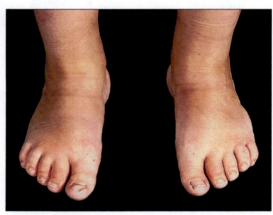

FIGURE 17.15 Bilateral ankle arthritis and dactylitis of the left fourth toe.

ARTHRITIS ASSOCIATED WITH OTHER CHRONIC DISEASES

INFLAMMATORY BOWEL DISEASE

- Arthritis occurs in 10–20% of inflammatory bowel disease patients with ulcerative colitis or Crohn disease.
- Treatment of underlying bowel disease typically improves the arthritis.
- Arthritis can become progressive and destructive, requiring intensive treatment.
- Sulphasalazine is often useful.
- Arthritis and growth failure may precede symptomatic bowel disease (**Fig. 17.16**).

CYSTIC FIBROSIS

- 5–10% of patients may develop an inflammatory arthropathy.
- It is commonest in teenagers and young adults.
- Arthritis usually responds to NSAIDs, rarely destructive.
- Hypertrophic osteoarthropathy: associated with severe lung disease.
- Diagnosed by plain x-ray; shows periosteal reactions of long bones.
- Ongoing arthritis may require immunosuppression with methotrexate; the drug is usually well tolerated

IMMUNODEFICIENCY

- Humoral and cellular deficiency syndromes may be associated with inflammatory arthritis.
- Rarely destructive or deforming. Treat with NSAIDs, physiotherapy and in some cases methotrexate.

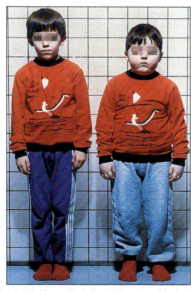

FIGURE 17.16 Growth failure in one of twin boys who presented with inflammatory arthritis of the knees. Colonoscopy showed severe inflammatory bowel disease.

ASSOCIATED SYNDROMES

Patients with Down, Turner and velocardiofacial (22q deletion) syndromes may all develop inflammatory arthritis requiring treatment.

SCLERODERMA

Scleroderma is characterised by thickened fibrotic skin and subcutaneous tissue. It is considered to be a vasculopathy with secondary changes in collagen and connective tissue.

SYSTEMIC SCLEROSIS

INCIDENCE

Systemic form of scleroderma also affects internal organs. It is rare, and occurs in <1 in 200,000 children per year, ten times less common than the localised form. However, it is the commonest form in adults.

DIAGNOSIS

Diagnosis is made on clinical grounds. The progressive form has widespread skin and internal organ involvement. Skin changes are typical on the face and limbs, with loss of subcutaneous tissues, hardening and tightening of the skin with telangiectasia and calcinosis. Joint contractures are common, especially of the hand (**Fig. 17.17**).

In the limited form there is oesophageal involvement and skin changes in the distal extremities. Raynaud and nail bed capillary changes are almost universal and may occur as part of overlap syndromes.

Involvement of kidneys, lungs or heart can be life threatening.

TREATMENT

- Local skin-softening treatments.
- Corticosteroids and immunosuppressives: methotrexate, mycophenolate mofetil, intravenous cyclophosphamide, although disease may be unresponsive in some patients.
- Raynaud: nifedipine, glyceryl trinitrate patches, iloprost if severe.
- Bosentan and ACE inhibitors, for cardiopulmonary and renal disease respectively, have improved prognosis.

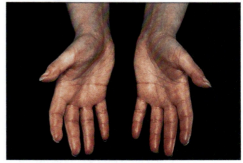

FIGURE 17.17 Severe sclerodactyly in a 15-year-old girl with systemic sclerosis.

PROGNOSIS

Mortality is 5–10% during childhood, but is improved with early treatment of complications such as pulmonary hypertension and renal disease.

LOCALISED SCLERODERMA (MORPHOEA)

INCIDENCE

Morphoea affects fewer than 1 in 200,000 children per year. It is very rare in adults.

DIAGNOSIS

Children may present with morphoea (round or oval patches of indurated, hyper- or hypopigmented skin), which may become widespread (diffuse form). Linear scleroderma usually affects limbs (upper and/or lower) or face (*en coup de sabre*) or trunk. The *en coup de sabre* lesion is associated with uveitis and cerebral involvement (seizures) (**Fig. 17.18**).

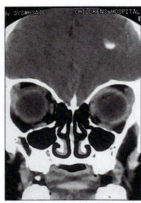

FIGURE 17.18 Intracerebral calcification shown on CT scan in a 5-year-old child with localised scleroderma of the face on the same side.

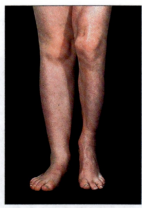

FIGURE 17.19 Severe localised scleroderma of the left leg in a 6-year-old girl showing tissue atrophy and local growth failure.

Disease may be severe, with thickening of superficial skin, loss of subcutaneous tissue, deformity of long bones, and failure of limb growth (**Fig. 17.19**). Contractures of joints are common.

TREATMENT/PROGNOSIS

Corticosteroids and immunosuppressives (e.g. methotrexate, mycophenolate mofetil) may halt progress of the disease. Physical therapies are essential to improve function.

Active disease occurs in many for 5–6 years; disease progress may be unrelenting despite treatment.

JUVENILE DERMATOMYOSITIS

INCIDENCE

Juvenile dermatomyositis (JDM) affects 2–3 cases per million children per year. The mean age of onset is 7 years; 25% of cases occur before the age of 4 years. There is no association with malignancy (unlike adult cases).

DIAGNOSIS

Diagnosis is based on clinical features, including a typical heliotrope rash (bluish- purple colour) over the eyelids with periorbital oedema (**Fig. 17.20**) and Gottron's papules – thickened erythematous, scaly rash over the MCP, PIP, distal interphalangeal joints (DIP), elbows and knees, which may be mistaken for psoriasis (**Fig. 17.21**).

Muscle enzymes are elevated, including creatinine kinase (CK), lactate dehydrogenase (LDH), aspartate aminotransferase (AST) and alanine aminotransferase (ALT).

The EMG is abnormal, with myopathic changes. There are MRI findings of muscle and fascia involvement and characteristic muscle biopsy appearance. Children show progressive proximal weakness of hip, shoulder, trunk and neck muscles. Palatal and oesophageal muscle involvement causes dysphagia and dysphonia and respiratory muscle weakness can lead to respiratory failure. Interstitial lung disease (ILD), may occur in 5–10%. Patients often have myalgia and irritability.

Erythematous nail-beds with dilated capillary loops are often seen; a generalised vasculopathy

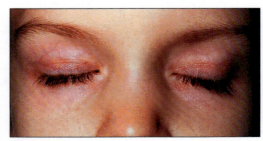

FIGURE 17.20 Typical heliotrope rash on the eyelids of a 7-year-old girl with juvenile dermatomyositis.

occurs in severe disease, with skin ulceration, gut involvement and CNS involvement. Calcinosis may be present at onset, or occurs later if disease is not controlled.

TREATMENT

High-dose long-term steroids (often intravenous followed by oral) are used with immunosuppression (e.g. methotrexate, ciclosporin, intravenous immunoglobulin [IVIg] or mycophenolate mofetil). Hydroxychloroquine may be useful for persistent severe rash. In resistant or severe disease children may need intravenous cyclophosphamide, or anti-TNF.

Physical therapies are essential to prevent contractures and improve function. Disease activity is monitored clinically – muscle strength, skin involvement, nail-bed capillary involvement, as well as muscle enzymes (though these may be helpful only in the early phases of the disease). MRI (**Fig. 17.22**) or ultrasound can be useful.

PROGNOSIS

The mortality rate of 33% prior to the use of corticosteroids is now reduced to 1–2%. Mortality is associated with severe disease (ulceration, ILD, gastrointestinal involvement). Poorer outcome occurs with late treatment, with loss of muscle, contractures and calcinosis. Skin disease is often difficult to control.

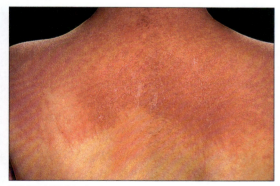

FIGURE 17.21 A photosensitive 'shawl' distribution rash in a 10-year-old girl with juvenile dermatomyositis.

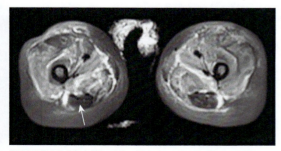

FIGURE 17.22 MRI of the thighs of a 3-year-old boy with juvenile dermatomyositis showing widespread muscle oedema due to inflammation.

VASCULITIDES

HENOCH SCHÖNLEIN PURPURA (IgA VASCULITIS)

See also Chapter 10 Renal Diseases, page 304.

INCIDENCE/PATHOGENESIS

Henoch Schönlein purpura (HSP) is the commonest vasculitis in childhood, with an incidence of 10–20.4 (mean 13.5) per 100,000 children.

The pathogenesis is unknown, a probable polygenic contribution. HSP nephritis may be due to immune complexes formed between polymeric galactose-deficient IgA and antiglycan IgG or IgA1. Disease may be a response to infection or immunisation in some individuals. Immune complexes are deposited in glomeruli with activation of mesangial cells resulting in glomerulonephritis.

CLINICAL PRESENTATION

HSP presents as a vasculitis with IgA-dominant immune deposits. It affects small vessels in the skin, gut and glomeruli. It is associated with arthritis and/or arthralgia. Intussusception, appendicitis, cholecystitis, pancreatitis, orchitis, gastrointestinal haemorrhage, ulceration, infarction or perforation can occur.

Classification criteria are palpable purpura (**Fig. 17.23**) in a predominantly lower limb distribution with at least one of:

- diffuse abdominal pain
- any biopsy showing IgA deposition (mandatory if rash is atypical)
- arthritis and/or arthralgia: pain, swelling decreased range of movement
- haematuria and/or proteinuria.

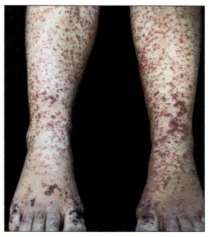

FIGURE 17.23 Typical (severe) palpable purpura of Henoch Schönlein purpura in a 13-year-old female without renal involvement.

Presentation is variable:

- 60% have arthritis and/or arthralgia: usually knees and ankles.
- 25–60% have renal involvement with nephritis (HSN).
- 68% have gastrointestinal involvement: intermittent colicky abdominal pain, vomiting, with or without haematemesis or melaena (check for faecal occult blood).
- 43% of patients: abdominal pain precedes rash by 1–14 days.
- 76% will develop HSN within 4 weeks of disease onset.
- 97% will develop HSN within 3 months of disease onset.

DIAGNOSIS

Diagnosis of HSP is clinical. Skin histology can be helpful and shows a leucocytoclastic cutaneous vasculitis with predominant IgA deposition. Renal involvement demonstrates focal and segmental proliferative glomerulonephritis, sometimes crescentic glomerulonephritis (**Fig. 17.24**). Serum IgA may be elevated. It is essential to measure BP and monitor urine dipstick for haematuria and proteinuria.

DIFFERENTIAL DIAGNOSIS

- Sepsis.
- Systemic vasculitides: systemic lupus erythematosus (SLE), polyarteritis nodosa (PAN), anticytoplasmic antibody (ANCA)-associated, and hypersensitivity.
- Familial Mediterranean fever (FMF).

TREATMENT

Treatment is symptomatic, including rest and analgesia. Prophylactic corticosteroids are used at the start, but do not prevent renal or gastrointestinal involvement. Corticosteroids are effective for renal, gastrointestinal involvement, severe facial and/or scrotal haemorrhagic oedema. Severe renal involvement may require immunosuppressive agents, antiproteinuric and antihypertensive agents (see Chapter 10 Renal Diseases, page 305).

PROGNOSIS

Prognosis is usually excellent. However, the severity of HSN is the main prognostic determinant, causing 1.6–3% of all childhood end-stage kidney disease in the UK. Some patients show a relapsing course: one-third have symptoms for up to a fortnight, one-third for up to 1 month and one-third with recurrence of symptoms within 4 months.

KAWASAKI DISEASE

INCIDENCE

Kawasaki disease (KD) is the second commonest vasculitis of childhood. It has a world-wide distribution, with a male preponderance. UK incidence is 8 in 100,000 children aged under 5 years, while in Japan the incidence is 138 in 100,000. KD is the leading cause of childhood acquired heart disease in developed countries.

PATHOGENESIS

KD has a pronounced seasonality, with occasional epidemics and clustering of cases. No single infectious agent has been found as a cause. The aetiology of KD remains unknown; it may result from an infection evoking an abnormal immunological response in genetically susceptible individuals.

DIAGNOSIS

Diagnosis requires 5/6 of the following criteria:

- Fever persisting for 5 days or more.
- Peripheral extremity changes (reddening of the palms and soles, indurative oedema and subsequent desquamation).
- A polymorphous exanthema (**Fig. 17.25**).

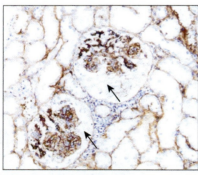

FIGURE 17.24 Immunohistochemistry of renal histology from a 16-year-old male with Henoch Schönlein purpura and heavy proteinuria, showing: diffuse mesangial matrix expansion and thickening of capillary walls; strong diffuse granular mesangial and capillary wall IgA deposition; fibrocellular crescentic change is also present in both the glomeruli (arrowed).

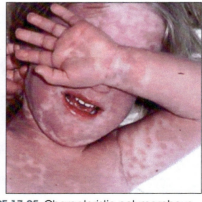

FIGURE 17.25 Characteristic polymorphous exanthema and reddening of the lips in a 4-year-old with Kawasaki disease. (Courtesy of Prof. N. Klein.)

Rheumatology

- Bilateral conjunctival injection or congestion.
- Lips and oral cavity changes (reddening or cracking of lips, strawberry tongue, oral and pharyngeal injection).
- Acute non-purulent cervical lymphadenopathy.
- Can be diagnosed <5 days, if coronary artery aneurysm (CAA) or dilatation are present (2-D echocardiography or angiography).

Symptoms and signs may present sequentially. Patients can develop coronary artery aneurysms (CAA): 15–25% in untreated cases, 4% with treatment. Other clinical features include arthritis, aseptic meningitis, pneumonitis, uveitis, gastroenteritis, meatitis and dysuria and otitis.

DIFFERENTIAL DIAGNOSIS

- Scarlet fever.
- Rheumatic fever.
- Streptococcal or staphylococcal toxic shock syndrome.
- Staphylococcal scalded skin syndrome.
- SJIA.
- Infantile polyarteritis nodosa.
- SLE.
- Adenovirus, enterovirus, EBV, CMV, parvovirus, influenza virus.
- *Mycoplasma pneumoniae* infection.
- Measles.
- Leptospirosis.
- *Rickettsiae* infection.
- Adverse drug reaction.
- Mercury toxicity (acrodynia).
- Lymphoma – particularly for IVIg resistant cases.

TREATMENT

IVIg 2 g/kg is given as a single infusion over 12 hours, preferably within the first 10 days of the illness. IVIg should be given even after 10 days if there are signs of persisting inflammation. IVIg resistance occurs in up to 20% of cases. A second dose of IVIg and/or corticosteroids should be considered. Severe cases including those deemed at high risk of IVIG resistance should have corticosteroids plus IVIG as primary therapy.

For fever, aspirin 30–50 mg/kg/day can be given in four divided doses; the dose of aspirin is reduced to 2–5 mg/kg/day when the fever settles, continued for a minimum of 6 weeks.

Refractory cases should be treated with infliximab (human chimeric anti-TNF-α monoclonal antibody). Patients with giant aneurysms require anticoagulation.

PROGNOSIS

Treatment with IVIg and aspirin reduces CAA from 25% for untreated cases to 4%. Clinical trials now suggest the addition of corticosteroids to IVIG as primary therapy for severe cases.

IVIg resistance is associated with a higher risk of CAA. The acute mortality rate due to myocardial infarction is <1% but the disease may contribute to the burden of adult cardiovascular disease and cause premature late-KD vasculopathy of the coronary arteries, an area of active ongoing research.

POLYARTERITIS NODOSA

INCIDENCE/PATHOGENESIS

PAN is a necrotising vasculitis associated with aneurysmal nodules along the walls of medium-sized muscular arteries. It affects approximately 2.0–9.0 per million and is the commonest systemic vasculitis after HSP and KD. Peak age of onset in childhood is 7–11 years, with often a male preponderance.

Pathogenesis is unknown; there is possible interaction between infection and aberrant host response. Genetic factors have not yet been defined. There is a well-recognised association of PAN and FMF (where FMF is common). A new monogenic form of PAN has recently been described, caused by deficiency of adenosine deaminase type 2 (DADA2).

CLINICAL PRESENTATION

Early in disease clinical manifestations can be non-specific: malaise, fever, weight loss, skin rash, myalgia, abdominal pain and arthropathy. Vasculitic skin lesions can include livedo reticularis (**Fig. 17.26**), skin nodules, superficial skin infarctions, deep skin infarctions and peripheral tissue (nose and ear tips) necrosis/gangrene.

Haematuria, proteinuria, hypertension, abdominal pain, gastrointestinal haemorrhage, perforation and pancreatitis can present. Neurological features such as focal defects, hemiplegia, visual loss, mononeuritis multiplex and organic psychosis may also be present.

Classification criteria for PAN in children are:

Histopathology or angiographic abnormalities (mandatory) plus 1 of criteria:

- skin involvement
- myalgia/muscle tenderness
- hypertension
- peripheral neuropathy
- renal involvement.

DIAGNOSIS

Diagnosis needs a high index of suspicion. Selective visceral digital subtraction catheter angiography (**Fig. 17.27**) shows abnormalities in medium vessel walls (e.g. aneurysms). Tissue biopsy (**Fig. 17.28**) demonstrates medium-vessel vasculitis.

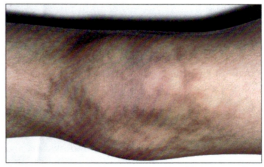

FIGURE 17.26 Livedo reticularis.

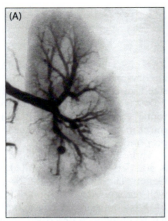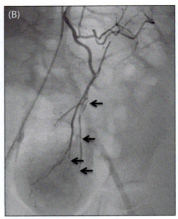

FIGURE 17.27 (A) Selective renal digital subtraction arteriography in an 8-year-old girl with polyarteritis nodosa. Large aneurysms, small aneurysms, renal, parenchymal perfusion defects, and calibre variation of intrarenal arteries are demonstrated. Perfusion defects in the renal cortex are also present; (B) selective mesenteric digital subtraction arteriography in a 6-year-old boy with partially treated polyarteritis nodosa. More subtle changes, including calibre variation and beading of medium-sized mesenteric arteries are demonstrated (arrowed) and these are unlikely to have been detected using non-invasive angiography such as CT angiography or MR angiography.

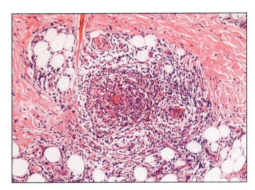

FIGURE 17.28 High-power view of a skin biopsy from a 4-year-old boy with polyarteritis nodosa. Biopsy shows a neutrophilic vasculitis affecting medium and small arteries in the deep dermis and subcutis. There is also an associated lobular panniculitis.

DIFFERENTIAL DIAGNOSIS

- HSP, ANCA associated vasculitides, KD.
- Autoimmune or autoinflammatory diseases:
  - JIA- particularly the systemic form.
  - JDM.
  - SLE.
  - undifferentiated connective tissue disease.
  - sarcoidosis.
  - Behçet disease.
- Infections:
  - bacterial, particularly streptococcal infections, and subacute bacterial endocarditis.
  - viral – particularly hepatitis B/C, CMV, EBV, parvovirus B19 and consider HIV.
- Malignancy: lymphoma, leukaemia and other malignancies can mimic PAN.
- Monogenic disease: autosomal recessive deficiency of adenosine deaminase type 2 (DADA2) caused by mutation in the *CECR1* gene.

TREATMENT

Induce remission, and after 3–6 months maintain remission for 18–24 months, using **induction therapy**: high-dose corticosteroid with an additional cytotoxic agent such as intravenous cyclophosphamide monthly for 3–6 months. Aspirin 1–5 mg/kg/d can be considered as an antiplatelet agent. Plasma exchange is used in life-threatening situations.

Once remission is achieved, **maintenance therapy** is established, with daily low-dose prednisolone and azathioprine for up to 18–24 months. Other maintenance agents include methotrexate, mycophenolate mofetil and ciclosporin.

In children unresponsive to treatment anti-TNF-alpha therapy or rituximab have been used. For mild predominantly cutaneous disease (see Chapter 10 Renal Diseases), corticosteroid alone may be appropriate, with careful monitoring of clinical and laboratory parameters as this is weaned.

PROGNOSIS

Permanent remission can be achieved. However, relapses can occur. If treatment is delayed or inadequate life-threatening complications can occur. The mortality rate of almost 100% prior to corticosteroid use is now reduced to 1.1–10%. Late morbidity can occur, possibly due to chronic vascular injury; this may result in premature atherosclerosis.

Rheumatology

ANTI-NEUTROPHIL CYTOPLASMIC ANTIBODY-ASSOCIATED VASCULITIDES

INCIDENCE/AETIOLOGY

The ANCA-associated vasculitides (AAV) are:

- Granulomatosis with polyangiitis (GPA, formerly Wegener granulomatosus).
- Microscopic polyangiitis (MPA).
- Eosinophilic granulomatosis with polyangiitis (EGPA; formerly Churg–Strauss syndrome).
- Renal limited vasculitis (previously referred to as idiopathic crescentic glomerulonephritis).

AAV is rare in children, with an incidence of <1 in 100,000. GPA is the commonest AAV seen in childhood.

PATHOGENESIS

It is not known why patients develop ANCAs. There are two main types, proteinase 3 (PR3) and myeloperoxidase (MPO) ANCA:

- PR3 ANCA is mainly associated with GPA.
- MPO ANCA is mainly associated with MPA.

A possible aetiology proposed is that ANCA activates cytokine-primed neutrophils, leading to bystander damage of endothelial cells and an escalation of inflammation with recruitment of mononuclear cells. Other factors may include genetic susceptibility.

CLINICAL PRESENTATION

Principal features of each of the AAV include:

- **GPA:** granulomatous inflammation involving the respiratory tract and necrotising vasculitis affecting small to medium vessels.
- **MPA:** necrotising vasculitis, with few or no immune deposits, affecting small vessels; necrotising arteritis involving small and medium-sized arteries may be present; pulmonary capillaritis often occurs. Clinically, it often presents with rapidly progressive pauci-immune glomerulonephritis, in association with perinuclear ANCA, MPO-ANCA) positivity.
- **EGPA:** eosinophil-rich and granulomatous inflammation involving respiratory tract; necrotising vasculitis affecting small to medium-sized vessels; association with asthma and eosinophilia.
- **Renal limited:** rapidly progressive glomerulonephritis, often with ANCA positivity (usually MPO-ANCA) but without other organ involvement.

Clinical features of GPA

- Upper respiratory tract:
  - epistaxis
  - otalgia, and hearing loss (conductive and/or sensorineural); chronic otitis media; mastoiditis
  - nasal septal involvement with cartilaginous collapse results in the characteristic saddle nose deformity (**Fig. 17.29**)
  - chronic sinusitis
  - glottic and subglottic polyps and/or large and medium-sized airway stenosis (**Fig. 17.30**).
- Lower respiratory tract manifestations include (singly or in combination):
  - granulomatous pulmonary nodules (**Fig. 17.31**) with or without central cavitation
  - pulmonary haemorrhage with respiratory distress (**Fig. 17.32**), frank haemoptysis and/or evanescent pulmonary shadows (on chest x-ray)
  - interstitial pneumonitis
- Renal involvement: typically a focal segmental necrotising glomerulonephritis, with pauci-immune crescentic glomerular changes (**Fig. 17.33**). The clinical manifestations associated with this lesion are:
  - hypertension
  - significant proteinuria
  - nephritic and/or nephrotic syndrome
  - other manifestations of acute kidney injury and chronic kidney disease.
- Ophthalmological disease: retinal vasculitis, conjunctivitis, episcleritis, uveitis, optic neuritis. Unilateral or bilateral proptosis may be caused by granulomatous inflammation affecting the orbit (pseudotumour) (**Fig. 17.29**).
- Malaise, fever, weight loss or growth failure, arthralgia and arthritis.
- Other manifestations include: peripheral gangrene with tissue loss (**Fig. 17.34**), and vasculitis of the skin, gut (including appendicitis, **Fig. 17.35**), heart, CNS (**Fig. 17.36**) and/or peripheral nerves (mononeuritis multiplex), salivary glands, gonads and breast.

DIAGNOSIS

- GPA: cytoplasmic staining pattern of ANCA by indirect immunofluorescence (IIF), and enzyme linked immunosorbent assay (ELISA) reveals specificity against PR3 (PR3 ANCA).
- MPA and renal limited AAV are typically associated with pANCA by IIF and with MPO ANCA specificity on ELISA.
- ANCA-negative forms of GPA, MPA, renal limited vasculitis, and CSS are well described in children.
- ANCA is probably unreliable for monitoring of disease activity in many GPA patients.
- Tissue diagnosis: renal (also skin, nasal septum, or other tissue) biopsy can be important diagnostically for diagnosing all of the AAV and can help stage the disease for therapeutic decision-making.

DIFFERENTIAL DIAGNOSIS

- Other primary systemic vasculitides.
- Chronic infections, including *Mycobacterium tuberculosis*, and atypical mycobacterial infections; other granulomatous infections.

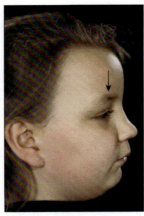

FIGURE 17.29 10-year-old girl with granulomatosis with polyangiitis. Note the typical saddle nose deformity, and orbital mass lesion from granulomatous inflammation (arrowed).

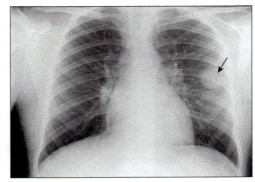

FIGURE 17.31 Chest x-ray from a 12-year-old girl with granulomatosis with polyangiitis, revealing pulmonary nodule (arrowed).

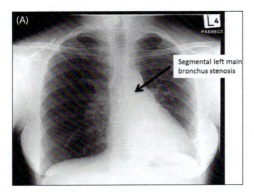

Segmental left main bronchus stenosis

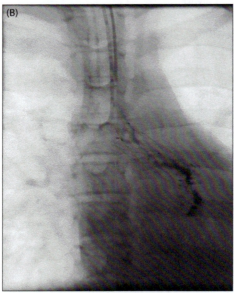

FIGURE 17.30 (A) Chest x-ray from a 14-year-old girl with granulomatosis with polyangiitis, demonstrating left main bronchus narrowing; (B) bronchogram performed in the same patient following insertion of a left main bronchial stent.

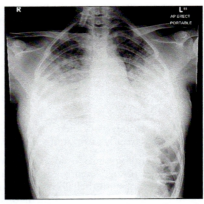

FIGURE 17.32 Diffuse alveolar hemorrhage in granulomatosis with polyangiitis (GPA). Chest x-ray from a 14-year-old girl with diffuse alveolar haemorrhage due to GPA with high titre PR3 antineutrophil cytoplasmic antibody (ANCA).

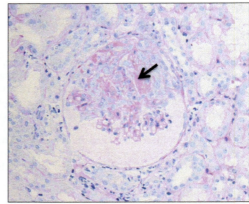

FIGURE 17.33 Renal biopsy from a 12-year-old girl with granulomatosis with polyangiitis, renal impairment, heavy proteinuria, and microscopic haematuria. Fibrocellular crescentic nephritis associated with glomerular necrotising tuft lesions (arrowed). Immunohistochemical staining with IgG, IgM, IgA, C1q and C3 was negative (pauci-immune focal segmental necrotising glomerulonephritis).

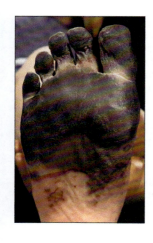

FIGURE 17.34 Peripheral gangrene in a 14-year-old girl with granulomatosis with polyangiitis (PR3 ANCA positive).

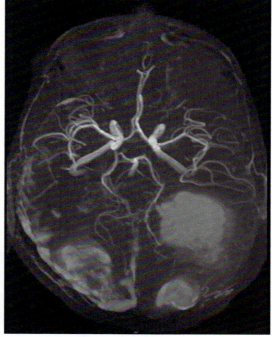

FIGURE 17.36 MRA of the brain performed following acute visual loss in a 12-year-old previously well female, with MPO ANCA positivity, but normal renal function. Multiple parieto-occipital haematomas are depicted. The intra- and extracranial large and medium-sized arteries were normal, and the final diagnosis was MPO ANCA positive small vessel vasculitis of the brain.

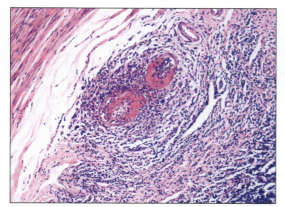

FIGURE 17.35 Fibrinoid necrosis of small vessels within the appendix of a 15-year-old girl who presented with acute appendicitis as a feature of granulomatosus with polyangiitis (PR3 ANCA positive).

- Immunodeficiencies including chronic granulomatous disease; transporter associated with antigen processing (TAP) deficiency.
- Sarcoidosis.
- Idiopathic orbital pseudotumour of the young.
- Orbital foreign body and other trauma including non-accidental injury.
- Cocaine abuse (associated with cartilaginous nasal destruction, sometimes hypertension).
- Malignancy.

TREATMENT

The initial aim of treatment is to induce remission, using corticosteroids, cyclophosphamide, plasma exchange (particularly for pulmonary capillaritis and/or rapidly progressive glomerulonephritis – 'pulmonary–renal syndrome'). To maintain remission, low-dose corticosteroids and azathioprine are used. For limited GPA corticosteroids and methotrexate are used for induction. In GPA cotrimoxazole is used as prophylaxis against opportunistic infection and as a possible disease-modifying agent, particularly with upper respiratory tract involvement. Newer agents such as mycophenolate mofetil and rituximab are increasingly used.

PROGNOSIS

There is considerable disease-related morbidity and mortality with progressive renal failure or aggressive respiratory involvement in AAV and therapy-related complications such as sepsis. Mortality for GPA from one recent paediatric series was 12% over a 17-year period of study inclusion. The largest paediatric series of patients with GPA reported 40% of cases with chronic kidney disease at 33 months of follow-up despite therapy. Mortality for MPA has been reported between 0 and 14%, while for CSS in children, the most recent series quotes a related mortality of 18%.

TAKAYASU ARTERITIS

INCIDENCE/PATHOGENESIS

Takayasu arteritis (TA) is a rare large-vessel vasculitis, with incidence less than 1 in 100,000 children. The pathogenesis is unknown, although genetic contribution in some children, and familial cases have been described.

CLINICAL PRESENTATION

TA is most common during third decade of life, but has been reported in young children and can occur even in children under the age of 2 years. Classification criteria for childhood TA are: angiographic abnormalities of the aorta or its main branches (also pulmonary arteries) showing aneurysm/dilatation (mandatory criterion), plus 1 out of the following criteria:

- Pulse deficit or claudication.
- Four limb blood pressure discrepancy.
- Bruits.
- Hypertension.
- Acute phase response.

Clinical features are usually non-specific: fever and acute phase response, initial florid inflammatory vasculitic phase followed by a later fibrotic phase of the illness. A proportion of children present in this late fibrotic/stenotic phase of the disease, usually with hypertension. Hypertension and/or its sequelae is the most common form of presentation in both children and adults. Common presentations include headache (84%), abdominal pain (37%), claudication of extremities (32%), fever (26%), weight loss (10%), hypertension (89%), absent pulses (58%) and arterial bruits (42%). Aortic and mitral valve involvement with the vasculitic process is recognised, as is myocardial involvement including the formation of ventricular aneurysms, sometimes with calcification.

DIAGNOSIS

A high index of suspicion is required. Clinical features plus findings on MRA (**Fig. 17.37**) are important diagnostically, and for monitoring disease progression catheter arteriography and CT angiography are sometimes required. In addition PET coregistered with CT angiography (PET-CT) can be helpful to detect large-vessel vasculitis, but carries a significant burden of radiation, so has limited value for monitoring disease progression.

DIFFERENTIAL DIAGNOSIS

- Other vasculitides including medium- and small-vessel vasculitis: KD; PAN; GPA is a recognised cause of aortitis.
- Infections:
  - bacterial endocarditis.
  - septicaemia without true endocarditis.
  - tuberculosis.
  - syphilis.
  - HIV.
  - borelliosis (Lyme disease).
  - brucellosis (very rare).
- Other autoimmune diseases: SLE; rheumatic fever; sarcoidosis.
- Non-inflammatory large-vessel vasculopathy of congenital cause:
  - fibromuscular dysplasia.
  - Williams syndrome.
  - Coarctation of the aorta.
  - Midaortic syndrome.
  - Ehlers–Danlos type IV.
  - Marfan syndrome.
  - Neurofibromatosis type 1.
- Other: post radiation therapy.

TREATMENT/PROGNOSIS

Treatment is with corticosteroid and cyclophosphamide induction followed by methotrexate. In some instances anti-TNF or anti-IL6 therapy may be beneficial.

TA is a relapsing and remitting disorder. The 5-year mortality rate in children has been reported as high as 35%. Prognosis is dependent upon the extent of arterial involvement and on the severity of hypertension.

Other vasculitides

Behçet disease, vasculitis secondary to infection, malignancy, drugs, vasculitis associated with other

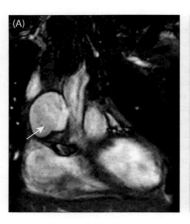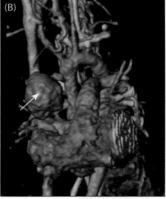

FIGURE 17.37 (A) MRA performed in a 13-year-old boy with Takayasu arteritis. Massive saccular aneurysm with narrow peduncle arising from the ascending aorta (arrowed); (B) three-dimensional construct of the same study. In addition, he had a left ventricular aneurysm (repaired twice) and aortic root dilatation with increased uptake in the wall demonstrated on FDG PET scanning (not shown). There was also a giant aneurysm of the right coronary artery (not shown).

connective tissue diseases and primary angiitis of the CNS are also seen in children, but are beyond the scope of this chapter.

SYSTEMIC LUPUS ERYTHEMATOSUS

INCIDENCE

The incidence of SLE is 1 in 3,000–10,000 children per year (Africans > Asians > Caucasians). Onset is common in girls over 12 years (rare under 8 years).

AETIOLOGY/PATHOGENESIS

SLE is an episodic, multi-system autoimmune disease with widespread inflammation of blood vessels and connective tissues, which continues into adulthood. It may be due to defects in apoptosis, which leads to polyclonal B-cell activation, immune complex formation and deposition. Dysregulated interferon-alpha pathway may also contribute to disease.

DIAGNOSIS

Onset is commonly insidious, with fatigue, rash and polyarthritis. Acute onset demonstrates serositis; CNS or renal involvement; malar or butterfly rash that is erythematous and photosensitive, but spares nasolabial folds. Rash also occurs in other sun-exposed sites. Discoid lesions can become thicker and cause scarring; lesions can occur alone (e.g. discoid lupus, **Fig. 17.38**). Vasculitic rashes occur, especially on fingertips (**Fig. 17.39**).

Arthritis is polyarticular and painful, but it is not often destructive. Renal involvement is demonstrated by proteinuria, albuminuria and casts in urine; renal involvement with glomerulonephritis requires percutaneous renal biopsy to confirm and grade severity. If there is severe renal involvement, renal dysfunction (elevated plasma creatinine with reduced glomerular filtration rate [GFR]) is seen.

CNS effects include seizures, chorea, depression or cognitive changes. CSF findings are non-specific, MRI findings may be supportive. ANAs are found in virtually all patients (95%) and more specific antibodies to double stranded DNA are found in >60%; anti-Sm antibodies, present in 20%, are very specific and anticardiolipin (antiphospholipid) antibodies are present in more than 25% and are associated with risk of thrombosis.

Risk of thrombosis is greatest in patients with lupus anticoagulant; the molecular basis for thrombosis risk is now identified as the autoantibody targeting domain 1 of beta 2 glycoprotein.

Patients with only anticardiolipin antibodies and thromboses or recurrent abortions have the primary antiphospholipid syndrome.

TREATMENT

- Mild disease: hydroxychloroquine, low-dose steroids and NSAID.
- Moderate disease: oral corticosteroids and immunosuppresive treatment such as azathioprine, methotrexate or mycophenolate mofetil.
- Severe disease (includes renal and CNS) requires high-dose corticosteroids with mycophenolate mofetil, rituximab (an anti-CD20 monoclonal antibody) or cyclophosphamide.
- Antiplatelet treatment with aspirin is required for antiphospholipid antibody positive patients.
- Thrombosis: need warfarin, cover initial warfarinisation with heparin until therapeutic INR is achieved to prevent 'paradoxical' thrombosis.

PROGNOSIS

The 5-year survival for SLE has improved to over 90%. However, CNS and renal involvement contribute significant morbidity. Deaths occur due to overwhelming disease or infections (especially fungal). There increased risk of cardiovascular disease long term, seen in adult cohorts.

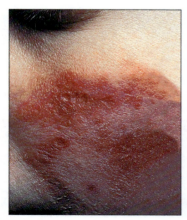

FIGURE 17.38 Typical malar rash in a 15-year-old showing some discoid lesions.

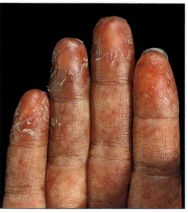

FIGURE 17.39 Severe vasculitis of the fingertips with scarring in a 13-year-old girl.

OVERLAP CONNECTIVE TISSUE DISEASE

- Incidence: uncommon, 1 in 50,000–100,000, mostly females.
- Diagnosis: patients develop clinical features of two different connective tissue diseases (CTD):
  - includes SLE, JDM (**Fig. 17.40**), JIA and scleroderma.
    - often ANA positive.
    - undifferentiated CTD: moderate features of several disorders, but insufficient to fulfill 1 diagnosis.
  - mixed CTD (MCTD): may be a subgroup of SLE.
    - MCTD: ribonucleoprotein positive, arthritis and lung involvement possible, renal and CNS involvement being absent or late (**Fig. 17.41**).

TREATMENT AND PROGNOSIS

As for the underlying CTD.

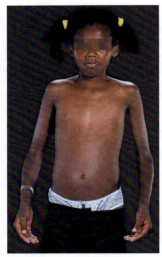

FIGURE 17.40 A 10-year-old girl with myositis, arthritis of wrists and elbows and scleroderma skin changes.

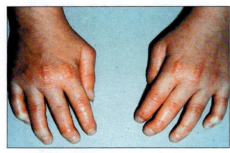

FIGURE 17.41 Polyarthritis, sclerodactyly and Gottron papules in a 13-year-old boy with mixed connective tissue disease who is antiribonucleoprotein antibody positive.

CHRONIC RECURRENT MULTIFOCAL OSTEOMYELITIS

INCIDENCE

Chronic recurrent multifocal osteomyelitis is rare, fewer than 1 in 200,000.

DIAGNOSIS

- Bone pain (sometimes with joint pain), swelling and fever.
- Bony swelling is metaphyseal and can affect several sites.
- Joints usually normal, can have an associated synovitis.
- X-rays: osteolytic metaphyseal lesions, osteitis, new bone formation (**Fig. 17.42**).
- Bone scan: often helpful, with increased uptake at sites of osteitis.
- Bone biopsy: chronic inflammation consistent with osteomyelitis but with negative cultures.
- Pustular rash: synovitis, acne, pustulosis, hyperostosis and osteitis (SAPHO) (**Fig. 17.43**).

TREATMENT

- Antibiotics usually have no effect.
- NSAIDs may improve symptoms.
- Corticosteroids may help resolve persistent lesions.
- Other treatments used include methotrexate, sulphasalazine, bisphosphonates and anti-TNF-α therapies.

PROGNOSIS

Remissions and painful relapses can continue into late adolescence. Pain can be severe and disabling. Bony overgrowth or loss of growth may cause leg-length discrepancy or joint deformity.

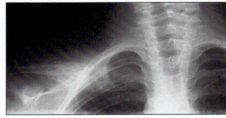

FIGURE 17.42 Clavicular osteitis in a 9-year-old boy with chronic recurrent multifocal osteomyelitis.

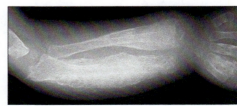

FIGURE 17.43 Extensive osteitis and new bone formation in an 11-month-old boy with SAPHO syndrome.

PERIODIC FEVER SYNDROMES/ AUTOINFLAMMATORY DISEASES

INTRODUCTION

The periodic fever syndromes are disorders of innate immunity, now usually referred to as autoinflammatory diseases. They are characterised by the following:

- Recurring episodes of fever and constitutional upset, but with normal health between attacks.
- Systemic inflammatory symptoms affecting:
  - serosal surfaces
  - joints
  - skin
  - eyes.
- Biochemical markers of inflammation: raised ESR, CRP and leucocytosis.
- Near normal life expectancy, except for risk of developing AA amyloidosis in later life.
- Seven major inherited syndromes are well described, but many new monogenic autoinflammatory diseases have recently been discovered (**Table 17.1**):
  - FMF.
  - TNF receptor-associated period syndrome (TRAPS).
  - mevalonate kinase deficiency (MKD) (also known as hyperimmunoglobulin D and periodic fever syndrome [HIDS]).
  - cryopyrin-associated periodic syndrome (CAPS) (subdivided into familial cold autoinflammatory syndrome [FCAS], Muckle Wells syndrome [MWS] and chronic infantile, neurological, cutaneous and articular syndrome/ neonatal onset multi-system inflammatory disease [CINCA/NOMID]).
  - pyogenic arthritis, pyoderma gangrenosum and acne (PAPA) syndrome.
  - deficiency of IL-1 receptor antagonist (DIRA).
  - Blau syndrome/early onset sarcoidosis (EOS).

Treatment is effective for most patients with FMF, CAPS and DIRA; good treatments are available for most of the other syndromes.

Disorders of unknown aetiology that share some features with the inherited syndromes include:

- periodic fever, aphthous stomatitis, pharyngitis and cervical adenitis (PFAPA) syndrome.
- Behcet disease.
- Chronic recurrent multifocal osteomyelitis (CRMO).
- SJIA.

FAMILIAL MEDITERRANEAN FEVER

INCIDENCE/AETIOLOGY

FMF is commonest in Middle Eastern populations; prevalence is 1 in 250–1,000. FMF occurs worldwide. It has a recessive inheritance, wih mutations in the *MEFV* gene on chromosome 16.

CLINICAL PRESENTATION

- Attacks occur irregularly, precipitated by minor physical or emotional stress, menstrual cycle or diet. Attacks resolve within 72 hours. Clinical features include
- fever
- aseptic peritonitis in 85%
- pleuritic chest pain in 40%
- erysipelas-like rash in 20%
- meningitic headache occurs rarely
- orchitis occurs rarely
- joint involvement is rare and generally mild affecting the lower limbs.
- neutrophil leucocytosis and a dramatic acute phase response occurs with attacks.
- protracted febrile myalgia (rare): severe muscle pain, may have vasculitic rash, usually responds to high-dose corticosteroids.

DIAGNOSIS

Diagnosis remains clinical: recurrent self-limiting attacks of fever and serositis, prevented by colchicine. It is supported by DNA analysis. Differential diagnosis is other periodic fever syndromes (**Table 17.1**).

TREATMENT

Colchicine is the prophylactic treatment of FMF (licensed in USA >4 years old):

- Continuous use reduces/prevents symptoms of FMF in at least 95%.
- Almost completely eliminates the risk of developing AA amyloidosis.
- Mechanism is poorly understood; children respond to 0.25–2 mg/d.

PROGNOSIS

The long-term outlook is excellent with life-long treatment. Prior to colchicine treatment 60% of Turkish patients developed AA amyloidosis. Destructive arthritis is very rare.

TABLE 17.1 Hereditary autoinflammatory diseases

Periodic fever syndrome	Gene	Mode of inheritance	Predominant ethnic groups	Usual age at onset	Potential precipitants of attacks	Distinctive clinical features	Typical duration of attacks	Typical frequency of attacks	Characteristic laboratory abnormalities	Treatment
FMF	MEFV Chromosome 16	Autosomal recessive (dominant in rare families)	Eastern Mediterranean	Childhood/ early adult	Usually none Occasionally menstruation, fasting, stress, trauma	Short severe attacks Colchicine responsive Erysipelas-like erythema	1–3 days	Variable	Marked acute phase response during attacks	Colchicine
TRAPS	TNFRSF1A Chromosome 12	Autosomal dominant, can be de novo	Northern European but reported in many ethnic groups	Childhood/ early adult	Usually none	Prolonged symptoms	More than 1 week, may be very prolonged	Variable, may be continuous	Marked acute phase response during attacks Low levels of soluble TNFR1 when well	Etanercept High-dose corticosteroids
HIDS	MVK Chromosome 12	Autosomal recessive	Northern European	Infancy	Immunisations	Diarrhoea and lymphadenopathy	3–7 days	1–2 monthly	Elevated IgD & IgA, acute phase response, and mevalonate aciduria during attacks.	Anti-TNF and anti IL-1 therapies
CAPS	NLRP3 Chromosome 1	Autosomal dominant or sporadic	Northern European	Neonatal/ infancy	Marked diurnal variation Cold environment but less marked than in FCAS	Severity spectrum including; urticarial rash conjunctivitis sensorineural deafness aseptic chronic meningitis deforming arthropathy	Continuous, often worse in the evenings	Often daily	Varying but marked acute phase response most of the time	Anti-IL1 therapies (mainly anakinra; canakinumab)

(Continued)

TABLE 17.1 *(Continued)* Hereditary autoinflammatory diseases

Periodic fever syndrome	Gene	Mode of inheritance	Predominant ethnic groups	Usual age at onset	Potential precipitants of attacks	Distinctive clinical features	Typical duration of attacks	Typical frequency of attacks	Characteristic laboratory abnormalities	Treatment
PAPA	*PSTPIP1* (*CD2BP1*) Chromosome 15	Autosomal dominant	Northern European (only 3 families reported)	Childhood	None	Pyogenic arthritis, pyoderma gangrenosum Cystic acne	Intermittent attacks with migratory arthritis	Variable, may be continuous	Acute phase response during attacks	Anti-TNF therapy or Anti IL-1 therapies
DIRA	*IL1RN* Chromosome 2	Autosomal recessive	Hispanic and European (few families reported)	Neonatal	None	Sterile multifocal osteomyelitis, periostitis and pustulosis	Continuous	Continuous	Marked acute phase response	IL-1ra
Blau syndrome	*NOD2* (*CARD15*) Chromosome 16	Autosomal dominant	None	Childhood	None	Granulomatous polyarthritis, iritis and dermatitis	Continuous	Continuous	Sustained modest acute phase response	Corticosteroids, anti-TNF, anti-IL1

TUMOUR NECROSIS FACTOR RECEPTOR-ASSOCIATED PERIODIC SYNDROME

INCIDENCE/AETIOLOGY

Tumour necrosis factor receptor-associated periodic syndrome (TRAPS) is rare, with an estimated prevalence of about 1 per million in Europe. It occurs in many ethnic groups, with presentation usually before the age of 4 years. TRAPS is caused by autosomal dominant, gene mutations in *TNFRSF1A* on chromosome 12.

CLINICAL PRESENTATION

Attacks are often far less distinct than in FMF, precipitated by minor stress, travel, menstrual cycle or diet. Prolonged attacks occur, lasting 1–3 weeks (symptoms are near continuous in 30%). 50% give no clear family history. Features include:

- Fever >95%.
- Arthralgia and myalgia in 80%, often with centripetal migration.
- Abdominal pain in 80%.
- Rash in 70%: erythematous, oedematous plaques, discrete reticulate or serpiginous lesions (**Fig. 17.44**).
- Headache, pleuritic pain, lymphadenopathy, conjunctivitis and periorbital oedema.
- Symptoms are accompanied by a marked acute phase response.

DIAGNOSIS

Diagnosis is from genetic testing. However, the difficulty is in interpretation of the significance of two common polymorphisms, R92Q (Caucasian) and P46L (African/Arab origin). Both are present in ~4% of the normal population but can be associated with a mild inflammatory syndrome. Differential diagnosis is other periodic fever syndromes (**Table 17.1**).

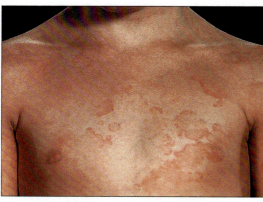

FIGURE 17.44 Erythema multiforme rash in a 7-year-old girl with tumour necrosis factor receptor-associated periodic syndrome.

TREATMENT

Acute attacks are treated with high-dose corticosteroids, but these do not reduce the frequency of attacks. Etanercept is useful in some patients, but infliximab and other monoclonal antibodies to TNF exacerbate attacks. IL-1 blockade seems to be most effective: recombinant IL-1 Ra (anakinra) is effective in ~ 80%, and long acting IL-1 blocking agents (canakinumab) may be used more frequently in future.

PROGNOSIS

Without treatment >25% develop AA amyloidosis. Patients have poor growth, interrupted schooling and poor fertility. Life-long treatment is needed, but there is a good long-term outlook.

MEVALONATE KINASE DEFICIENCY/HYPERIMMUNOGLOBULIN D PERIODIC FEVER SYNDROME

INCIDENCE/AETIOLOGY

MKD/HIDS is extremely rare. Most patients are North European, many in Holland (it was called 'Dutch fever'), but can occur in other ethnicities. The disease is caused by an autosomal recessive gene, with mutation of MVK, the enzyme acting after HMG CoA reductase.

CLINICAL PRESENTATION

Onset of MKD/HIDS is below 1 year of age. Children experience irregular attacks, that may be precipitated by vaccination, minor trauma, surgery or stress. Attacks last 4–7 days. Fever, unilateral or bilateral cervical lymphadenopathy, abdominal pain with vomiting and diarrhoea, headache, arthralgia, large joint arthritis, erythematous macules and papules and aphthous ulcers are common. A history of high fevers or a full attack with vaccination is often obtained.

DIAGNOSIS

- High serum IgD, IgE and IgA (not sensitive nor specific).
- Presence of mevalonic acid in the urine during attacks.
- Genetic confirmation.

TREATMENT/PROGNOSIS

Etanercept is useful in some patients, but IL-1 blockade seems to be the most effective treatment anecdotally. Recombinant IL-1 Ra (anakinra) can either be used continuously or to abort attacks.

Symptoms may partially improve with age. AA amyloidosis is seen, but is less common than in FMF, TRAPS or CAPS.

CRYOPYRIN-ASSOCIATED PERIODIC SYNDROME

CAPS includes a spectrum of conditions ranging from mild to severe, and includes three syndromes:

- FCAS.
- MWS.
- CINCA/NOMID.

INCIDENCE/AETIOLOGY

CAPS is extremely rare, with an incidence of probably <1 in 500,000. CAPS is due to mutations in NLRP3/CIAS1 on chromosome 1q44, that encodes the key component of IL-1 activation complex: the inflammasome. A dominant inheritance occurs in about 75% of patients with FCAS and MWS, whereas CINCA is usually due to *de novo* mutations.

CLINICAL PRESENTATION

Onset is in early infancy, often from birth; there is no sex bias. Children present with a characteristic appearance of flattened nasal bridge and bossing of the skull (**Fig. 17.45**).

- FCAS: attacks of fever, urticarial rash, arthralgia and conjunctivitis are precipitated by exposure to cold or damp conditions.
- MWS: daily attacks (afternoon/evenings), there may be some cold exacerbation. Acute symptoms include fever, urticarial rash, arthralgia and myalgia, conjunctivitis, headache and fatigue. Rash can be persistent (**Fig. 17.46**). Deafness occurs later and is often missed in the early stages.
- CINCA/NOMID: continuous inflammation with additional severe chronic aseptic meningitis, raised intracranial pressure, uveitis, deafness and arthropathy.

DIAGNOSIS

- FCAS and MWS have mutations in *NLRP3*.
- Clinical diagnosis for CINCA/NOMID: mutations are found in only 50%.
  Differential diagnosis (see **Table 17.1**).

TREATMENT

Treatment is IL-1 blockade with anakinra or with two other licensed therapies: the fully human anti IL-1beta antibody canakinumab; or IL-1 Trap (rilonacept).

PROGNOSIS

- ~25% develop AA amyloidosis.
- Complications of chronic CNS inflammation: severe in CINCA, less in MWS.
- 40% sensorineural deafness; blindness due to optic atrophy or uveitis; developmental delay.
- CINCA arthropathy: cartilage and bony overgrowth (patella), joint destruction can occur.
- MWS and CINCA: 17% clubbing of the finger nails.

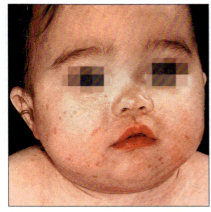

FIGURE 17.45 Typical facial features of chronic infantile, neurological, cutaneous and articular syndrome (CINCA) in a child at 11 months, showing flattened nasal bridge and hydrocephalus.

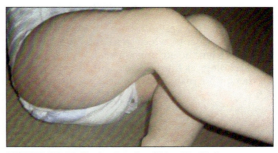

FIGURE 17.46 Typical rash of Muckle Wells syndrome in a 2-year-old boy. The rash completely resolved within 24 hours of receiving the first dose of canakinumab (monoclonal antibody against interleukin-1 beta).

PERIODIC FEVER, APHTHOUS STOMATITIS, PHARYNGITIS AND ADENITIS

PFAPA was first described in 1987 (as Marshall syndrome). It has an unknown aetiology, and the epidemiology is poorly described. PFAPA is the commonest periodic fever syndrome in childhood. It is unlikely to be due to a single gene.

- **Diagnosis** is clinical, in the absence of evidence of recurrent upper respiratory tract infections or cyclic neutropenia:
  - regular recurrent fever of early onset.
  - oral aphthous ulcers.
  - cervical lymphadenopathy.
  - pharyngitis.
- **Treatment**:
- single dose of corticosteroid (1–2 mg/kg) given at the start of an attack.
  - tonsillectomy: approximately 50% success reported.
  - colchicine or anakinra may be useful but have an unpredictable response.
- **Prognosis** is good; most outgrow their symptoms by adolescence.

OTHER DISEASES

There are many other emerging and recently described genetic autoinflammatory diseases (see **Table 17.1**), beyond the scope of this chapter.

CHRONIC PAIN SYNDROME

- Can be localised or diffuse, pain needs to have lasted at least 3 months.
- Includes forms similar to adult fibromyalgia.
- Overlaps with chronic fatigue syndrome and postviral fatigue syndrome.
- All of these conditions have major psychological components, which are either aetiological or result from the inciting illness.
- Psychological intervention and, usually, physiotherapy are mandatory in these conditions.

COMPLEX REGIONAL PAIN SYNDROME

INCIDENCE

This was previously called reflex sympathetic dystrophy or algodystrophy. It is uncommon, <1 in 50,000, predominantly in females over 8 years of age.

DIAGNOSIS

Diagnosis is clinical, possibly an exaggerated response to minor trauma or minor pathology. It has psychosocial features. Early on there is soft tissue swelling, sweating and oedema; later on children develop cold skin, increased hair growth, allodynia (severe skin hypersensitivity to light stimuli) and pseudoparalysis.

Untreated there is atrophy of skin and undergrowth of bone (**Fig. 17.47**). Bone scans may show increased uptake in the early phases and reduced uptake later on with disuse of the limb. X-rays may show osteoporosis with long-standing disease.

TREATMENT/PROGNOSIS

Intensive physiotherapy and psychological input are essential. Skin massage and desensitisation can be helpful; analgesia and sympathetic nerve blocks are often unhelpful in children.

Patients improve significantly with treatment, but recurrences do occur. Any delay in diagnosis causes prolonged morbidity and disability and many patients persist with various symptoms into their adult years. Psychosocial issues may predispose patients to chronicity and poor treatment response.

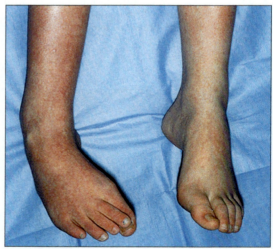

FIGURE 17.47 Long-standing reflex sympathetic dystrophy in a 13-year-old, showing skin colour changes and flexion posture of the right foot.

JOINT HYPERMOBILITY SYNDROME

INCIDENCE

This is common: children have a greater range of normal joint mobility than adults and 5–10% of normal children have either localised or generalised hypermobility (up to 10% of which becomes symptomatic). Genetic syndromes include Marfan syndrome and Ehlers–Danlos syndrome.

DIAGNOSIS

The joints commonly affected include the knees, ankles, elbows, wrists (**Fig. 17.48**) and feet. Recurrent minor 'sprains', subluxation/dislocation lead to recurrent arthralgias and occasional joint effusions. 'Growing pains' are commonly related to hypermobility. Adolescents may present with back pain.

TREATMENT/PROGNOSIS

Treatment is with physiotherapy, with specific muscle strengthening and joint protection measures, such as supportive shoes and insoles. Anti-inflammatories and analgesics are often unhelpful.

Prognosis is generally good; many improve with age and function is usually maintained.

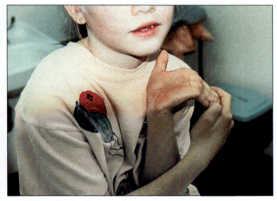

FIGURE 17.48 Hyperextension of the metacarpopharyngeal joints of the hands in a 9-year-old girl with benign joint hypermobility syndrome.

FURTHER READING

Cassidy J, Petty R, Laxer R, Lindsley C (eds). *Textbook of Paediatric Rheumatology*, 6th edn. Philadelphia: Saunders, 2011.

Cobb JE, Hinks A, Thomson W. The genetics of juvenile idiopathic arthritis: current understanding and future prospects. *Rheumatology* (Oxford) 2014;53(4):592–9.

De Benedetti F, Brunner HI, Ruperto N, et al. Randomized trial of tocilizumab in systemic juvenile idiopathic arthritis. *N Engl J Med* 2012;367(25):2385–95.

Foster H, Brogan PA. *The Oxford Handbook of Paediatric Rheumatoloy*. Oxford: Oxford University Press, 2012.

Hinks A, Cobb J, Marion MC, et al. Dense genotyping of immune-related disease regions identifies 14 new susceptibility loci for juvenile idiopathic arthritis. *Nat Genet* 2013;45(6):664–9.

Lovell DJ, Giannini EH, Reiff A, et al.; Pediatric Rheumatology Collaborative Study Group. Etanercept in children with polyarticular juvenile rheumatoid arthritis. *N Engl J Med* 2000;342(11):763–9.

Magni-Manzoni S, Malattia C, Lanni S, Ravelli A. Advances and challenges in imaging in juvenile idiopathic arthritis. *Nat Rev Rheumatol* 2012;8(6):329–36.

Prakken B, Albani S, Martini A. Juvenile idiopathic arthritis. *Lancet* 2011;377(9783):2138–49.

Ringold S, Weiss PF, Beukelman T, et al. 2013 update of the 2011 American College of Rheumatology recommendations for the treatment of juvenile idiopathic arthritis: recommendations for the medical therapy of children with systemic juvenile idiopathic arthritis and tuberculosis screening among children receiving biologic medications. *Arthritis Care Res* (Hoboken) 2013;65(10):1551–63.

Ruperto N, Brunner HI, Quartier P, et al. Two randomized trials of canakinumab in systemic juvenile idiopathic arthritis. *N Engl J Med* 2012;367(25):2396–406.

Schulert GS, Grom AA. Macrophage activation syndrome and cytokine-directed therapies. *Best Pract Res Clin Rheumatol* 2014;28(2):277–92.

van Dijkhuizen EH, Wulffraat NM. Early predictors of prognosis in juvenile idiopathic arthritis: a systematic literature review. *Ann Rheum Dis* 2014; 74(11):1996–2005.

Watts R, Conaghan P, Denton C, Foster H, Isaacs J, Muller-Ladner U (eds). *Oxford Textbook of Rheumatology*, 4th edn. Oxford: Oxford University Press, 2012.

Neonatal and General Paediatric Surgery

Lewis Spitz and Joe Curry

OESOPHAGEAL ATRESIA

INCIDENCE AND TYPES

Oesophageal atresia occurs in 1 in 4,500 live births.

- Proximal atresia with distal tracheo-oesophageal fistula –85% (**Fig. 18.1**).
- Isolated oesophageal atresia –7% (**Fig. 18.2**).
- H-type tracheo-oesophageal fistula without atresia –4%.
- Atresia with proximal tracheo-oesophageal fistula –1%.
- Atresia with proximal and distal fistula –3%.

RISK CLASSIFICATION

The Waterston risk grouping (1962) has recently been superseded and an updated classification proposed as follows:

Group I: infants with birthweight >1,500 g and no major congenital cardiac defect (98.5% survival).

Group II: birthweight <1,500 g or a major cardiac defect (82% survival).

Group III: birthweight <1,500 g and major cardiac defect (50% survival).

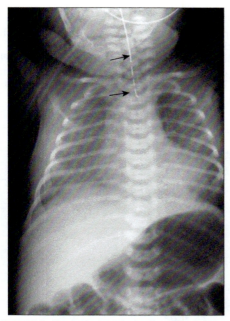

FIGURE 18.1 Oesophageal atresia with distal tracheo-oesophageal fistula. X-ray of chest and abdomen showing a radio-opaque catheter in the upper blind oesophageal pouch and gas in the gastrointestinal tract.

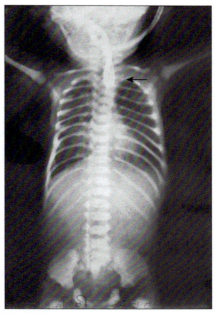

FIGURE 18.2 Oesophageal atresia without tracheo-oesophageal fistula. X-ray of chest and abdomen showing a radio-opaque catheter in the upper oesophagus and the complete absence of gas in the bowel.

ASSOCIATED ANOMALIES

Congenital cardiac malformations are the single most common anomalies and are responsible for the majority of deaths. Cardiac defects occur in 25–40% of patients and, of these, ventricular septal defects and tetralogy of Fallot are the most common. The VATER association of defects is well-recognised (V = vertebral, A = anorectal, TE = tracheo-oesophageal, R = radial and/or renal anomalies) with the term 'VACTERL' used to denote also cardiac and limb defects.

PRENATAL DIAGNOSIS

The possibility of an oesophageal atresia is often heralded by the presence of polyhydramnios. The absence of a detectable stomach 'bubble' on prenatal ultrasound scan provides confirmatory evidence for the presence of an isolated atresia without tracheo-oesophageal fistula. In addition, the upper oesophageal pouch may be seen to be dilated and obstructed on the ultrasound scan.

POSTNATAL DIAGNOSIS

In the presence of polyhydramnios, all newborn infants should have a nasogastric tube passed. An oesophageal atresia (**Figs 18.1, 18.2**) should be suspected when the infant is 'excessively mucusy' at birth. The advent of coughing and cyanosis coinciding with the first feed is a consequence of delayed diagnosis.

DIAGNOSIS

Inability to advance a No.8–10F nasogastric tube by mouth beyond 10 cm from the lower gum margin and an x-ray showing the tip of the tube in the upper thorax provides confirmation of the diagnosis. The presence of gas within the gastrointestinal (GI) tract is indicative of a distal tracheo-oesophageal fistula.

TREATMENT

Optimal treatment is ligation of the tracheo-oesophageal fistula and primary oesophageal anastomosis. Occasionally, primary anastomosis is not possible and delayed repair is required. In rare circumstances, oesophageal replacement is necessary.

CONGENITAL DIAPHRAGMATIC HERNIA

INCIDENCE

This occurs in 1 in 4,500 live births, but probably as high as 1 in 2,500 gestations. The herniation of abdominal contents occurs through a defect in the pleuroperitoneal canal (foramen of Bochdalek), which fails to close during intrauterine development.

PATHOPHYSIOLOGY

Herniation occurs more frequently on the left side (4:1) and causes compression of the ipsilateral developing lung and shift of the mediastinal structures to the opposite side. This is associated with hypoplasia of the ipsilateral and, to a lesser extent, of the contralateral lung. In addition, there is thickening of the musculature of the pulmonary arterioles with resultant pulmonary hypertension, which can lead to persistent fetal circulation with right to left shunting through the patent foramen ovale and ductus arteriosus.

DIAGNOSIS

Detection of a diaphragmatic hernia can be made on prenatal scan (**Fig. 18.3**) at around 20 weeks of gestation. It is important to exclude lethal chromosomal defects at an early stage and to evaluate the heart for congenital cardiac anomalies. The first sign of a diaphragmatic hernia may be late in gestation, at birth or at any stage later on, even into adult life.

CLINICAL PRESENTATION

Respiratory distress is usually present at birth (with respiratory rate >40/min, heart rate >160/min, subcostal recession and cyanosis). There are decreased breath sounds on the ipsilateral side, the heart sounds are shifted to the contralateral side and the abdomen is flat or even scaphoid.

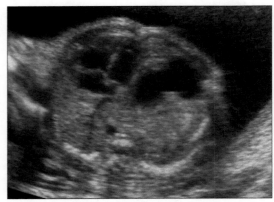

FIGURE 18.3 Congenital diaphragmatic hernia. Prenatal ultrasound scan showing the presence of intestine in the chest.

DIAGNOSIS

Plain chest and abdominal x-ray will reveal loops of intestine in the chest, shift of the mediastinal structures to the contralateral side and an absence of bowel gas shadows in the abdomen (**Figs 18.4, 18.5**). In late presenting cases or when the diagnosis is doubtful, upper GI contrast studies will show contrast-filling intestinal loops within the pleural cavity.

TREATMENT

Emergency repair is no longer practised. The infant with respiratory distress requires urgent resuscitation and stabilisation prior to surgery. This consists of endotracheal intubation, gentle mechanical ventilation and elective sedation and paralysis. In refractory cases high-frequency oscillating ventilation, nitric oxide and extracorporeal membrane oxygenation (ECMO) may be used. Operative repair consists of reduction of the herniated contents back into the abdomen and closure of the diaphragmatic defect with or without a prosthetic patch.

PROGNOSIS

The overall mortality for diaphragmatic hernia has not changed significantly over the past few decades. Survival rate remains around 50% but most infants succumb prenatally or prior to surgery, due to failure of stabilisation of cardiorespiratory function.

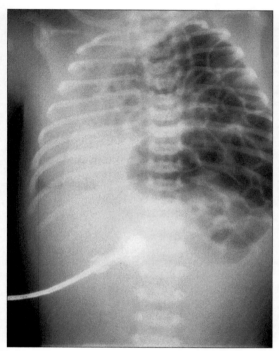

FIGURE 18.4 Congenital diaphragmatic hernia. X-ray of the chest and abdomen showing intestinal gas shadows in the left chest, a shift of the mediastinum to the right and absence of bowel in the abdomen.

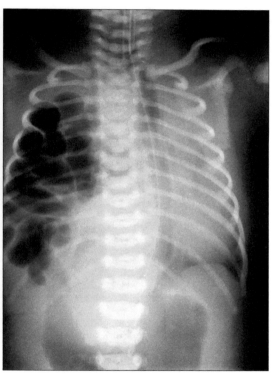

FIGURE 18.5 Congenital diaphragmatic hernia. X-ray of the chest and abdomen showing a right-sided diaphragmatic hernia, which is less common than left-sided hernia.

NEONATAL INTESTINAL OBSTRUCTION

See **Table 18.1** for overview.

TABLE 18.1 Intestinal obstruction in the neonate (**Figs 18.6, 18.7**)

Mechanical	
Intraluminal	– Meconium ileus – Meconium obstruction of the newborn
Intramural	– Atresia: duodenal, intestinal – Anorectal anomalies – Hirschsprung's disease
Extraluminal	– Malrotation – Duplication – Hernia – Cysts – Tumours

Paralytic ileus
Septicaemia
Necrotising enterocolitis
Symptomatology
Bile-stained vomiting
Abdominal distension
Failure to pass meconium

Oedema and/or erythema of the anterior abdominal wall indicates peritonitis, perforation or gangrenous intestine.

MECONIUM ILEUS

INCIDENCE

Meconium ileus occurs in 1 in 2,500.

AETIOLOGY

Meconium ileus is a manifestation of cystic fibrosis, which is a genetic defect involving the long arm of chromosome 7, the commonest mutation being a single amino acid substitution, ΔF508 and is inherited as an autosomal recessive characteristic with 25% transmission. Meconium ileus occurs in 10–15% of infants with cystic fibrosis.

PATHOPHYSIOLOGY

Due to the pancreatic exocrine deficiency, the meconium becomes tenacious and sticky and cannot be propelled by peristalsis through the GI tract. The resultant intraluminal obstruction causes proximal dilatation, which may culminate in volvulus with or without atresia, or perforation with meconium peritonitis.

CLINICAL PRESENTATION

The infant is usually born already with a distended abdomen (**Fig. 18.8**). Bilious vomiting occurs soon after birth and it may be possible to palpate the distended loops of intestine impacted with meconium through the abdominal wall. No meconium will be passed and a small amount of mucus may follow rectal probing.

DIAGNOSIS

The plain abdominal x-ray shows dilated loops of intestine of varying calibre (**Fig. 18.9**) and, unless there is an atresia or volvulus, an absence of air–fluid levels. Calcification indicates the prior occurrence of an intestinal perforation. A 'ground-glass' appearance of impacted meconium may be seen on the plain x-ray. In meconium peritonitis, the abdomen may be opaque due to the presence of ascites.

Chromosomal analysis will reveal the ΔF508 defect in 90% of cases. Sweat test with pilocarpine iontophoresis is diagnostic when the volume of sweat obtained is over 100 g and the sodium and chloride content is in excess of 60 mEq/l.

TREATMENT

For uncomplicated meconium ileus, a carefully performed gastrografin enema may relieve the intraluminal obstruction (**Fig. 18.10**). For complicated meconium ileus and when gastrografin enema fails to relieve the obstruction, surgery is required (**Fig. 18.11**). The procedure consists of either enterotomy with washout of the obstructing meconium or resection and reanastomosis of the intestine.

PROGNOSIS

The prognosis for meconium ileus is near 100% survival from the meconium obstruction. Lifelong replacement of pancreatic enzymes is required due to the presence of pancreatic insufficiency, as is physiotherapy to improve the drainage of bronchial secretions and intensive antibiotic management of respiratory infections.

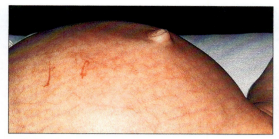

FIGURE 18.6 Neonatal intestinal obstruction: infant with a distended abdomen.

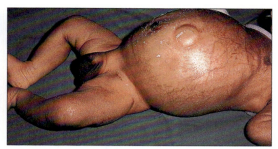

FIGURE 18.7 Neonatal intestinal obstruction. Oedema and erythema of the abdominal wall indicative of perforation with peritonitis.

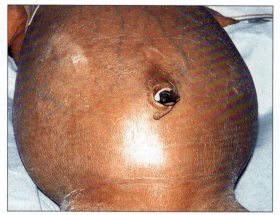

FIGURE 18.8 Meconium ileus. Infant with abdominal distension present at birth.

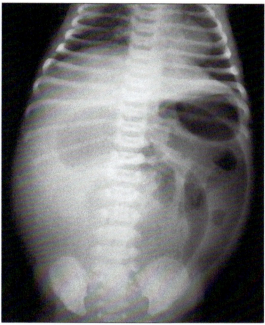

FIGURE 18.9 Meconium ileus. Abdominal x-ray showing dilated loops of intestine of varying calibre and an absence of air–fluid levels.

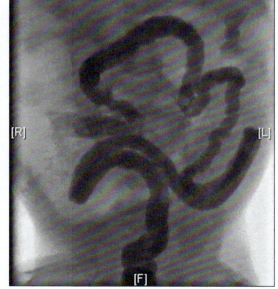

FIGURE 18.10 A carefully performed gastrografin enema may relieve the intraluminal obstruction.

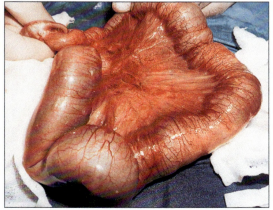

FIGURE 18.11 Meconium ileus. Operative appearance of the intestine showing dilated small intestine distended with impacted meconium.

DUODENAL ATRESIA

INCIDENCE AND TYPE

Duodenal atresia occurs in 1 in 7,500.

- Duodenal atresia – in continuity, with fibrous connection, or with gap.
- Duodenal web – perforated and/or windsock.
- Duodenal stenosis.

ASSOCIATED ANOMALIES

These include Down syndrome (30%), cardiac malformations, malrotation and atresias involving other parts of the alimentary canal, especially oesophageal atresia and anorectal anomalies.

PRENATAL DIAGNOSIS

The presence of polyhydramnios should alert the clinician to the diagnosis of a proximal GI obstruction. Prenatal ultrasound scan will show the typical 'double-bubble' of duodenal atresia.

CLINICAL PRESENTATION

Bilious vomiting is the most prominent symptom when the obstruction is below the level of the ampulla of Vater (two-thirds of cases). In higher obstructions, the vomitus is clear but persistent. There is usually upper abdominal distension and visible gastric peristalsis may be seen.

DIAGNOSIS

Plain abdominal x-ray will reveal the 'double-bubble' diagnostic of duodenal atresia (**Fig. 18.12**). In incomplete obstructions, a contrast study may be required to reveal the partial duodenal obstruction.

TREATMENT

Duodenoduodenostomy.

INTESTINAL ATRESIA

INCIDENCE AND TYPES

Intestinal atresia occurs in 1 in 6,000.

- Type 1 – atresia in continuity.
- Type 2 – atresia with fibrous connection.
- Type 3 – atresia with gap in mesentery.
- Type 4 – multiple atresias.

AETIOLOGY

There is intrauterine vascular insufficiency to the involved segment of intestine (e.g. strangulation, intussusception, volvulus). Intestinal atresia is usually an isolated anomaly, although additional anomalies may be found in up to 10% of cases.

PRENATAL DIAGNOSIS

The presence of an intestinal atresia may be suspected on prenatal ultrasound scan by the presence of dilated or echogenic bowel.

CLINICAL PRESENTATION

Bilious vomiting is usually the first sign of an intestinal atresia. The degree of abdominal distension is proportional to the level of the obstruction, with massive distension sufficient to cause respiratory embarrassment occurring in low obstructions. A small amount of meconium may be passed but, in general, only mucus may be present in the rectum and no air is ever passed.

DIAGNOSIS

Plain abdominal x-ray shows dilated loops of proximal intestine with an absence of gas distally (**Fig. 18.13**). It is not possible to differentiate small from large intestine on plain x-ray and occasionally it may be necessary to perform contrast studies to document the level of the obstruction.

TREATMENT

Surgical management consists of excising a portion of the grossly dilated proximal intestine and a small section of distal bowel (**Fig. 18.14**) and performing an end-to-end single-layer seromuscular intestinal anastomosis.

Neonatal and general paediatric surgery

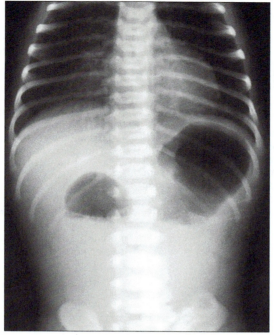

FIGURE 18.12 Duodenal atresia. Abdominal x-ray showing the typical 'double-bubble'.

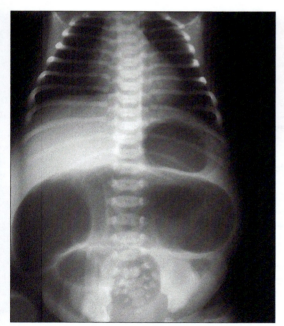

FIGURE 18.13 Intestinal atresia. Abdominal x-ray showing large dilated loops of obstructed proximal small intestine.

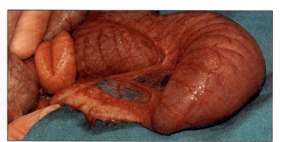

FIGURE 18.14 Intestinal atresia. Operative appearance, showing dilated proximal and collapsed distal bowel.

ANORECTAL ANOMALIES

INCIDENCE

Anorectal anomalies occur in 1 in 3,000 live births. Anorectal anomalies arise out of failure to complete the final stages in the development of the hindgut.

ASSOCIATED ANOMALIES

Most frequent are anomalies of the urinary system (dysplastic kidney, hydronephrosis, vesicoureteric reflux, neuropathic bladder), which occur in 66% of high anomalies and 33% of low lesions. Other commonly encountered associated anomalies include vertebral defects (particularly sacral), cardiac malformations, oesophageal atresia and limb deformities (VACTERL association).

DIAGNOSIS

See **Fig. 18.15**.

ANATOMICAL TYPES

The number and variety of abnormalities is vast but a few basic principles in diagnosis and treatment should be adhered to (**Table 18.2** [19.2]) (**Figs 18.16–18.21**).

TREATMENT

- High anomaly – colostomy followed later by posterior sagittal anorectoplasty.
- Low anomaly – local perineal procedure either as an anoplasty or limited posterior sagittal repair.

PROGNOSIS

The outlook for normal continence will depend on the height of the lesion and associated spinal abnormalities. In general the higher the lesion and the more affected is the sacral spine the less likely there is to be normal faecal continence.

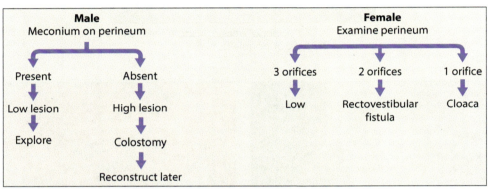

FIGURE 18.15 Diagnosis of anorectal anomalies.

TABLE 18.2 Commonest anatomical varieties of anorectal anomalies

	High (supralevator)	Low (translevator)
MALE	Rectourethral fistula	Covered anus
FEMALE	Cloacal or recto-Vaginal fistula	Ectopic anus or anovestibular fistula

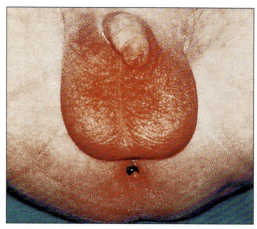

FIGURE 18.16 Low anorectal anomaly in a male infant, showing a spot of meconium on the perineum.

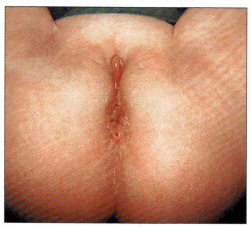

FIGURE 18.19 Low anterior ectopic anus, located immediately posterior to the fourchette, in a female infant.

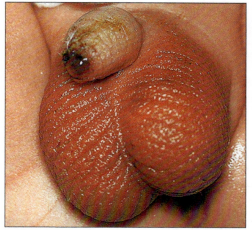

FIGURE 18.17 A high anorectal anomaly in a male infant, showing a 'flat' perineum and meconium in the urine.

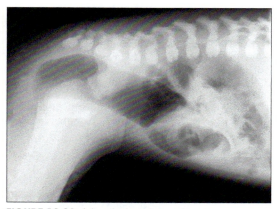

FIGURE 18.20 A low lesion shown by an invertogram, with bowel gas well below the pelvic muscles.

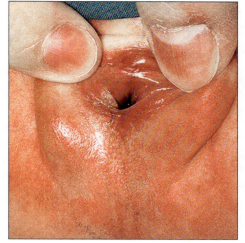

FIGURE 18.18 High anorectal anomaly in a female infant with a single opening on the perineum (a cloacal anomaly).

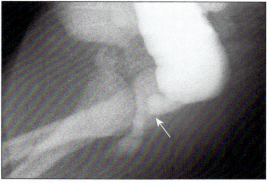

FIGURE 18.21 Rectourethral fistula. A distal colonogram showing the terminal rectum entering the bladder outlet in the region of the prostatic urethra.

HIRSCHSPRUNG DISEASE

INCIDENCE

Hirschsprung disease occurs in 1 in 5,000 live births. This condition is characterised by the absence of ganglion cells in the distal intestine. The anorectal region is always affected, with 75% of cases being confined to the rectosigmoid area and 10% including the entire colon (total colonic aganglionosis), extending for a greater or lesser extent into the small bowel.

GENETICS

There is a definite familial pattern of inheritance. Males are affected four times as frequently as females. There is a 25% risk of inheritance in total colonic aganglionosis where the male to female ratio is 1:1. One of the genes responsible for Hirschsprung disease has been isolated on the RET proto oncogene.

CLINICAL PRESENTATION

Delayed passage of meconium, in excess of 24 hours after birth, should arouse the suspicion of Hirschsprung disease. There is usually abdominal distension (**Fig. 18.22**) and bilious vomiting, which may be relieved following rectal probing or washout, only for the symptoms to recur shortly afterwards. Chronic intractable constipation may only occur in later childhood (**Fig. 18.23**).

DIAGNOSIS

The plain abdominal x-ray shows dilated loops of intestine with an absence of gas in the rectum (**Fig. 18.24**). A contrast enema may show a contracted rectum with dilated bowel proximally, but in the neonatal period this feature may be absent. Anorectal manometry reveals failure of relaxation of the internal anal sphincter in response to

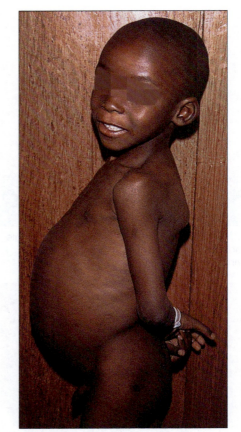

FIGURE 18.23 Hirschsprung disease in an older child with a distended abdomen and thin limbs reflecting poor nutritional status.

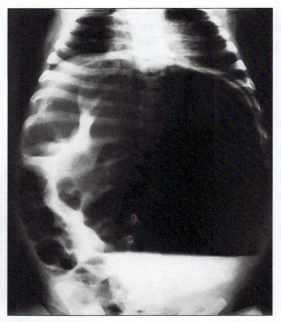

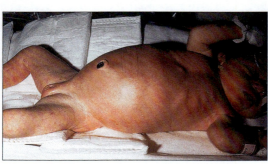

FIGURE 18.22 Hirschsprung disease: appearance of an infant showing a distended abdomen with dilated loops of bowel visible.

FIGURE 18.24 Hirschsprung disease: abdominal x-ray showing hugely distended loops of intestine.

proximal distension. The definitive diagnosis is on histopathological examination of a rectal suction biopsy (**Figs 18.25, 18.26**). Typically, this will show an absence of ganglion cells with large nerve trunks present in the submucosa. Histochemistry shows a proliferation of acetylcholinesterase fibres in the submucosa and particularly in the lamina propria.

TREATMENT

Definitive treatment consists of either excising (Swenson) or bypassing (Duhamel, Soave) the aganglionic intestine. This may be carried out as a two- or three-stage procedure with an initial colostomy in normally ganglionic intestine or as a one-stage primary procedure. Primary definitive surgery performed entirely through the anal canal is now widely practised although the long-term results are not yet known.

COMPLICATIONS

The most feared complication is the development of enterocolitis, which is characterised by profuse diarrhoea and toxicity in combination with gross abdominal distension and, if untreated, can culminate in hypovolaemic shock.

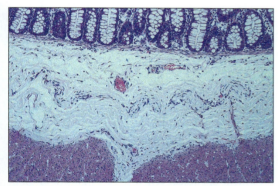

FIGURE 18.25 Hirschsprung disease: rectal biopsy (H&E) showing absence of ganglion cells and large nerve trunks in the submucosal layer.

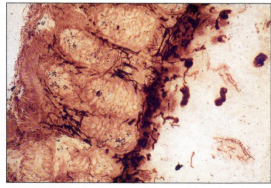

FIGURE 18.26 Hirschsprung disease: histochemistry of rectal biopsy showing increased acetylcholinesterase positive nerve fibres in the submucosa and in the lamina propria.

MALROTATION

AETIOLOGY

Failure of the intestine (midgut) to rotate normally in the first 12 weeks of development results in an abnormally mobile midgut with a short narrow-based mesentery that has the propensity to twist, causing life-threatening midgut volvulus.

PRENATAL DIAGNOSIS

The condition is not detectable on prenatal ultrasound scan unless complicated by intrauterine volvulus.

CLINICAL PRESENTATION

Bile-stained vomiting may be the only symptom. This alone should lead to investigations to confirm or refute the diagnosis of malrotation. The infant's abdomen is usually flat and undistended (**Fig. 18.27**). In the presence of volvulus, there will be additional signs such as blood-stained nasogastric aspirate and/or bloody mucosy stools and hypovolaemic shock in cases with advanced intestinal necrosis.

In older children, malrotation may present with gastro-oesophageal reflux (see Chapter 9 Gastroenterology, page 278) with the occasional bilious vomit, symptoms suggestive of anorexia nervosa or recurrent abdominal pain.

DIAGNOSIS

The diagnosis may be suspected on plain abdominal x-ray by the absence of intestinal gas in the presence of bilious vomiting, especially in the neonatal period. A contrast upper GI study will reveal the abnormally rotated duodenum with a 'corkscrew' pattern in the case of midgut volvulus (**Fig. 18.28**). An ultrasound scan may show abnormal orientation of the superior mesenteric vessels, with the artery anterior or lateral to the vein.

TREATMENT

Urgent surgical intervention, following rapid and intense fluid and electrolyte imbalance resuscitation, is required to prevent volvulus. The procedure consists of straightening the duodenal loop, widening the base of mesentery of the small intestine by dividing fibrous adhesions and placing the intestines in a non-rotated position, with the small bowel on the right side and the caecum and large bowel on the left side of the abdomen (**Fig. 18.29**). Where volvulus has already occurred, the intestines should be de-rotated and inspected for viability. In extreme cases (no viable bowel) it is advisable to resect frankly gangrenous intestine and to carry out a 'second-look' laparotomy 24 hours later. It may then be possible to salvage sufficient intestine for normal GI function.

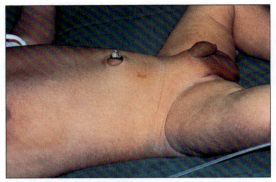

FIGURE 18.27 Malrotation: clinical appearance of an infant showing an undistended abdomen in the presence of bile-stained vomiting.

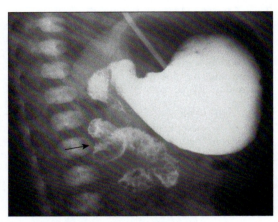

FIGURE 18.28 Malrotation: lateral upper gastrointestinal contrast study showing 'corkscrew' appearance of the duodenum signifying a volvulus.

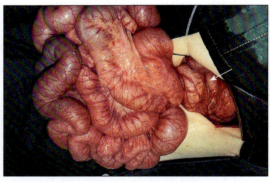

FIGURE 18.29 Malrotation: operative appearance of the twist in the mesentery of the midgut. The intestine is viable.

DUPLICATIONS OF THE ALIMENTARY TRACT

INCIDENCE/AETIOLOGY

Duplications can occur anywhere in the alimentary tract, from the mouth to the anus. They most commonly occur in the small bowel mesentery. Duplications comprise a mucosal lining, frequently of an area remote from the site of duplication, and a muscular wall. They may be cystic or tubular in form.

The neurenteric canal theory of origin of duplication is generally accepted with failure of the canal to resorb totally.

CLINICAL PRESENTATION

Cystic duplications (**Fig. 18.30**) cause symptoms from pressure on the adjacent intestine. The most common clinical features are those of intestinal obstruction in association with a palpable mass. Tubular duplications (**Fig. 18.31**) cause symptoms from peptic ulceration due to an acid-secreting mucosal lining. The ulceration develops in the adjacent normal intestine that is unable to resist acid peptic digestion.

DIAGNOSIS

An ultrasound scan will reveal the cystic nature of the mass. In tubular duplication, a technetium pertechnetate scan may reveal the presence of ectopic gastric mucosa. The presence of split vertebra in the upper thoracic spine provides additional diagnostic support.

TREATMENT

Excision of the duplication with or without the adjacent intestine and end-to-end anastomosis is the treatment of choice. Where long lengths of intestine are involved or when the site of duplication is in a critical area (duodenum), stripping of the mucosal lining is the best option.

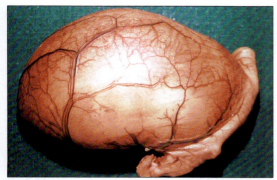

FIGURE 18.30 Cystic duplication.

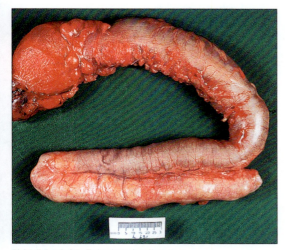

FIGURE 18.31 Tubular duplication.

NECROTISING ENTEROCOLITIS

INCIDENCE

Neonatal necrotising enterocolitis (NEC) occurs predominantly in the stressed premature infant and is currently one of the most common neonatal surgical emergency conditions.

AETIOLOGY

Although not completely clear, it would appear that certain factors (e.g. prematurity, the presence of intraluminal substrate [breast milk is protective] and micro-organisms [*Klebsiella*, *E coli*, *Clostridia*]) are commonly present. Other contributing factors, such as hypoxia, hypovolaemia, hyperviscosity, hypotension and hypothermia, may be important. The most frequently affected parts of the GI tract are the terminal ileum and caecum and the splenic flexure of the colon. The final common pathway in the pathogenesis of the condition is an ischaemic process.

PATHOLOGY

The mesenteric ischaemia leads progressively from mucosal ulceration through to full-thickness necrosis and perforation with peritonitis.

CLINICAL PRESENTATION

The first sign of the onset of NEC is reluctance of the infant to feed. This is followed rapidly by bilious vomiting or nasogastric aspirate, the passage of blood and mucus in the stool and abdominal distension (**Fig. 18.32**). Erythema and/or oedema of the anterior abdominal wall is indicative of impending intestinal gangrene with perforation. In severe cases, the infant becomes shocked and hypovolaemic.

DIAGNOSIS

The hallmark of the diagnosis is the finding of pneumatosis intestinalis on plain abdominal x-ray. Free air (pneumoperitoneum) is indicative of perforation. Gas in the portal venous system may be a sign of advanced disease (**Figs 18.33–18.35**).

TREATMENT

Immediate resuscitation is required in all cases. Conservative treatment consists of nasogastric aspiration, broad-spectrum antibiotics and complete GI rest for 7–10 days, during which total parenteral nutrition is administered.

Indications for surgery are intestinal perforation, intestinal obstruction or failure to respond to conservative measures. Late indication for surgery is stricture formation.

Operative procedures comprise resection with primary anastomosis or resection with stoma formation.

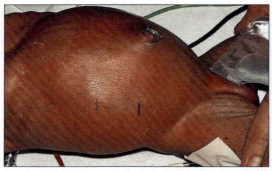

FIGURE 18.32 Premature infant with necrotising enterocolitis, displaying a distended abdomen, with redness and oedema of the abdominal wall.

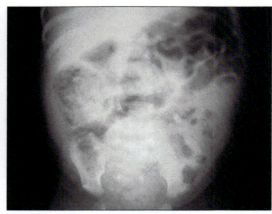

FIGURE 18.33 Necrotising enterocolitis: plain x-ray showing pneumatosis intestinalis (gas in the bowel wall).

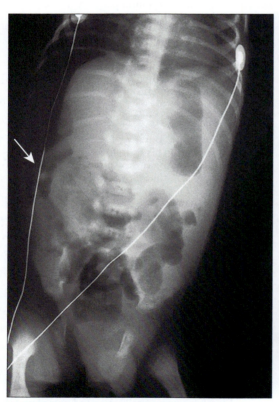

FIGURE 18.34 Necrotising enterocolitis: plain x-ray showing pneumoperitoneum indicative of a perforation.

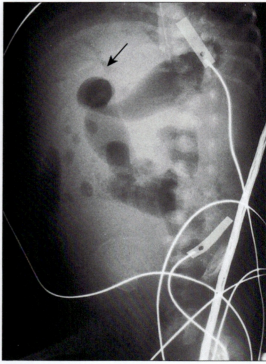

FIGURE 18.35 Necrotising enterocolitis: plain x-ray showing portal venous gas.

EXOMPHALOS

INCIDENCE/AETIOLOGY

Exomphalos occurs in 1 in 5,000 live births and is failure of the physiological umbilical hernia to reduce fully into the abdominal cavity by the 12th week of gestation.

CLINICAL PRESENTATION

The infant is born with an obvious defect in the umbilicus. The anomaly can be detected early in intrauterine life on ultrasound scan. The covering of the sac comprises an outer layer of amnion and an inner layer of peritoneum, with intervening layers of Wharton's jelly.

Exomphalos may be divided into two categories:

- Minor – defect <5 cm (**Fig. 18.36**).
- Major – defect >5 cm (**Fig. 18.37**).

Major exomphalos is associated with a high incidence of associated anomalies, e.g. cardiac, GI, genitourinary. It is also associated with the chromosomal anomaly, Beckwith syndrome (exomphalos, gigantism, macroglossia and hypoglycaemia).

INVESTIGATIONS

- Monitoring of blood glucose levels.
- Cardiac ECHO.

TREATMENT

Prenatal counselling should be offered, especially for larger exomphalos, including exclusion of a chromosomal anomaly; cardiac ECHO and detection of associated defects.

Immediately postnatal, the sac must be covered with plastic wrap to prevent excessive fluid and heat loss. Minor lesions are amenable to primary closure of the defect. Major lesions may be treated by surgical application of a silo (preformed or surgically applied), with gradual progressive reduction of the contents into the abdomen or application of an escharic agent.

PROGNOSIS

Small lesions and larger exomphalos without associated anomalies have a good prognosis. Large exomphalos with other major associated anomalies have a poor prognosis.

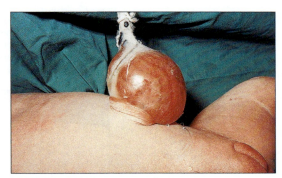

FIGURE 18.36 Minor exomphalos.

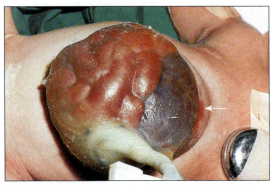

FIGURE 18.37 Major exomphalos including liver (arrow).

GASTROSCHISIS

INCIDENCE

Gastroschisis occurs in 1 in 3,000 live births. The incidence appears to have increased in recent years. The term denotes an extrusion of part of the intestine through a defect to the right of an intact umbilicus.

PRENATAL DIAGNOSIS

The lesion is usually recognised on routine antenatal scan (**Fig. 18.38**). As it is not accompanied by any other major congenital anomaly, no further prenatal investigations are necessary.

DIAGNOSIS

The diagnosis is self-evident at birth (**Fig. 18.39**). The lesion with the extruded bowel, which may be grossly thickened and oedematous, should be covered with plastic wrap to prevent fluid and heat loss.

TREATMENT

Emergency repair of the defect should be undertaken as soon as possible after birth, when the bowel is generally pliable and easily reduced into the peritoneal cavity. If the extruded intestine is thickened and matted it will be necessary to place the bowel in a silo as a temporary measure.

PROGNOSIS

Prognosis is excellent, except in infants with associated intestinal atresia or short-bowel syndrome.

UMBILICAL HERNIA

CLINICAL PRESENTATION

The hernia occurs through a defect in the umbilical cicatrix and usually contains omentum only (**Fig. 18.40**). Umbilical hernia is extremely common in infancy and particularly in black infants. These hernias tend to resolve spontaneously by the time the children reach the age of 5 years. Incarceration is extremely unlikely except in the large truncated variety (**Fig. 18.41**).

TREATMENT

Surgery is undertaken for large truncated hernias in infancy or following failure to close spontaneously after the age of 5 years. The operative procedure consists of closure of the neck of the hernial sac and repair of the fascia surrounding the defect.

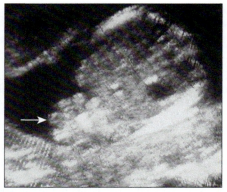

FIGURE 18.38 Gastroschisis: prenatal scan showing intestinal loops outside the peritoneal cavity of the fetus (arrow).

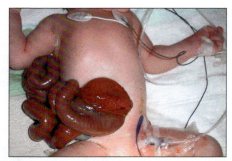

FIGURE 18.39 Gastroschisis: appearance of the infant at birth with a large amount of intestine extruding through a defect in the abdominal wall just to the right of the umbilical cord.

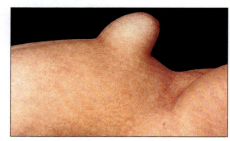

FIGURE 18.40 Umbilical hernia of moderate size.

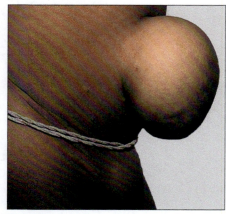

FIGURE 18.41 Umbilical hernia: large, truncated.

UMBILICAL ANOMALIES

INCIDENCE

A number of defects can occur at the umbilicus. Each requires precise diagnosis as their treatment differs considerably:

- Umbilical granuloma: due to failure of the umbilical cord to separate completely. Application of silver nitrate to the granulation tissue will result in its resolution (**Fig. 18.42**).
- Umbilical polyp: due to persistence of a remnant of the vitello-intestinal duct at the umbilicus. It is covered by mucosa that requires formal excision (**Fig. 18.43**).

- Patent vitello-intestinal duct. There is a fistula at the umbilicus through which intestinal content is evacuated. There is a distinct risk of prolapse of the intestine through the fistula or volvulus around the 'band'. Urgent surgery is required to excise the fistula from the umbilicus to the ileum and restore intestinal continuity by end-to-end anastomosis (**Fig. 18.44**).
- Patent urachus. This is a communication between the bladder dome and the umbilicus that may produce a persistent urinary leak. It is important to exclude a bladder outlet obstruction (e.g. posterior urethral valves) before attempting closure of the urachal remnant (**Fig. 18.45**).

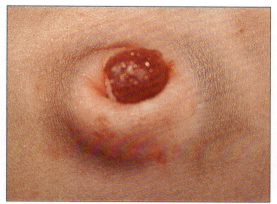

FIGURE 18.42 Umbilical granuloma: an infected remnant of the umbilical cord that has failed to separate completely.

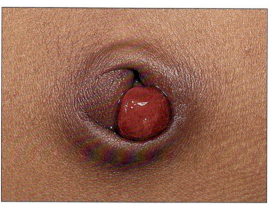

FIGURE 18.43 Umbilical polyp: mucosal remnant of the vitello-intestinal duct at the umbilicus.

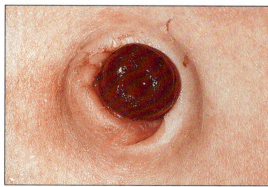

FIGURE 18.44 Patent vitello-intestinal duct due to persistence of the duct, which allows discharge of faeces.

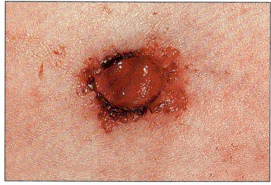

FIGURE 18.45 Patent urachus causing a urinary discharge from the orifice of the duct.

GASTROINTESTINAL HAEMORRHAGE

The presence of blood in the stool is an alarming symptom, which is promptly brought to the attention of the doctor. It is important to determine the nature and quantity of blood loss and to search for additional physical signs such as hypovolaemic shock, anaemia or bilious vomiting. Swallowed maternal blood may lead to the appearance of blood in the vomitus or in the stool. To differentiate between maternal and fetal blood, the Apt test is used. Mixing the material with sodium hydroxide will colour adult haemoglobin brown while fetal haemoglobin remains pink.

DIAGNOSIS

The age of the patient may be an important determinant of the likely cause of haemorrhage:

- Age <2 years: volvulus, NEC, intussusception, Meckel's diverticulum, Cow milk protein allergy.
- Age >2 years: oesophageal varices, peptic ulceration, colonic polyps, inflammatory bowel disease.

A diagnostic scheme for children presenting with rectal bleeding is shown in **Fig. 18.46**.

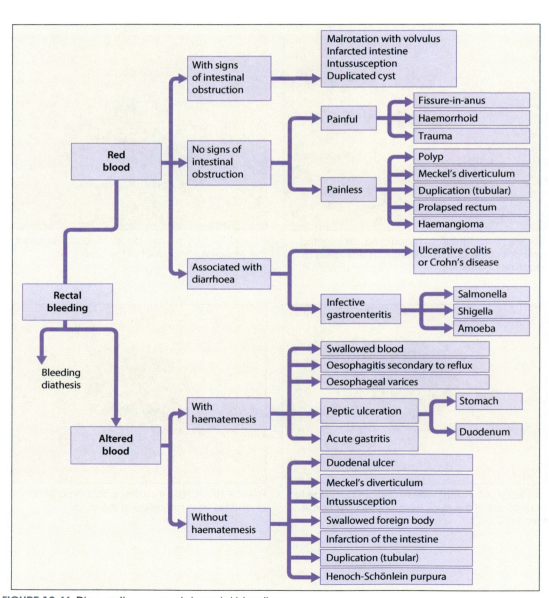

FIGURE 18.46 Diagnostic approach to rectal bleeding.

MECKEL DIVERTICULUM

INCIDENCE

Meckel diverticulum represents persistence of the intestinal end of the vitello-intestinal duct. It is present in 2% of the population, is located around 60 cm (2 feet) from the ileocaecal junction and may remain asymptomatic throughout life (**Fig. 18.47**).

CLINICAL PRESENTATION

Symptoms arise out of complications with GI bleeding, due to the presence of ectopic gastric mucosa causing ulceration in the adjacent ileal mucosa (**Fig. 18.48**). Haemorrhage can be significant and is dark red in colour. The most frequent age at which GI bleeding occurs is 6–24 months. Intestinal obstruction may be due to kinking of the intestine by a fibrous band arising at the mesenteric attachment, or intussusception with the Meckel diverticulum at its apex, or volvulus around a band connecting the Meckel diverticulum to the umbilicus. Diverticulitis can mimic acute appendicitis.

DIAGNOSIS

In the presence of ectopic gastric mucosa, the Meckel scan will detect uptake of technetium, which localises in the gastric mucosa (**Fig. 18.49**).

TREATMENT

Operative management consists of resection of the Meckel diverticulum together with a segment of the adjacent ileum and end-to-end anastomosis or wedge-resection and closure of the defect.

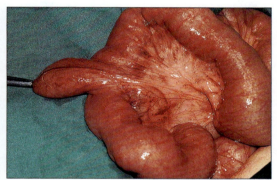

FIGURE 18.47 Typical appearance of a Meckel diverticulum originating on the antimesenteric border of the distal ileum.

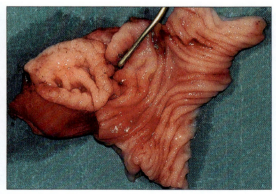

FIGURE 18.48 Opened Meckel diverticulum showing typical ectopic gastric mucosa leading to ulceration at the junction with the ileum. The ulcer may bleed or perforate.

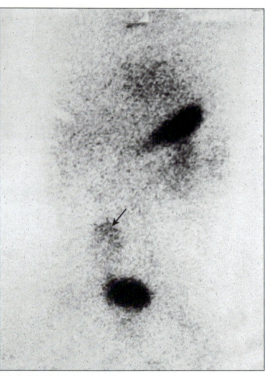

FIGURE 18.49 Technetium (Tc99) isotope scan showing simultaneous appearance of isotope in the stomach, Meckel diverticulum and bladder.

PYLORIC STENOSIS

INCIDENCE

Pyloric stenosis occurs in 1 in 400. The pyloric muscle undergoes hypertrophy creating gastric outlet obstruction. A family history is common. Male to female ratio is 4:1.

CLINICAL PRESENTATION

The onset of vomiting usually commences at 2–4 weeks of age. The vomiting is projectile and non-bilious leading to weight loss, dehydration and electrolyte disturbance characterised by hypochloraemic metabolic alkalosis. Visible gastric peristalsis may be seen on the abdomen. The diagnosis is based on clinical examination with the palpation of the typical olive-shaped pyloric 'tumour' in the right upper quadrant of the abdomen. Ultrasound assessment of the pylorus shows thickened pyloric musculature measuring >17 mm in length and >4 mm thickness (**Figs 18.50, 18.51**).

TREATMENT

Electrolyte disturbance is corrected with half normal saline and potassium. Myotomy (open or laparoscopic) of the pyloric muscle preserving the mucosal layer is curative with infants usually discharged within 24 hours after surgery (**Fig. 18.52**).

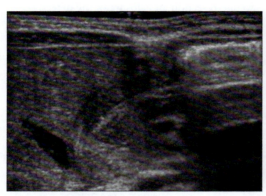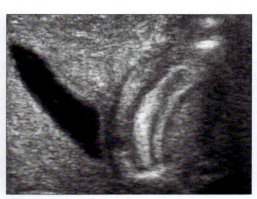

FIGURES 18.50, 18.51 Ultrasound scan showing thickened pyloric musculature.

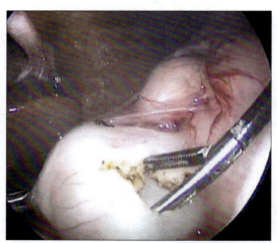

FIGURE 18.52 Operative view of pyloromyotomy showing split thickened pyloric muscle down to, but not including mucosa.

Neonatal and general paediatric surgery

INTUSSUSCEPTION

INCIDENCE

Intussusception occurs in 1 in 250 infants. An intussusception consists of invagination of one part of the intestine into the adjacent bowel. This causes an incomplete obstruction which, if unrelieved, leads to complete obstruction together with impairment of the vascularity to the invaginated (intussusceptum) bowel, initially venous congestion but ultimately ischaemic necrosis. The ileocaecal region is the most common site but any portion of the intestinal tract may be involved.

Peak incidence is 6–9 months of age, with a seasonal variation of increased incidence in spring and early summer and again in mid-winter.

PATHOPHYSIOLOGY

Over 95% of cases of intussusception in the age range 3–24 months do not have a recognisable leading pathological point and are assumed to occur as a result of an enlarged Peyer patch, secondary to an enteral infection. Leading points occur in 5% of cases and comprise polyps, Meckel diverticulum, duplications and tumours.

CLINICAL PRESENTATION

The cardinal signs of intussusception include colicky abdominal pain, during which the infant draws up his/her legs and goes pale, vomiting (initially of food only but, as the obstructive element develops, becoming bilious and eventually faeculent) and the passage of 'redcurrant jelly'-like stools *per rectum* are. It may be possible to palpate a 'sausage-shaped' mass in the right upper quadrant of the abdomen.

DIAGNOSIS

Diagnosis is by history, clinical examination and with investigations. Plain abdominal x-ray shows an absence of gas in the right iliac fossa and may show a soft tissue mass of the apex of the intussusception (**Fig. 18.53**).

Ultrasonography: shows the intussusception with a 'doughnut' appearance (**Figs 18.54, 18.55**).

Contrast radiography: shows the apex of the intussusception in the colon (meniscus sign) and seepage of contrast around the intussusception (coiled spring sign) (**Fig. 18.56**).

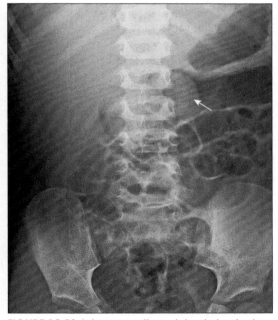

FIGURE 18.53 Intussusception: plain abdominal x-ray showing obstructed small intestinal loops and an 'empty' right iliac fossa and flank. The arrow shows a soft tissue mass of the apex of the intussusception.

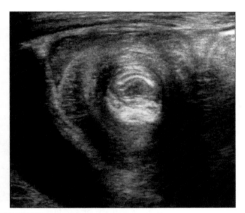

FIGURE 18.54 Ultrasound scan of an intussusception showing 'doughnut' appearance.

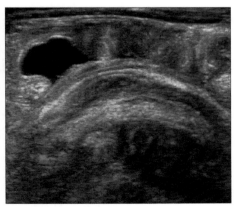

FIGURE 18.55 Ultrasound scan showing 'pseudokidney' appearance of an intussusception.

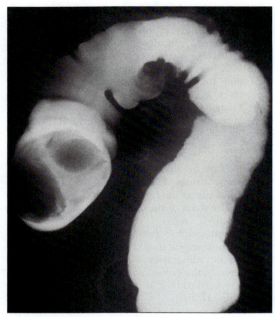

FIGURE 18.56 Intussusception: barium enema showing an intraluminal obstruction in the right transverse colon.

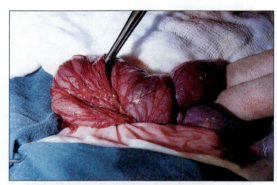

FIGURE 18.57 Intussusception: operative appearance of an ileocolic intussusception.

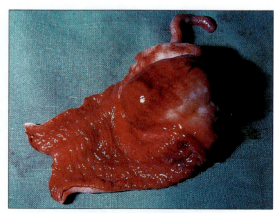

FIGURE 18.58 Intussusception with a duplication cyst as the leading point.

TREATMENT

Resuscitation as required is an essential first priority. Non-operative reduction uses air or contrast (hydrostatic) under fluoroscopic or ultrasound control. Contraindications for non-operative reduction are the presence of shock/toxicity, evidence of necrotic intestine or perforation.

Operative treatment consists of reduction of a viable intussusception (**Fig. 18.57**) or resection and primary anastomosis for necrotic intestine or to resect a pathological leading point (**Fig. 18.58**).

SACROCOCCYGEAL TERATOMA

INCIDENCE AND TYPES

Sacrococcygeal teratoma occurs in 1 in 40,000 live births.

- Stage I: external sacrococcygeal mass (46%).
- Stage II: mostly external but with presacral extension (35%).
- Stage III: mostly presacral but with external element (9%).
- Stage IV: entire presacral in location (10%).

The tumour consists of derivatives of all three germ cell elements: ecto-, endo- and mesoderm.

PRENATAL DIAGNOSIS

The presence of a large sacrococcygeal teratoma can be detected on prenatal ultrasound scan. The mode of delivery may be dictated by the size of the lesion, with elective caesarean section recommended for large lesions capable of causing dystocia or bleeding or rupture during delivery.

CLINICAL PRESENTATION

There may be a visible sacrococcygeal tumour at birth (**Figs 18.59, 18.60**). Rectal examination will determine the extent of presacral extension.

DIAGNOSIS

Plain x-ray may reveal calcification in the mass (**Fig. 18.61**).

TREATMENT

Resection of the tumour *en bloc* with the coccyx is performed soon after birth. Incidence of malignancy:

- 1% at birth.
- 30% at 6 months of age.
- α-fetoprotein levels elevated in malignancy.

PROGNOSIS

Urinary and anorectal neuropathy may be present.

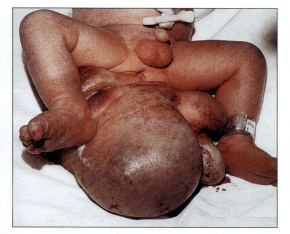

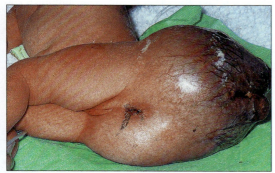

FIGURES 18.59, 18.60 Clinical appearance of infants with massive sacrococcygeal - teratomas.

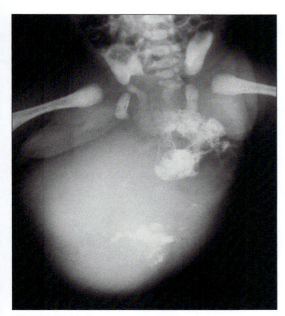

FIGURE 18.61 Sacrococcygeal teratoma: x-ray showing calcification in the mass.

APPENDICITIS

INCIDENCE

Appendicitis is one of the most common causes of acute abdominal pain in children.

CLINICAL PRESENTATION

The classical presentation is with acute onset of vague periumbilical pain that rapidly radiates and localises in the right iliac fossa, where it is continuous in nature. The pain is invariably accompanied by anorexia and nausea, which usually culminates in vomiting. There is usually constipation, but diarrhoea may develop when there is pelvic appendicitis. Most children have a low-grade pyrexia of 38–39°C. Physical examination reveals localised tenderness in the right lower quadrant of the abdomen, ranging from pain on deep palpation in the earlier stages to guarding and rigidity later in the course of the disease. Rebound tenderness causes intense distress and should not be attempted. Infants under the age of 2 years generally present with perforated appendicitis and peritonitis.

DIAGNOSIS

Clinical features typical of appendicitis include:

- Leukocytosis of $10–15 \times 10^9/l$.
- Plain x-ray of abdomen may rarely show a faecolith (**Fig. 18.62**).
- Ultrasound scan may rarely show thickening of the wall of the appendix and free fluid in the right iliac fossa.
- MRI scan in difficult cases.
- Diagnostic laparoscopy.

TREATMENT

For children in whom the diagnosis is not in doubt, the decision to proceed immediately on clinical findings to appendicectomy should be made (**Fig. 18.63**). Where the diagnosis is in doubt, a period of active observation in hospital should be undertaken. The diagnosis of appendicitis will become clear within 24–48 hours.

In patients with perforated appendicitis and peritonitis, a period of active resuscitation with intravenous fluids, nasogastric decompression and intravenous antibiotics are essential prior to appendicectomy. In the presence of an established mass conservative treatment with antibiotics alone and delayed appendecectomy may be appropriate.

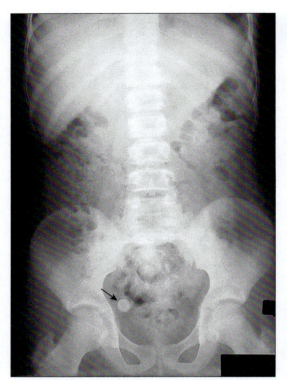

FIGURE 18.62 Appendicitis: plain abdominal x-ray showing a faecolith in the right iliac fossa (arrow).

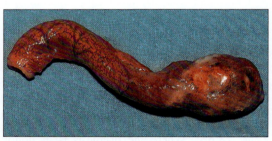

FIGURE 18.63 Appendicitis: operative specimen of an acute appendicitis.

NECK LESIONS

During childhood, a variety of lesions occur in the neck. These are remnants of embryonic structures that have failed to resorb completely during development.

CYSTIC HYGROMA

Cystic hygroma are multi-cystic malformations of the lymphatic system and comprise innumerable small cystic spaces or larger single cysts.

INCIDENCE

The majority of cystic hygromas are located in the neck, but they also occur in the axilla, abdomen and groin. They appear as soft, cystic, discrete non-tender masses that are transilluminable. They vary in size from a few centimetres in diameter to lesions that encase the entire neck (**Figs 18.64, 18.65**). These latter lesions are particularly hazardous, in that rapid enlargement can develop as a result of inflammation; this can cause acute respiratory distress from compression of the airway, or dysphagia from compression of the oesophagus.

DIAGNOSIS

Diagnosis is on clinical examination followed by ultrasonography to confirm the cystic nature of the lesion and also the extent of involvement. CT or MRI will define the lesion more accurately and may be helpful in planning surgical excision.

TREATMENT

Spontaneous regression of the cystic hygroma is excessively rare. Injection sclerotherapy is now the main treatment of choice (e.g. hypertonic saline, bleomycin, doxycycline, OK-432). Surgical excision is reserved for persistent disease or recurrence and may prove difficult due to 'infiltration' of the cysts between vital structures (e.g. carotid artery, internal jugular vein, phrenic nerve, cranial nerves). It is important NOT to sacrifice vital structures but to accept that recurrences will occur, which can then be treated on their merits.

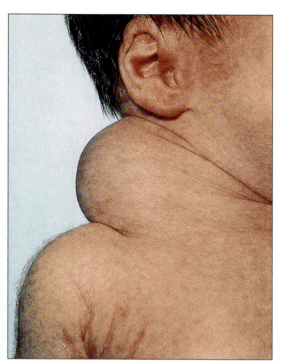

BRANCHIAL SINUS/CYST

These arise out of failure of obliteration of the second pharyngeal pouch. Complete retention of the pouch leads to the development of a branchial fistula with an external opening in the lower one-third of the neck at the anterior border of the sternomastoid muscle (**Fig. 18.66**). The fistula extends from this tiny opening, which constantly produces mucus, through the subcutaneous tissue and platysma muscle, beneath the digastric muscle, over the hypoglossal and glossopharyngeal nerves and between the bifurcation of the carotid artery, to enter the lateral wall of the pharynx. Incomplete obliteration leaves remnants of the tract; these enlarge to form branchial cysts that are located deep to the sternomastoid muscle in the anterior triangle of the neck.

TREATMENT

Excision of the lesion and the associated tract is performed.

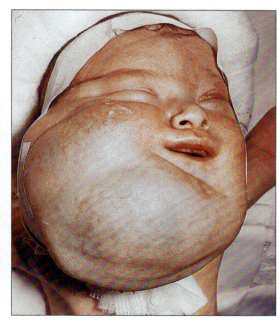

FIGURE 18.65 Massive cystic hygroma, extending from the temporal region across the parotid and cheek to cross the midline of the neck. The lesion caused respiratory embarrassment necessitating the tracheostomy.

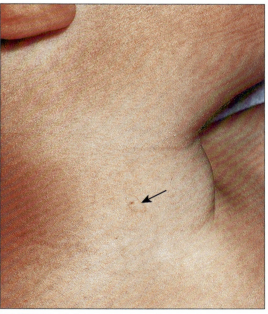

FIGURE 18.66 Branchial sinus. There is a tiny opening on the right side of the neck, anterior to the junction between the upper two-thirds and lower one-third of the sternomastoid muscles (arrow).

PREAURICULAR SINUS

This occurs anterior to the tragus of the ear and may contain hair and other skin appendages (**Fig. 18.67**). They may be asymptomatic but are prone to infection, which will only respond to wide excision.

TREATMENT

Elective excision of uninfected sinuses is recommended.

SACRAL SINUSES

These occur mostly below the level of the natal cleft.

DIAGNOSIS

This is based on clinical examination and an appreciation of the depth of the sinus.

TREATMENT

For sinuses below the natal cleft and in the midline no treatment is needed and parents are reassured. High lesions (**Fig. 18.68**), those aside the midline or with abnormal overlying skin should have MRI assessment to rule out spinal pathology.

DERMOID CYSTS

These occur at lines of embryonic fusion. The cyst wall contains sebaceous glands, hair follicles, connective tissue and papillae.

DIAGNOSIS

The most common location is the lateral supraorbital region (**Fig. 18.69**), and in the midline of the neck. They must be differentiated from thyroglossal cysts, which contains mucoid material, in contrast to the sebaceous content of dermoid cysts.

TREATMENT

Treatment is complete excision.

THYROGLOSSAL CYSTS/FISTULAE

Thyroglossal cysts and fistulae arise out of remnants of the thyroglossal tract that fails to involute, following descent of the thyroid gland from the region of the foramen caecum of the tongue to its final position in the lower midline of the neck. Complete failure of migration leads to the development of a lingual thyroid. When the thyroid descends fully but remnants of the tract remain, a thyroglossal cyst may develop.

DIAGNOSIS

The thyroglossal cyst is characteristically midline in location at approximately the level of the hyoid bone (**Fig. 18.70**) (see Chapter 19 Otorhinolaryngology, page 592). The non-inflamed cyst is smooth and not tender and moves with swallowing and protrusion of the tongue. Inflammation results in a red, tender, well-localised swelling in the midline of the neck which, following drainage, produces a mucoid discharge. Ultrasound examination is essential to confirm the presence of the normal thyroid gland.

TREATMENT

Excision of the cyst and the thyroglossal tract upwards to the base of the tongue, including the central portion of the hyoid bone is performed.

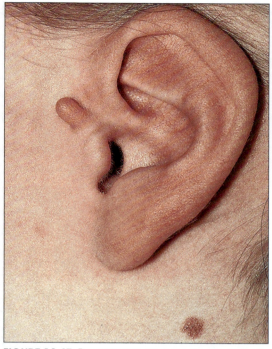

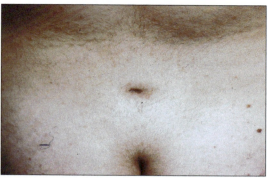

FIGURE 18.68 Typical appearance of a sacral sinus in the lower midline of the back overlying the sacrum.

FIGURE 18.67 Preauricular sinus located anterior to the tragus of the ear. They may be marked with a remnant of cartilaginous tissue.

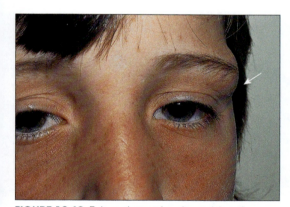

FIGURE 18.69 External angular dermoid cyst affecting the left lateral upper eyebrow.

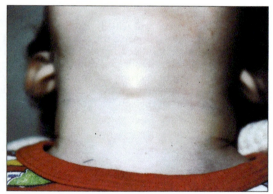

FIGURE 18.70 Classical appearance of a thyroglossal cyst in the midline of the neck overlying the hyoid bone.

INGUINAL HERNIA

INCIDENCE

Inguinal hernia occurs in 1–2 per 100 live births, but may be as high as 20–30% in premature infants. Male infants are four times more frequently affected than females and the right side twice as often as the left.

CLINICAL PRESENTATION

An inguinal hernia in a child comprises the protrusion of part of the intestine into the patent processus vaginalis. The hernia may be complete when it extends down into the scrotum or incomplete when it stops short in the groin. In infancy, the first presentation may be as an incarcerated hernia, but generally there is an intermittent swelling in the groin and/or scrotum, which is noticed by the parents during bathing or changing of the nappy (**Figs 18.71, 18.72**). In female infants, there is a bulge in the groin that may extend into the labia and may contain an ovary (**Fig. 18.73**).

DIAGNOSIS

Clinical presence of a hernia or a good history provided by the parents is diagnostic.

TREATMENT

In infancy there is a significant risk of irreducibility and urgent surgery is generally recommended. At all ages, a simple herniotomy (open or laparoscopic) is all that is required.

Irreducible hernias will usually reduce spontaneously or with 'taxis' following the administration of the analgesia. A strangulated hernia requires urgent resuscitation followed by surgical reduction of viable contents, resection of necrotic intestine, followed by herniotomy. The ipsilateral testis may be congested due to obstruction of the venous return.

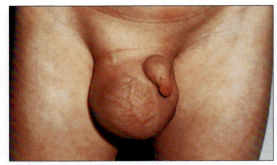

FIGURE 18.71 Uncomplicated right inguinal hernia.

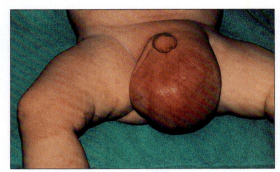

FIGURE 18.72 Incarcerated left inguinal hernia.

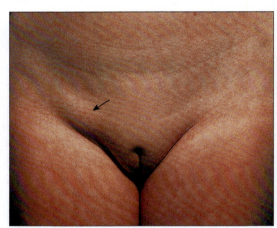

FIGURE 18.73 Right inguinal hernia in a girl (arrow).

Neonatal and general paediatric surgery

HYDROCOELE

Failure of the processus vaginalis to undergo obliteration leads to the development of an inguinal hernia. When the communication between the peritoneal cavity is very narrow, the passage of peritoneal fluid only is possible and this results in the formation of a hydrocoele, which may occupy the tunica vaginalis and surround the testis or may occur as a localised swelling anywhere along the cord.

CLINICAL PRESENTATION

A scrotal hydrocoele appears as a soft, non-tender, fluid-filled sac that is transilluminable. The swelling may fluctuate somewhat in size and it is possible to palpate a normal cord above the swelling. A hydrocoele of the cord presents as a well-circumscribed, fluid-filled mass in the inguinal region (**Figs 18.74, 18.75**).

TREATMENT

The majority of scrotal hydrocoeles regress spontaneously within the first 2 years of life. Operative correction is as for an inguinal hernia, with ligation and division of the patent processus vaginalis and evacuation of fluid from the scrotum.

UNDESCENDED TESTIS

The testes develop in the mesonephric ridge on the posterior abdominal wall. Descent occurs in two phases, both of which involve the gubernaculum:

- In the first phase (10–15 weeks) the gubernaculum enlarges and anchors the testis close to the inguinal region.
- In the second phase (28–35 weeks), the gubernaculum migrates out of the inguinal canal across the pubic region and into the scrotum. The processus vaginalis develops as a peritoneal outpouching within the gubernaculum and creates a space into which the testis descends.

INCIDENCE

An 'empty' scrotum is present in 2–4% of mature newborn male infants and in 20–30% of premature infants (**Fig. 18.76**). 'Spontaneous' descent can occur up to 6 months of age and by the age of 1 year the incidence is around 1%.

TYPES OF MALDESCENT

- Retractile testis is a normal testis that retracts into the inguinal canal by an actively contracting cremaster muscle. No surgery is required.
- Ectopic testis is a testis that has descended normally through the external inguinal ring and then taken an abnormal course – prepubic, perineal, femoral.
- Incompletely descended testis that has come to rest along a normal pathway of descent (e.g. intra-abdominal, at the internal ring or within the inguinal canal).

CLINICAL PRESENTATION

Absence of the testis is found at routine examination.

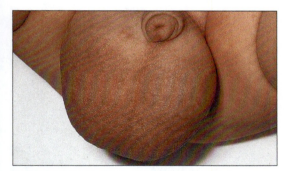

FIGURE 18.74 Hydrocoele: bilateral scrotal swellings.

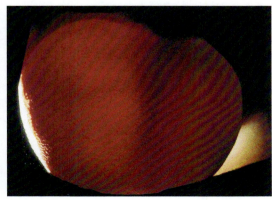

FIGURE 18.75 Hydrocoele: transillumination depicting fluid in the scrotal sac.

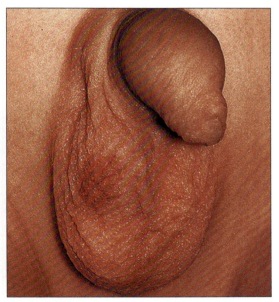

FIGURE 18.76 Left undescended testis with an empty left scrotum.

INDICATIONS FOR SURGERY

- To preserve spermatogenesis – degenerative changes occur around the age of 1 year.
- To treat an associated indirect inguinal hernia.
- To prevent torsion, which is more common in the undescended testis.
- To reduce the incidence of trauma.
- To place the testis in a position where the diagnosis of malignancy can be made early. Surgery does not change this risk.
- For psychological reasons.

OPERATIVE PROCEDURE

Orchidopexy is the mobilisation of the testis and spermatic cord and fixation of the testis within the scrotum. It is recommended that the optimal age for orchidopexy is between 6 and 12 months.

TORSION OF THE TESTIS

Testicular torsion occurs when the spermatic cord twists and occludes the blood supply to the testis and epididymis (**Figs 18.77, 18.78**).

CLINICAL PRESENTATION

There are two common varieties:

- **Extravaginal**, due to twisting of the spermatic cord outside the tunica vaginalis secondary to inadequate fixation of the testis within the scrotum. This type usually occurs prenatally and the infant is born with an enlarged, non-tender testis. The testis is non-viable but it is vital to perform a contralateral orchidopexy as soon as possible to protect this testis.
- **Intravaginal**, due to abnormal suspension of the testis and epididymis within the tunica vaginalis ('bell-clapper anomaly'). The testis lies horizontally and the twist occurs towards the midline. Peak incidence is in older children.

DIAGNOSIS

Children present with an acute onset of severe pain in the scrotum. The testis is swollen and acutely tender and is often elevated within the scrotum. There is frequently associated nausea and vomiting. Torsion of the testis can often be differentiated on clinical examination from torsion of a testicular appendage, which appears as a tender nodule at the upper pole of the testis. Doppler ultrasound scan and/or radio-isotope tests, if immediately available, may help to differentiate torsion from acute epididymo-orchitis. If in doubt it is best to treat as a torsion.

TREATMENT

Urgent surgical exploration with untwisting of the torsion is necessary. If viable, the testis is anchored within the scrotum whereas a necrotic testis should be excised. It is mandatory to anchor the contralateral testis.

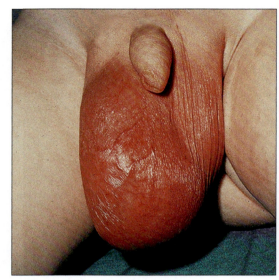

FIGURE 18.77 Torsion of the right testis showing a swollen, erythematous, right scrotal swelling.

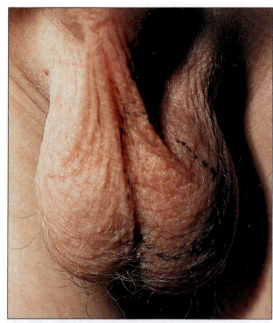

FIGURE 18.78 Torsion of a testicular appendage, which presents as a painful, tender nodule on the upper part of the scrotum above a normal testis. If the diagnosis is in doubt, it is safer to explore the scrotum.

PHIMOSIS

Phimosis is the inability to retract the foreskin over the glans. It is physiological in the early years of life (**Fig. 18.79**).

CLINICAL PRESENTATION

Pathological phimosis rarely occurs before the age of 6 years. The foreskin is scarred and whitish in appearance and the opening is severely narrowed resulting in non-retractability (**Fig. 18.80**). During micturition there may be ballooning of the foreskin and dribbling may occur after voiding. Following an erection, the narrowed foreskin may remain around the glans, constricting its blood supply and culminate in a paraphimosis. The paraphimosis is an extremely painful swelling of the glans that requires emergency treatment either in reduction of the foreskin or a dorsal slit if reduction is not possible.

TREATMENT

Pathological phimosis is an absolute indication for circumcision. Preputial adhesions are common in the first few years of life and normally resolve spontaneously – they do not constitute an indication for circumcision.

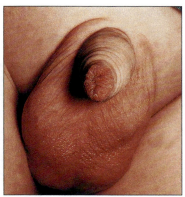

FIGURE 18.79 Non-retractable foreskin – a normal phenomenon.

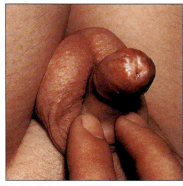

FIGURE 18.80 Phimosis showing evidence of scarring of the foreskin resulting in non-retractability – a pathological condition.

BILIARY ATRESIA

INCIDENCE/AETIOLOGY

Biliary atresia occurs in 1 in 12,000. The aetiology is unknown but many theories have been postulated, including a genetic susceptibility, metabolic, infective and anatomical factors such as an abnormally long common channel at the junction of the biliary and pancreatic ducts.

CLINICAL PRESENTATION

Prolonged jaundice occurs in the first few weeks of life. In addition, the stools are greyish in colour.

INVESTIGATIONS

Investigations include: elevated conjugated serum bilirubin; hepatobiliary radionuclide imaging (DISIDA scan); ultrasound scan; endoscopic retrograde cholangiopancreatography (ERCP); laparoscopy; percutaneous liver biopsy; operative cholangiography.

DIFFERENTIAL DIAGNOSIS

- Neonatal hepatitis, α-1-antitrypsin deficiency.
- Types of anomalies (**Fig. 18.81**):
  - Type 1: atresia of the common bile duct, which may be associated with a dilatation of the common hepatic duct at the porta hepatis (5%).
  - Type 2: atresia of the common hepatic duct with residual patency of the right and left hepatic ducts (3%).
  - Type 3: atresia of the whole of the extrahepatic biliary system (92%).

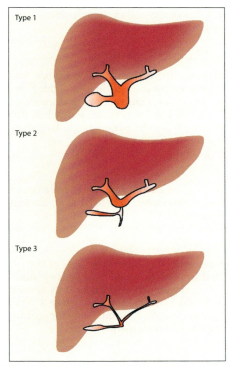

FIGURE 18.81 Three types of biliary atresia.

TREATMENT

Exploration of the extrahepatic biliary system and hepaticojejunostomy is performed with a Roux-en-Y loop.

PROGNOSIS

The success rate is greatest when drainage of the biliary system is achieved within the first 3 months of life. Liver transplantation is a viable option for children who fail to respond to portoenterostomy or who develop intractable liver cirrhosis at a later age.

CHOLEDOCHAL CYST

A choledochal cyst is a dilatation of the biliary system, which may affect the extrahepatic and/or the intrahepatic bile ducts (**Figs 18.82, 18.83**).

CLASSIFICATION

- Type I: cystic dilatation of the extrahepatic bile ducts with or without dilatation of the intrahepatic ducts.
- Type II: fusiform dilatation of the extrahepatic ducts with or without dilatation of the intrahepatic ducts, which are fusiformly dilated.
- Type III: miscellaneous:
  - diverticulum of common bile duct.
  - intraduodenal choledochocele.
  - intrahepatic dilatation alone (Caroli).

AETIOLOGY

The aetiology is unknown, but two factors appear to be implicated:

- Weakness of the wall of the bile duct.
- Distal obstruction.

CLINICAL PRESENTATION

In infancy, obstructive jaundice occurs with pale stools or a palpable mass in the right hypochondrium. **In older children**, mild jaundice occurs, which may be intermittent, an abdominal pain or a palpable mass. Rarely, ascending cholangitis or pancreatitis are present.

DIAGNOSIS

Diagnosis is based on abdominal ultrasonography; DISIDA scintigraphy; CT/MRI scan; barium meal examination; ERCP.

TREATMENT

The treatment of choice is excision of the cyst and gall bladder and Roux-en-Y hepaticojejunostomy. Internal drainage procedures, such as cystoduodenostomy and cystojejunostomy, carry a significant postoperative complication rate for cholangitis, pancreatitis and malignancy.

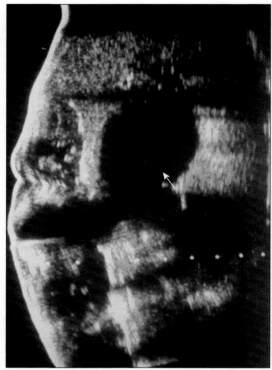

FIGURE 18.82 Choledochal cyst: ultrasound scan revealing the cystic lesion inferior to the liver.

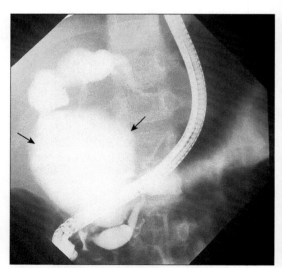

FIGURE 18.83 Choledochal cyst: endoscopic retrograde cholangiogram showing the cystic dilatation of the common bile duct.

VASCULAR MALFORMATIONS

HAEMANGIOMA

CAPILLARY HAEMANGIOMA

Diagnosis

These are intradermal haemangiomas that vary in severity from 'salmon patch', which is a minor cosmetic deformity comprising a pinkish discolouration level with the surrounding skin surface and which blanches on pressure, to a 'port wine stain'. The port wine stain is dark purple in colour and is located most frequently on the face in the area of distribution of the fifth cranial nerve (**Fig. 18.84**). There is no tendency for this type of haemangioma to regress spontaneously. Sturge–Weber syndrome is an occasional associated malformation. (See also Chapter 6 Dermatology, page 135 and Chapter 7 Ophthalmology, page 159.)

Treatment

Treatment is the judicious use of cosmetics to cover up the 'salmon patch', while laser therapy is currently the treatment of choice for 'port wine stains'.

STRAWBERRY HAEMANGIOMA

Clinical presentation

These are the most common form of haemangioma. They appear initially as a tiny red spot in the first few days or weeks of life. This is followed by rapid growth for the next 5–9 months, when the lesion becomes much more extensive, bright red in colour and raised above the surface of the surrounding skin with a well-defined margin (**Figs 18.85, 18.86**).

Treatment

They tend to undergo spontaneous resolution over the next 5 years, during which there is gradual and progressive fading and contraction of the lesion. In most instances, specific treatment is not necessary but various modalities have been advocated such as steroids and more recently propanolol.

Associated complications

Large and extensive haemangiomas may occasionally be complicated by congestive cardiac failure due to shunting of blood via numerous arteriovenous fistulae within the lesion, or the development of Kasabach–Merritt syndrome with disseminated intravascular coagulation and bleeding due to platelet trapping within the haemangioma.

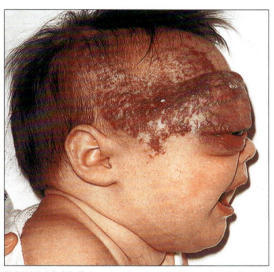

FIGURE 18.85 Extensive haemangioma involving the right eye and forehead.

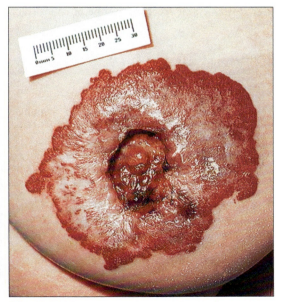

FIGURE 18.86 Haemangioma of the buttock with central ulceration and fading of the lesion in the immediate area of the ulcer.

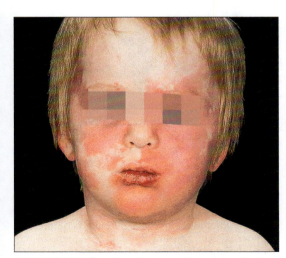

FIGURE 18.84 Capillary haemangioma (port wine stain) affecting the face.

CONGENITAL VASCULAR MALFORMATIONS

CLINICAL PRESENTATION

Usually involving the extremities or the head and neck region, these lesions appear as extensive spongy subcutaneous swellings with an overlying cutaneous capillary component (**Fig. 18.87**).

TREATMENT

They are less prone to spontaneous resolution, which may be slow and prolonged and are more likely to continue to grow and produce major disfigurement. Attempts to induce resolution by systemic high-dose prednisolone gives variable results. Other treatments include intralesional injections of steroid or sclerosing agents or compression of the lesion if its position permits.

KLIPPEL–TRENAUNAY SYNDROME

See also Chapter 6 Dermatology.

CLINICAL PRESENTATION

This syndrome affects one or more limbs and comprises haemangiomas, soft tissue hypertrophy, often to an alarming degree, bony overgrowth and varicosities on the surface (**Fig. 18.88**). The bone overgrowth often produces inequality in leg length.

TREATMENT

Treatment is generally symptomatic and the use of a graduated elastic stocking may be of considerable benefit.

LYMPHOEDEMA

CLINICAL PRESENTATION

Due to a primary abnormality of the lymphatic (hypoplasia or aplasia), the condition almost exclusively affects the lower limb(s).

- **Lymphoedema** may be present at birth when it usually affects both feet and lower limbs and has a tendency to resolve spontaneously by the age of 2 years.
- **Lymphoedema praecox** appears in early adolescence and affects one or both legs. Girls are more commonly affected except in Milroy's congenital familial lymphoedema (2% of all cases) in which the sexes are equally affected.

DIAGNOSIS

The involved limb is swollen to a greater or lesser extent, the skin is thickened and there is non-pitting subcutaneous tissue oedema.

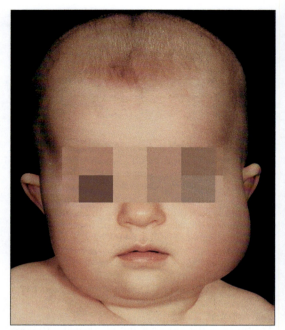

FIGURE 18.87 Haemangioma of the left parotid region – spontaneous resolution occurred.

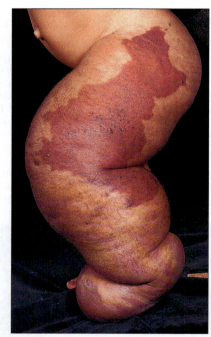

FIGURE 18.88 Klippel–Trenaunay malformation involving the lower extremity.

TREATMENT

Treatment consists of prevention of infection by meticulous foot care and hygiene, elevation of the legs at night and the use of a graduated compression support stocking during the day. A sequential peristaltic pump applied to the leg overnight is extremely useful in reducing the swelling. Surgery is reserved for extreme cases.

SPINA BIFIDA

See also Chapter 8 Neurology, page 226 and Chapter 21 Orthopaedics and Fractures, page 647.

INCIDENCE

Incidence varies greatly between regions but, in general, the overall incidence is continuing to decline from a peak of 3–4 per 1,000 births in 1970–80 to less than 1–2 per 1,000 births at the present time.

EMBRYOLOGY

Spina bifida esults from the failure of the neural groove to close fully by the end of the third week of intrauterine life.

AETIOLOGY

Aetiology is multifactorial, with both genetic and environmental factors:

- **Genetic**: polygenetic inherited predisposition with the incidence in affected siblings being approximately ten times the incidence in the general population.
- **Environmental**: geographical (e.g. high incidence in South Wales and Northern Ireland compared with other regions in the UK); dietary factors (e.g. potato blight, folic acid deficiency, and higher incidence in social class 5 [unskilled labour]).

CLINICAL PRESENTATION

- Local lesion, the extent of which varies:
  - spina bifida occulta (**Fig. 18.89**).
  - skin-covered lesion such as lipoma of the cauda equina (**Fig. 18.90**).
  - meningocoele – lesion covered by meninges.
  - myelomeningocoele – open lesion leaking CSF (**Fig. 18.91**).
  - rachischisis – central canal open to the surface.
- Hydrocephalus is present in over 80% of myelomeningocoele and 50% of meningocoele (**Fig. 18.92**). The hydrocephalus occurs secondary to an Arnold–Chiari malformation, which comprises caudal displacement of the cerebellar tonsils into the foramen magnum, obstructing the drainage of CSF out of the ventricles.
- Musculoskeletal effects. Partial or complete paralysis of the muscles below the lesion is almost invariable. In addition, deformities such as talipes equinovarus, dislocation of the hips and genu recurvatum are common.
- Sensory disturbances occur in skin distal to the lesion and predispose to trophic effects on the ankles and heels.
- Neuropathic bladder.
- Anal sphincter dysfunction.

PREVENTION

Folate is administred before and during pregnancy.

TREATMENT

Treatment includes surgical closure of the local lesion, management of the associated hydrocephalus and the neuropathic bladder, methods to improve bowel control and orthopaedic management of musculoskeletal deformities.

Intra-uterine closure of the defect is associated with a reduced incidence of hydrocephalus and improved leg function. It is undergoing investigation in a research trial.

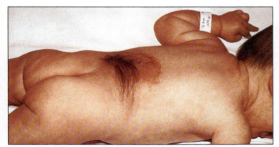

FIGURE 18.89 Spina bifida occulta with a hairy patch overlying the bony defect.

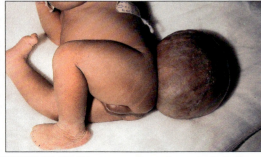

FIGURE 18.90 Skin-covered meningocoele in the lumbosacral region.

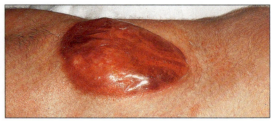

FIGURE 18.91 Myelomeningocoele showing the centrally exposed neural tissue.

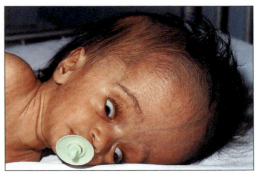

FIGURE 18.92 Hydrocephalus (untreated) showing the typical 'sunset' sign of the eyes.

CONJOINED TWINS

INCIDENCE

The frequency of conjoined twins is around 1 in 250,000 live births. 60% die during gestation or at birth. Females predominate in the ratio of 3:1.

AETIOLOGY

Two theories are proposed: 1. secondary fusion between two originally separate monovular embryonic disks at around 13–15 days gestation; or 2. failure of complete separation of the embryonic disk.

CLASSIFICATION

This is on the basis of site of union together with the suffix 'pagus' meaning fixed.

Thoracopagus (**Fig. 18.93**)	40%
Omphalopagus	33%
Pygopagus	19%
Ischiopagus (**Fig. 18.94**)	6%
Craniopagus	2%

DIAGNOSIS

Prenatal ultrasound is capable of detecting the abnormality as early as 12 weeks gestation. Detailed scanning at 20 weeks will determine accurately the extent of union and indicate the shared organs. Fetal echocardiography is necessary to exclude fused hearts. After birth more detailed CT/MRI scans will be valuable in planning the separation.

TREATMENT

- Non-operative management – for fused hearts of cerebral fusion; all will die.
- Emergency separation – when one twin is dead or dying threatening the survival of its twin; 25–30% survival.
- Planned separation – ideally at 2–4 months of age; 90% survival.

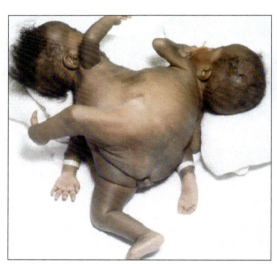

FIGURE 18.93 Ischiopagus twins.

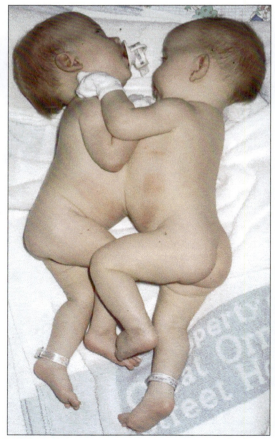

FIGURE 18.94 Thoracopagus conjoined twins.

FURTHER READING

General

Coran AG, Adzick NS, Krummel TM, Laberge J-M, Shamberger RC, Caldemone AA (eds). *Pediatric Surgery*, 7th edn. Elsevier/Saunders, 2012.

Davenport M, Pierro A. *Paediatric Surgery*. Oxford; Oxford University Press, 2009.

Puri P (ed). *Newborn Surgery*, 3rd edn. Hodder Arnold, 2011.

Oesophageal atresia

Spitz L. Esophageal atresia – lessons I have learned in a 40 year experience. *J Pediatr Surg* 2006;41:1635–40.

Congenital diaphragmatic hernia

Tovar JA. Congenital diaphragmatic hernia. *Orphanet J Rare Dis* 2012;7:1.

Neonatal bowel obstruction

Juang D, Snyder CL. *Surg Clin North Am* 2012;92:685–711.

Duodenal atresia

Kay S, Yoder S, Rothenberg S. Laparoscopic duodenoduodenostomy in the neonate. *J Pediatr Surg* 2009;44:906–8.

Anorectal anomalies

Pena A. *Atlas of Surgical Management of Anorectal Malformations*. New York: Springer Verlag, 1990.

Hirschsprung disease

Langer JC. Hirschsprung disease. *Curr Opin Pediatr* 2013;25:368–74.

Malrotation

Lampl B, Levin TL, Berdon WE, Cowles RA. Malrotation and midgut volvulus: a historical review and current controversies in diagnosis and management. *Pediatr Radiol* 2009;39:359–66.

Duplications of the alimentary tract

Stern LE, Warner BW. Gastrointestinal duplications. *Semin Pediatr Surg* 2000; 9:135–40.

Necrotising enterocolitis

Pierro A, Hall N. Surgical treatments of infants with necrotizing enterocolitis. *Semin Neonatol* 2003;8:223–32.

Exomphalos/Gastroschisis

Christisan-Lagar ER, Kelleher CM, Langer JC. Neonatal abdominal wall defects. *Semin Fetal Neonat Med* 2011;16:164–72.

Weber TR, Au-Fliegner M, Downard C, Fishman S. Abdominal wall defects. *Curr Opin Pediatr* 2002;14:491–7.

Umbilical anomalies

Beasley SW. Vitellointestinal (omphalomesenteric) duct anomalies. In: Spitz L, Coran AG (eds). *Pediatric Surgery*, 7th edn. Boca Rato: CRC Press, Taylor and Francis Group, 2013, pp. 445–57.

Pyloric stenosis

Hall NJ, Pacilli M, Eaton S, *et al*. Recovery after open versus laparoscopic pyloromyotomy for pyloric stenosis: a double-blind multicentre randomised controlled trial. *Lancet* 2009;373:390–8.

Intussusception

Applegate KE. Intussusception in children: evidence-based diagnosis and treatment. *Pediatr Radiol* 2009;39:S140.

Kaiser AD, Applegate KE, Ladd AP. Current success in the treatment of intussusception in children. *Surgery* 2007;142:469.

Teratomas in infants and children

Barksdale EM Jr, Obokhare I. Teratomas in infants in children. *Curr Opin Pediatr* 2009;21:344–9.

Flake AW. Fetal sacrococcygeal teratoma [review]. *J Pediatr Surg* 1993;2:113–20.

Appendicitis

Hernanz-Schulman M. CT and US in the diagnosis of appendicitis: an argument for CT. *Radiology* 2010;255:3.

Morrow SE, Newman KD. Current management of appendicitis. *Semin Pediatr Surg* 2007;16:34–40.

Gastrooesophageal reflux

Pacilli M, Chowdhury MM, Pierro A. The surgical treatment of gastro-esophageal reflux in neonates and infants. *Semin Pediatr Surg* 2005;14:34–41.

Undescended testis

Hutson JM, Balic A, Nation T, Southwell B. Cryptorchidism. *Semin Pediatr Surg* 2010;19:215–24.

Biliary atresia

Davenport M, Caponcelli E, Livesey E, *et al*. Surgical outcome in biliary atresia: etiology affects the influence of age at surgery. *Ann Surg* 2008;247:694.

Davenport M, De Ville de Goyet J, Stringer MD, *et al*. Seamless management of biliary atresia in England and Wales (1999–2002). *Lancet* 2004;363:1354.

Choledochal cyst

Liem NT, Hien PD, Dung LA, Son TN. Laparoscopic repair for choledochal cyst: lessons learned from 190 cases. *J Pediatr Surg* 2010;45:540–4.

Vascular malformation

Milliken JB, Fishman SJ, Burrow PE. *Vascular Anomalies: Hemangiomas and Malformations*. New York: Oxford University Press, 2011.

Spina bifida

Adzick NS. Fetal melomeningocele: natural history, pathophysiology, and in-utero intervention. *Semin Fetal Neonat Med* 2010;15:9–14.

Conjoined twins

Spitz L, Kiely E, Pierro A. Conjoined twins. In: Coran AG, Adzick NS, Krummel TM, Laberge J-M, Shamberger RC, Caldamone AA (eds). *Pediatric Surgery*, 7th edn. Philadelphia: Elsevier Saunders, 2012.

Further reading

19 Otorhinolaryngology

Chris Jephson and C. Martin Bailey

OTITIS MEDIA WITH EFFUSION ('GLUE EAR')

DEFINITION/INCIDENCE

Otitis media with effusion (OME) is defined as the presence of fluid (serous, mucoid or mucopurulent) in an inflamed middle ear cleft without acute signs or symptoms (**Figs 19.1, 19.2**).

The incidence of OME in children is high, with a prevalence of 5–10% unilaterally and 20% bilaterally under 6 years of age. It is more common in certain racial groups such as native Americans, Inuit, Aborigines and Maori. The male to female ratio is 2:1.

PATHOGENESIS

Aetiological factors may include eustachian tube dysfunction, viral and bacterial acute otitis media, craniofacial abnormalities and allergy. Other associated factors include the season of the year, adenoidal hypertrophy, dairy-product diet, bottle feeding, day-care attendance, reflux disease and passive smoking.

CLINICAL PRESENTATION

The usual presentation is with hearing loss, which if persistent may lead to speech and learning disability with behavioural problems. These symptoms may be associated with recurrent acute otitis media, or the child may be asymptomatic.

DIAGNOSIS

Common findings on pneumatic otoscopy include dullness, loss of the light reflex, reduced mobility and retraction of an atrophic tympanic membrane over the ossicles, with a visible air–fluid meniscus. Tympanometry is a sensitive test and will demonstrate fluid in the middle ear. Hearing loss can be demonstrated by age-appropriate testing, and can be shown to be conductive in those children old enough to perform a pure tone audiogram (usually 4 years and over).

TREATMENT

OME is generally self-limiting, and so a period of active monitoring for at least 3 months should precede any treatment. Decongestants, antibiotics and antihistamines are of no proven benefit, but intranasal steroid therapy may be effective when there is an underlying rhinitis.

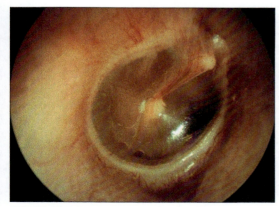

FIGURE 19.1 Normal tympanic membrane.

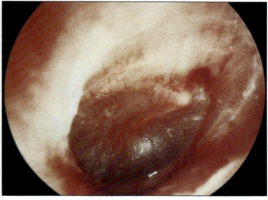

FIGURE 19.2 Otitis media with effusion (glue ear).

Grommet (ventilation tube) insertion (**Fig. 19.3**) remains the most efficacious treatment for persistent hearing loss. Adenoidectomy has been shown to have an additive effect in the resolution of OME when combined with grommets. Hearing aids can be offered as an alternative to surgical intervention. NICE guideline CG60 offers specific advice for treating OME in patients with Down syndrome and in patients with cleft lip and palate.

COMPLICATIONS

Local complications of OME include tympanosclerosis, perforation, ossicular erosion, retraction pocket formation and cholesteatoma. Tympanosclerosis (**Fig. 19.4**) is the result of hyaline degeneration and dystrophic calcification and produces characteristic 'chalk patches' in the tympanic membrane; it may also occur with repeated grommet insertion and attacks of acute otitis media. Perforations are most commonly of the central type, but can be marginal and these are more likely to be associated with cholesteatoma. Tympanic membrane retraction pockets (**Figs 19.5, 19.6**) can be of the pars tensa or flaccida and result from negative middle ear pressures secondary to eustachian tube dysfunction. Ossicular erosion (most commonly affecting the long process of the incus) may result if the tympanic membrane becomes draped over the ossicles. Cholesteatoma may arise in a retraction pocket.

PROGNOSIS

50% resolve spontaneously within 3 months and 95% within 1 year.

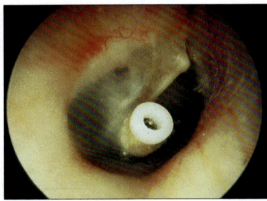

FIGURE 19.3 Grommet (ventilation tube) *in situ* in right tympanic membrane.

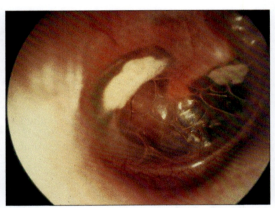

FIGURE 19.4 Tympanosclerotic plaque and otitis media with effusion.

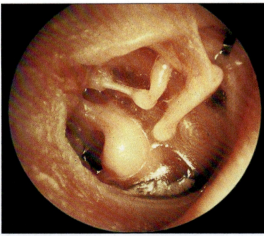

FIGURE 19.5 Retraction of the tympanic membrane onto the ossicles.

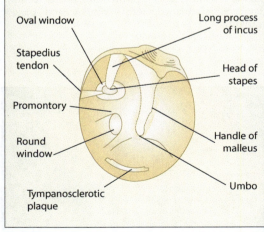

FIGURE 19.6 Line diagram demonstrating features shown in **19.5**.

Oval window
Stapedius tendon
Promontory
Round window
Tympanosclerotic plaque
Long process of incus
Head of stapes
Handle of malleus
Umbo

ACUTE OTITIS MEDIA

DEFINITION/INCIDENCE

Acute otitis media (AOM) is defined as an acute infection of the middle ear cleft (**Figs 19.7, 19.8**). Fifty percent of children under 5 years of age will have at least one episode of AOM, and 50% of episodes occur in those under 5 years of age. Males are affected more frequently than females, lower socio-economic groups are more affected and the prevalence is higher in the winter months.

PATHOGENESIS

AOM may be bacterial in origin with *Haemophilus influenzae*, *Streptococcus pneumoniae* and *Moraxella catarrhalis* being the commonest pathogens; often, however, it is of viral aetiology. Associated factors include adenoidal hypertrophy, Eustachian tube dysfunction, allergy, immunodeficiency, cleft palate and some craniofacial syndromes.

CLINICAL PRESENTATION

Clinical features include rapid onset of otalgia, pyrexia and systemic malaise. If perforation has occurred, ototorrhoea may also be present.

DIAGNOSIS

The tympanic membrane is erythematous and often bulging under pressure. The hyperaemia may extend onto the canal wall.

TREATMENT

Analgesia should be given, and an antibiotic added if symptoms persist beyond 24 hours. Amoxicillin is the initial treatment of choice. In cases of incomplete resolution, the immunocompromised or in the presence of a complication, myringotomy with grommet insertion is necessary, along with a sample for microbiology.

COMPLICATIONS

- **Mastoiditis** occurs when the infection within the middle ear cleft involves the mastoid portion of the temporal bone where it may cause osteitis, erosion and suppuration. The features include fever and inflammatory swelling behind the ear with auricular protrusion (**Fig. 19.9**). Treatment is with intravenous high-dose broad-spectrum antibiotics with antipseudomonal and staphylococcal activity. Occasionally a cortical mastoidectomy is necessary.

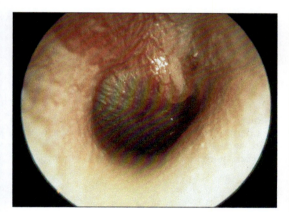

FIGURE 19.7 Early acute otitis media.

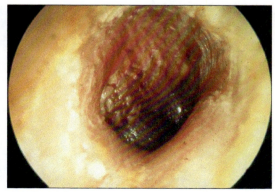

FIGURE 19.8 Acute otitis media with bulging of the tympanic membrane.

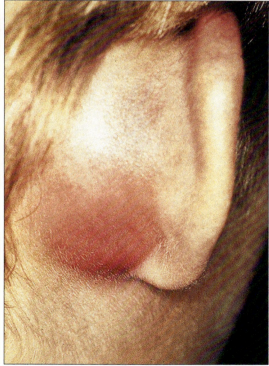

FIGURE 19.9 Acute mastoiditis showing postauricular swelling, erythema and protrusion of the pinna.

- **Labyrinthitis** may occur due to infection extending into the labyrinth via the round or oval window. Vertigo and associated hearing loss can last weeks to months. Treatment is with antibiotics, steroids and labyrinthine sedatives.
- **Sigmoid sinus thrombosis** is uncommon and results from thrombophlebitis developing adjacent to the middle ear cleft in the sigmoid sinus. The classical sign is a spiking 'picket-fence' pyrexia in a patient with AOM or mastoiditis (without any evidence of an abscess elsewhere). The thrombus requires prompt evacuation via a cortical mastoidectomy.
- **Meningitis**. Early recognition and treatment is mandatory.
- **Brain abscess.** Abscesses of the temporal lobe are twice as common as cerebellar abscesses. Spread is mainly via venous channels and preformed anatomical pathways. Treatment requires neurosurgical drainage of the abscess together with a mastoidectomy, and appropriate antibiotic therapy. Brain abscess formation is estimated to occur in less than 1% of cases of AOM in the paediatric population. The incidence is increased in certain racial groups (e.g. native Americans, Inuit, Australian aborigines, Maoris) and in lower socioeconomic groups.

CHOLESTEATOMA

DEFINITION/INCIDENCE

Cholesteatoma is defined as the presence of keratinising squamous epithelium within the middle ear or temporal bone. Continuing desquamation causes the cholesteatoma to enlarge, with consequent erosion of bone and the risk of intracranial complications. It may be congenital or acquired. Incidence is 0.3–1.6/10,000 per year.

CLINICAL PRESENTATION

- **Congenital cholesteatoma** is characterised by the presence of keratinising squamous epithelium behind an intact tympanic membrane (**Fig. 19.10**) in a patient without a history of otitis media. These patients are often asymptomatic and present with a whitish mass seen on otoscopy behind the tympanic membrane, usually in the anterosuperior quadrant (where a squamous epithelial cell rest may persist at the site of the primitive epidermoid body).
- **Acquired cholesteatoma** typically arises in a patient who has chronic suppurative otitis media (CSOM) with an attic or posterior marginal tympanic membrane perforation (see below). Tympanic membrane perforation or retraction with discharge is the characteristic presentation. Conductive hearing loss due to the perforation and ossicular erosion is usual; less commonly, vertigo may occur due to erosion of the horizontal semicircular canal and, rarely, facial nerve paralysis can develop due to pressure and inflammation from the cholesteatoma.

TREATMENT

Cholesteatoma requires surgical extirpation by means of a mastoidectomy. In children, the disease is often more aggressive than in adults and so prompt surgery is required to reduce the long-term morbidity.

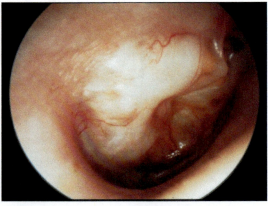

FIGURE 19.10 Congenital cholesteatoma behind an intact tympanic membrane.

CHRONIC SUPPURATIVE OTITIS MEDIA

DEFINITION

CSOM is defined as chronic inflammation of the mucosa of the middle ear in the presence of a tympanic membrane perforation of at least 6 weeks duration, resulting in otorrhoea and hearing loss.

CLINICAL PRESENTATION

Otoscopy reveals a perforation with chronic inflammation of the middle ear. There is a conductive hearing loss and intermittent discharge. The perforation can be central (**Fig. 19.11**) or marginal (**Fig. 19.12**). There can also be an associated cholesteatoma (**Fig. 19.13**). Discharge may be precipitated by an upper respiratory tract infection, or by water getting into the ear following bathing or swimming.

TREATMENT

Initial treatment should include microscopy and suction toilet of the ear, microbiological culture of the discharge and appropriate topical antibiotic ear drops. Audiometry should be done once the discharge has settled. Simple perforations can be repaired by myringoplasty; more advanced disease may require mastoidectomy, with or without tympanoplasty to reconstruct the tympanic membrane and ossicular chain.

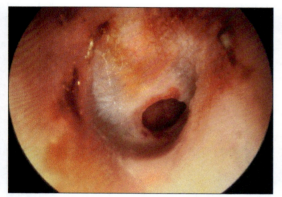

FIGURE 19.11 Chronic otitis media: central tympanic membrane perforation.

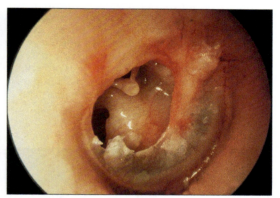

FIGURE 19.12 Chronic otitis media: posterior marginal tympanic membrane perforation.

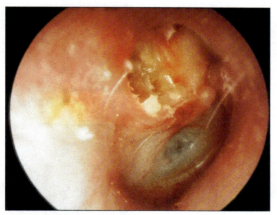

FIGURE 19.13 Acquired cholesteatoma arising from an attic retraction pocket.

OTITIS EXTERNA

DEFINITION

Inflammation of the skin of the external auditory canal (**Fig. 19.14**), most commonly due to bacterial or fungal infection (**Fig. 19.15**).

CLINICAL PRESENTATION

Symptoms include pain, irritation, discharge and hearing loss. Acute otitis externa is the most common form, with many predisposing factors, including local trauma, irritants, meatal exostoses, a discharging perforation, dermatological conditions and swimming (particularly in tropical waters, spas and hot pools). Skin conditions such as dermatitis or psoriasis are less common aetiologies. The common organisms include *Pseudomonas aeruginosa*, *Staphylococcus aureus*, *Proteus* and *Escherichia coli*. Furunculosis may produce a particularly severe otitis externa secondary to *S aureus* infection of the hair follicles located in the cartilaginous portion of the ear canal. In the typical case, there will be a short history of severe otalgia with a localised area of swelling, erythema and pus formation. Recurrent episodes are associated with staphylococcal carrier status.

TREATMENT

This includes meticulous aural toilet, bacteriological swabs and, if necessary, the use of wicks with antibiotic/antifungal/steroid drops. If cellulitis spreads beyond the canal onto the auricle, systemic antibiotics are necessary. It is important to keep the ear dry and continue treatment for several days after the acute episode has settled. Furunculosis may require incision and drainage.

AURAL POLYPS

Most polyps are benign (**Fig. 19.16**) and consist of granulation tissue arising as a result of infection such as otitis media, otitis externa or the presence of foreign material such as a grommet. Occasionally, there may be an underlying cholesteatoma. A differential diagnosis of rhabdomyosarcoma, glomus tumour or facial nerve neuroma should be considered. The decision to remove or biopsy the polyp will depend upon the history and the age of the patient. A CT scan will be useful in some cases. Treatment includes aural toilet, removal of the polyp and antibiotic ear drops.

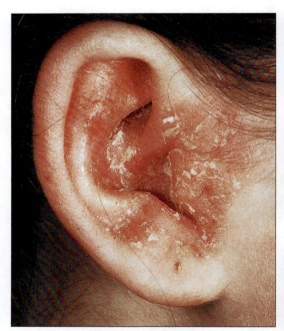

FIGURE 19.14 Bacterial otitis externa with involvement of the pinna.

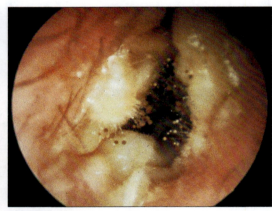

FIGURE 19.15 Fungal otitis externa.

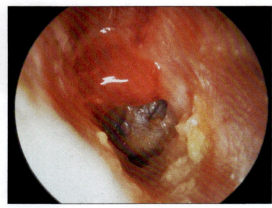

FIGURE 19.16 Benign aural polyp.

AURAL FOREIGN BODIES

CLINICAL PRESENTATION

Foreign bodies in the ear (**Fig. 19.17**) are common in the 2–4 year age group. Inert foreign bodies may cause local pain as a result of secondary infection. Some foreign bodies, such as button batteries, vegetable material and insects produce an intense reaction with ulceration and otitis externa. There may be tympanic membrane perforation and, occasionally, ossicular disruption.

TREATMENT

Removal under a microscope is required, which frequently can only be achieved safely under general anaesthesia in children.

CONGENITAL ANOMALIES OF THE EAR

PREAURICULAR SINUS AND ABSCESS

CLINICAL PRESENTATION

Preauricular sinuses (**Fig. 19.18**) arise from the inclusion of ectodermal elements between the six mesenchymal hillocks during embryological development of the pinna. They lie in close proximity to the anterior, ascending limb of the helix, running a tortuous branching course that is usually superficial to the temporalis fascia. These sinuses are often asymptomatic but can become infected and discharge, occasionally with abscess formation.

TREATMENT

Preauricular sinuses that become recurrently infected require excision, with meticulous dissection to ensure complete removal. Abscesses require initial incision and drainage, followed by wide surgical excision of the sinus tract after an interval.

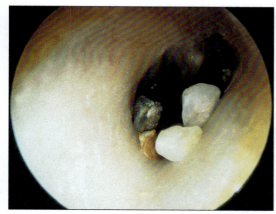

FIGURE 19.17 Multiple foreign bodies in the ear canal (stones).

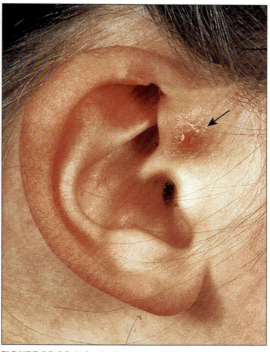

FIGURE 19.18 Infected preauricular sinus.

Preauricular sinus and abscess

EXTERNAL EAR ANOMALIES

CLINICAL PRESENTATION

These range from minor abnormalities such as 'bat ears', as a result of abnormal folding of the cartilage, through varying degrees of microtia (**Fig. 19.19**), to complete absence of the pinna (anotia) with atresia of the external auditory meatus. Such anomalies can occur in isolation or in combination with other craniofacial or genetic syndromes, and there may be not only a cosmetic deformity but also a conductive hearing loss. The facial nerve may follow an abnormal course with these congenital ear anomalies.

TREATMENT

The cosmetic treatment of microtia is either by autologous tissue reconstruction or by a bone-anchored prosthesis from about the age of 10 years. The functional hearing loss should be addressed with a bone-conducting hearing aid from birth, which can be converted to a bone-anchored hearing aid from the age of approximately 5 years.

MIDDLE EAR ANOMALIES

CLINICAL PRESENTATION

These vary from minor, isolated ossicular abnormalities to major deformities of the middle ear cleft associated with microtia and meatal atresia, and result in a conductive hearing loss.

TREATMENT

The results of attempted surgical correction for these major anomalies are poor. The treatment of choice is therefore amplification via conventional air-conduction hearing aids if the external auditory meatuses are present, or a bone-conduction hearing aid if they are not.

INNER EAR ANOMALIES

CLINICAL PRESENTATION

Anomalies of the cochlea, vestibule, semicircular canals, aqueducts and internal auditory meatus can occur in isolation or in combination with various syndromic and non-syndromic conditions. The usual presentation is one of severe bilateral sensorineural hearing loss, which in some cases may be progressive.

TREATMENT

These children will need full audiological evaluation, appropriate amplification, speech and language therapy, support from a teacher of the deaf, and genetic counselling. Some are suitable for cochlear implantation, whereby the auditory nerve endings are electrically stimulated in response to sound.

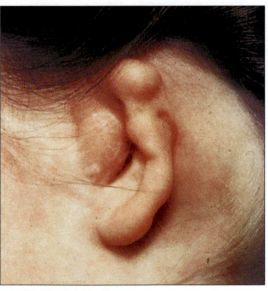

FIGURE 19.19 Microtia.

NASAL POLYPS

Polyps are uncommon in children under the age of 4 years. When present they are often associated with conditions such as cystic fibrosis (**Fig. 19.20**), Young syndrome, Kartagener syndrome or immune deficiency syndromes.

CLINICAL PRESENTATION

Symptoms are nasal obstruction, discharge and anosmia. Many patients have a secondary sinusitis. The polyps arise from the ethmoid air cells and look like a bunch of pale, pearly grapes.

DIAGNOSIS

A CT scan will demonstrate the extent of disease if surgical treatment is planned. A sweat test, RAST test, serum immunoglobulins including IgG subclasses and ciliary function tests may be useful.

TREATMENT

The aim is to treat the underlying cause by medical means. Polyps are responsive to both topical nasal steroids and systemic steroids. Surgical treatment is reserved for those children who fail to respond to adequate medical treatment and comprises polypectomy with or without endoscopic intranasal ethmoidectomy. There is a high rate of recurrence despite total surgical clearance of polyps and medical treatment must be continued postoperatively.

RHINOSINUSITIS

DEFINITION

This is an inflammation of the nose and paranasal sinuses characterised by nasal congestion and one or more of discharge, facial pain or pressure and loss of smell. Acute rhinosinusitis is an infection with complete resolution of symptoms in less than 12 weeks. Chronic rhinosinusitis is associated with low-grade symptoms present for over 12 weeks.

PATHOGENESIS

The ethmoid and maxillary sinus buds are present at birth: the frontal and sphenoid sinuses develop by the age of 6 and 7 years respectively. The maxillary sinuses are fully developed by 6 years, the sphenoid sinuses by 8–10 years and the frontal sinuses by the age of 10–12 years. Causative bacteria include *Streptococcus pneumoniae*, *Haemophilus influenzae* and *Staphylococcus aureus*.

Immunodeficiency, abnormal ciliary function, immunosuppression, malignancy, radiotherapy and anatomical abnormalities are all predisposing factors.

CLINICAL PRESENTATION

Symptoms of sinusitis include nasal obstruction, rhinorrhoea, anosmia, postnasal drip, cough, facial pain and headaches. Systemic symptoms of acute infection may be present.

DIAGNOSIS

Nasal swabs are of little value. Plain sinus x-rays are no longer felt to be a useful investigation. CT is the investigation of choice if complications develop or surgical treatment is contemplated.

TREATMENT

Acute rhinosinusitis should be treated with a combination of an antibiotic and a topical decongestant to facilitate drainage. When unusual organisms are suspected and a specimen for culture is needed, a maxillary sinus lavage ('antral washout') could be undertaken. Chronic rhinosinusitis is relatively uncommon in children and is usually associated with other medical problems. Treatment is complex but can involve endoscopic sinus surgery.

COMPLICATIONS

Acute rhinosinusitis may be complicated by periorbital cellulitis (**Fig. 19.21**), subperiosteal abscess (**Fig. 19.22**), orbital abscess, cavernous sinus thrombosis, cerebral abscess and optic neuritis. Treatment of these complications in children requires prompt referral to the paediatric otolaryngology team, a CT scan of the sinuses and brain, an ophthalmological and, if necessary, neurosurgical opinion.

NASAL MASS

The differential diagnosis of a nasal mass is as shown in **Table 19.1**.

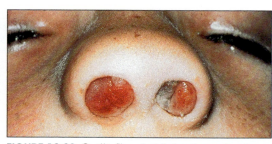

FIGURE 19.20 Cystic fibrosis: bilateral nasal polyps in a child.

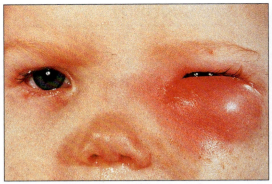

FIGURE 19.21 Periorbital cellulitis and subperiosteal abscess in a 9-month-old child.

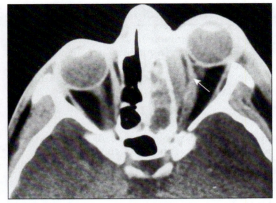

FIGURE 19.22 Periorbital cellulitis and subperiosteal abscess: axial CT scan of the child in 19.21 demonstrating the subperiosteal abscess.

TABLE 19.1 Differential diagnosis of a nasal mass

Congenital	Acquired
• Glioma	**Inflammatory**
• Meninogoencephalocoele	• Abscess
• Epidermoid cyst	• Polyp
• Dermoid cyst	• Antrochoanal polyp
• Chordoma	• Mucocoele
• Craniopharyngioma	
• Thornwald cyst	**Benign**
	• Haemangioma
	• Lymphangioma
	• Lipoma
	• Angiofibroma
	• Neuroblastoma
	• Neurofibroma
	• Papilloma
	Malignant
	• Lymphoma
	• Rhabdomyosarcoma
	• Thyroid carcinoma
	• Nasopharyngeal carcinoma

NASAL GLIOMA AND MENINGOEN-CEPHALOCOELE

DEFINITION

Nasal gliomas and meningoencephalocoeles are rare congenital nasal swellings resulting from herniation of cerebral tissue through the anterior skull base during fetal development. The difference between the two is that at birth, nasal gliomas do not have an intracranial connection whereas meningoencephalocoeles maintain an intracranial connection.

CLINICAL PRESENTATION

Presentation in the paediatric population is with nasal obstruction, feeding difficulties and in some cases a visible mass in the nose (**Fig. 19.23**).

DIAGNOSIS

Any polypoid mass within the nose should raise the suspicion of a possible intracranial connection: simple excision may result in CSF leak or recurrence, and a CT or MRI scan is mandatory. Because of its intracranial connection a meningoencephalocoele will increase in size with crying, straining or coughing and is pulsatile, unlike a glioma.

TREATMENT

These lesions usually require complete excision via an endoscopic intranasal approach. A large skull base defect may need neurosurgical repair. The prognosis is excellent.

JUVENILE NASOPHARYNGEAL ANGIOFIBROMA

DEFINITION/INCIDENCE

A juvenile nasopharyngeal angiofibroma (JNA) is a benign vascular neoplasm that affects young males; it arises in the region of the sphenopalatine foramen and expands into the pterygopalatine fossa and nasopharynx. Incidence is approximately 1 in 15,000 males, peaking at 7–14 years of age.

CLINICAL PRESENTATION

Patients present with recurrent epistaxis and progressive nasal obstruction. Rarely, patients present with unilateral visual disturbance. Examination reveals a mass in the nasopharynx.

DIAGNOSIS

A CT scan with contrast (**Fig. 19.24**) or an MRI scan should be performed but biopsy should be avoided, as it may result in torrential haemorrhage.

TREATMENT

This includes selective preoperative embolisation, followed by surgical resection via an open approach (mid-facial degloving) or increasingly via an endoscopic approach. Very large lesions and recurrences can be treated with radiotherapy. Prognosis is excellent when there is total microscopic clearance of tumour.

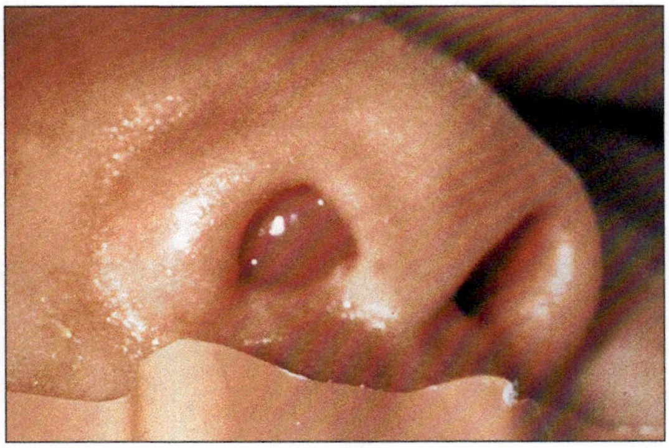

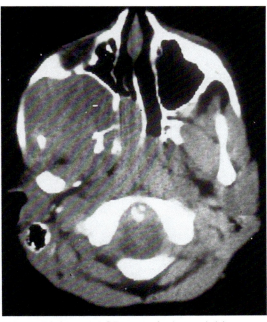

FIGURE 19.23 Nasal glioma in an infant.

FIGURE 19.24 Axial CT scan of a large right postnasal angiofibroma.

NASAL FOREIGN BODIES

CLINICAL PRESENTATION

Nasal foreign bodies (**Fig. 19.25**) are common in 2–5-year-old children, and present with a history of unilateral, purulent, malodorous discharge or with nasal obstruction. Button batteries may cause rapid ulceration. Foreign bodies may be multiple and bilateral.

DIFFERENTIAL DIAGNOSIS

The differential diagnosis includes rhinosinusitis, adenoiditis, sinonasal malignancy and unilateral choanal atresia.

TREATMENT

Retrieval using an angled hook, drawing the object from behind forwards under direct vision, is the most efficacious method of removal. The first attempt, under appropriate restraint, is generally the most successful because thereafter compliance is reduced. Inappropriate instrumentation, such as using forceps for retrieving a bead, may force the foreign body deeper into the nasal cavity or even into the lower airways. Foreign bodies can erode into the submucosa or become impacted under the turbinates, making clinical detection difficult. A CT scan may be required to detect the foreign body, followed by examination under general anaesthesia to remove it.

CHOANAL ATRESIA

DEFINITION

Choanal atresia is a congenital malformation where there is a failure to develop a communication between the nasal cavity and the nasopharynx. It can be unilateral and more rarely, bilateral.

INCIDENCE

This has been estimated at 1 in 8,000 live births, with females affected twice as often as males. Other congenital anomalies occur in over 50% of patients, and up to 30% may have the CHARGE association. The ratio of unilateral to bilateral cases is 2:1, and less than 10% are membranous, the rest being bony or mixed bony/membranous.

CLINICAL PRESENTATION

Bilateral choanal atresia presents at birth as an emergency with respiratory distress, as neonates are obligate nasal breathers. Unilateral atresia often presents later with nasal obstruction and unilateral mucopurulent discharge: there is absence of air flow, and inability to pass a size 8 French gauge nasal catheter beyond 5 cm into the nose.

DIAGNOSIS

Diagnosis is by CT scan (**Fig. 19.26**). Examination of the postnasal space under general anaesthetic confirms the diagnosis.

TREATMENT

Neonates with bilateral choanal atresia will require a taped-in oral airway and orogastric feeding tube until surgical correction is undertaken, usually within the first week of life. Surgery for unilateral atresia is performed electively when the diagnosis is made, usually at an older age. The repair is usually undertaken via a transnasal approach under

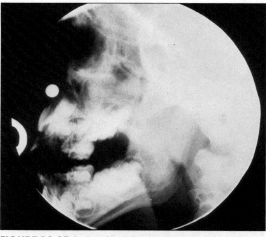

FIGURE 19.25 Lateral neck x-ray demonstrating the position of a foreign body, a ballbearing 'cannon ball' in the nose.

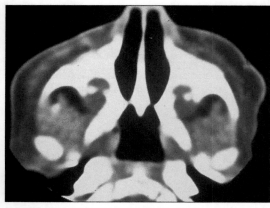

FIGURE 19.26 Bilateral choanal atresia: axial CT scan.

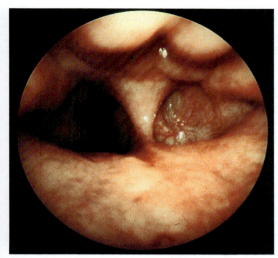

FIGURE 19.27 Unilateral choanal atresia: nasopharyngeal endoscopic view.

endoscopic control (**Fig. 19.27**), and the transpalatal approach has been largely abandoned. Stenting may be required for 6–8 weeks and subsequent dilatations are often necessary.

PROGNOSIS

The outcome is excellent in almost all cases with normal growth, development and function of the nose.

TONSILLITIS (ACUTE, CHRONIC AND RECURRENT)

INCIDENCE

It is common for a child to have at least two episodes of tonsillitis during childhood, especially during the nursery or school-entry year.

PATHOGENESIS

This may be viral due to the EBV, adenovirus or respiratory syncytial virus (RSV); or bacterial due to *Streptococcus pyogenes*, *Streptococcus pneumoniae*, *Staphylococcus aureus* or *Haemophilus influenzae*. The immunocompromised are more susceptible.

CLINICAL PRESENTATION

Acute tonsillitis (**Fig. 19.28**) is usually bilateral and presents with a sore throat, fever, abdominal pain, dysphagia, otalgia and tender cervical lymphadenopathy. Chronic tonsillitis is defined as lasting 6 weeks or more. Features associated with chronic tonsillitis include dysphagia, halitosis, tonsillar hypertrophy or fibrosis, debris-filled tonsillar crypts, persistent cervical lymphadenopathy and poor general health.

DIAGNOSIS

Throat swabs are helpful in prolonged/resistant infections, when an unusual organism is suspected or in the immunocompromised. A full blood count, monospot and EBV-titres may be useful. Differential diagnosis includes toxoplasmosis and infectious mononucleosis.

TREATMENT

Intravenous or oral penicillin for 5 days is the treatment of choice in acute infections (erythromycin in cases of penicillin sensitivity). For beta-lactamase-resistant infections, amoxicillin–clavulanate may be necessary. Rehydration, antipyretic and analgesic therapy is required. Tonsillectomy is recommended for recurrent, chronic or complicated tonsillitis. Recurrent tonsillitis may justify tonsillectomy if there are seven or more episodes during a 1-year period, five per year over 2 years, or three per year for 3 years or longer (SIGN guideline 117).

COMPLICATIONS

These include rheumatic fever, peritonsillar cellulitis or abscess, retropharyngeal or parapharyngeal abscess, septicaemia and upper airway obstruction.

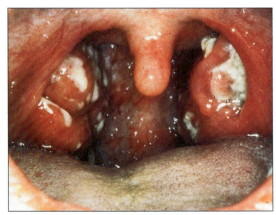

FIGURE 19.28 Acute follicular tonsillitis.

PERITONSILLAR ABSCESS (QUINSY)

DEFINITION

This is a unilateral collection of pus outside the capsule of the tonsil, following an acute or acute-on-chronic infection.

CLINICAL PRESENTATION

Quinsy should be suspected if there is fluctuating pyrexia, persistent unilateral sore throat and trismus following an adequate course of antibiotic in a child with tonsillitis.

TREATMENT

Incision and drainage, together with intravenous antibiotics are needed; usually this demands a general anaesthetic but needle aspiration under local anaesthesia may be sufficient in some older patients. Recurrent quinsy requires interval tonsillectomy, 4–6 weeks after the infection has resolved.

RETROPHARYNGEAL ABSCESS

DEFINITION

This is an abscess arising in a retropharyngeal (prevertebral) lymph node, from which pus may track down inferiorly into the mediastinum. Causes include trauma secondary to a foreign body, tonsillitis, adenoiditis, cervical osteomyelitis or dental infection.

CLINICAL PRESENTATION

Pyrexia, odynophagia, stiff neck and signs of upper airway obstruction are usual.

DIAGNOSIS

A lateral neck x-ray is the initial investigation of choice. A CT scan can help surgical planning.

TREATMENT

Incision and drainage is performed under general anaesthesia with intravenous antibiotic cover.

OBSTRUCTIVE SLEEP APNOEA

DEFINITION

Airway obstruction causing sleep-disordered breathing encompasses a spectrum ranging from primary snoring through to obstructive sleep apnoea (OSA). OSA is the temporary cessation (apnoea) or reduction (hypopnoea) of airflow during sleep caused by an obstruction. OSA can be mild, moderate or severe depending upon the number of hyponoeas and apnoeas per hour.

INCIDENCE

Prevalence of paediatric OSA could be as high as 1–5%. The incidence is higher in boys and in the black and Hispanic populations.

PATHOGENESIS

In children, this is usually the result of hypertrophy of the lymphoid tissues of the Waldeyer ring (**Figs 19.29, 19.30**). Retrognathia, macroglossia, midfacial hypoplasia and generalised hypotonia may also contribute.

CLINICAL PRESENTATION

OSA in children presents with snoring, mouth breathing, a disturbed sleep pattern with frequent waking, witnessed episodes of respiratory obstruction, impaired growth and behavioural problems. In severe cases, sternal recession, pectus excavatum and ultimately cor pulmonale may result.

DIAGNOSIS

Diagnosis is largely clinical. Parents will often present video recordings of their children asleep, which aids the diagnosis. Polysomnography is required when the history is unclear or if central sleep apnoea is suspected.

TREATMENT

Adenotonsillectomy cures the vast majority of affected children, but not necessarily those with craniofacial abnormalities or other comorbidities. In these cases a nasopharyngeal airway and/or continuous positive airway pressure (CPAP) may be used in addition to adenotonsillectomy. It is now very unusual to perform a tracheostomy for OSA, but it may be required in extreme cases.

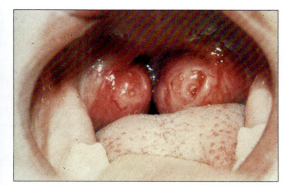
FIGURE 19.29 Tonsillar hypertrophy in a child with obstructive sleep apnoea.

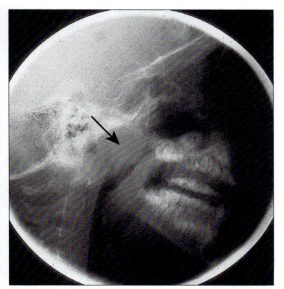
FIGURE 19.30 Lateral neck x-ray showing adenoidal hypertrophy.

DROOLING

PATHOGENESIS

Drooling occurs due to lack of oromotor control associated with a poor swallow reflex in children with cerebral palsy and other neurological conditions.

CLINICAL PRESENTATION

There is excessive drooling that requires multiple changes of clothing or bibs, with skin excoriation around the lips and chin. The dribbling may also interfere with school.

TREATMENT

There are several treatment strategies. If posture is thought to contribute, physiotherapy can be beneficial. Speech and language therapy can improve lip closure, jaw elevation and tongue control. Anticholinergic drugs (hyoscine patches or oral glycopyrrolate) reduce saliva production but are associated with side-effects. Botulinum toxin injection offers temporary relief, but needs repeating every few months. Surgical options include submandibular duct transposition and submandibular gland excision with or without parotid duct ligation.

LARYNGOMALACIA

DEFINITION/INCIDENCE

Laryngomalacia is the collapse of the supraglottis on inspiration. The collapse may be partial or complete. The exact incidence is unknown, but laryngomalacia is the commonest cause of stridor in neonates and infants, accounting for 35–40% of cases.

PATHOGENESIS

It is thought to be due to laxity of the immature laryngeal tissue allowing collapse of the supraglottic structures on inspiration, but the exact cause is unknown. The epiglottis tends to be long and omega-shaped, the aryepiglottic folds tend to be tall and tightly tethered to the epiglottis, and there may be excessive mucosa and submucosa over the arytenoids.

CLINICAL PRESENTATION

Stridor is usually inspiratory and variable. Onset is generally a few days after birth and the stridor is worse with effort (e.g. when feeding or crying). Difficulty with feeds, reflux and vomiting are common; failure to thrive occurs in severe cases. Other signs include tachypnoea, subcostal recession, tracheal tug and pectus excavatum.

DIAGNOSIS

Examination of the larynx, either with a flexible fibreoptic nasendoscope or with a rigid laryngoscope, is necessary for all but the very mildest cases. On endoscopy, an omega-shaped epiglottis, short aryepiglottic folds, redundant arytenoid mucosa and collapse of supraglottic tissues into the laryngeal introitus with inspiration are diagnostic.

TREATMENT

Mild laryngomalacia can be observed and most cases will resolve by the age of 18–24 months. Those who show signs of failure to thrive should undergo endoscopic aryepiglottoplasty to trim the redundant supraglottic tissues.

RECURRENT RESPIRATORY PAPILLOMATOSIS

INCIDENCE

The incidence of recurrent respiratory papillomatosis (RRP) is 7 per million in the USA, with a bimodal age distribution; 66% of cases involve those under 16 years of age.

PATHOGENESIS

RRP is caused by the human papilloma virus (HPV) types 6 and 11 (**Fig. 19.31**). The characteristic papillomas are benign exophytic proliferations of keratinised stratifed squamous respiratory epithelium. The papillomas can occur anywhere in the aerodigestive tract, but typically present in the larynx, especially on the vocal cords.

CLINICAL PRESENTATION

Children with RRP present at an average age of 4 years with symptoms dependent upon the location and severity of the disease. Symptoms include a progressively hoarse voice, abnormal cry, stridor, respiratory distress and exercise intolerance. The younger the child, the more aggressive the clinical course. HPV 11 behaves more aggressively than HPV 6.

DIAGNOSIS

Diagnosis is by endoscopic examination. A biopsy is needed to confirm the diagnosis. Typing of HPV using the polymerase chain reaction (PCR) may be useful in the future.

TREATMENT

The aim of treatment is to maintain a good airway and adequate voice while awaiting spontaneous remission without causing long-term scarring of the larynx. This is achieved by 'debulking' the papillomas on a regular basis. Powered instruments

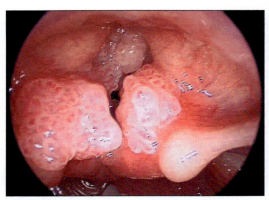

FIGURE 19.31 Endoscopic view of recurrent respiratory papillomatosis of the supraglottis and glottis.

("microdebrider") have superseded CO_2 laser vaporisation as the treatment of choice as this causes less laryngeal scarring. Current adjunctive therapies include intralesional cidofovir, which remains controversial but has proved useful in florid disease. Tracheostomy is occasionally necessary in severe cases, but tends to cause tracheobronchial spread of papillomas and so should be avoided if at all possible.

PROGNOSIS

There is no effective systemic or surgical treatment to eradicate HPV. The disease tends to remit after a number of years, but can progress to adulthood. Malignant transformation is rare (<1%). It is hoped that with the advent of quadrivalent HPV vaccination, RRP will become a disease of the past.

SUBGLOTTIC STENOSIS

DEFINITION/INCIDENCE

Subglottic stenosis (SGS) is a narrowing of the airway at the level of the subglottis. SGS is mostly acquired, but can also be congenital. The incidence of SGS is difficult to estimate. Acquired SGS has reduced with increased awareness of the role of intubation: currently about 1–2% of intubated neonates develop an acquired SGS.

PATHOGENESIS

The narrowest portion of a child's airway is the subglottis, where the airway immediately below the vocal cords is enclosed within the cricoid cartilage. Acquired SGS occurs following periods of intubation when the pressure of the endotracheal tubing in this area can lead to ischaemia, ulceration and infection, which can in turn lead to stenosis (**Figs 19.32, 19.33**). Congenital SGS is much less common and can occur in isolation or in conjunction with a syndrome.

CLINICAL PRESENTATION

Inspiratory stridor is the most common presenting symptom and may resemble recurrent croup. The child may present with failure to extubate following neonatal intubation and ventilation.

DIAGNOSIS

The investigation of choice is microlaryngoscopy and bronchoscopy. At this point the severity of the stenosis can be measured. Current staging is based on the percentage of lumen occluded, in a system proposed by Myer and Cotton (**Table 19.2**).

TREATMENT

Treatment depends upon the grade of stenosis and may include endoscopic or open surgery. For the failed neonatal extubation, a cricoid split procedure may be suitable. Grade I stenosis may need no treatment if symptoms are mild. More severe grades may require laryngotracheal reconstruction using a costal cartilage graft (with or without a covering tracheostomy).

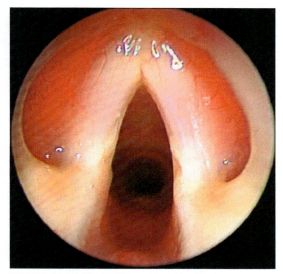

FIGURE 19.32 Normal larynx: endoscopic view.

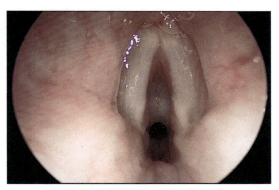

FIGURE 19.33 Acquired subglottic stenosis: endoscopic view.

TABLE 19.2 Myer–Cotton Grading of subglottic stenosis

Grade	% of subglottic lumen occluded
I	0–50
II	51–70
III	71–99
IV	>99

LARYNGEAL AND TRACHEOBRONCHIAL FOREIGN BODIES

CLINICAL PRESENTATION

Inhaled foreign bodies are most common in toddlers. Objects tend to lodge at the carina or in the right main bronchus (**Fig. 19.34**), as it branches off the trachea at a less acute angle than the left main bronchus. The inhalation may be witnessed; if not, coughing spasms, choking or respiratory obstruction may be evident. Stridor if present may be inspiratory, expiratory or biphasic depending upon the level of the foreign body. Occasionally, the episode may be asymptomatic, and these children may present with recurrent or chronic respiratory infections or with an irritable airway mimicking asthma. Classically with bronchial obstruction, there will be reduction of air entry to the affected lung segments with expiratory rhonchi.

DIAGNOSIS

Diagnosis is by history and clinical examination. The bronchial foreign body may have a ball-valve effect, causing air trapping and hyperinflation of the affected lung. Inspiratory and expiratory chest x-rays may give clues as to the location of a foreign body and show any hyperinflation, mediastinal shift (**Fig. 19.35**) or atelectasis. Frequently, however, there may be little to suggest the presence of a bronchial foreign body after the initial episode of coughing/choking.

TREATMENT

With symptoms, signs or suspicion of foreign body inhalation, bronchoscopy should be performed by an experienced surgical, anaesthetic and nursing team. Distal foreign bodies occasionally require flexible endoscopy for retrieval and, very rarely, a thoracotomy may be required.

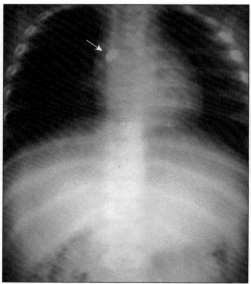

FIGURE 19.34 Peanut in the right main bronchus, demontrated by a chest x-ray.

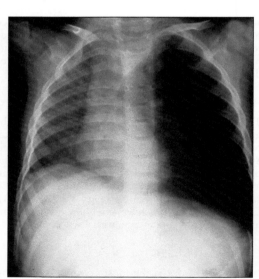

FIGURE 19.35 Hyperinflation of the left lung with mediastinal shift to the right due to air trapping by a foreign body in the left main bronchus.

BRANCHIAL SINUSES, FISTULAE AND CYSTS

DEFINITION

These are rare embryological anomalies that arise from incomplete fusion of the branchial arches, resulting in a sinus, cyst or fistula. The commonest is a second branchial cleft sinus or fistula, followed by first branchial cleft sinus or fistula and finally fourth branchial pouch sinus. The details of these anomalies are shown in **Table 19.3**.

CLINICAL PRESENTATION

First and second branchial cleft sinuses present with a congenital opening to the skin that intermittently discharges mucoid or mucopurulent fluid; occasionally, an abscess may develop. Branchial cysts usually lie deep to the anterior border of the sternomastoid at the junction of its upper and middle thirds

(**Fig. 19.36**). Fourth branchial pouch sinuses do not have an external opening and present with recurrent neck abscesses which may have undergone a number of incision and drainage procedures.

DIAGNOSIS

Ultrasound will give valuable information about the size and position of a cyst and can show the pathway of a sinus or fistula. To further assess the sinus tract a sinogram or CT scan can be performed. If a fourth branchial pouch sinus is suspected, endoscopic examination of the piriform fossa is required.

TREATMENT

For first and second arch anomalies, surgical excision of the entire tract is curative. In the case of fourth pouch sinuses, surgical excision has been superseded by endoscopic ablation of the sinus opening in the piriform fossa.

TABLE 19.3 Branchial sinuses and fistulae

Type	Internal opening	External opening	Pathway of tract
I	Middle ear/external auditory canal	Preauricular, cheek, angle of mandible	Lateral or medial to facial nerve
II	Tonsillar fossa	Along anterior border of sternomastoid	Between external and internal carotid, above cranial nerves IX, X and XI
IV	Piriform fossa	None	From piriform fossa to upper lobe of thyroid gland

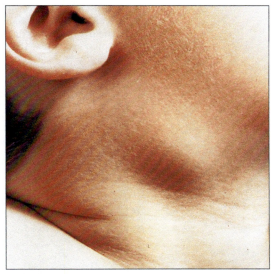

FIGURE 19.36 Second branchial arch cyst in an 8-year-old boy.

PAEDIATRIC HEAD AND NECK MASSES

PATHOGENESIS

Head and neck masses in children are common. They are usually due to reactive lymphadenopathy associated with upper respiratory tract infections, and are usually self-limiting. Congenital head and neck masses include thyroglossal duct cysts, dermoid cysts, branchial anomalies, haemangiomas and vascular malformations. 5% of paediatric malignancies arise in the head and neck region, the most common types of which are lymphoma and sarcoma.

DIAGNOSIS

It is important to establish whether the lump is congenital or acquired, acute or chronic, rapid or slow growing, painful or painless, midline or lateral, solitary or multiple. Also to be determined are its size; shape; whether it is smooth or irregular, solid or cystic; its mobility (i.e. fixation to skin or underlying tissue); any change in colour of the overlying skin; any functional disability; whether it transilluminates; and any other local or systemic features. Consideration of the above should lead to the appropriate differential diagnosis.

Ultrasound will give information regarding tissue density, size, location, depth and often diagnosis. CT and MRI scans can give additional information but require a general anaesthetic in most small children. Serology, FBC, Mantoux test, thyroid function tests and chest x-ray may be contributory. An ENT opinion should be obtained as soon as possible. Fine needle aspiration cytology (FNA) is not often used in children; ultrasound guided core biopsy or open biopsy is preferable.

THYROGLOSSAL DUCT CYST

INCIDENCE

Thyroglossal duct cysts make up 70% of congenital head and neck masses. Males and females are affected equally.

PATHOGENESIS

During development, the thyroid descends from the tongue at the foramen caecum into the lower neck. The tract usually disappears after descent, but a remnant may persist anywhere along its course, enlarge and present as a cyst. The tract has an intimate relationship with the body of the hyoid bone.

CLINICAL PRESENTATION

A thyroglossal duct cyst usually presents in the first two decades of life as a solitary midline cystic neck swelling (**Fig. 19.37**). It may be of variable size, may become infected to form an abscess and may discharge forming a sinus. The cyst lifts with protrusion of the tongue and can be attached to the hyoid.

DIAGNOSIS

Thyroid ultrasound to demonstrate the cyst and ascertain the presence of normal thyroid tissue is mandatory – a thyroglossal cyst may very rarely contain the only functioning thyroid tissue.

TREATMENT

Wide surgical excision is the treatment of choice because of the risk of infection and abscess formation, and because of the rare possibility of malignancy arising in a thyroglossal cyst. An abscess requires incision and drainage, followed by excision of the cyst when the infection has completely resolved. Definitive excision of the tract should consist of an extended Sistrunk procedure to remove the cyst, tract, body of the hyoid, and a core of tissue leading towards the foramen caecum at the tongue base.

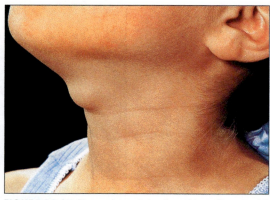

FIGURE 19.37 Thyroglossal duct cyst in a 7-year-old boy.

PROGNOSIS

Excision of the cyst alone carries a recurrence rate of up to 50%. Wide excision using an extended Sistrunk procedure has a recurrence rate of less than 5%.

OROPHARYNGEAL AND OESOPHAGEAL FOREIGN BODIES

INCIDENCE

These can occur in any paediatric age group. Fish, lamb and chicken bones are common foreign bodies. Small objects such as fish bones tend to lodge in the oropharynx, particularly in the tonsil, base of tongue and the valleculae. Larger foreign bodies such as coins are typically found at the cricopharyngeal level.

CLINICAL PRESENTATION

Older children may be able to localise a foreign body above the cricopharyngeus. Younger children present with drooling, dysphagia or irritability. Examination may reveal cricoid tenderness and, occasionally, surgical emphysema is present. A normal lateral neck x-ray does not exclude a foreign body. The x-ray may demonstrate a radio-opaque foreign body (**Fig. 19.38**), prevertebral soft tissue swelling, retropharyngeal or mediastinal air. Further imaging with a contrast swallow or CT may be helpful.

TREATMENT

If there is suspicion of an ingested or inhaled foreign body, an urgent otolaryngological opinion should be obtained. Surgeons should have a low threshold for endoscopy to exclude an ingested foreign body. A spiking temperature ('picket fence' type) should suggest the possibility of complications such as a retropharyngeal abscess, perforated viscus, mediastinitis or septicaemia.

If such a complication is suspected, the child should be placed nil-by-mouth, blood cultures obtained and a contrast swallow or CT scan considered. The child should be placed on high-dose systemic antibiotics with anaerobic and gram-negative cover.

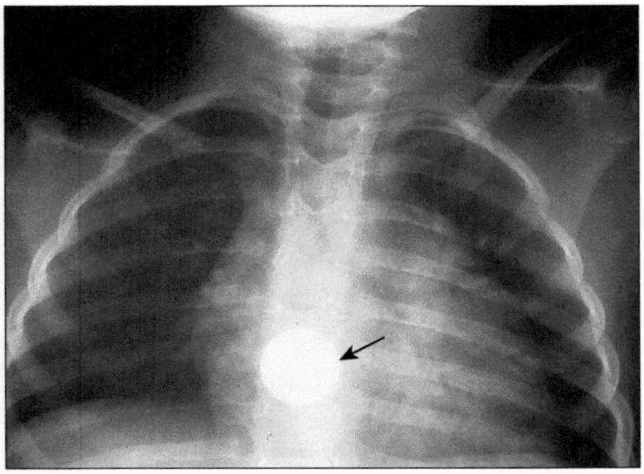

FURTHER READING

Bajaj Y, Cochrane LA, Jephson CG, *et al*. Laryngotracheal reconstruction and cricotracheal resection in children: recent experience at Great Ormond Street Hospital. *Int J Pediatr Otorhinolaryng* 2012;76(4):507–11.

Bajaj Y, Ifeacho S, Tweedie D, *et al*. Branchial cleft anomalies in children. *Int J Pediatr Otorhinolaryng* 2011;75 (8):1020–3.

Gaddikeri S, Vattoth S, Gaddikeri MD, *et al*. Congenital cystic neck masses: embryology and imaging appearances, with clinicopathological correlation. *Curr Prob Diagnost Radiol* 2014;43(2):55–67.

Gleeson M, Browning GG, Burton MJ, *et al*. *Scott-Brown's Otorhinolaryngology, Head and Neck Surgery*, 7th edn. London: Hodder Arnold, 2008.

Graham JM, Scadding GK, Bull PD. *Pediatric ENT*. Berlin: Springer, 2007.

Léauté-Labrèze C, Dumas de la Roque E, Hubiche T, Boralevi F, Thambo JB, Taïeb A. Propranolol for severe hemangiomas of infancy. *N Engl J Med* 2008;358(24):2649–51.

National Institute for Health and Clinical Excellence. Clinical guideline CG60 Surgical management of OME. 2008. www.nice.org.uk

Rosenfield RM, Kay D. Natural history of untreated otitis media. *Laryngoscope* 2003;113:1645–57.

Scottish Intercollegiate Guidelines Network. Guideline 117 Management of sore throat and indications for tonsillectomy. 2010. www.sign.ac.uk

Tweedie D, Bajaj Y, Ifeacho S, *et al*. Peri-operative complications after adenotonsillectomy in a UK pediatric tertiary referral centre. *Int J Pediatr Otorhinolaryng* 2012;76(6):809–15.

FIGURE 19.38 Chest x-ray demonstrating a radio-opaque foreign body (coin).

20 Plastic Surgery

Loshan Kangesu, Jonathan A. Britto, Neil Bulstrode, David Dunaway, Paul Morris, Branavan Sivakumar, Gill Smith and Guy Thorburn

CLEFT LIP AND ALVEOLUS +/− PALATE

INCIDENCE

Cleft lip may be unilateral or bilateral (**Figs 20.1, 20.2**). The defect often extends into the alveolus (gum). In just over one-half of the cases the defect extends into the palate. In the UK, the overall incidence is approximately 0.8 in 1000 (42% unilateral and bilateral cleft lip and alveolus; 42% unilateral cleft lip and palate; 16% bilateral cleft lip and palate). There is racial heterogeneity with rates higher in Chinese and lower among Afro-Caribbean.

AETIOLOGY/PATHOGENESIS

These common facial clefts result from a failure of fusion of the central (frontonasal) and lateral (maxillary) embryological processes that form the midface. The aetiology is unknown for the majority of families but is probably multi-factorial with environmental and genetic factors. There is only a 30% concordance rate among identical twins. Recognised environmental factors are maternal diabetes, alcohol and drugs (phenytoin, steroids) and known syndromes (5–15%) e.g. Van der Woude and ectodactyly, ectodermal dysplasia clefting (EEC) syndrome.

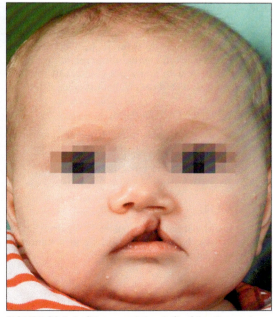

FIGURE 20.1 Left incomplete cleft of the lip and alveolus (gum).

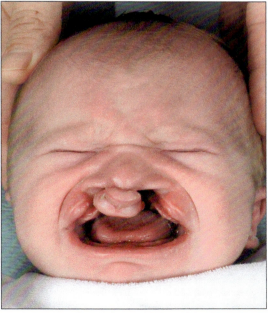

FIGURE 20.2 Complete bilateral cleft lip and palate.

CLINICAL PRESENTATION

Up to 70% of cleft lips are diagnosed in the second trimester antenatal scan, the others are diagnosed at birth.[1]

DIAGNOSIS

The palate must be examined in all cases on cleft lip and alveolus.

DIFFERENTIAL DIAGNOSIS

The cleft itself is obvious but it is important to exclude associated anomalies. Less common types are where there is hypoplasia of either the lateral segment as in hemifacial micosomia or the central segment as in medical facial dysplasia. In this group rarely there may be pituitary dysfunction.

TREATMENT

In the healthy infant cleft lip repair is undertaken at 3–4 months and cleft palate repair at 8–10 months. The alveolar defect requires a bone graft at 8–10 years. Maxillary advancement may be done in 10–30% of cases during late adolescence. Many patients request septorhinoplasty, which is usually the final procedure in late adolescence.

PROGNOSIS

The overall prognosis is good. About 10–30% of children may need secondary surgery for speech difficulty caused by velopharyngeal insufficiency. Revision of the lip repair may also be required. Long-term studies on psychological wellbeing show mild or no concerns in the majority of patients but there is some evidence of lower physical and intellectual capacity or school achievement.

CLEFT PALATE (ISOLATED)

INCIDENCE

Unlike cleft lip and alveolus there is no racial variation. The incidence is about 0.6 in 1000.

AETIOLOGY/PATHOGENESIS

There is failure of fusion of the palatal shelves that are part of the paired maxillary processes. The aetiology is unknown for the majority of families but there are associated genetic and environmental factors. Associated syndromes have been identified in up to 13% of cases and an addition 25–30% having Robin sequence, which is an association of cleft palate with mandibular retrognathia and breathing difficulties. This group also have feeding problems with a higher than normal occurrence of gastro-oesophageal reflux and aspiration in infancy. Commonly associated syndromes are 22q deletion (velo-cardio-facial/DiGeorge), Stickler, fetal alcohol and van der Woude.

CLINICAL PRESENTATION

The diagnosis should be made on the postnatal check by visual inspection. However, the practice of examining the palate with the finger has resulted in 28% being missed on the first day in one study. Any neonate who feeds poorly or has nasal regurgitation should have their palate inspected. Rare variants of cleft palate such as submucous cleft palate will present with poor speech characterised by velopharyngeal incompetence.

DIAGNOSIS

The diagnosis is made by visual inspection (**Fig. 20.3**). The defect cannot be seen on routine antenatal scans but has been demonstrated by research techniques. A submucous cleft palate is characterised by a bifid uvula, a thin membrane in the midline of the palate and a bony defect in the hard palate that is detected on palapation (**Fig. 20.4**).

DIFFERENTIAL DIAGNOSIS

The diagnosis is quite obvious. However, it is important to consider:

- associated anomalies especially cardiac
- genetic causes listed above.

TREATMENT

In the healthy infant cleft palate is repaired in the first year, usually at 8–10 months and a minimum weight of 6 kg is advisable.

PROGNOSIS

The overall prognosis is good. Most patients with cleft palate achieve normally intelligible speech. Up to 25% of patients will require secondary surgery either for complications such as fistula (10%) or the development of velopharyngeal incompetence due to poor soft palate lift or length. Patients with associated anomalies or syndromes have a poorer outcome.

CONGENITAL MELANOCYTIC NAEVI

INCIDENCE

This varies from 10–20 in 1000 for congenital melanocytic naevi (CMN) of any size. Giant CMN are defined as more than 20 cm in their widest diameter of the projected adult size (PAS) (formerly the definition was >5% body surface area) are rare, at 0.05 in 1000.[2]

AETIOLOGY/PATHOGENESIS

The majority of CMN are dermal or compound melanocytic naevi with naevus cells extending deeper into the dermis than in acquired naevi. Melanocytes are found frequently within skin appendages within the adventitia of eccrine ducts and hair follicles in the midreticular dermis as well as within blood vessels, nerves, smooth and striated muscle and fat.[3]

CLINICAL PRESENTATION

The lesions are brown or black papular lesions present at birth; smaller paler lesions may not be apparent immediately. Most grow hair that is usually more coarse and darker (but may be lighter) than scalp hair. Satellite lesions may be present. There is a slightly higher incidence in females. There are associations with abnormal neurodevelopment and maternal ill health and smoking during pregnancy.[4]

DIAGNOSIS

There is usually an obvious clinical diagnosis (**Fig. 20.5**).

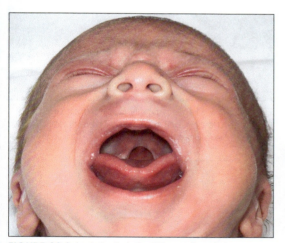

FIGURE 20.3 Isolated cleft of the soft palate.

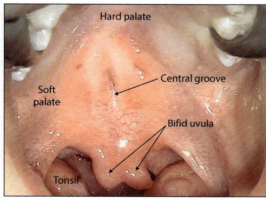

FIGURE 20.4 Submucous cleft palate with bifid uvula.

Hard palate

Soft palate

Central groove

Bifid uvula

Tonsil

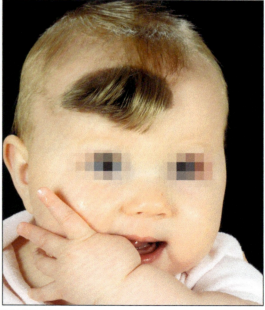

FIGURE 20.5 Congenital melanocytic naevus of the forehead that was treated by excision and skin graft at 12 months. (Courtesy of the Department of Medical Photography, Broomfield Hospital.)

DIFFERENTIAL DIAGNOSIS

Other pigmented lesions of childhood:

- Blue/black macular pigmented lesions such as Mongolian spot around the base of the back and buttock, naevus of Ito around the upper trunk and naevus of Ota around the face.
- Café-au-lait patch (as seen in neurofibromatosis).
- Acquired compound naevi (develop from 6 months of age of the junctional, dermal and compound naevi).
- Carney syndrome (an autosomal dominant multiple neoplasia syndrome with spotty skin pigmentation, cardiac myxoma, endocrine tumours and melanotic schwannomas.
- Epidermal naevus syndrome.

TREATMENT

The majority do not require intervention. Lesions may be excised for cosmetic purposes from about 1 year of age. Surgical techniques include simple excision, multi-staged excision, excision and resurfacing with tissue expanded skin and excision and resurfacing with skin grafts.

PROGNOSIS

Many lesions become paler.[2-5] The overall risk of malignant melanoma is 0.7–2.4% in childhood but this risk is almost exclusively in patients with larger giant CMN greater than 60 cm PAS and with satellite lesions (14% risk). Surgery does not remove the risk of malignancy because the melanoma may arise outside the CMN (such as within the CNS).

CRANIOSYNOSTOSIS

INCIDENCE

Craniosynostosis (CSS) is the premature fusion of the cranial sutures, which are the adaptive 'joints' between the skull bones resulting in distinct head shapes. Traditionally, the CSS have been divided into non-syndromic and syndromic forms. However, contemporary knowledge about the causes of this group of conditions lends better division into 'single suture' (**Fig. 20.6**) and 'multisutural' or 'complex' CSS (**Fig. 20.7**). The common single suture synostoses are sagittal synostosis (0.2–0.33 per 1000, male predominant) and unicoronal synostosis (0.125 per 1000, female predominant). The most common syndromic synostoses are the 'Crouzon-Pfeiffer' group

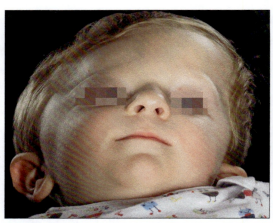

FIGURE 20.6 Plagiocephaly due to right unilateral single suture coronal synostosis. There is no threat to brain development.

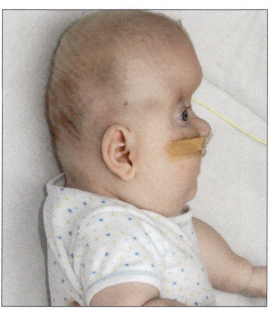

FIGURE 20.7 Apert syndrome with multisuture or complex synostosis. There are risks to the airway, vision and increased intracranial pressure.

(0.0165 per 1000), and the more clinically and genetically distinct Apert syndrome (0.0155 per 1000).

The management of this heterogeneous group of challenging conditions is firmly multi-disciplinary, and relies upon careful assessment and problem based, rather than time based and protocol based clinical intervention.

AETIOLOGY/PATHOGENESIS

The cranial sutures form in normal development *in utero,* where the radiating ossification plates of the foetal skull bones meet over site specific dura mater (covering the brain), to allow complex molecular events to determine suture formation. Where this process of suture formation/ossification is deranged, CSS results. There are many causative factors, including metabolic disease (mucopolysaccharidosis), hormonal disease (thyroid disease), and chromosomal anomaly relating to other named developmental syndromes. A family of genetic mutations in the fibroblast growth factor receptor genes, *FGFR1, FGFR2* and *FGFR3* are causative in the Crouzon and Pfeiffer syndromes (the Crouzon–Pfeiffer group are overlapping), Apert syndrome and coronal synostosis (uni- and bicoronal synostosis). Other genes are implicated in allied syndromes featuring CSS, such as Antley–Bixler syndrome and Saethre–Chotzen syndrome. Most of the genetic pathways leading to CSS result in accelerated differentiation of the osteoblast cells that promote ossification and skeletal maturity.

CLINICAL PRESENTATION

True CSS normally presents at birth. The single suture forms cause recognisable head shape deformity without midface retrusion. Complex, syndromic CSS (Apert syndrome, the Crouzon–Pfeiffer group) are diagnosed at birth, or at prenatal diagnosis by fetal ultrasound. The head shapes of severe bicoronal synostosis (brachycephaly) combined with posterior suture fusion (turribrachycephaly) are recognisable. Midface retrusion may be an early or delayed feature, but is often severe, leading to prominent eyes and a small nasopharynx.

- Early breathing difficulty may be compounded by choanal stenosis requiring early airway intervention to support life. Threats to breathing may be neurological (from central sleep apnoeas) or at many levels in the airway from a deviated septum, a constricted nasopharynx or tracheal stenosis.
- Prominent eyes within the shallow orbit may lead to ocular surface exposure requiring topical lubricants at best or dislocation of the eye onto the cheek at worst, leading to urgent surgery.
- A major concern is the potential for raised intracranial pressure (ICP). Airway compromise is additive to this problem, which is not caused simply by volume reduction in a CSS skull. Raised ICP is quantified by visual electrophysiology studies, or by direct measurement, and can be treated by supporting the airway or cranial vault surgery. Ventricular dilatation and hydrocephalus pose particular challenges.

Other challenges to an infant and child with syndromic CSS include feeding and nutritional difficulties, hearing impairment (there is fusion of the ossicles of the middle ear), and the impact of coincident extracranial features such as cardiac anomalies, gastrointestinal features and peripheral limb abnormalities. Intellectual impairment is a feature in complex CSS, and may be compounded by raised ICP, hearing loss, visual impairment and hydrocephalus. Complex multi-system challenges are particularly common in Apert syndrome, in which the problems of complex CSS and midface retrusion can be accompanied by cleft palate (70%), severe digital syndactyly in hands and feet and cardiac anomalies. Two specific genetic mutations in *FGFR2* are causative to this unique syndrome.

DIAGNOSIS

Single suture CSS is diagnosed by clinical appearance, supported where necessary in marginal cases by CT scan (plain x-ray is seldom valuable). Single suture CSS is rarely associated with a 'functional' problem such as raised ICP. Unicoronal synostosis causes orbital asymmetry (not midface retrusion) such that squint surgery may be required after corrective craniofacial surgery is undertaken (12–15 months). Some forms of coronal CSS are associated with FGFR or TWIST mutations, and genetic analysis is undertaken to provide further information to families about clinical risk and patterns of inheritance.

Complex syndromic CSS is also a clinical diagnosis, supported by genetic analysis for the range of causative known genes, or new genetic causes. Special investigations and analysis quantify the various risks to the airway, ICP, vision, nutrition, hearing and other multi-system challenges. CT and MRI scans are useful to assess the brain, head and face and in surgical planning.

DIFFERENTIAL DIAGNOSIS

Deformational (positional) posterior plagiocephaly: a common problem since the 'back to sleep' practise to reduce cot death.[6]

Single suture CSS

- Sagittal synostosis (scaphocephaly) – usually isolated, male > female, frontal and occipital bossing, temporal indrawing, long thin skull.
- Metopic synostosis (trigonocephaly) – usually isolated, male > female, central forehead ridge and bilaterally flat temples.
- Unicoronal synostosis (anterior asymmetrical plagiocephaly) – isolated or familial, female > male, orbital asymmetries and squints. No midface retrusion, normal rounded occiput.
- Lambdoid synostosis – very rare cause of posterior plagiocephaly.

Complex CSS

- Crouzon syndrome – coronal synostosis, brachycephaly or turribrachycephaly. Clinically (not radiologically) normal hands and feet. No cleft palate, midface retrusion.
- Pfeiffer syndrome – coronal synostosis, brachycephaly or turribrachycephaly. Mild digital anomalies and radial deviation of the great toe and thumb. No cleft palate, midface retrusion.
- Apert syndrome – coronal synostosis, brachycephaly or turribrachycephaly. Range of complex complete syndactylies. Cleft palate (70%), midface retrusion, hypertelorism. Range of extracraniofacial multi-system features.

TREATMENT

The treatment of single suture synostosis is largely for the normalisation of appearance and involves cranial or cranio-orbital surgery. Sagittal synostosis is treated by cranioplasty optimally at 6 months, the other single suture CSS by fronto-orbital surgery at 12–15 months.

Complex CSS is treated in each case in a highly bespoke manner, based upon regular multi-disciplinary assessment. For some children the first step in treatment may be a PEG for nutritional support, or nasopharyngeal airway support, while in others urgent cranio-fronto-facial advancement surgery or cranioplasty may be required to defend vision or against raised ICP. The key is regular, multi-disciplinary and targeted assessment for the anticipation of clinical problems or the evaluation of intervention.

PROGNOSIS

The outcome of surgery for single suture synostosis is very good at bringing a craniofacial difference (with statistical significance) towards a postoperative appearance within the normal range. Secondary surgery for appearance change is not often required.

Children with complex CSS receive a high level of care for functional outcome across many disciplines, and contemporary care relieves these young people from severe functional impairment. In later childhood and adolescence, functional challenges often give way to aesthetic concerns and appearance difference, and surgical strategies are directed towards this. Many will go on to independent lives in adulthood, with jobs and rewarding social relationships.

EPIDERMOLYSIS BULLOSA

INCIDENCE

Epidermolysis bullosa (EB) comprises a collection of rare genetically inherited skin disorders (genodermatoses) with skin fragility as the predominant feature.

AETIOLOGY/PATHOGENESIS

Genetic abnormalities produce defects in the adhesion molecules that normally maintain adherence of the epidermis to the dermis allowing easy separation at the dermoepidermal junction. There are multiple subtypes that are broadly categorised into three main groups according to the level at which separation occurs: EB simplex, where cleavage is within the basal keratinocytes; junctional EB, where the defect is within the lamina lucida; and dystrophic EB, where cleavage occurs at the level of the superficial papillary dermis. There are dominant and recessive subtypes, the latter being those more likely to come to the attention of the plastic surgeon due severe progressive scarring of the hands.

CLINICAL PRESENTATION

Children presents to the dermatologist as blistering with minimal trauma (Nikolsky sign). Long standing ulcers may occur at sites of repetitive trauma. The age at presentation largely depends on type and EB simplex may present late. Referral to the plastic surgeon may be either in relation to the acquired hand deformities or the presence of skin malignancy. The latter is usually aggressive invasive squamous cell carcinoma.

Hand deformities present with pseudosyndactyly affecting all the digits, adduction contracture of the first web and flexion contractures of the digits. When left untreated, these features combine and cause a mitten hand where all digits are cocooned in scar. (**Fig. 20.8**).

Pain or the heaping up of an edge in long-standing ulcers, especially over bony prominences, may reflect malignant change within that lesion. All patient's wounds are regularly screened and parents/patients themselves are warned to watch for changes that may warrant biopsy.

DIAGNOSIS

A skin biopsy taken from a blister formed deliberately by shear forces will show cleavage of the superficial layers of the skin from those deeper in the dermis. Immunofluorescent staining will identify the adhesion molecules that are deficient. Gene testing of a family may identify the specific mutation. If the gene mutation has been identified in a known EB patient, prenatal diagnosis in the mother's subsequent pregnancies may be obtained from chorionic villus sampling. If the exact mutation is unknown, then prenatal testing is from amniocentesis, which prevents the option of early termination.

The diagnosis of skin malignancy in a patient with EB is extremely difficult and requires a specialist pathologist with an interest in the condition.

DIFFERENTIAL DIAGNOSIS

- Non-accidental injury.
- Bullous disorders.

TREATMENT

Treatment is largely supportive. It requires a multidisciplinary team with a specialist interest in EB headed by a dermatologist.

Dressing materials need to be absorbent, bacteriostatic or bacteriocidal and non-adherent and held in place with bandages, as tape will damage the skin. Physiotherapy maintains the range of motion in those joints where pain rather than scarring is the limiting factor. Splintage may reduce the speed of deterioration.

Severe anaemia may necessitate transfusion although chronic anaemia is well tolerated. Nutrition is a major issue since mucosal involvement may cause oesophageal stricture requiring oesophageal dilatation or gastrostomy feeding. Also, dental review is required as decay is universal in these patients.

Anaesthesia is a major undertaking for any procedure as these patients may have limited mouth opening, loose teeth, difficult airways, poor venous access, inability to protect their eyes due to eyelid contractures, fragile skin to hold a face mask to and require lifting and not sliding on and off the operating table.

Surgical correction of hand deformities requires careful consideration of functional benefit. Sadly, the initial deformities will recur with time due to the ongoing disease process. When resecting malignant tumours in the EB patient, there is frequently histopathological field change extending far beyond the clinically apparent area of involvement, often requiring re-excision. Deep involvement is common and amputation may be the only option for tumour clearance. Regional metastases to the local lymph node basin are also common and require lymph node block dissection.

Bone marrow transplantation and gene therapy are currently experimental treatments that hold the hope of lasting cure.

PROGNOSIS

Prognosis depends on type. Most EB simplex patients will have a normal lifespan. There is a high mortality in junctional EB in the first year of life, but beyond that most would expect to live into adulthood. Recessive dystrophic EB carries a longer-term toll of disability with severe hand and foot deformities developing before adulthood, the risk of other joint deformities, osteopenia, malnutrition, severe overwhelming infection and cardiomyopathy, all of which contribute to the morbidity associated with this condition.

With improved nutritional support, most dystrophic EB patients will live into adulthood but die young of locally and regionally aggressive squamous cell carcinoma that arise within their chronic wounds.

Hand surgery may provide a temporary improvement in function but recurrence is universal and the timing of this recurrence is more closely related to patient compliance with splintage and the underlying disease severity than the skill of the surgeon.

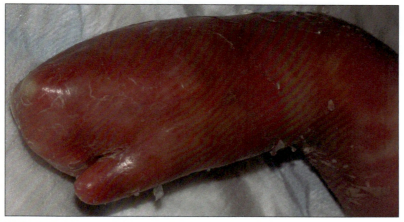

FIGURE 20.8 The pseudosyndactyly (mitten hand) caused by the scar tissue.

EXTRAVASATION

INCIDENCE

This occurs when a substance harmful to the interstitial soft tissues leaks out into them rather than passing into the lumen of a vein as intended. Failure of intravenous devices in hospitalised children is reported as between 11–58%, with an estimated one-quarter of these associated with an extravasation injury (**Fig. 20.9**).

AETIOLOGY/PATHOGENESIS

The substance may be vesicant or dessicant in nature. The adverse consequences depend on the volume and toxicity of the extravasation fluid and the timing and nature of any treatment instituted to limit damage to the local tissues. Local toxicity can lead to soft tissue and skin necrosis and tendon adhesions with secondary joint contractures. The effect of large volumes can create compartment syndromes and lead to digital loss. Neonates are most commonly affected with the dorsum of the hand the most frequent site of injury.

CLINICAL PRESENTATION

There is abnormal swelling around the site of an intravenous line. This is usually, but not invariably, associated with a malfunction to the running of the line. If the patient is able to they will complain of pain locally. Later the skin locally or the digits distally may become discoloured – red, blue or white. The signs of compartment syndrome are identical to those from other causes.

DIAGNOSIS

This relies on maintaining a high index of suspicion in the vulnerable and monitoring intravenous lines regularly with the area around kept visible. Where swelling occurs, infusion must be stopped promptly.

DIFFERENTIAL DIAGNOSIS

- Infiltration (where a non-vesicant solution enters the interstitial tissues).
- Pressure sore (where pressure is externally applied).
- Vascular injury.

TREATMENT

Prompt washout of all suspected extravasation injuries with the technique described by Gault should be instituted.[7] The cannula should be left *in situ* and any fluid within it withdrawn. The area should be infiltrated through the cannula with hyaluronidase and local anaesthetic multiple small stab incisions created around the affected area. The area should be washed out through the cannula with large volume of normal saline, the cannula removed, wounds dressed and reviewed regularly. The injury must be documented thoroughly, including ideally with photographs and measurements.

PROGNOSIS

The prognosis depends on the severity of the initial injury and the speed and competence with which it is treated. Prompt aggressive treatment avoids or minimises long-term serious sequelae.

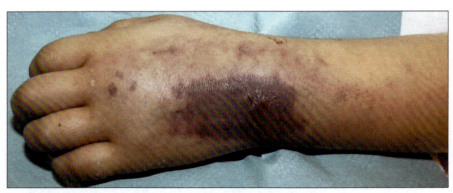

FIGURE 20.9 Early damage to the skin following extravasation.

HEMIFACIAL MICROSOMIA

INCIDENCE

Hemifacial microsomia (HFM) is a congenital condition resulting in the underdevelopment of one, or more rarely both, sides of the face (between 5 and 30%). It is the second most common congenital craniofacial anomaly after cleft lip and palate with an incidence between 1 in 3,000 and 1 in 6,000 live births. Other terms for hemifacial microsomia include craniofacial microsomia, Goldenhar syndrome, lateral facial dysplasia, 1st and 2nd arch syndrome and otomandibular dysostosis.

AETIOLOGY/PATHOGENESIS

The precise cause of hemifacial microsomia is unknown. The condition results in underdevelopment of facial structure derived from the first and second branchial arches. It is generally a sporadic condition, although rarely familial cases have been reported.

CLINICAL PRESENTATION

HFM has a very variable presentation in both its severity and facial structures involved. Commonly underdeveloped structures are the mandible and maxilla, the orbit and ear (**Figs 20.10, 20.11**). The soft tissues of the affected side face are also commonly underdeveloped. The Vth, VIIth and XIIth cranial nerves may be absent or hypoplastic. Macrostomia and cleft lip and palate are also associated with hemifacial microsomia.

The wide variety of anomalies has caused confusion with classification. The OMENS classification is now most commonly used to describe the degree to which the most commonly involved structures are involved (orbit, mandible, ear, nerve and soft tissues).[8] Functional problems associated with HFM include upper airway obstruction, speech and feeding difficulties along with hearing and visual problems on the affected side.

HFM is also commonly associated with extracranial anomalies (e.g. cardiac, renal and cervical spine anomalies).

DIAGNOSIS

Diagnosis is on history and clinical examination. Underlying bony and soft tissues anomalies may be confirmed and further delineated by CT and MRI.

Differential diagnosis

- Acquired conditions – hemifacial atrophy, Parry–Romberg syndrome.
- Unilateral overgrowth – facial hemihypertrophy, mandibular condylar hyperplasia.
- Bialteral inherited conditions – Treacher–Collins syndrome, Nager syndrome.

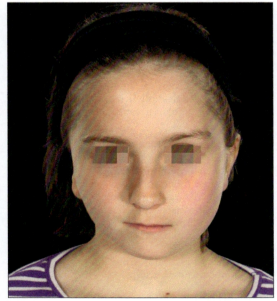

FIGURE 20.10 Right hemifacial microsomia with ear deformity.

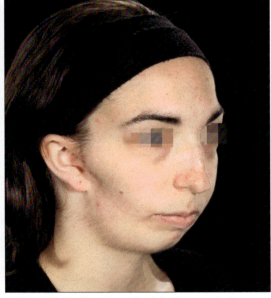

FIGURE 20.11 Right hemifacial microsomia in an older patient.

Hemifacial microsomia

TREATMENT

Treatment is directed towards managing functional problems arising from anatomical deformity and correcting asymmetry and undergrowth. In early life treatment is directed towards function. Upper airway support may required and in the most severe cases a tracheostomy may be required. Management should be within a multi-disciplinary team.

Growth enhancing procedures to treat facial asymmetry including distraction osteogenesis, functional orthodontics and costochondral grafting to the mandible may be undertaken in infancy and childhood.

Definitive treatment of facial asymmetry cannot usually be completed until adolescence or early adulthood because abnormal growth potential undoes the effects of early surgery. Definitive surgery often includes osteotomies of the mandible and maxilla along with soft tissue augmentation of the affected side.

PROGNOSIS

Long-term prognosis is generally good. In mild and moderately affected individuals an almost complete correction of the defect and functional problems can usually be achieved. More severely affected individuals generally suffer some functional deficit associated with an incomplete correction of their asymmetry.

MICROTIA AND EAR RECONSTRUCTION

INCIDENCE

Microtia, or small ear, can be unilateral or bilateral. The incidence of unilateral microtia in Caucasians is 1 in 6–8000 births, in Japan 1 in 4000 births and among Navajo Indians 1 in 1000 births. It affects the right side more than the left and can be associated with HFM. Bilateral microtia can be part of the presentation of Treacher–Collins syndrome.

AETIOLOGY/PATHOGENESIS

The aetiology is unknown. There is an association with a family history of twinning in patients with microtia. There is a theory stating that it may be caused by a deficiency or embolism in the stapedial artery in the early weeks of gestation.

CLINICAL PRESENTATION

Microtia is normally discovered at birth. The external ear is deficient and deformed and there are also varying degrees of conductive hearing loss with external auditory canal stenosis and atresia (**Fig. 20.12**).

Patients with HFM and Treacher–Collins syndrome will need assessment of jaw deformity affecting function, breathing and feeding.

DIAGNOSIS

Clinical examination includes full hearing assessment. Patients with hemifacial microsomia should also be investigated for renal deformities.

DIFFERENTIAL DIAGNOSIS

- Isolated.
- HFM/Goldenhar.
- Treacher–Collins syndrome.

TREATMENT

Treatment is within a multi-disciplinary team, involving audiological physicians and scientists, surgeons (ENT, craniofacial, oral and maxillofacial) and orthodontists.

- Microtia (external ear):
  - none.
  - bone-anchored prosthesis.
  - Medpore framework.
  - carved rib cartilage framework placed in a subcutaneous pocket from 9 years onwards (**Figs 20.13, 20.14**).
- Hearing deficit:
  - hearing aids.
  - bone conduction hearing aid.
  - bone-anchored hearing aid.

PROGNOSIS

The prognosis is excellent when treated in multi-disciplinary units dedicated to the treatment of this condition. Patient reported outcome measures have shown good satisfaction with surgical intervention.

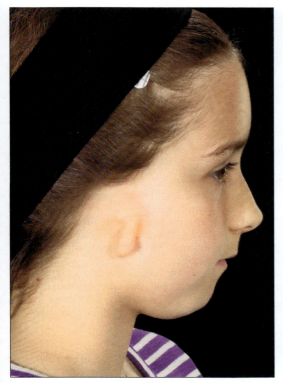

FIGURE 20.12 Patient with lobular microtia.

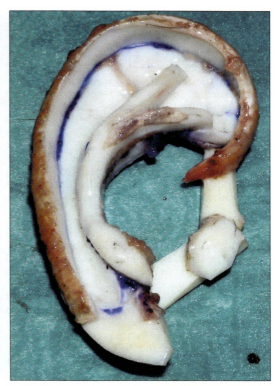

FIGURE 20.13 An ear framework carved and built up from costal cartilage.

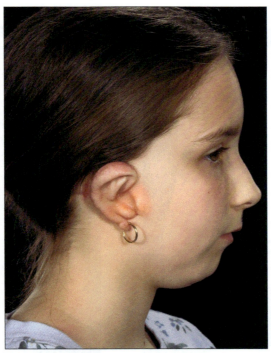

FIGURE 20.14 Same patient after surgery, the framework was in a subcutaneous pocket.

PROTEUS SYNDROME

INCIDENCE

Proteus syndrome is extremely rare, fewer than 200 confirmed affected individuals worldwide. The suggested prevalence is less than 1 case per 1,000,000 live births (0.001:1000).[9] Hans-Rudolf Wiedemann named the syndrome in 1983 after the Greek sea god Proteus, who had the ability to change his body shape.

Joseph Merrick, the unfortunate individual who was paraded as the Elephant Man in Victorian England, is now thought to have had Proteus syndrome rather than neurofibromatosis.[10]

AETIOLOGY

Proteus syndrome occurs sporadically with a mosaic distribution; the causative event occurs early in fetal development, but not in all cells in the body. Various genes have been associated including a tumour suppressor gene, *PTEN*. Recently researchers identified a specific gene mutation present in 26 of 29 patients who met strict clinical criteria for the disorder in AKT1 kinase in a mosaic state gene.[11,12] This implicated the activation of the PI3k-AKT pathway in the characteristic findings of overgrowth and tumour susceptibility.

CLINICAL PRESENTATION

Proteus syndrome is characterised by abnormal overgrowth of bone, blood vessels, lymphatics and soft tissues. It presents in early childhood with lipomas, vascular malformations (capillary, venous and lymphatic malformations), epidermal naevi and often asymmetric overgrowth of limbs and digits. Deep lines and overgrowth of soft tissues on the soles of the feet causing cerebriform thickening is also a characteristic feature (**Figs 20.15, 20.16**).

DIAGNOSIS

Diagnosis is based on clinical presentation characterised by asymmetrical overgrowth with general and specific criteria categorised into A, B and C (see **Table 20.1**). The general diagnostic criteria of mosaic distribution, sporadic occurrence and progressive course, must all be present.[12]

The diagnosis of Proteus syndrome requires all three general criteria, plus one criterion from category A, or two criteria from category B, or three criteria from category C. (Adapted from Biesecker, 2006).[12]

DIFFERENTIAL DIAGNOSIS

Conditions associated with overgrowth that should be considered in the differential diagnosis include:

- Klippel–Trenaunay syndrome – combined vascular malformations of capillaries, veins and lymphatics associated with limb hypertrophy.

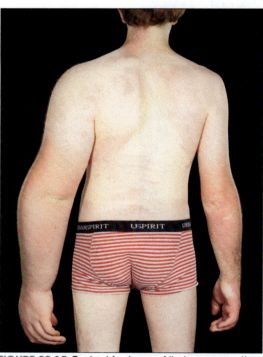

FIGURE 20.15 Typical features of limb overgrowth and capillary malformations (port wine stain) in Proteus syndrome.

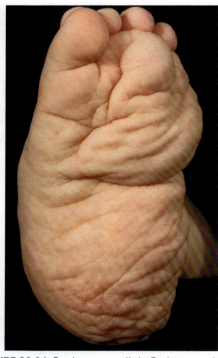

FIGURE 20.16 Foot overgrowth in Proteus syndrome.

Plastic surgery

- Maffucci syndrome – benign enlargement of cartilage (enchondroma) with multiple haemangiomas.
- Neurofibromatosis – autosomal dominant inherited disorder causing overgrowth of nerve tissue, i.e. neurofibromas.

TREATMENT

The condition should be managed by identifying early any serious medical problems, use of prophylactic and symptomatic treatment combined with providing psychological support. A multi-disciplinary team approach is required that includes dermatologists, plastic and orthopaedic surgeons, paediatricians, geneticists and psychologists.

Treatment options are individualised to the patient's needs and range from medical support for predisposition to thrombosis, pulsed dye laser for capillary malformations and surgical resection for overgrowth or bleeding vascular malformations.

PROGNOSIS

Although data on long-term survival are not currently available, complications are likely to contribute to premature death. Prompt attention to complications and early detection of potential problems may significantly reduce overall morbidity and mortality.

TABLE 20.1 Diagnostic criteria for Proteus syndrome

GENERAL CRITERIA

Mosaic distribution

Progressive course

Sporadic occurrence

SPECIFIC CRITERIA

Category A

Cerebriform connective tissue nevus[1]

Category B

Linear epidermal nevus[2]

Asymmetric, disproportionate overgrowth of two of:[3] limbs, skull, external auditory canal, vertebrae or viscera

Specific tumors in the first decade of life:

- Bilateral ovarian cystadenomas[4]
- Monomorphic parotid adenomas[5]

Category C

Dysregulated adipose tissue[6]

Vascular malformations:[7] capillary, venous and/or lymphatic

Lung bullae[8]

Facial phenotype:[9] long face, dolichocephaly, down-slanted palpebral fissures, low nasal bridge, wide or anteverted nares, open mouth at rest

RADIAL LONGITUDINAL DEFICIENCY

INCIDENCE

Radial longitudinal deficiency (RLD) is also known as radial dysplasia or 'radial club hand'. Its overall incidence ranges from 1 in 30,000 to 1 in 100,000 live births. The incidence of unilateral cases equals that of bilateral.

AETIOLOGY/PATHOGENESIS

The aetiology of most cases of RLD is unknown. However, some environmental factors have been implicated in the past including drugs, radiation, poor nutrition and viruses. A well known associated drug teratogen is thalidomide – a sedative used by some pregnant women during the 1950s and early 60s.

CLINICAL PRESENTATION

Most patients with RLD will have a shortened forearm with a radial bow, severe radial deviation of the hand at the wrist, and hypoplasia or aplasia of the thumb (**Figs 20.17, 20.18**). Bayne and Klug categorised RLD into four types based on the amount of radius present. Type I is characterised by mild radial shortening. Cases with a hypoplastic (or 'miniature') radius are considered type II, partial absence of the radius constitutes type III, and total absence type IV. Associated conditions are common and can effect almost any organ system. These include blood dyscrasias such as Fanconi anaemia and thrombocytopenia-absent radius, heart conditions such as Holt–Oram syndrome and multi-system disorders such as VACTERL association.

DIAGNOSIS

Prenatal diagnosis is possible through ultrasound screening. Clinical and radiographic evaluation of the newborn will enable severity grading and treatment planning. As associated anomalies are common, detection of the limb abnormality should prompt investigation for other conditions, which are present in approximately 40% of unilateral and 77% of bilateral cases.

DIFFERENTIAL DIAGNOSIS

Underdevelopment of the radius can be easily established through clinical and radiographic examination of the upper limb. It is important to look for anomalies along the length of the upper limb including abnormalities of the elbow, wrist, thumb and digits, as well as associated conditions affecting other organ systems as mentioned above.

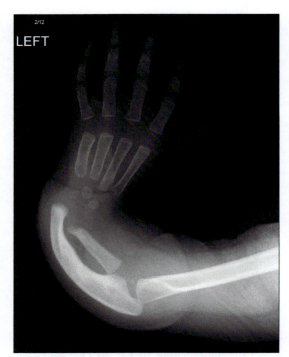

FIGURE 20.17 Radiograph of a child with type II radial longitudinal deficiency.

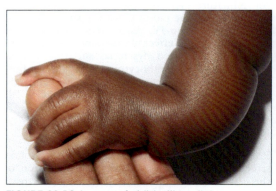

FIGURE 20.18 Image of child with radial longitudinal deficiency – demonstrating a short forearm, radial deviation at the wrist and an absent thumb.

TREATMENT

Treatment for these patients begins with manual stretching exercises and splintage from birth. The mainstay of surgical treatment is a technique known as centralisation, where the carpus is moved onto the central portion of the distal ulna, as a means of correcting radial deviation and wrist subluxation. In cases of severe radial deviation, centralising the wrist can be difficult at the time of surgery, due to tight and unforgiving soft tissue contractures. Therefore precentralisation soft tissue distraction is now recommended in the majority of severe cases and in late-presenting patients with significant fixed deformities of the wrist. As the entire radial side of the upper limb can be hypoplastic in this condition, affected children may lack a functional thumb. This may necessitate thumb reconstruction in the form of index finger pollicisation in later life.

PROGNOSIS

Generally children with congenital upper limb abnormalities such as radial deficiency adapt well to their disability. Outcomes of treatment vary according to the severity of the condition. Centralisation procedures effectively increase overall limb length, create a more aesthetically acceptable upper extremity and improve wrist positioning for finger function and thumb reconstruction. However, regardless of treatment ulnar growth is compromised in the majority to around 50–60% of normal.

VASCULAR ANOMALIES

The term vascular anomalies encompasses benign vascular lesions that can be either vascular tumours or malformations.[13,14] The commonest tumour is the infantile haemangioma or strawberry birthmark. Les common lesions are rapidly-involuting congenital haemangioma (RICH), non-involuting congenital haemangioma (NICH), kaposiform haemangioendothelioma/tufted angioma and infantile myofibroma. Vascular malformations are classified by their vessel type into capillary, venous, lymphatic, and arteriovenous malformations. Mixed types are very common.

CAPILLARY MALFORMATIONS IN LATER CHILDHOOD

INCIDENCE

Capillary malformations are rare, occurring in 3–5 per 1000 births.[15] They are commonly known as port wine stains and many occur on the face.

AETIOLOGY/PATHOGENESIS

The lesions are commonly isolated and consist of dilated capillaries; studies have indicated a lack of vasoconstrictor innervation. With time the surrounding soft tissue and even bone can hypertrophy causing further deformity and the need referral for plastic surgery.

CLINICAL PRESENTATION

The lesions or patches are present at birth and grow with the child, but some are diagnosed later as they become more obvious. Initially they are a pale pink but become darker turning blue/purple with time and into adulthood. Nodules may appear on the involved skin. These are usually either pyogenic granuloma, which bleed easily, or nodules of hypertrophic skin (that do not bleed) and there is even a higher incidence of squamous cell carcinoma in adults on involved skin especially in sun exposed areas.

DIAGNOSIS

The diagnosis is clinical. In the neonate and infant the areas blanch easily but later on there is fixed staining, which is thought to be due to haemosiderin deposition.

DIFFERENTIAL DIAGNOSIS

Capillary malformations may occur with other vascular anomalies or in recognised patterns or associated with limb hypertrophy in a number of syndromes:

- Klippel–Trenaunay (associated with lymphatic and venous malformation and
- Cutis mamorata telengiectasia congenita (associated with limb hypertrophy, where the colour often fades).
- Sturge–Weber (the malformation is in the distribution of a branch of the facial nerve and there are associated eye (glaucoma) and brain anomalies (seizures).
- Parkes–Weber (association with arteriovenous malformations).
- Proteus (see above).
- Capillary malformation–arteriovenous malformation (a rare condition with both malformations, a positive family history and associated with *RASA1* gene mutations).[16]

TREATMENT

In childhood, the primary effective treatment is thermocoagulation with one of the vascular lasers, the pulsed dye being the most popular. The lesions fade but may recur. Surgery is indicated for soft tissue and bone hypertrophy that occurs especially during puberty and treatment is therefore best planned in late teenage (**Figs 20.19, 20.20**). Camouflage has a role at all ages.

PROGNOSIS

The lesions are permanent and overall management involves helping patients to live with the deformity; psychological support is important.

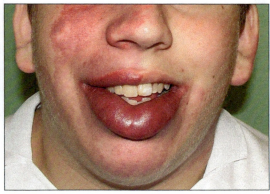

FIGURE 20.19 A teenager with facial (non-syndromic) capillary malformation and secondary lip hypertrophy.

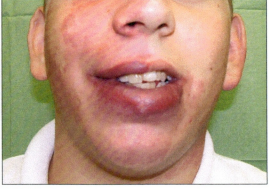

FIGURE 20.20 The same patient after his first lip reduction procedure. One more operation was done when he was older.

INFANTILE HAEMANGIOMA

INCIDENCE

Infantile haemangioma (IH) is relatively common. The true incidence is not known as many smaller IH never require medical attention, but it is estimated to affect up to 10% of Caucasian babies. IH is 2–4 times more common in girls than boys. It is more common in premature births.

AETIOLOGY/PATHOGENESIS

The aetiology is unknown.

CLINICAL PRESENTATION

At birth there is either nothing seen, or occasional a small red dot or mark on the skin. The lesion becomes apparent over the first 6 weeks of life. There is then a proliferative phase for 6–12 months. The appearance varies according to how superficial the IH lies, and how large it is. More superficial IH tends to have a slightly raised and bright red surface in infancy. Deeper IH will tend to be more palpable than visible, but may have overlying bluish discolouration or telangiectasia. The area is warm, non-pulsatile and compressible. Although IH tends to involute, there is considerable variation in how rapidly and at what age involution occurs. As a rule of thumb, 50% involute by age 5 years, and 80% by age 8 years old. Deeper lesions can leave a fibro-fatty residuum; superficial or ulcerated lesions can leave skin changes with loss of elasticity and dermal atrophy.

DIAGNOSIS

Diagnosis is typically made based on the history, and assisted by clinical examination. Doppler ultrasound and MRI can assist with diagnosis. IH demonstrates high flow on Doppler. GLUT-1 staining is positive on histology.

DIFFERENTIAL DIAGNOSIS

- Pyogenic granuloma.
- NICH.
- RICH.
- Kaposiform haemangioendothelioma.
- Tufted angioma.
- Arteriovenous malformation.

TREATMENT

The majority of cases require no treatment, and will involute over time. The indications for treatment are: ulceration, bleeding and pain (typically only large IH, often perineal); obstruction or predicted obstruction of key functional area (e.g. airway, vision, hearing); distortion of key area (e.g. nose, lips); later treatment of residuum. Since 2008, propanolol has become the mainstay of medical treatment (**Figs 20.21, 20.22**).[17] Surgery has an occasional selective role in early treatment, and wider role in treatment of residuum. Pulsed dye laser can be useful for residual telangiectasia.

PROGNOSIS

The prognosis of IH is usually good. Early identification of problematic IH is important, as is reassuring parents of children with simpler lesions so that unnecessary treatment can be avoided.

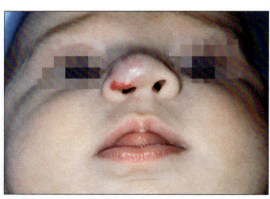

FIGURE 20.21 Infantile haemangioma of the nose.

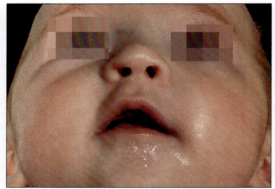

FIGURE 20.22 Same child as in **20.21** 2 months after oral β-blocker therapy. (Courtesy of the Department of Medical Photography, Broomfield Hospital.)

ACKNOWLEDGEMENTS

The authors are indebted to Mr M. Moses, Craniofacial Fellow and Mr J. Volcano from the Department of Medical Illustration, GOSH for preparing several of these images.

REFERENCES

1 Demircioglu M, Kangesu L, Ismail A, *et al.* Increasing accuracy of antenatal ultrasound diagnosis of cleft lip with or without cleft palate, in cases referred to the North Thames London Region. *Ultrasound Obstet Gynecol* 2008;31(6):647–51.

2 Kinsler V, Bulstrode N. The role of surgery in the management of congenital melanocytic naevi in children: a perspective from Great Ormond Street Hospital. *J Plast Reconstr Aesthet Surg* 2009;62(5):595–601.

3 Newton Bishop J. Melanocytic naevi and melanoma. In: Harper JOA, Prose N (eds). *Textbook of Paediatric Dermatology.* Oxford: Blackwell, 2006, pp. 1105–21.

4 Kinsler VA, Birley J, Atherton DJ. Great Ormond Street Hospital for Children Registry for congenital melanocytic naevi: prospective study 1988–2007. Part 1– epidemiology, phenotype and outcomes. *Br J Dermatol* 2009;160(1):143–50.

5 Kinsler VA, Birley J, Atherton DJ. Great Ormond Street Hospital for Children Registry for Congenital Melanocytic Naevi: prospective study 1988-2007. Part 2 – evaluation of treatments. *Br J Dermatol* 2009;160(2):387–92.

6 Jones BM, Hayward R, Evans R, Britto J. Occipital plagiocephaly: an epidemic of craniosynostosis? *Br Med J* 1997;315(7110):693–4.

7 Gault DT. Extravasation injuries. *Br J Plast Surg* 1993;46:91–6.

8 Vento AR, LaBrie RA, Mulliken JB. The O.M.E.N.S. classification of hemifacial microsomia. *Cleft Palate Craniofac J* 1991;28:68–76.

9 Cohen M. Proteus syndrome: an update. *Am J Med Genet C Semin Med Genet* 2005;137C(1):38–52.

10 Tibbles JA, Cohen MM, Jr. The Proteus syndrome: the Elephant Man diagnosed. *Br Med J (Clin Res Ed)* 1986;293(6548):683–5.

11 Lindhurst MJ, Sapp JC, Teer JK, *et al.* A mosaic activating mutation in AKT1 associated with the Proteus syndrome. *N Engl J Med* 2011;365:611–19.

12 Biesecker L. The challenges of Proteus syndrome: diagnosis and management. *Eur J Hum Genet* 2006;14(11):1151–7.

13 Mulliken JB, Glowacki J. Hemangiomas and vascular malformations in infants and children: a classification based on endothelial characteristics. *Plast Reconstr Surg* 1982;69: 412–22.

14 Enjolras O. Classification and management of the various superficial vascular anomalies: hemangiomas and vascular malformations. *J Dermatol* 1997;24(11):701–10.

15 Alper JC, Holmes LB. The incidence and significance of birthmarks in a cohort of 4,641 newborns. *Pediatr Dermatol* 1983;1(1):58–68.

16 Orme CM, Boyden LM, Choate KA, Antaya RJ, King BA. Capillary malformation –arteriovenous malformation syndrome: review of the literature, proposed diagnostic criteria, and recommendations for management. *Pediatr Dermatol* 2013;30(4):409–15.

17 Leaute-Labreze C, Dumas de la Roque E, Hubiche T, Boralevi F, Thambo JB, Taïeb A. Propanolol for severe hemangiomas of infancy. *N Engl J Med* 2008;358:2649–51.

21 Orthopaedics and Fractures

Deborah M. Eastwood

Children change as they grow: their musculoskeletal system is designed to withstand and indeed adapt to the changing forces and stresses that occur as a baby progresses through from infancy to skeletal maturity. This process can be both 'painful and ungainly' and hence the cause of considerable concern to parents and often to clinicians. The aim of this chapter is to help the reader to identify what is normal, what is abnormal and what will change with growth and over time thus giving you the confidence to recognise the cases where there is cause for concern. A good history and complete examination with a knowledge of growth and development are the keys to making the correct diagnosis. It is always helpful to plot the heights of the child and his/her parents on a growth chart (**Fig. 21.1**).

Assess the presence/absence of the 5 Ss:

- Symmetry.
- Stiffness.
- Symptoms.
- Skeletal dysplasias.
- Systemic disorder.

Symmetrical, asymptomatic problems in an otherwise normal child are usually no cause for concern.

NORMAL VARIATIONS OF GAIT AND POSTURE

Most differences in gait patterns are usually just variations of normal (i.e. mean ±2 standard deviations) rather than a pathological condition. The foot progression angle is defined as the angle of the foot in relation to an imaginary straight line that the patient is walking; it represents the sum total of the shape of the bones in the leg and the muscular forces acting on them (**Fig. 21.2**).

INTOEING

An intoeing gait is a very common cause of parental concern and childhood 'tripping' (**Table 21.1**) It is rarely a cause of orthopaedic concern. The intoeing may orginate from one of three sites:
- The hip/thigh – femoral neck anteversion (**Fig. 21.3**).
- The tibia – internal tibial torsion.
- The foot – metatarsus adductus (**Fig. 21.4**).

TABLE 21.1 Intoeing

Cause of intoeing	Typical age at presentation	Age at resolution	Treatment required	Type
Metatarsus adductus	Infant	2–3 y	Occasionally	Physiotherapy and/or casting
Tibial torsion	Toddler	4–6 y	Occasionally Very rarely	Gait education Tibial osteotomy
Femoral neck anteversion	Child	8–11 y	Occasionally Very rarely	Gait education Femoral osteotomy

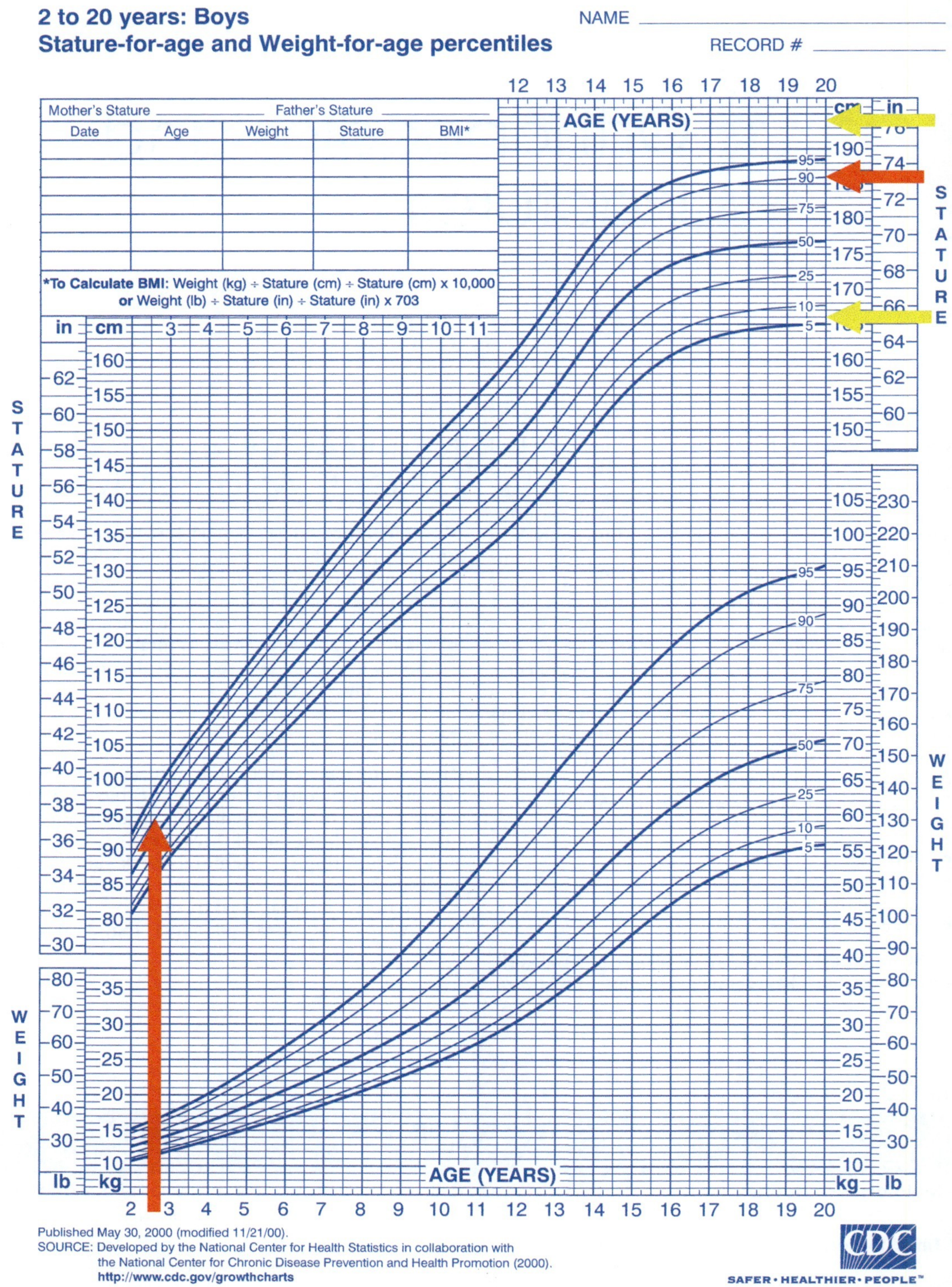

2 to 20 years: Boys
Stature-for-age and Weight-for-age percentiles

NAME _____

RECORD # _____

FIGURE 21.1 Growth chart for boys depicting a red arrow that represents the child's height age 2.5 years. The yellow arrows represent father's height and mother's height; the child's predicted height at skeletal maturity (the short red arrow) is at the mid-parental height given a correction for gender.

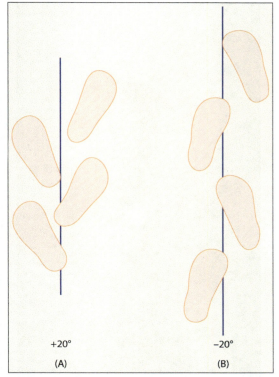

+20°

(A)

−20°

(B)

FIGURE 21.2 Foot progression angle demonstrating (A) extoeing and (B) intoeing gait patterns. The cause of the gait abnormality is identified on clinical examination. (From Williams *et al.* (eds), *Bailey and Love's Short Practice of Surgery*, CRC Press 2013, with permission.)

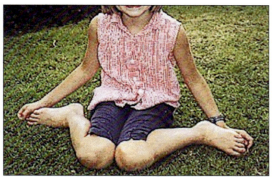

FIGURE 21.3 Child showing increased hip internal rotation ability and the 'w'-sitting posture characteristic of femoral neck anteversion. Such children often have an intoeing gait pattern.

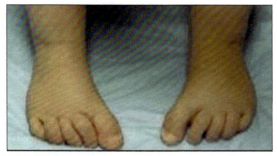

FIGURE 21.4 Metatarsus adductus – if the curved lateral border of the forefoot is correctible/flexible, by pushing on the medial border, no treatment is required; if it is stiff, then physiotherapy stretches and/or casting may be required.

EXTOEING

A tendency to ex-toe is less common. It is usually due to an external rotation contracture of the infant hip or tibial torsion in the older child. In the infant it may be a cause of a late start to walking.

Spontaneous resolution is common but occasionally corrective tibial osteotomies are required in the older child.

TIP-TOE WALKING

This often represents a stage that children pass through as they develop a normal walking pattern. A neurological abnormality must be excluded in bilateral cases and in unilateral cases, a dislocated hip or congenital anomaly creating a leg length difference must be considered (**Fig. 21.5**).

Treatment

Spontaneous improvement is likely but in some families there is a history of idiopathic toe-walking and these cases may require further treatment with physiotherapy or release of the Achilles tendon if this is tight.

BOWLEGS AND KNOCK KNEES (GENU VARUM AND GENU VALGUM)

Normal growth charts show that any individual child can go from a significant degree of bow legs in infancy to definite knock knees as a toddler and yet still turn out to have normal leg alignment by the age of 7–8 years (**Fig. 21.6**). Clinical examination usually confirms the diagnosis but sometimes a standing leg alignment radiograph helps to exclude a pathological cause and allows the deformity to be quantified (**Fig. 21.7**).

Treatment

No treatment is required if a pathological condition has been excluded; spontaneous improvement is expected (unless bow legs/knock knees run in the family: look at mother and father!). If the deformity is noticeable in later childhood and/or progressive or asymmetrical an underlying cause should be identified and treatment offered to ensure normal alignment. Prior to skeletal maturity, surgical treatment may be relatively simple using guided growth techniques (**Figs 21.8, 21.9**).

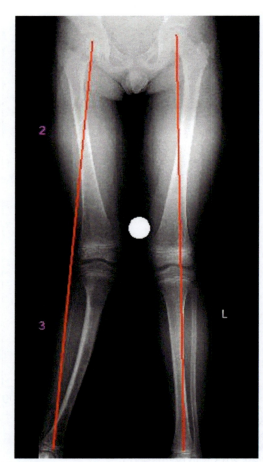

FIGURE 21.7 Standing leg alignment radiograph documenting genu valgum (knock knees). The mechanical axis is a line that links the centre of the hip to the centre of the ankle: it should pass through the centre of the knee. In this example the line from hip to ankle passes lateral to the middle of the knee joint. On the patient's left the line is within the central half of the knee and thus normal; on the right the line is outside the knee joint and thus very abnormal. The underlying diagnosis is R fibula hemimelia.

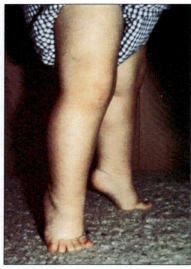

FIGURE 21.5 Child demonstrating a tip-toe gait; note that her knees are straight. A child with toe walking and flexed knees might have a neurological cause for the gait pattern.

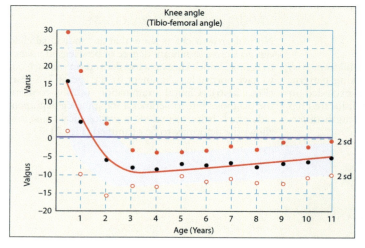

FIGURE 21.6 Graph depicting the change from genu varum to genu valgum to normal alignment during the first few years of life. (From Williams *et al.* (eds), *Bailey and Love's Short Practice of Surgery*, CRC Press 2013, with permission.)

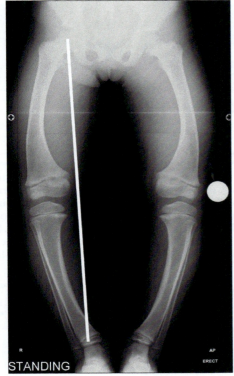

FIGURE 21.8 AP leg alignment radiograph demonstrating bow legs. Two plates have been inserted on the lateral aspect of the limb, spanning the growth plate or physis and hence tethering growth on this side. Unimpeded growth occurs on the opposite side of the limb and over time the deformity corrects.

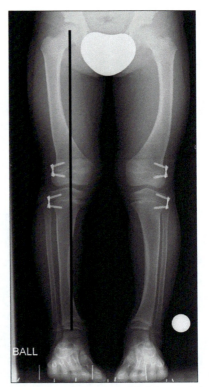

FIGURE 21.9 Same child as in 21.8 1 year later demonstrating correction of deformity and the mechanical axis now passes through the centre of the knee. The underlying diagnosis was hypophosphataemic rickets.

FLAT FEET

All children under 3 years have fat and flat feet: the medial longitudinal arch has not yet developed. Many children continue to have flat feet, perhaps associated with their normal joint laxity.

Flat feet may be more common in conditions (such as trisomy 21) where ligamentous laxity is more obvious. Most adults do **not** have flat feet although genetic factors (both family and racial) influence this. The majority of flat feet are asymptomatic: they do **not** predispose the child to backache or arthritis in later life.

The natural history of flat feet is for spontaneous improvement and the painless, flexible flat foot needs **no** treatment. Orthoses **do not** alter the natural history of the condition but can alleviate symptoms such as tired/achy calves or feet, **if** they arise.

The flexible flat foot may look quite abnormal and this causes parental concern. (**Fig. 21.10**). The symptomatic, rigid flat foot is usually the result of a tarsal coalition or inflammation and appropriate medical or surgical treatment may be required. Clinical examination and appropriate imaging differentiates between the flexible and the rigid foot (**Table 21.2**) (**Figs 21.11, 21.12**).

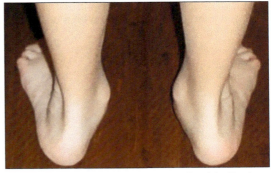

FIGURE 21.10 Flexible flat foot showing hindfoot valgus and the 'too many toes' sign when viewed from behind.

TABLE 21.2 Differentiation between the flexible and rigid foot

Type	Characteristics
Flexible	On tip-toe the arch is restored and the heel corrects into varus; subtalar joint movements are full and pain free
Rigid	On tip-toe the arch fails to return; subtalar joint movements are restricted and often painful

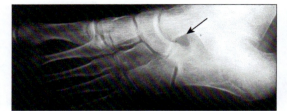

FIGURE 21.11 Oblique radiograph of the foot showing a calcaneonavicular coalition. The arrow points to the almost complete bony fusion: there is no space between the two bones on this view.

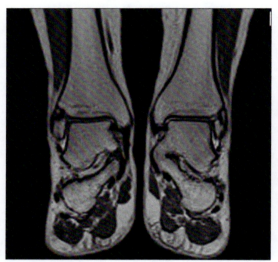

FIGURE 21.12 A coronal CT scan demonstrating a talocalcaneal coalition on the left: on the right there is a joint space between the talus and the calcaneum.

CONGENITAL AND DEVELOPMENTAL ABNORMALITIES OF THE LOWER LIMB

POSTURAL ABNORMALITIES (THE MOULDED BABY)

Many babies are subjected to moulding pressures whilst *in utero*. At birth they have 'postural deformities': the foot will tend to lie in either calcaneovalgus (up and out) (**Figs 21.13A, B**) or equinovarus (down and in). Torticollis and plagiocephaly (**Fig. 21.14**) are also common, as are asymmetric hip movements which may raise the possibility of a dislocated hip.

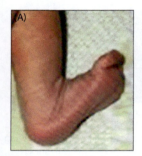
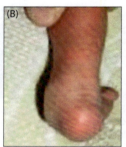

FIGURE 21.13 (A) An infant foot lying in a calcaneovalgus position viewed from the side; (B) from behind.

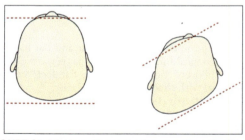

FIGURE 21.14 Line diagram of a plagiocephalic head secondary to intrauterine moulding.

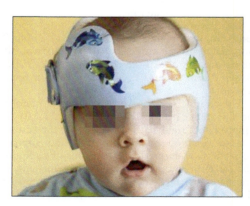

FIGURE 21.15 A child wearing a helmet to aid correction of this moulding abnormality.

Orthopaedics and fractures

A careful examination will exclude significant abnormalities; postural problems improve with time and/or some stretching exercises. Occasionally plagiocephaly is treated with a helmet (**Fig. 21.15**).

CONGENITAL TALIPES EQUINOVARUS DEFORMITY ('THE CLUB FOOT')

AETIOLOGY/INCIDENCE

The foot with a congenital talipes equinovarus (CTEV) points 'down and in' (**Fig. 21.16**). It is always present at birth and can often be detected on antenatal scans although it is not easy/accurate to judge the severity of the condition *in utero*. The false positive rate is approximately 15%.

Clubfeet may be postural, idiopathic, syndromic or neuromuscular in origin. For idiopathic feet, the incidence is 1–2/1000 and 50–60% are bilateral; boys are more frequently affected. There is a small increased risk with affected siblings or a family history.

TREATMENT

- All idiopathic feet respond well to the Ponseti treatment regime: a system that involves weekly foot manipulations and application of above-knee plaster casts that sequentially correct all aspects of the foot deformity (in reverse order: 'CAVE', **Table 21.3**) (**Figs 21.17, 21.18**).
- An Achilles tendon release performed in clinic under local anaesthetic is often required to gain full correction. 95% of idiopathic feet avoid a major surgical procedure. The child wears a system of 'boots and bars' at night time and naptime for the first few years of life (**Fig. 21.19**).

TABLE 21.3 Ponseti treatment regime

Description	Site of the deformity
Equinus	Hindfoot
Varus	Subtalar joint
Adduction	Midfoot and forefoot
Cavus	Pronation of the first ray

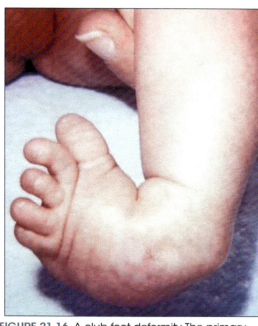

FIGURE 21.16 A club foot deformity. The primary pathology can be considered to be a subluxation of the talonavicular joint; treatment aims at stretching the tight soft tissues to allow the joint to 'relocate'.

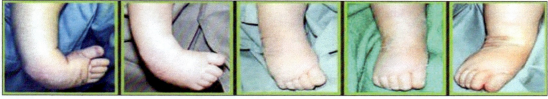

FIGURE 21.17 A series of photographs of the club foot deformity being corrected with weekly manipulations and casting.

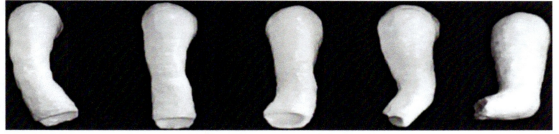

FIGURE 21.18 The shape of the casts mirrors the improving club foot position.

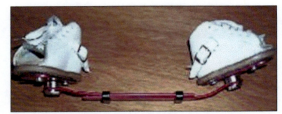

FIGURE 21.19 The 'boots and bars' that the children wear for some part of the day/night for the first 4 years of life to maintain the club foot correction.

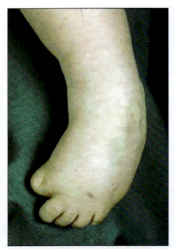

FIGURE 21.20 A congenital talipes equinovarus deformity secondary to amniotic band syndrome. Note the 'amputated' tip of the great toe and the relatively featureless appearance of the skin/soft tissues.

PROGNOSIS

- Relapse or recurrence can be treated with further casting and/or a tibialis anterior tendon transfer. The foot may always be small with a wasted calf when compared to the contralateral normal side and there may be a small leg length difference.
- Multiple recurrences/relapses suggest a non-idiopathic aetiology and a neurological cause should be sought.
- The results of treatment of the non-idiopathic/syndromic club foot (**Fig. 21.20**) are not so good but it is still worthwhile attempting the Ponseti technique as it may lessen the surgery required.

CONGENITAL VERTICAL TALUS

AETIOLOGY/INCIDENCE

- Congenital vertical talus (CTV) is much rarer than CTEV deformities. In CVT the child has a rocker-bottom foot: the foot may appear 'flat' with a bony lump (the talar head) taking up the arch of the foot. Up to 50% of cases are associated with other abnormalities and classified as syndromic feet (**Figs 21.21, 21.22**).

TREATMENT

- A modified Ponseti technique is used to manipulate the foot into position although overall the results are less successful than with a club foot and surgical treatment is often required.

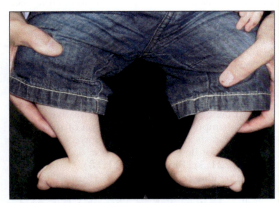

FIGURE 21.21 Bilateral congenital vertical talus foot deformities in a child with arthrogryposis: the feet have a 'rocker-bottom' appearance.

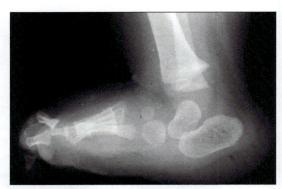

FIGURE 21.22 A lateral x-ray of a foot demonstrating the radiological features of the rocker bottom foot which occurs in congenital vertical talus (hindfoot equinus with a dorsiflexed midfoot and a subluxed talonavicular joint). (From Williams *et al.* (eds), *Bailey and Love's Short Practice of Surgery*, CRC Press, 2013, with permission.)

DEVELOPMENTAL DYSPLASIA OF THE HIP

AETIOLOGY/INCIDENCE

Developmental dysplasia of the hip (DDH) describes the spectrum of hip instability ranging from the irreducibly dislocated hip to the hip that is correctly located but associated with a shallow ('dysplastic') acetabulum.

The incidence of neonatal instability may be as high as 20 cases per 1000 births, whereas the incidence of dislocated hips is about 2 cases per 1000 live births. Many hips that are unstable at birth will stabilise spontaneously.

- The quoted risk factors vary but the following should always be noted:
  - Female.
  - Breech position.
  - Family history.
- All babies are examined at birth and at various subsequent timepoints (NIPE programme) looking for signs of hip instability, subluxation and dislocation (**Table 21.4, Fig. 21.23**). Asymmetric thigh skin folds on their own are not a risk factor; soft tissue 'clicks' are common and not now

TABLE 21.4 Questions to ask on a neonatal hip examination

1. Is the hip dislocated?	If so, is it reducible?	Ortolani positive
	If not ….	Ortolani negative
2. Is the hip dislocatable?	Does it sublux/dislocate?	Barlow positive
3. Is the hip clinically normal?	If so, does it have risk factors requiring further investigations?	Ultrasound scan for diagnosis

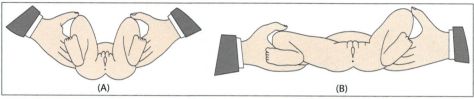

FIGURE 21.23 Neonatal hip examination. (A) Line diagram of a child with hips and knees flexed to 90° about to undergo a neonatal hip examination; (B) limited abduction in flexion of the baby's left hip. Note the fingers on the lateral proximal thigh at the level of the greater trochanter. Once limitation of abduction has been identified, the examiner can use this finger to lift up on the trochanter to see if the hip will reduce (Ortolani test: positive if the hip reduces). The hips must be flexed to at least 90° before the hips are abducted: less flexion and the limitation of abduction is much less obvious.

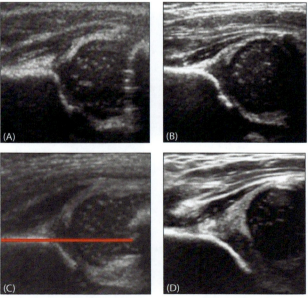

FIGURE 21.24 (A) a normal ultrasound scan; (B, C) scans showing progressive dysplasia, i.e. a 'shallow' acetabulum with less than 50% of the femoral head lying within the acetabulum (the red line defines the Morin Index: the percentage of the femoral head 'contained' within the acetabulum); (D) the femoral head is subluxed and the acetabulum severely dysplastic. (From Sewell M *et al.*, *BMJ* 2009;339:4454, with permission.)

considered to be a risk factor. It is important however, to maintain a high index of suspicion as early detection is the key to successful treatment.

- If the clinical examination is unclear and/or there are risk factors for DDH an ultrasound scan should be performed (**Figs 21.24, 21.25**).

TREATMENT

Neonatal presentation

- Dislocated and/or unstable joints must be reduced and held in joint by the simplest means possible. In the infant, treatment should be commenced between 2 and 6 weeks of age. A Pavlik harness (or similar splint) is worn for essentially 24 hours per day for a period of 6–8 weeks depending on how quickly the dysplasia resolves and the stability improves (**Fig. 21.26**). Some clinicians wean the baby out of the splint – others do not. If early treatment fails, the hip is treated as below as a 'late presenting' hip.

Late presentation

- Unfortunately, in many parts of the UK and around the world, diagnosis is delayed and the child presents later in infancy with restricted hip movements or, after walking age, with a limp. The clinical signs are:
- A leg length difference (Galeazzi sign positive) (**Fig. 21.27**).
- The short leg lies in external rotation.
- Limited abduction in flexion; in unilateral cases a difference in the arc of movement of 20° or so between the left and right legs may be significant (**Fig. 21.28**).
- Beware the bilateral cases: the gait pattern is waddling but the signs on examination are symmetrical and thus harder to identify (**Fig. 21.23**). After the age of 4–5 months, x-rays are the investigation of choice (**Figs 21.29, 21.30**).

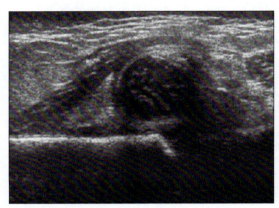

FIGURE 21.25 An ultrasound scan showing a femoral head lying outside the acetabulum (a dislocated hip); such a scan is **not** incompatible with a seemingly normal clinical examination.

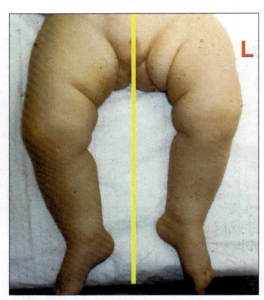

FIGURE 21.27 A child (under anaesthetic) demonstrating a short left leg, asymmetrical skin creases and a widened perineum suggestive of a dislocated left hip. The Galeazzi sign would have been positive on the left leg.

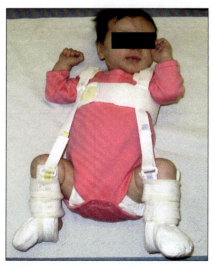

FIGURE 21.26 A baby wearing a Pavlik harness: the hips should be flexed to a right angle and the anterior straps should lie across the baby's thigh.

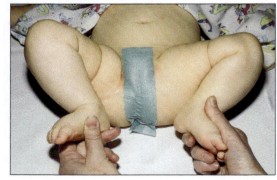

FIGURE 21.28 Clinical photo of a child (under anaesthetic – hence no fingers on the thighs) demonstrating limitation of abduction of the right hip.

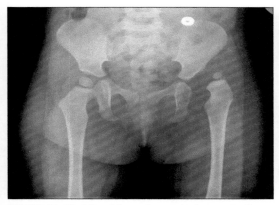

FIGURE 21.29 AP pelvic radiograph demonstrating a dislocated left hip representing a late presentation of developmental dysplasia of the hip. The ossific nucleus (within the cartilaginous anlage) is smaller on the left than on the right, the proximal femur is laterally displaced and the bony acetabulum is abnormally shaped; the acetabular index is high).

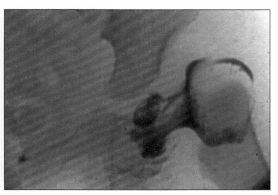

FIGURE 21.30 Arthrogram of the left hip: dye has been injected into the joint to outline the cartilaginous femoral head.

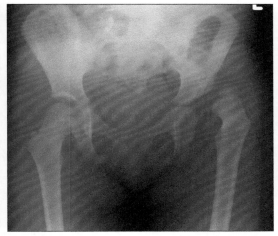

FIGURE 21.31 Plain radiograph of a pelvis showing a dislocated left hip in a 4.5-year-old girl.

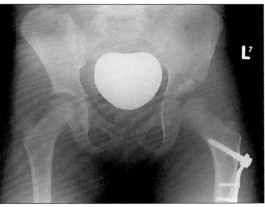

FIGURE 21.32 Same child as in **21.31** 2 years following open reduction and a femoral osteotomy. The hip is reduced, Shenton's line is intact and the hip is stable. The ossific nucleus has grown but the acetabular index has not improved significantly – a pelvic osteotomy may be required.

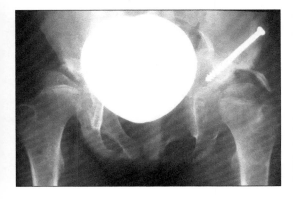

FIGURE 21.33 AP pelvic radiograph of a teenager with a poor outcome following surgical treatment for bilateral late presenting developmental dysplasia of the hip: both hips remain subluxed and 'uncovered'. They will develop degenerate change (osteoarthritis) in early adult life.

- The longer the hip has been 'out', the more aggressive the treatment to relocate it.
- Under the age of 12 months, a closed reduction and soft tissue release might be enough.
- After walking age, an open reduction is usually required and with increasing delay it would be increasingly likely that additional femoral (**Figs 21.31, 21.32**) and/or pelvic osteotomies would be required.
- The more surgery that is needed, the less likely the child is to have an excellent outcome: early detection is therefore very important. Long-term follow-up is required to ensure that the hip continues to develop during childhood and adolescence to minimise the risks of the hip developing degenerative change in later life (**Fig. 21.33**).

LEG LENGTH DISCREPANCIES

AETIOLOGY/CLINICAL PRESENTATION

- Limb length discrepancies (which can affect the upper limbs too) may be secondary to a wide variety of congenital and acquired causes and the 'surgical sieve' may help you think of all the possible causes (**Table 21.5**).
- Congenital abnormalities are classified according to an internationally recognised system illustrated in **Table 21.6**.
- A small difference may not be associated with any problems in childhood or indeed in adult life. The skill lies in identifying the cause and ascertaining if the discrepancy is progressive or not; if it is progressive, it is possible to predict at essentially any age (via a downloaded 'app' or by using standard graphs) what the discrepancy will be at skeletal maturity if the condition is left untreated. If the lower leg discrepancy is predicted to be more than 2–2.5 cm at the end of growth, treatment is advised.
- The discrepancy is measured clinically by standing the child up with a block under the foot on the shorter leg until the pelvis is levelled: the difference is 'checked' on a standing leg length radiograph (**Fig. 21.34**).

TABLE 21.5 Congenital and acquired causes of limb length discrepancy

Congenital	Acquired
Generalised: e.g. skeletal dysplasia	Traumatic
Localised: failure of formation of a limb	Infective
	Metabolic
	Neoplastic
	Vascular
	Inflammatory

TABLE 21.6 Congenital leg length discrepancies

Category	Description	Example
I	Failure of formation of parts • Transverse • Longitudinal	Congenital amputation Fibular hemimelia
II	Failure of differentiation	Vertebral body fusion; radioulnar synostosis
III	Duplication	Extra digits
IV	Overgrowth	Gigantism; macrodactyly
V	Undergrowth	
VI	Congenital constriction band syndrome	Often affects hands/feet with poor formation of the digits
VII	Generalised skeletal abnormalities	Skeletal dysplasia, e.g. achondroplasia

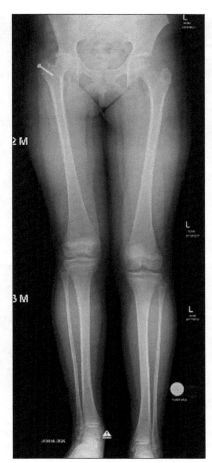

FIGURE 21.34 Standing AP limb length and alignment radiograph; the child has a short right leg secondary to poor development of the proximal femur following osteomyelitis as an infant. She is a standing on a 3 cm block and her pelvis is level. She is due for an epiphyseodesis.

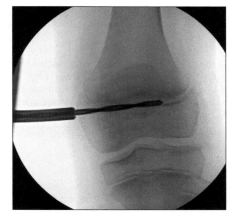

FIGURE 21.35 Intra-operative radiograph of a left knee demonstrating the technique of a 'drill epiphyseodesis' of the distal femoral physis; the name of this surgical technique is incorrect as it is the physis (the growth plate) that is being damaged not the epiphysis. The drill bit must pass along the physis causing enough damage to stop it growing.

TREATMENT

- Treatment may involve the following options:
- Controlling/slowing down the growth of the longer leg via a temporary or permanent epiphyseodesis ('fusion' of the growth plate) (**Fig. 21.35**).
- Formal limb lengthening treatment with an external fixator frame applied to the leg – the most basic advice would be that it takes 30 days in the frame for every 1 cm of length that is gained and only 5–7 cm should/could be gained at any one treatment session. Deformity in terms of angulation and rotation can be corrected at the same time (**Fig. 21.36**).
- Operative shortening of the longer limb: unusual.
- Rarely, amputation and prosthetic limb use.
- A combination of the first two approaches and the use of orthotic supports.

Treatment choice is multi-factorial and of course is defined by the function and comfort of the shorter leg and a holistic assessment of the child and any other associated problems.

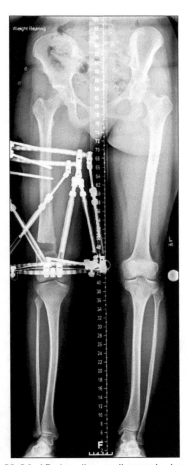

FIGURE 21.36 AP standing radiograph demonstrating leg length and alignment: the right femur has undergone an osteotomy with application of an external fixator to support the limb while the deformity is corrected and the femur lengthened.

FIBULA HEMIMELIA

AETIOLOGY/INCIDENCE

This is the most common major congenital lower limb deformity (1:20–30,000 live births) (**Figs 21.37, 21.38**). It is characterised by the following features, which highlight the fact that this is due to a 'field defect' during embryonic/fetal life:

- Absent or deficient lateral rays of the foot.
- Tarsal coalitions.
- Ball and socket ankle joint.
- Deficient or absent fibula.
- Short and angulated tibia (apex anterior bow to be distinguished from the less troublesome apex posterior bow).
- Absent/deficient knee ligaments.
- Deficient formation of the femoral lateral condyle.
- Short and externally rotated femur.
- Coxa vara and/or hip instability.

Not all the features may be present and usually those at the top of the list are more severe/more obvious than those at the bottom.

- The diagnosis is made on clinical suspicion/examination and on plain radiographs.

TREATMENT

- For this and for all other limb deficiencies is guided by the principles outlined above for the management of a limb length discrepancy. The overall principle is to try to obtain a well-aligned limb of suitable length but with functioning, stable and comfortable joints. In certain circumstances, surgery is associated with complications that adversely affect the outcome: joint instability and/or stiffness may lead to pain and poor function (**Fig. 21.39**).

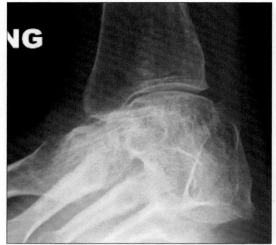

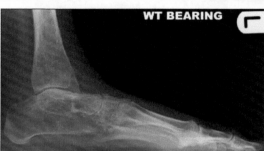

FIGURE 21.38 AP (A) and lateral (B) radiographs of the ankle/foot of an older child with the same condition: an absent fibula, an absent 5th ray of the foot; a ball and socket ankle joint; and a tarsal coalition are noted. The coalition is between the talus and the calcaneum so no subtalar joint movement is possible.

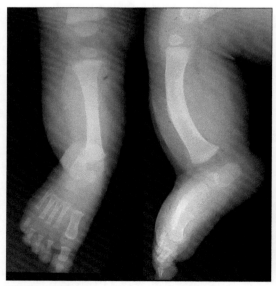

FIGURE 21.37 AP and lateral radiographs of a young child with fibula hemimelia. There is no fibula present on the right lower leg but there are five toes.

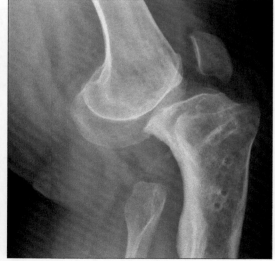

FIGURE 21.39 Lateral radiograph of a knee and tibia following tibial lengthening in a case of fibula hemimelia; the surgery was complicated by subluxation of the knee joint and permanent stiffness. Not all surgery leads to an improvement in function.

PROXIMAL FEMORAL FOCAL DEFICIENCY

- Proximal femoral focal deficiency (PFFD) (**Figs 21.40, 21.41**) is much less common than fibula hemimelia (1 in 50,000 live births). The same features as were listed above for fibula hemimelia may be present, but the severity is in the reverse order so that the development of the hip and proximal femur are most affected (as the name implies). Without a functioning or reconstructable hip joint, limb function is destined to be poor with or without an artificial limb to provide length.

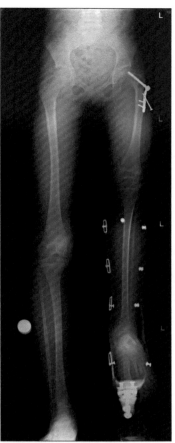

FIGURE 21.41 A child (aged 11 years) with proximal femoral focal deficiency who has undergone hip surgery to stabilise the joint and who wears an extension prosthesis; she has elected to keep her foot and she has refused limb lengthening surgery. (There is a loose screw at the site of her previous femoral osteotomy!)

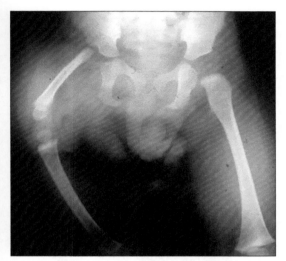

FIGURE 21.40 AP radiograph of both legs of a 6-month-old child showing an underdeveloped proximal femur on the right. The fibula is also absent. The whole of the right leg is about the same length as the left thigh (femur). This is an example of proximal femoral focal deficiency.

CONGENITAL TIBIAL DEFICIENCY

- This is the rarest of the 'classical' lower limb congenital anomalies (1 in 1,000,000 live births). The foot may be relatively well preserved but depending on the severity of the tibial deficiency there may be no functioning ankle or knee joint. The fibula is often deceptively large and it may be mistaken for the tibia. The foot looks like a club foot as there is no 'support' for it at ankle level (**Fig. 21.42**).

TREATMENT

- Ultrasound scans can identify the cartilaginous portions of the tibial remnants; if the proximal tibia is present and if the quadriceps is present, attached and functioning, then a below knee amputation may be possible otherwise, currently, the treatment of choice is a through knee amputation and artificial limb fitting (**Fig. 21.43**).

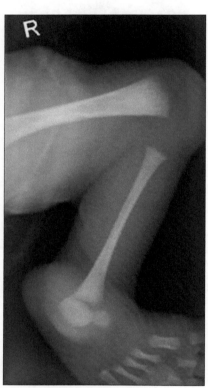

FIGURE 21.42 Lateral radiograph of an infant with an absent tibia: the fibula looks 'large' and may be mistaken for the tibia; the clue is the significant foot deformity and the fibula lies 'behind' the femur, i.e. not articulating with it.

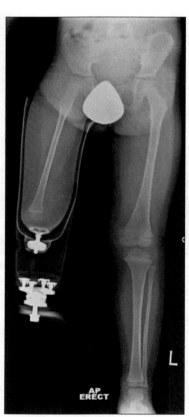

FIGURE 21.43 Same child as in **21.42** aged 4.5 years following a through knee amputation. He is wearing his 'cheetah' artificial limb.

COMMON CONGENITAL TOE PROBLEMS

Curly toes: medial deviation of the 3rd, 4th and/or 5th toes are of no clinical significance. Symptoms are rare but cosmetic concerns are common. The curly toes are treated easily by flexor tenotomy, but the more the toes are treated, the less individual toe movement the child has (**Fig. 21.44**).

Laterally deviated tips of the 2nd and/or 3rd toes are also common and similarly essentially asymptomatic. Surgical treatment is rarely required and should be delayed until late childhood so that growth is not disturbed.

Over-riding 5th toes (**Figs 21.45, 21.46**) may develop symptoms where they rub on shoes; surgical correction is simple and reliable.

Syndactyly (webbing) of the lesser toes is a cosmetic problem; separation can be considered but surgery is more extensive than patients realise.

Ingrowing toenails are a frequent cause of pain and sometimes become infected. Basic advice about nail care and footwear is usually all that is needed but sometimes wedge excision of the lateral nail edge is necessary with phenolisation of the nail bed to prevent regrowth.

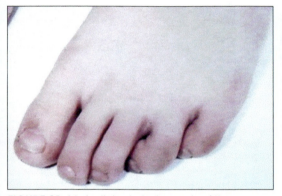

FIGURE 21.44 A clinical photograph of the forefoot of a young child with curly 4th and 5th toes.

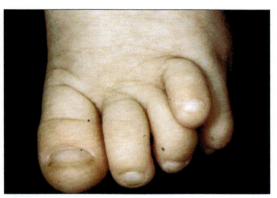

FIGURE 21.45 An 'over-riding' 4th toe is usually due to a short metatarsal, which is often associated with an underlying syndrome.

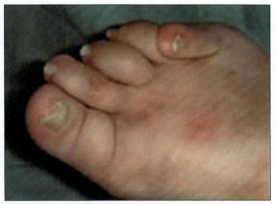

FIGURE 21.46 An over-riding 5th toe is often due to a congenital malformation of the toe; surgical treatment is simple and reliable giving a good cosmetic result.

OTHER CONGENITAL/ ACQUIRED LOWER LIMB PROBLEMS

BLOUNT DISEASE

In this condition there is disordered growth in the posteromedial tibial physis.

- The aetiology is unknown but the infantile form is more common in those of Afro-Caribbean origin. The adolescent onset disease affects all ethnic origins.
- Risk factors include early walking and obesity. The child presents with progressive and often severe tibia vara with significant intoeing. There are classical features on radiography (**Fig. 21.47**).

- Treatment is surgical and, following correction of limb alignment via an osteotomy, an epiphyseodesis of the remaining physis may be necessary to prevent recurrence of deformity. The osteotomy may be stabilised with a plate and screws or with an external fixator device: the latter can be used to correct leg length and it is arguably the most accurate way of correcting limb alignment and joint congruity (**Fig. 21.48**).
- It is possible that the guided growth techniques applied earlier in the pathological process may reduce the need for such extensive surgery (**Figs 21.49, 21.50**).

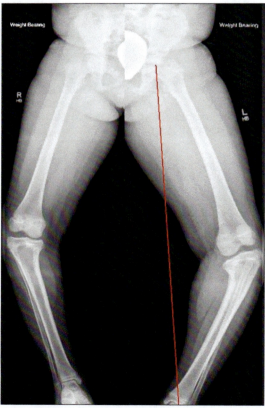

FIGURE 21.47 AP limb alignment view demonstrating bilateral severe bow legs (note the position of the mechanical axes, the radiographs have been 'stitched' together as both legs would not fit on one film), secondary to Blount disease: a condition caused by poor function of the posteromedial part of the proximal tibial physis and epiphysis.

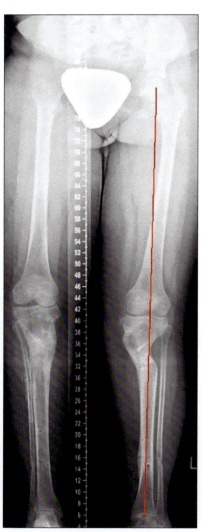

FIGURE 21.48 The same patient as in **21.47** following correction of deformity using an external fixator frame; the left leg has a correct mechanical axis (despite the crooked tibia) and this is the important factor. The right leg has a straighter tibia but actually has some residual deformity in terms of mechanical axis.

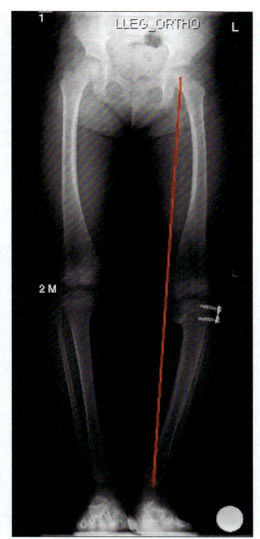

FIGURE 21.49 AP alignment radiograph of a young child with Blount disease. The mechanical axis is medial to the knee; a plate has been inserted recently to tether growth on the lateral side and allow the 'diseased' posteromedial portion of the proximal tibial physis to continue to grow and correct the deformity.

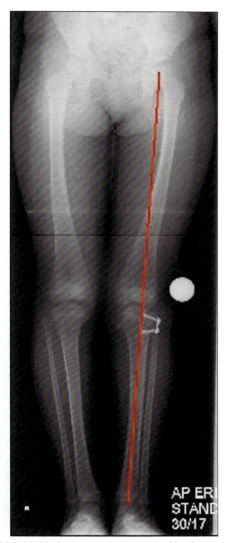

FIGURE 21.50 Similar radiograph to **21.49** taken 12 months later; the mechanical axis is now correct, the screws in the plate have diverged demonstrating that growth has occurred medially.

CONGENITAL PSEUDARTHROSIS OF THE TIBIA

This rare condition presents clinically with an antero-lateral bow (defined by where the apex of the bow is) of the tibia with or without a fracture (**Fig. 21.51**). Classic radiographic changes are noted and up to 50% of cases are thought to be associated with neurofibromatosis. Once fractured the tibia is reluctant to heal and long-term orthotic treatment may be necessary, with subsequent surgical procedures designed to obtain bony union and restore leg length.

POSTEROMEDIAL TIBIAL BOW

Of the uncommon things, this is quite common and it may present as a calcaneovalgus foot deformity but close inspection will show that the problem is in the tibia (apex of the deformity is posteromedial) rather than in the foot. The deformity resolves with time but the child may be left with a short leg that would require leg equalisation treatment (lengthening one leg vs. shortening the other) (**Figs 21.52, 21.53**).

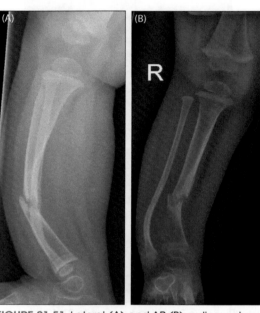

FIGURE 21.51 Lateral (A) and AP (B) radiographs of a child's right tibia/fibula showing a bowed tibia with an anterolateral apex which is a cause for concern: the diagnosis is tibial pseudarthrosis associated with neurofibromatosis.

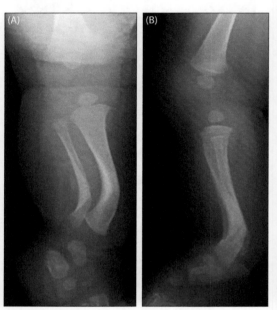

FIGURE 21.52 AP (A) and lateral (B) radiographs of a child's tibia/fibula showing a bowed tibia with a posteromedial apex, which is not such a cause for concern: the bow usually straightens spontaneously but the leg is often a few centimetres short.

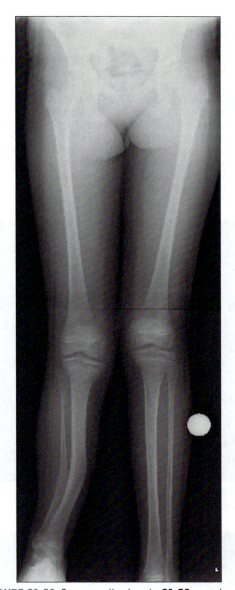

PES CAVUS (THE HIGH ARCHED FOOT)

In contrast to the flat foot, a high arched foot is almost always a warning sign of an underlying neurological abnormality, particularly if there is a progressive change in shape of the foot (**Fig. 21.54**). Spina bifida, tethered cord syndrome and the peripheral neuropathies (hereditary sensory motor neuropathies types 1, 2) should be considered. Investigations should be conducted as necessary with spinal MR and/or neurophysiological testing.

Treatment includes:

- Physiotherapy stretches/orthotic supports: both aim to prevent further joint/soft tissue contractures and maintain function and comfort.
- Surgical treatment may be required: the timing depends on the aetiology.

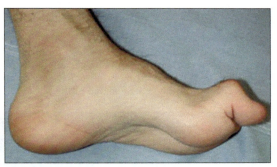

FIGURE 21.53 Same patient as in **21.52** aged 10 years. She has more than the usual amount of residual bowing and the leg is 5 cm short; correction of deformity and leg lengthening will be performed.

FIGURE 21.54 A lateral clinical photograph of a high-arched (cavus) foot with clawing of the great toe. This type of foot is often seen in older children or adolescents; a neuropathic cause must be sought and excluded.

CLASSIC CAUSES OF LOWER LIMB PAIN

GROWING PAINS

These must be a diagnosis of exclusion but they are a legitimate cause of parental distress and children's pain. They are defined as:

- Pain lasting for >3 months.
- Symptom-free intervals.
- Pain at the end of the day or waking the child at night that is not necessarily joint related.
- Symptoms tend to be symmetrical and equally severe but they may alternate from limb to limb.
- Symptoms that are unilateral may require more investigation to exclude rarities such as tumours and infections.
- Treatment involves reassurance, explanation and conservative measures.

KNEE PAIN

Osgood–Schlatter disease

- Tenderness and swelling are localised to the tibial apophysis, either unilaterally or bilaterally.
- Pain is often asymmetrical, exacerbated by exercise and/or by prolonged periods of sitting with the knees bent.
- Symptoms are frequently precipitated by growth or a minor injury.
- Conservative treatment consisting of relative rest, reassurance and analgesia is usually helpful.

Anterior knee pain syndrome

- Symptoms of ill-defined pain around the front of the knee, with giving way and clicking, exacerbated by prolonged sitting or by activity, are often present in both knees of teenage girls.

- Patellofemoral crepitus may be detected on examination with discomfort on patellofemoral compression.
- Patella maltracking (see Patellofemoral subluxation) must be excluded.

Patellofemoral subluxation

- This usually presents in adolescent girls.
- Treatment is usually conservative with physiotherapy to strengthen the quadriceps muscle.
- It may be associated with ligamentous laxity.
- Surgical reconstruction is required in cases of persistent subluxation/dislocation and loss of function (**Figs 21.55, 21.56**).

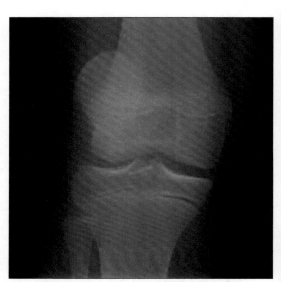

FIGURE 21.55 AP radiograph of the right knee showing the patella subluxed laterally.

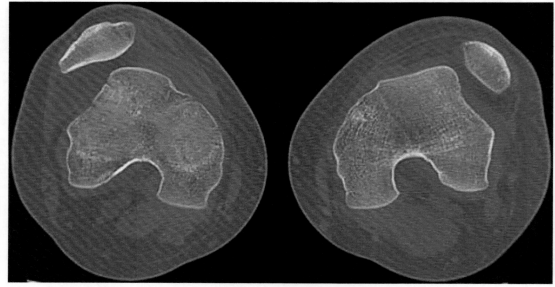

FIGURE 21.56 Transverse CT cuts through the distal femora showing both patellae are displaced. In this case, persistent subluxation and pain necessitated surgical relocation and rebalancing of the surrounding soft tissues.

Other conditions include:

- Osteochondritis dissecans.
- Discoid meniscus.

FOOT PAIN

Kohler disease

- Presents with dorsal forefoot pain and swelling in young children.
- The radiological appearances (of increased density and/or fragmentation of the navicular bone, **Fig. 21.57**) resolve spontaneously and without sequelae.

Sever disease

Enthesopathy of the calcaneal apophysis (**Fig. 21.58**).

- Presents with heel pain related to activity.
- Tightness in the calf muscle complex may be a contributing factor.

Freiberg osteochondrosis

- Presents with forefoot pain.
- Avascular change is seen in the second metatarsal head on x-ray.
- It may be asymptomatic and can present at any age as an incidental finding on radiography.
- Occasionally it remains symptomatic because of changes within the joint.
- Bony spurs and osteochondral fragments may need excision.

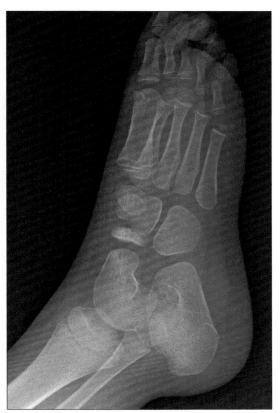

FIGURE 21.57 Oblique radiograph of the foot showing increased density in the navicular in keeping with a diagnosis of Kohler disease.

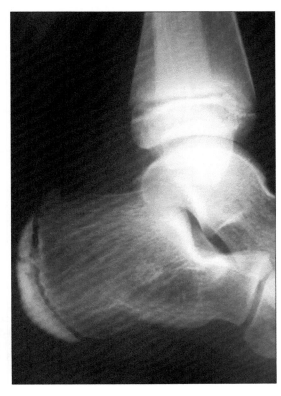

FIGURE 21.58 Lateral radiograph of the foot showing fragmentation of the calcaneal apophysis: this is in fact a normal radiographic appearance. The child may have heel pain and the diagnosis may be Sever disease but the parents must be reassured that the x-ray changes are within normal limits.

THE CHILD WITH A (PAINFUL) LIMP

Children may limp because of pain, weakness, deformity or to gain attention, and the causes vary from sepsis to a spinal tumour and from a leg-length discrepancy to a shoe that rubs. It is essential to exclude serious causes such as a tumour and to distinguish the rare but important cases of sepsis, Perthes disease and a slipped upper femoral epiphysis from the much more common stubbed toe, minor fractures, bruised legs or transient synovitis. Many conditions, such as sepsis and juvenile arthritis, can present at any age but certain hip conditions are more likely in particular age groups.

HISTORY

The following points will help distinguish these conditions:

- Symptom onset: sudden or gradual?
- Duration of symptoms.
- Concurrent events: recent viral infection, trauma, new shoes, new sport?
- General health: is the child well or ill?
- Examination:
  - must include all joints and soft tissues.
  - a brief neurological examination.
  - measurement of leg length,
  - pain on movement or on weight bearing?
- Investigations:
  - plain radiographs should usually include both anteroposterior and 'frog' lateral views of the pelvis.
  - further imaging such as MRI may be required to exclude tumour or other causes.

BONE AND JOINT INFECTION (OSTEOMYELITIS AND SEPTIC ARTHRITIS)

The pathology leading to osteoarticular infection must be clearly understood by any doctor involved in the management of children (**Figs 21.59, 21.60**). Prompt, accurate diagnosis can still save lives and preserve joint and limb function. The following comments refer to acute or acute-on-chronic infections.

- There is no substitute for regular assessment and continuity of care.
- Diagnosis is often based on clinical assessment supported by haematological results.
- Radiographic features should be minimal if the diagnosis is being made promptly (**Fig. 21.61**).
- Management is guided by the site and severity of the infection and local hospital protocols but must adhere to certain principles:
  - intravenous antibiotics are required initially.
  - the affected limb must be rested.
  - appropriate analgesia must be prescribed.
  - the presence of pus in the joint, the soft tissues or in the bone requires surgical drainage (**Fig. 21.62**).
  - with an improvement in clinical and haematological parameters, intravenous therapy can be changed to oral therapy.

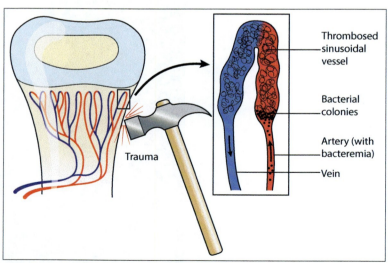

FIGURE 21.59 Diagram depicting the effects of minor trauma to the metaphysis of a long bone: the haematoma and thrombosis in the blood vessels allows passing bacteria to be 'trapped' in the region and encourages colonisation and the development of an osteomyelitis. (From Williams *et al.* (eds). *Bailey and Love's Short Practice of Surgery*, CRC Press, 2013, with permission.)

FIGURE 21.60 Diagrammatic representation of what might happen if an abscess forms within the metaphysis: pus may 'discharge' into the joint (a secondary septic arthritis) or out through the cortical bone, lifting the periosteum and causing a subperiosteal abscess. (From Williams *et al.* (eds). *Bailey and Love's Short Practice of Surgery*, CRC Press, 2013, with permission.)

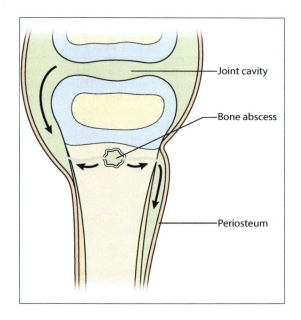

— Joint cavity

— Bone abscess

— Periosteum

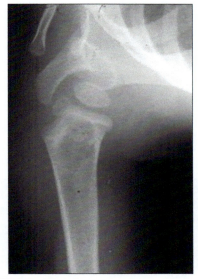

FIGURE 21.61 AP radiograph of a proximal humerus demonstrating a lytic area within the metaphysis compatible with infection. The child responded promptly to intravenous antibiotics: no surgery was required. It usually takes 7–10 days for such features to become apparent on a plain radiograph.

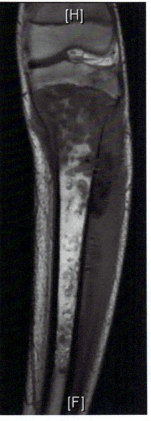

[H]

[F]

FIGURE 21.62 MRI of a tibia demonstrating widespread involvement of the bone and the soft tissues with methicillin resistant *Staphylococcus aureus* infection; multiple surgical procedures were required to gain control of the infective process.

TRANSIENT SYNOVITIS VS. SEPTIC ARTHRITIS

Many clinicians feel that there is a qualitative difference between these two conditions. Transient synovitis remains a diagnosis of exclusion; it should not be considered in a child <2 years of age.

Four clinical predictors have been identified, that help differentiate between septic arthritis and transient synovitis:

- History of fever.
- Non-weight bearing status.
- Erythrocyte sedimentation rate > 40 mm/h.
- White cell count >12×10^9/l.
- With all 4 factors present, the predictive probability of joint sepsis is >90%. C-reactive protein >20 mg/l is also a predictive factor.

Ultrasound scans help delineate the extent of the joint effusion (**Fig. 21.63**).

LEGG–CALVÉ–PERTHES DISEASE (OFTEN CALLED PERTHES DISEASE)

This condition is characterised by the development of avascular necrosis (AVN) of the femoral head, which leads to its collapse; as the blood supply returns, healing occurs albeit with some deformity. The radiographic appearances are very dramatic (**Figs 21.64, 21.65**).

- It is rare and affects boys predominantly.
- Most common between the ages of 4 and 8 years.
- The aetiology is unknown although a variety of factors have been implicated.
- Up to 10% of patients may develop bilateral disease (**Fig. 21.66**).

Treatment aims to minimise femoral head deformity and, hence, reduce the likelihood of secondary acetabular dysplasia and degenerative change.

- Non-surgical methods maximise range of movement to maintain the shape of the femoral head.
- Surgical methods attempt to contain the head better within the acetabulum to prevent secondary deformity.

The prognosis is better in the younger children and those with less severe involvement.

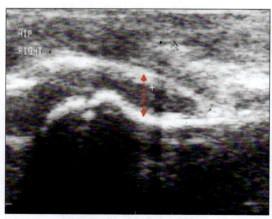

FIGURE 21.63 Ultrasound scan of the right proximal femur demonstrating a joint effusion. The red dotted line shows how far the fluid has displaced the capsule from the surface of the bone. (From Williams *et al.* (eds). *Bailey and Love's Short Practice of Surgery*, CRC Press, 2013, with permission.)

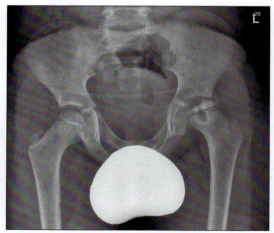

FIGURE 21.64 AP pelvic radiograph showing Perthes disease of the left hip with 'whole head' involvement, i.e. all the epiphysis is affected. It looks sclerotic and it has lost height, i.e. collapsed when compared with the normal right side. A metaphyseal cyst is also seen.

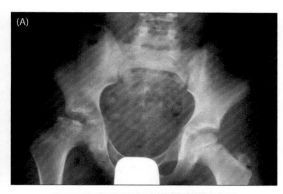

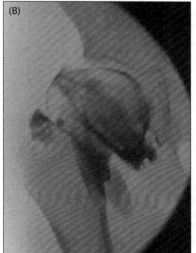

FIGURE 21.65 AP pelvic radiograph (A) showing Perthes disease of the right hip: the process is in the fragmentation phase and the epiphysis appears to be in pieces; (B) an arthrogram outlines the cartilaginous head and confirms that this is still spherical.

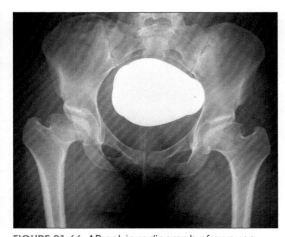

FIGURE 21.66 AP pelvic radiograph of a young adult who had had bilateral Perthes disease as a child. Both femoral heads are oval but the acetabulae have grown to 'match' the femoral heads. These are 'second-rate' hips and will cause symptoms in adult life.

SLIPPED UPPER FEMORAL EPIPHYSIS

AETIOLOGY/INCIDENCE

This is a rare (5 per 100,000) but important condition where the head of the femur (the epiphysis) literally slips off the neck (the metaphysis). A prompt diagnosis is associated with a significantly better prognosis; surgical treatment is necessary.

Boys are more frequently affected than girls and classically patients are overweight. Children often present with pain in/around their knee or with relatively non-specific symptoms of discomfort around the groin area and an intermittent limp or altered posture/gait pattern (externally rotated foot progression angle).

Subtle radiographic changes may be more visible on a frog-lateral view of the hips than on the AP view: thus both must be requested (**Fig. 21.67**).

Other conditions such as hypothyroidism and renal failure also increase the risk of a slip. Patients who have undergone radiotherapy treatment may be at increased risk if the treatment has weakened the physis and/or been responsible for pituitary

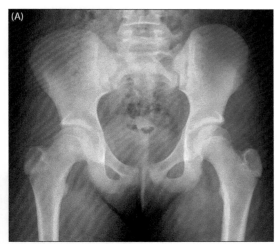

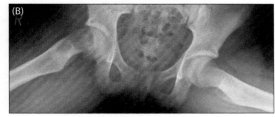

FIGURE 21.67 AP pelvic radiograph (A) of an adolescent patient complaining of right groin pain. A line drawn up the edge of the neck should 'cut off' a portion of the femoral head as it does on the patient's left. On the right the femoral head (epiphysis) has slipped off the metaphysis; (B) the changes are sometimes easier to see on the 'frog-lateral' view.

hormonal changes. If the slip happens acutely, this is just like a fracture and it must be treated urgently to protect the blood supply to the femoral head: loss of the blood supply can lead to AVN, which is synonymous with a poor quality hip in young adult life (**Fig. 21.68**).

TREATMENT

The pin/screw is inserted up the femoral neck into the epiphysis to 'fix' the head onto the neck: the further the head has slipped off the neck, the more difficult this is technically (**Fig. 21.69**).

Other options include a more aggressive surgical procedure to restore more normal anatomy via an osteotomy: however, the risks of damage to the blood supply are greater with this approach.

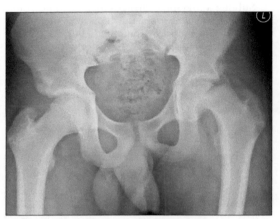

FIGURE 21.68 AP pelvic radiograph of an adolescent patient complaining of acute left groin pain. He is unable to walk and has essentially sustained a pathological fracture of his femoral neck; this is, however, called an acute, severe slip of the upper femoral epiphysis.

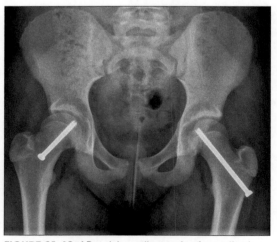

FIGURE 21.69 AP pelvic radiograph of a patient who complained of bilateral groin pain; both epiphyses had slipped, the left more than the right and both were 'pinned *in-situ*' to stabilise the situation.

UPPER LIMB ABNORMALITIES

NEONATAL BRACHIAL PLEXOPATHY

Damage to the brachial plexus during delivery of a child can occur in several high risk situations:

- A large-for-dates baby and/or born to a diabetic mother.
- Abnormal intrauterine positions such as a transverse lie or a breech presentation.
- A prolonged labour and/or a forceps delivery.

The child presents with a paralysed arm of varying severity and with the complete lesion there may also be a Horner syndrome. The diagnosis is clinical initially; other causes of a 'pseudo-paralysis' such as a clavicular fracture or sepsis of the shoulder joint may need to be excluded actively.

Ideas on the timing of further investigation (neurophysiological testing and MRI) are changing and it would be sensible to know what the referral protocols are for your nearest Brachial Plexus Unit.

All infants should receive prompt physiotherapy designed to stretch the functioning muscles and maintain a normal range of passive joint movement to prevent the development of muscle contractures and joint deformity.

TORTICOLLIS

The child presents with a 'cock-robin' head tilt due to a tight sternocleidomastoid muscle that pulls the affected side down and tilts the head round. Torticollis is often considered to be secondary to a sternomastoid 'tumour', perhaps caused by a muscle tear during delivery especially if forceps were used; in reality, a tumour is rarely found.

The tight muscle responds to stretching supervised by a physiotherapist and tricks such as placing interesting objects on the other side of the baby's cot to encourage head turning. Untreated, the head tilt leads to a noticeable asymmetry in facial growth and hence appearance and thus surgical release is merited any time after the age of 18–24 months (**Fig. 21.70**). A squint with diplopia may encourage a child to adopt the cock-robin posture: in such a case there is no true tightness of the muscle.

Torticollis that is noted at birth may be due to an abnormality of the cervical spine and should be referred immediately. One that develops later and acutely, often with pain, minor trauma and/or an upper respiratory tract infection must be assessed for atlantoaxial rotatory instability.

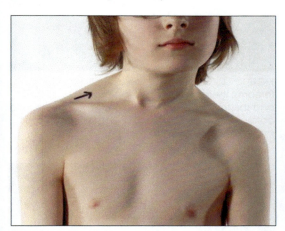

FIGURE 21.70 Clinical photograph of a child with a 'cock-robin' head posture secondary to a torticollis. This is often considered to be secondary to a sternomastoid tumour, which is never more than a benign haematoma-type swelling within the muscle. By the time the child is this age, the muscle is contracted and unresponsive to physiotherapy. If left untreated, facial asymmetry results so surgical release is indicated.

CONGENITAL UPPER LIMB ANOMALIES

RADIAL CLUB HAND

- This longitudinal deficiency affects approximately 1 in 30,000 live births. It is diagnosed clinically, confirmed radiologically. Radial club hand is often associated with abnormalities of others systems:
- TAR syndrome (**Figs 21.71, 21.72**).
- Holt–Oram syndrome (**Fig. 21.73**).

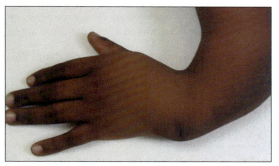

FIGURE 21.71 Clinical photograph of a child with an absent radius and thrombocytopenia (TAR syndrome); the thumb is often well developed.

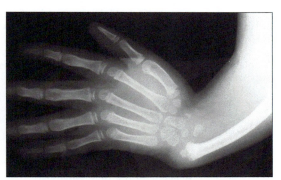

FIGURE 21.72 AP radiograph of the arm of the same child as in **21.71** showing an absent radius but well-developed thumb.

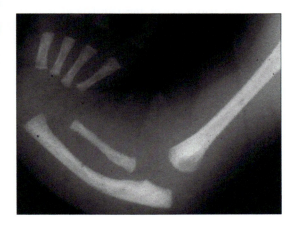

FIGURE 21.73 AP radiograph of a forearm of a child with Holt–Oram syndrome and a radial club hand; the radius is under-developed, the thumb is absent and there is significant deviation of the hand with respect to the forearm. (From Williams et al. (eds). Bailey and Love's Short Practice of Surgery, CRC Press, 2013, with permission.)

- Function is often surprisingly good. Treatment options may depend on the quality of the thumb (often poor) and whether or not the condition is bilateral:
- Pollicisation of the index finger remains a popular treatment.
- Wrist position and instability are managed by the surgical procedures of centralisation and soft tissue rebalancing.
- Forearm lengthening may also be considered.
- Physiotherapy and splinting are often essential parts of the management plan.

ULNAR CLUB HAND

- Rare and often associated with other limb abnormalities (**Fig. 21.74**).
- Surgical options include making a 'one bone forearm'.
- Procedures to maximise function of the digits.

RADIOULNAR SYNOSTOSIS

Failure of separation of the cartilage anlage of the forearm occurs *in utero* (**Fig. 21.75**). Clinically the forearm loses pronation/supination movement and the hand on the end of the arm is effectively stuck in one position. The condition is often bilateral.

Careful assessment of function is required before treatment is considered. Surgery can exchange one fixed position for another but it cannot regain movement. In bilateral conditions, one hand may be placed in some pronation and the other in some supination.

CONGENITAL DISLOCATION OF THE RADIAL HEAD

This may be associated with a radioulnar synostosis (**Fig. 21.75**) or not (**Fig. 21.76**). It can be an isolated finding and is often asymptomatic, but if pain and/or stiffness interfere with function, surgical excision can be considered.

Surgical relocation of the radial head is rarely successful

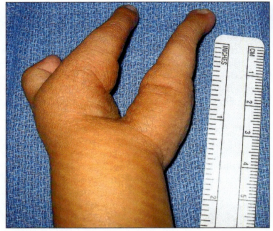

FIGURE 21.74 Clinical photograph of a cleft hand (ectrodactyly): in this case part of the ulnar club hand anomaly.

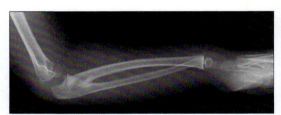

FIGURE 21.75 Lateral radiograph of a child's forearm: there is a proximal radioulnar synostosis and the radial head is dislocated. It is impossible to obtain a 'good' lateral view as the synostosis limits pronation/supination movement.

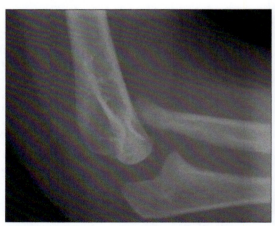

FIGURE 21.76 Lateral radiograph of the elbow showing a congenital anterior dislocation of the radial head: the proximal portion of the radius is malformed and the head deficient.

OTHER MINOR UPPER LIMB ABNORMALITIES

Trigger thumb is a common anomaly, often present from birth although perhaps not noticed until some months later. The tip of the thumb is held in the flexed position: sometimes the child or their parent can straighten it but with active flexion the thumb gets stuck again. The condition is analogous to trigger fingers in adults but there is no association with synovitis or joint problems. If the problem persists past 1 year of age, surgical release of the A1 pulley of the flexor tendon sheath solves the problem (**Fig. 21.77**).

Polydactyly of the hands or feet is one of the common, uncommon conditions. There is an association with other medical conditions such as renal disease or more widespread skeletal problems (**Fig. 21.78**).

Pseudarthrosis of the clavicle is rare; it always affects the right side (except in dextrocardia) and presents from birth with a non-tender lump. It is often mistaken for a simple fracture but when it does not heal, the diagnosis is clear (**Fig. 21.79**).

Symptoms are unusual in childhood but become more noticeable with time. Operative treatments are designed at reducing the 'fracture' and obtaining fixation across the pseudarthrosis so that it is encouraged to heal. Cosmetic concerns may also lead to surgery.

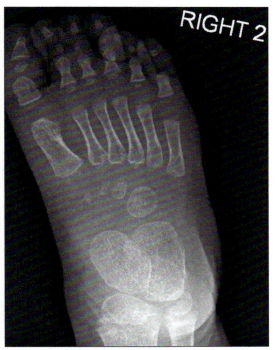

FIGURE 21.78 AP radiograph of a foot showing 6 well-formed digits: polydactyly is a common congenital anomaly.

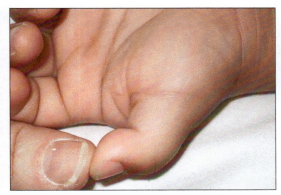

FIGURE 21.77 Clinical photograph of a trigger thumb: the thumb is flexed at the interphalangeal joint and cannot be straightened. Surgical release of one of the tendon pulleys cures the problem.

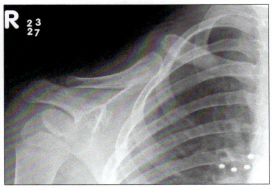

FIGURE 21.79 Radiograph showing a pseudarthrosis of the clavicle (always on the right unless there is dextrocardia!). It presented in late childhood and was of cosmetic concern only.

Sprengel shoulder is a rare problem where the embryonic descent of the shoulder from the cranial end of the embryo fails, leaving the scapula in the root of the neck rather than on the posterior wall of the chest (**Figs 21.80, 21.81**). Symptoms include difficulty with certain overhead movements. Cosmetic concerns are common; surgical repositioning of the scapula is possible.

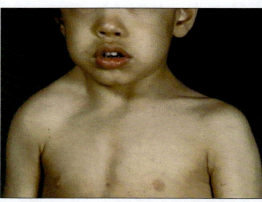

FIGURE 21.80 Clinical photograph of a child with a 'lump in the neck', which represents the failed embryological descent of the right scapula to its normal place on the posterior chest wall, a Sprengel shoulder.

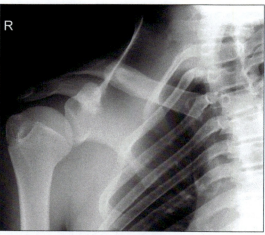

FIGURE 21.81 AP radiograph showing a high riding right scapula in keeping with a Sprengel shoulder.

EXAMPLES OF GENERALISED CONDITIONS AFFECTING THE MUSCULOSKELETAL SYSTEM

BENIGN JOINT HYPERMOBILITY SYNDROME

All children are lax jointed: this is normal. Joint laxity is maximal at birth, declining rapidly during childhood, less rapidly during the teens, and slowly during adult life.

Women are more lax jointed than men and there is wide ethnic variation. The quick clinical test for joint laxity developed by Beighton is helpful. A child who scores five or more is hypermobile and when hypermobility becomes symptomatic, the 'hypermobility syndrome' is said to exist. Symptoms in children include joint and back pains, occasionally subluxations or frank dislocations, ligament muscle and tendon injuries after mild trauma and fasciitis.

On the other hand most children are asymptomatic and violinists, flautists and pianists (of all ages) with lax finger joints suffer less pain than their less flexible peers. Gymnasts/ballet dancers also have supple joints but in addition they have good muscle strength and co-ordination. Symptomatic children can be helped greatly by experienced physiotherapists.

ARTHROGRYPOSIS

This descriptive term simply means stiff joints. Several hundred different causes have been established. A full neurological assessment is indicated as treatment and prognosis may be affected if an underlying cause can be identified.

The generalised type of the condition (arthrogryposis multiplex congenita) is generally much more disabling than the distal form (**Fig. 21.82**). Some forms of the condition are genetic (distal arthrogryposis) but most are spontaneous. The infant joints have not moved *in utero* and the skin and soft tissues classically are 'featureless', lacking skin creases and muscle bulk.

Physiotherapy and splinting are the mainstays of early treatment; some improvement in passive range of movement is common but active control may be more difficult to establish. Surgical options are available for particular individual problems but must be considered in the light of the child's overall functional abilities.

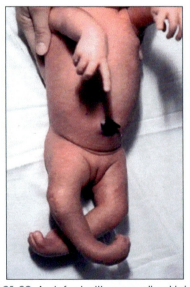

FIGURE 21.82 An infant with generalised joint contractures in keeping with a diagnosis of arthrogryposis multiplex congenita.

NEUROMUSCULAR CONDITIONS WITH ORTHOPAEDIC CONCERNS

CEREBRAL PALSY

This results from a non-progressive injury to the developing brain, which classically affects the motor cortex alone. There may be other areas affected: the larger the insult to the motor cortex, the greater the risk of associated damage. Although the damage is non-progressive, its effects on the musculoskeletal system are progressive and these vary depending on the type of tonal abnormality exhibited by the child: spastic vs. hypotonic vs. dystonic.

Such changes are progressive with growth but equally importantly they tend to stabilise when growth is complete at skeletal maturity (around 14 in girls and 16 in boys).

Children are often classified according to the GMFCS (Gross Motor Function Classification System), which allows the treating team to predict, with some accuracy, the likelihood that the child will be able to function independently as a young adult. It must be remembered that a child does not have to be able to walk to function independently and treatment should not be directed at 'getting the child to walk' at any cost. There may be considerable differences in treatment aims for the GMFCS I–III children compared to their non-walking GMFCS IV/V counterparts.

As with other neuromuscular abnormalities the orthopaedic care must be seen as a small (but important!) part of the multi-disciplinary management plan. Treatment is aimed at preventing deformity and maximising function; a wide range of orthopaedic techniques may be used if/when appropriate but in association with good physiotherapy and orthotic devises. The aims of treatment may include:

- Control of spinal deformity (**Figs 21.83, 21.84**).
- Maintaining joint position.
- Control of muscle balance to prevent contractures.

Current controversy centres around the 'need' to screen hips and instigate early (and perhaps repeated) surgical treatment for hips that are beginning to sublux as indicated by limited hip abduction and increasing migration percentage on well-positioned plain AP pelvic radiographs (**Figs 21.85, 21.86**).

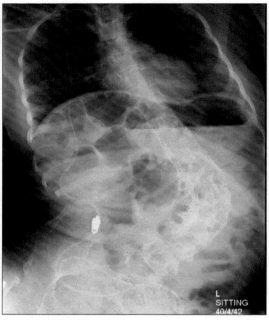

FIGURE 21.83 AP radiograph of a spine in a child with total body involvement spastic cerebral palsy: there is severe, long spinal curve.

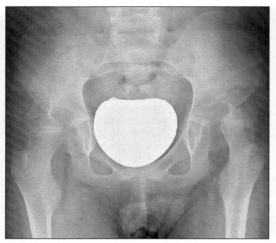

FIGURE 21.85 AP pelvic radiograph of a girl with spastic cerebral palsy, GMFCS level 4: both hips are subluxed and painful, the femoral necks show significant valgus deformity (i.e. they are straight).

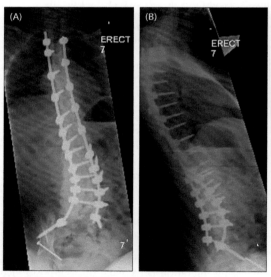

FIGURE 21.84 AP (A) and lateral (B) spinal radiographs of the child in **21.83** following correction of the deformity and spinal fusion. The child is now better balanced and can be sat more comfortably in her wheelchair allowing her to maximise her upper limb function.

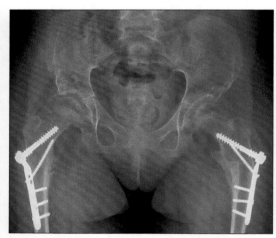

FIGURE 21.86 The same child as in 21.85, 2 years after bilateral staged hip reconstructions: the hips are pain-free and in-joint.

SPINA BIFIDA

World-wide, despite programmes of folate supplementation, antenatal screening and the possibility of termination of the pregnancy, many babies are born with spina bifida and there continues to be a significant burden of childhood disability secondary to myelomeningocoeles and their sequelae.

The severity of the clinical picture is very varied and alterations in neurological function raise the possibility of a tethered cord and/or Arnold–Chiari malformation and hydocephalus. Investigations include an ultrasound scan in infancy or a MRI later in childhood.

The child requires a multi-disciplinary team approach to management. Orthopaedic management is dictated/directed by the level of the lesion, associated problems including the intellectual impairment and the function achievable. Joints are often flaccid rather than contracted and splinting an insensate limb to provide joint stability is fraught with difficulties. Immobilisation following surgery may lead to further disuse osteoporosis and pathological fractures in the recovery period (**Fig. 21.87**).

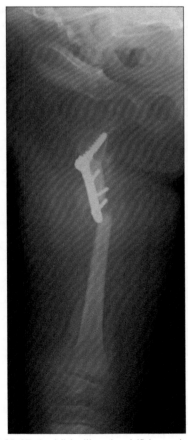

FIGURE 21.87 A child with spina bifida underwent an operative procedure to relocate his right hip; in the postoperative period he sustained two fractures, one proximally and one distally. Both healed with abundant callus but he was left with a stiff knee that severely limited his independent mobility.

THE SPINE

CONGENITAL DEFORMITIES

By definition these problems are present at birth: they represent failures of formation (a hemivertebra) or of segmentation of vertebral bodies (unilateral or bilateral bar). The clinical result is usually a scoliosis and treatment is based on the potential for curve progression. When a kyphosis results, progressive neurological deficit is common. Bracing is ineffective for congenital vertebral deformities.

SCOLIOSIS

AETIOLOGY/INCIDENCE

- Scoliosis is a curvature of the spine in 3 dimensions: the 's' shape may be most visible on the x-ray but the rib hump is what often concerns the patient and her mother (**Figs 21.88–21.90**). The aetiology may be idiopathic, neuromuscular, syndrome-related or congenital, and this, as well as the age of onset, affects the natural history.
- The majority of curves are defined as adolescent idiopathic scoliosis (AIS). It is most common in girls and there may be a family history. Recent developments suggest that there is a genetic link to the likelihood for curve progression: if the curve starts earlier in infancy or childhood, the prognosis is worse, mainly because there is more time to grow and hence more time for the curve to progress. Curves are usually pain free so that a painful scoliosis should raise an alarm and may provoke further investigation. Scoliosis curves are measured on an AP x-ray and assessed in terms of the Cobb angle.

TREATMENT

In general terms this is dictated by the size of the curve and the risk of progression:

- Curves of <25° can be watched.
- 25–45° curves are braced.
- Curves >45° and/or progressive may merit surgical treatment.

The aim is to delay spinal surgery if possible as the standard treatment involves spinal fusion leading to limited further growth (from the non-fused areas only) and some disproportionate short stature. More recent techniques with a variety of 'growing rods' have allowed some growth potential to be maintained even when treatment is started early.

The choice of treatment method is influenced by the aetiology; neuromuscular curves have a different prognosis and hence management plan compared with idiopathic curves or those associated with conditions such as osteogenesis.

Scoliosis

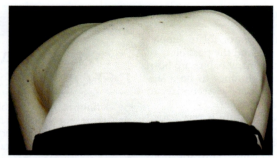

FIGURE 21.88 The Adams forward bend test highlights the rotational component of a scoliosis and allows the 'rib hump' to be visualised. (From Williams *et al.* (eds). *Bailey and Love's Short Practice of Surgery*, CRC Press, 2013, with permission.)

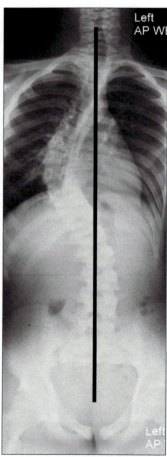

FIGURES 21.89 AP radiograph of the spine of a boy aged 15 years demonstrating an idiopathic scoliosis which is **much** more commonly seen in girls.

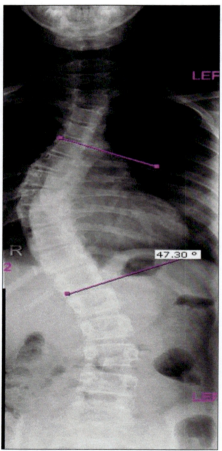

FIGURE 21.90 The scoliosis is described in terms of the apex of the curve: this lower thoracic curve, apex convex to the right, measures 47° and may warrant surgical treatment. (From Williams *et al.* (eds). *Bailey and Love's Short Practice of Surgery*, CRC Press, 2013, with permission.)

SCHEUERMANN DISEASE (KYPHOSIS)

The term kyphosis refers to the round backed posture common to all thoracic spines; the normal kyphosis is 20–50°. Kyphotic curves in excess of this may be postural or structural. Structural kyphosis is most commonly secondary to Scheuermann disease, which presents as progressive kyphosis in adolescence and is characterised radiologically by vertebral wedging of 5° or more at three adjacent levels and vertebral end-plate changes. The aetiology is unknown.

Treatment ranges from physiotherapy and bracing to surgery, depending on the degree of deformity, progression and symptoms.

SPONDYLOLISTHESIS

Spondylolysis refers to a defect in the pars interarticularis of the vertebra. The defect may be congenital or acquired (e.g. trauma) (**Fig. 21.91**).

Spondylolisthesis occurs when the upper vertebra slips forward on the lower; it is graded according to the percentage slip, measured by relating the slipped vertebra to the one below. Mild slips are often asymptomatic and do not require treatment.

Treatment options include physiotherapy, bracing and surgery. The choice depends on the degree of slip and symptoms. Mechanical back pain may respond to conservative methods but the development or threat of neurological involvement usually requires surgical intervention.

BACK PAIN

- It is taught that children do not suffer from back pain and thus if present there must be a worrying cause for it and pain is one of the 'red flag' signs for spinal pathology (**Fig. 21.92**). Although historically this may have been true, back discomfort in the adolescent or prepubertal child is actually quite common and can be treated with advice regarding posture, physiotherapy and analgesic medication.
- Red flag symptoms and signs for spinal pathology include:
  - Systemic illness, fever or weight loss.
  - Progressive neurological deficit.
  - Unrelenting or night pain.
  - Spinal deformity.

In the presence of such signs/symptoms investigations to find the underlying cause must take place.

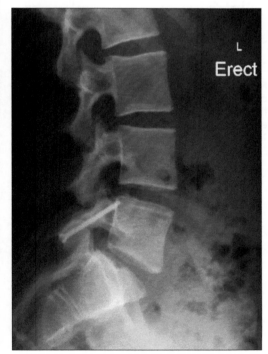

FIGURE 21.91 Lateral radiograph of the spine showing a screw fusion of a pars interarticularis defect, otherwise known as a spondylolysis. There had been no slip at the defect and hence no spondylolisthesis.

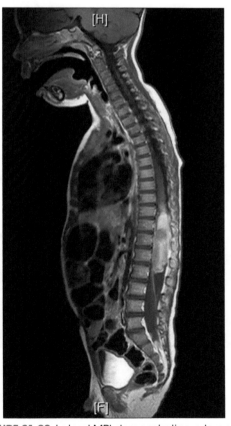

FIGURE 21.92 Lateral MRI demonstrating a large astrocytoma of the lower cord. The child presented with back pain that was waking him regularly from sleep. Night pain is a 'red flag' sign.

TRAUMA

Children have a reputation for bouncing rather than breaking when they fall and certainly there are specific fracture patterns that only happen in the immature skeleton:

- Buckle fractures (**Fig. 21.93**).
- Greenstick fractures (**Fig. 21.94**).
- Injuries to the physis or growth plate (**Fig. 21.95**).
- Children's ligaments are stronger than their bones so avulsion fractures are more common than ruptured ligaments in this age group.
- The growth plates may be mistaken for fractures so radiographs must be reviewed carefully and matched to the history and the physical signs (**Fig. 21.96**).

Fractures in children heal rapidly and remodel with growth so that some degree of malalignment at the fracture site can be accepted:

- Deformity in the plane of movement of the adjacent joint will remodel:
  - if the fracture is close to the joint and
  - if there is time enough for it to do so (>2 years of growth remaining).
- Rotational malalignment does not improve with growth.
- Fractures that involve the joint surface (intra-articular injuries) and or the growth plate (physis) do not 'remodel' (**Fig. 21.97**).
- Guidelines have been developed for most long bone fractures that help define what an acceptable fracture reduction is at various age groups (**Fig. 21.98**).

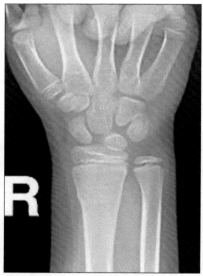

FIGURE 21.93 An AP radiograph of the wrist of a child demonstrating a buckle fracture of the radial metaphysis: the fracture line is barely visible but the cortex is not completely smooth and is 'buckled'.

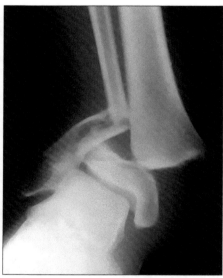

FIGURE 21.95 A Salter–Harris type 2 fracture of the distal tibial physis with considerable displacement: the fracture needs to be reduced carefully to ensure no damage is done to the growth plate. There is no involvement of the joint.

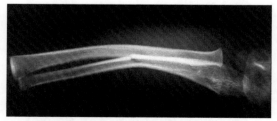

FIGURE 21.94 AP radiograph of the forearm demonstrating a greenstick fracture of the ulna. The bone is intact and may need to be broken in order to improve the deformity.

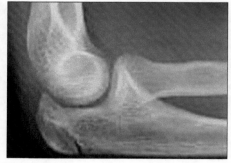

FIGURE 21.96 The physes can be mistaken for fractures: in this lateral radiograph of the elbow in a teenager approaching skeletal maturity, the remnants of the physis were reported as a fracture. Clinical examination confirmed no tenderness at this point and the history of trauma was minimal.

Orthopaedics and fractures

As with adults certain basic principles must be adhered to and resuscitation ('save a life before a limb') is the key to good trauma management. A fracture can be defined as a soft tissue injury complicated by a break in the bone, so it is most important to take note of the neurovascular status of the limb distal to the injury and to care for any open wounds (**Fig. 21.99**). Prevention of infection is an essential part of any trauma protocol.

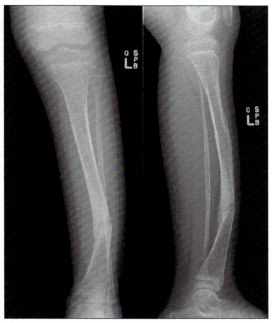

FIGURE 21.98 AP and lateral radiographs of a fracture of the tibia: it has healed with some deformity, which is unlikely to remodel completely. The fibula has remained intact.

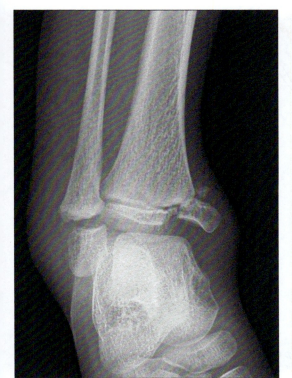

FIGURE 21.97 AP radiograph of the ankle demonstrating a significant physeal injury with disruption of the physis and the joint surface.

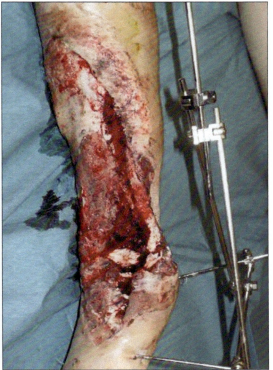

FIGURE 21.99 A major open injury to the lower leg of a 5-year-old child: ATLS principles ensured that the airway, breathing and circulation were managed in conjunction with the major soft tissue injury. Joint stiffness and physeal damage are inevitable with this injury, infection is not!

SPECIFIC PAEDIATRIC INJURIES

PHYSEAL INJURIES

These are classified according to the Salter–Harris system (**Fig. 21.100**), which is based on:

- The severity of the injury to the germinal cell layer of the physis that is responsible for growth (see **Figs 21.95, 21.97, 21.99**).
- Displacement at the articular surface (see **Fig. 21.97**).

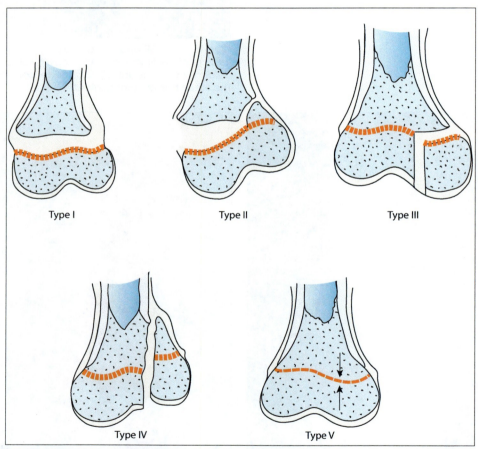

FIGURE 21.100 Salter–Harris classification of growth plate injuries. Type I: shear through physeal plate; type II: partial shear through physeal plate and partial metaphyseal fracture (commonest injury – around 70%); type III: partial physeal separation with an intra-articular epiphyseal fracture; type IV: plane passes from joint surface through physis and metaphysis; type V: compression of articular surface and impaction of epiphyseal bone into metaphyseal bone.

The physis is radiolucent on plain radiography and the extent of the injury has to be gauged by looking at the displacement/position of the metaphyseal and epiphyseal portions that are ossified. Additional imaging techniques may be required in order to visualise the fracture fully (**Figs 21.101, 21.102**).

TREATMENT

In general terms, the more severe the injury (SH types III and IV) the more likely it is that the fracture will require an operative procedure to obtain an accurate reduction of the physis and the joint surface and minimise the risk of future growth disturbance and joint incongruity.

PULLED ELBOW

In young children, it is relatively easy to sublux the radial head if, for example, the child is pulled by the hand. The child may cry and then be noted to have a limp arm with the elbow flexed and the forearm pronated.

Reduction is easy and often inadvertent. One hand cups the distal humerus at the elbow and the other hand holds the child's hand. The forearm is then supinated, a click may be heard as the radial head relocates and the child may cry but movement improves and becomes more comfortable. Normal function returns promptly. Recurrence is not unusual, but the children do grow out of this tendency eventually.

FRACTURES AROUND THE ELBOW

Elbow fractures are common in childhood and associated with both acute problems such as neurovascular injury and compartment syndrome, and chronic deformity and malfunction secondary to malunion and/or growth arrest.

SUPRACONDYLAR FRACTURES OF THE HUMERUS

These are classified according to the mechanism of injury and the degree of displacement. 98% are due to falls on the outstretched hand and associated with an extension force (**Fig. 21.103**).

The Gartland classification 1–4 dictates the need for closed reduction and the insertion of percutaneous pins to stabilise the position (**Fig. 21.104**). A careful neurovascular assessment of the hand must

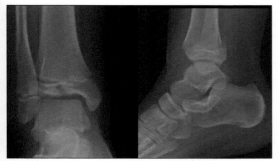

FIGURE 21.101 AP and lateral radiographs suggesting relatively minor displacement of the distal tibial physeal fracture.

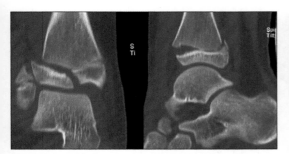

FIGURE 21.102 The 3-dimensional nature of the injury and the displacement can be clarified on further imaging, as with this CT scan.

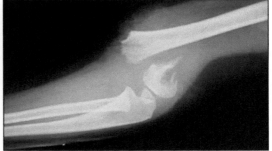

FIGURE 21.103 A lateral radiograph of a severely displaced supracondylar fracture of the humerus: the proximal fragment may have 'button-holed' through the biceps muscle and the brachial artery and/or the median nerve may become entrapped between the fracture fragments, either as a result of the injury or the attempts to reduce the fracture.

be made pre- and post-treatment and the following symptoms should raise the possibility of a compartment syndrome:

- Anxiety.
- Analgesic requirement.
- Agitation.

Management of the pink but pulseless hand remains controversial but the orthopaedic team must be notified in all cases where the pulse is 'missing'.

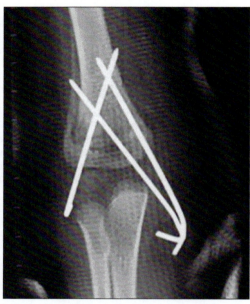

FIGURE 21.104 AP radiograph of a reduced and stabilised supracondylar fracture of the humerus. The arm is in plaster. The growth plate is not affected.

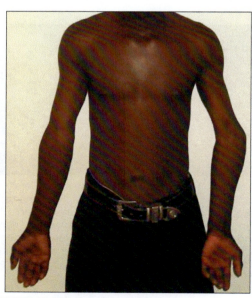

FIGURE 21.105 Cubitus varus is an unsightly deformity secondary to a poorly reduced fracture and not due to growth disturbance. A corrective osteotomy is sometimes required.

Malunion (cubitus varus) is less common than it was due to improved reduction and fixation techniques. The deformity does not improve with time (**Fig. 21.105**); it is usually asymptomatic but causes concern cosmetically.

Treatment is by a corrective osteotomy. Neurovascular injury is a risk of surgery. The deformity of the malunion is exchanged for a scar and an improved but not necessarily perfect position. Patient/family expectations must match what surgical correction can deliver!

MEDIAL EPICONDYLE FRACTURES OF THE HUMERUS

- Commonly associated with posterior dislocation of the elbow.
- Failure of the joint to stay reduced may indicate that the epicondyle is trapped within the joint.
- An open reduction of the joint may be required with subsequent fixation of the epicondyle.

LATERAL CONDYLE FRACTURES OF THE HUMERUS

These fractures have a reputation for leading to a non-union with joint instability. Thus all but the truly undisplaced fractures should be stabilised by closed or open means.

RADIAL HEAD FRACTURES

- Minor angulation may be accepted.
- Angulation of >30° may be associated with progressive subluxation of the radial head with continued growth; certainly angulation of 45–60° merits treatment.

PITFALLS AROUND FOREARM FRACTURES

It is a basic tenet of orthopaedic management that a x-ray taken to delineate the extent of an injury must include the joint above and the joint below, i.e. the whole bone. A failure to do so means the following injuries are all too frequently missed:

- Monteggia fracture: fracture of the ulna with radial head subluxation (**Figs 21.106, 21.107**).
- Galeazzi fracture: fracture of the radius with distal radioulnar subluxation.

A failure to assess the 'match' between the proximal and distal parts of the fracture can represent malrotation at the fracture site and if healing takes place in this position, there will be a significant loss of forearm movement in pronation and supination.

BUCKLE FRACTURES

Torus or buckle fractures of the distal radius and/or ulna are common. They require little if any treatment as long as the diagnosis is certain:

- Removeable back slabs or wrist splints or a tubigrip bandage may be sufficient.
- Local hospital protocols may suggest that no follow-up of these fractures is required.

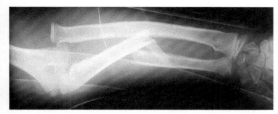

FIGURE 21.106 Lateral radiograph of a forearm fracture in which the fractured ulna and dislocated radial head are very obvious.

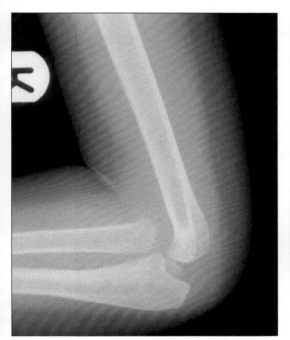

FIGURE 21.107 Lateral radiograph of a forearm injury, where no ulnar injury was seen and the radial head dislocation was 'missed': the ulnar injury was initially a greenstick injury.

LOWER LIMB INJURIES

FRACTURES OF THE PROXIMAL FEMUR

These are rare and usually due to high-velocity trauma (**Figs 21.108, 21.109**).

AVN, malunion and growth arrest are feared complications. Urgent appropriate surgical management is required.

An acute slipped capital femoral epiphysis should be treated similarly (see **Fig. 21.68**).

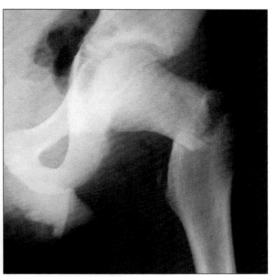

FIGURE 21.108 AP radiograph of a fractured neck of femur: in the elderly this is due to minor trauma, in a child a result of major trauma.

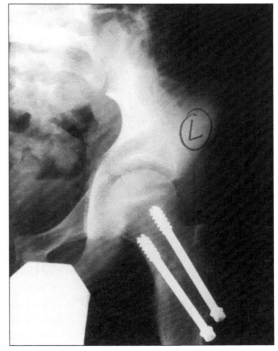

FIGURE 21.109 A prompt and accurate reduction is required to ensure a good result: as with an acute slipped capital femoral epiphysis, this is an orthopaedic emergency.

FRACTURES OF THE FEMORAL SHAFT

This is a reasonably common injury. Treatment depends on the age of the patient and the exact site, comminution of the fracture. Methods range from overhead gallows traction in the infant, to straight traction in the child, to intramedullary flexible nails in the older child and standard adult techniques in the adolescent. Cast treatment is appropriate in selected cases; it may be used to supplement other techniques if fracture stability remains a concern and/or patient compliance with partial weight bearing is impossible. External fixation techniques may be required in open fractures or in the multiply injured patient.

FRACTURES OF THE PATELLA

The normal variant of a bipartite patella is frequently misdiagnosed as a fracture. Fractures should be tender to the touch and associated with evidence of some soft tissue swelling. Some avulsion type fractures are associated with sporting injury or seen in patients with neuromuscular disability. A high riding patella with a lack of knee extension power may represent a 'sleeve fracture' where the patella tendon has pulled over the distal pole of the patella with a large piece of articular cartilage, which may be poorly visualised on the x-ray.

OTHER AVULSION INJURIES

- Tibial spine avulsion injury (anterior cruciate ligament).
- Injury to the tibial apophysis (patella tendon).
- Avulsion of the hamstrings from the ischial tuberosity.

The avulsed bone fragment enlarges over time leading to radiographic features in the chronic injury that may suggest new bone formation and raise the possibility of a tumour (**Fig. 21.110**). A careful history, examination and interpretation of the x-ray and appropriate further imaging should clarify the issues.

FRACTURES OF THE TIBIA/FIBULA

One particular type of minimally displaced proximal tibial fracture is worthy of mention.

The **Cozen fracture** is an essentially undisplaced proximal metaphyseal fracture that is associated with the development of deformity (knock knee) over the first 6–12 months postinjury (after the removal of the plaster cast). This is not a malunion and careful explanation about the risk of this deformity occurring prior to treatment, helps to ensure that the family are not too upset when they see it happening. Spontaneous improvement is usual over the next 12 months; occasionally surgical treatment is required.

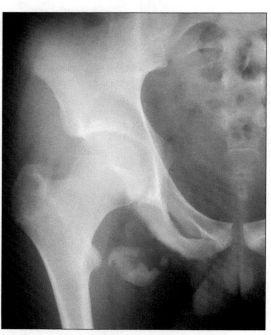

FIGURE 21.110 AP radiograph of the right hip showing 'an ossified mass' in the groin area. There was a history of a severe thigh strain 3 months previously; at that time the hamstring muscles were avulsed from the bone and the bone fragment has 'grown' over time.

PATHOLOGICAL FRACTURES

A fracture occurs as a result of an abnormal force applied to a normal bone; this is the 'normal' situation in traumatic injuries. A pathological fracture occurs under two circumstances:

- When a normal force is applied to an abnormal bone.
- When an excessive force is applied to a normal bone in abnormal circumstances, such as those that occur in cases of non-accidental injury.

ABNORMAL BONES

Pathological fractures through abnormal bone may occur at various stages of childhood due to a variety of causes:

- At birth, due for example, to osteogenesis imperfecta.
- In childhood, secondary to generalised poor bone density, for example in neuromuscular conditions (**Fig. 21.111**) or fibrous dysplasia.
- In conditions of localised poor quality bone formation, for example through simple bone cysts (**Fig. 21.112**) or benign or malignant tumours.

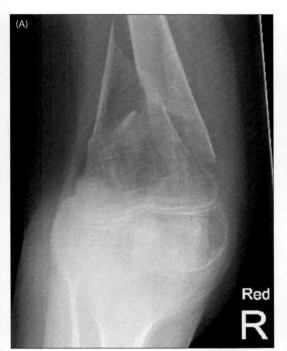

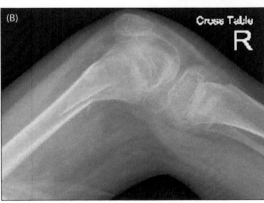

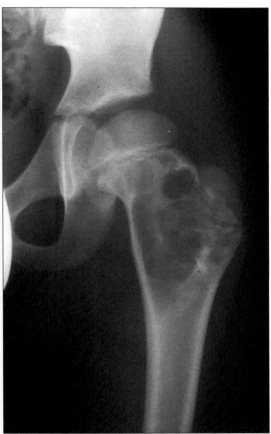

FIGURE 21.112 87 AP radiograph of the left proximal femur: there is a large simple bone cyst occupying most of the femoral neck. If this were to fracture, a poor outcome is likely thus it is wise to treat this cyst before it fractures.

FIGURE 21.111 86a,b AP (A) and lateral (B) radiographs of the knee of a child with severe cerebral palsy; his leg fractured during physiotherapy treatment. His tone and spasm meant the knee flexed and could not be straightened easily. Immobilisation in this position would lead to a very contracted knee joint.

NON-ACCIDENTAL INJURY

When excessive force is applied directly to a normal bone, fractures occur; the injury in a young child is often non-accidental. Such cases are unfortunately more common than we would like to admit and can affect children of all ages and from all walks of life. A high index of suspicion is required when the following features are associated with a fracture or soft tissue injury to the musculoskeletal system:

- Inappropriate and/or inconsistent history.
- Delay in presentation.
- Fracture in the non-walking child.
- Presence of multiple bruises of different ages (particularly in the non-walking child).
- There is no excuse for not examining any child fully and in cases of a poorly explained fracture, an examination to look for other injuries or concerns may save the life of the child. Child Protection Policies are an inherent part of NHS practice and you must be familiar with your local guidelines and referral protocols.
- Some injuries are considered 'classical' and have a high specificity for non-accidental injury, but care must be taken with every injury in every child:
  - Fractures in children below walking age.
  - Posterior rib fractures.
  - Scapular fractures.
  - Metaphyseal 'corner' fractures.
  - Multiple fractures at different stages of healing.

FURTHER READING

Benson M, Fixsen J, MacNicol M, Parsch K (eds). *Children's Orthopaedics and Fractures*, 3rd edn. Springer, 2010.

Caird MS, Flynn JM, Leung YL, Millman JE, D'Italia JG, Dormans JP. Factors distinguishing septic arthritis from transient synovitis of the hip in children. A prospective study. *J Bone Joint Surg* (Am) 2006;88(6):1251–7.

Dartnell J, Ramachandran M, Katchburian M. Haematogenous acute and subacute paediatric osteomyelitis: a systematic review of the literature. *J Bone Joint Surg Br* 2012;94(5):584–95.

Kocher MS, Mandiga R, Zurakowski D, Barnewolt C, Kasser JR. Validation of a clinical prediction rule for the differentiation between septic arthritis and transient synovitis of the hip in children. *J Bone Joint Surg* (Am) 2004;86-A(8):1629–35.

Morrissey RT, Weinstein SL (eds). *Lovell and Winter's Paediatric Orthopedics*, 6th edn. Lippincott, Williams, Wilkins, 2005.

Perry DC, Harper AR, Bruce CE. A limping child. *Br Med J* 2011;342:d3565.

Sewell MD, Rosendahl K, Eastwood DM. Developmental dysplasia of the hip. *Br Med J* 2009;339:b4454.

Solomon L, Warwick DJ, Nayagam S (eds). *Apley's Concise System of Orthopaedics and Fractures*, 3rd edn. CRC Press, 2005.

Wenger DR, Rang M. *The Art and Practice of Children's Orthopaedics*. Raven Press, 1992.

Wenger DR, Rang M, Pring ME. *Rang's Children's Fractures*. Lippincott, Williams, Wilkins, 2005.

CONGENITAL URINE FLOW ANOMALIES

HYDRONEPHROSIS/ DILATATION

DEFINITION

Hydronephrosis denotes dilatation of the urinary collecting system of the kidney – the pelvicalyceal system. Ureteronephrosis refers to dilatation of the ureter. The degree of dilatation is assessed on ultrasound by measuring the diameter of the renal pelvis at the renal parenchymal–pelvic junction in the anterior-posterior plane and that of the ureter behind the bladder. A diameter ≤8 mm for the renal pelvis and <5 mm for the ureter is deemed normal. Hydroureteronephrosis can result from impairment to the flow of urine or the retrograde reflux of urine.

SIGNIFICANCE

In previous decades, the management of hydronephrosis was straight forward as children presented with symptoms, such as infection or pain, which warranted surgery. Today, antenatal ultrasound identifies a congenital anomaly of the urinary tract, primarily hydronephrosis, in 1 in 350 pregnancies. Long-term natural history studies have shown that dilatation often improves or resolves spontaneously; hydronephrosis does not equate with obstruction and the need for surgery.

ANTENATAL HYDRONEPHROSIS/ DILATATION

In utero, hydronephrosis is defined as fetal renal pelvic diameter ≥5 mm in the 2nd and ≥7 mm in the 3rd trimester. When antenatal hydronephrosis is discovered, it is essential to confirm the diagnosis after birth (**Fig. 22.1**). Knowledge of the prenatal evaluations during the progression of pregnancy

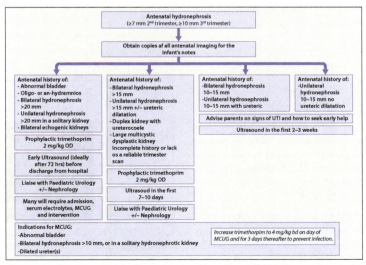

FIGURE 22.1 Flow diagram of assessment of newborn with antenatal hydronephrosis (adapted with permission from Smeulders N. and Paul A. Hydronephrosis. In: Wilcox D, Godbole P, Coopper C [eds]. www.pediatricurologybook.com). MCUG: micturating cystourethrogram; UTI: urinary tract infection.

forms the starting point of the assessment of the newborn, and should include the degree of uni- or bilateral hydronephrosis, ureteric dilatation, renal size and parenchymal appearance, size of the fetal bladder and the amniotic fluid volume in relation to gestational age. Fetal urine production commences around the 10th week of pregnancy and accounts for the majority of amniotic fluid by the 2nd trimester. The likelihood of significant postnatal pathology correlates to the severity of antenatal hydronephrosis.

PELVIURETERIC JUNCTION ANOMALY (PUJA)

INCIDENCE

The incidence of pelviureteric junction (PUJ) anomaly (PUJA) is 1 in 1500 live births, accounting for almost one-half of all antenatally diagnosed hydronephrosis. PUJA is bilateral in 10–20%, left to right ratio is 2:1, male to female ratio is 2:1.

AETIOLOGY/CLINICAL PRESENTATION

The majority are primary and congenital in origin, although the problem may not become apparent until much later in life. The lack of an anatomical blockage combined with abnormal smooth muscle and neural arrangements at the PUJ have lead to the concept of a 'functional obstruction' with impaired peristalsis of urine across the PUJ. While spontaneous improvement is seen in many, others will suffer progressive renal loss if left untreated.

Alternatively, or additionally, extrinsic compression of the PUJ by aberrant vessels crossing to the lower pole of the kidney can result in acute distension of the renal pelvis – typically intermittent – causing renal angle or loin pain accompanied by nausea and vomiting. Pyelonephritis/pyonephrosis, haematuria and hypertension are less common presentations.

DIAGNOSIS

Serial imaging is pivotal in the assessment of PUJA. The diagnosis of PUJA can be suspected on ultrasound when this shows renal pelvic dilatation without ureteric dilatation and a normal urinary bladder (**Fig. 22.2**). Diuretic renography with mercaptoacetyltriglycine (MAG3) is the most popular functional imaging modality in PUJA today, providing information on differential renal clearance through the extraction of tracer from the blood as well as the excretion through the urinary tract by the disappearance of tracer (**Fig. 22.3**). Assessment of drainage is controversial: while good drainage is easy to define, impaired drainage does not necessarily indicate obstruction. Instead this may reflect poor hydration, poor overall renal function, on-going filling of a capacious pelvicalyceal system, a full bladder or gravity – a further acquisition after change in posture

and micturition is therefore essential. Even then, sequential renography documenting changes in differential function may be needed to identify those with obstruction, defined by Koff and Campbell as a restriction to urine flow, which if left untreated will cause progressive renal deterioration (**Fig. 22.4**).

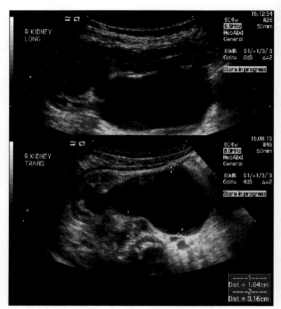

FIGURE 22.2 Ultrasound: longitudinal and transverse view of right hydronephrotic kidney. Distance 1 indicates the renal pelvic diameter in the anterior-posterior plane (AP pelvis) and distance 2 the extra-renal pelvic diameter.

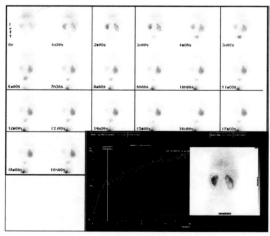

FIGURE 22.3 MAG3 renogram: equal split differential function. While prompt drainage is observed from the left kidney, there is continuous accumulation of tracer in the hydronephrotic right kidney even after change in posture and micturition.

TREATMENT

For those presenting with pain or infection, the aim of treatment is the resolution of symptoms, whereas for asymptomatic PUJA the goal is the prevention of renal loss balanced against unnecessary surgery and its complications. Approximately 25% of antenatal hydronephrosis due to a PUJA will require surgery, usually within the first few years of life. The gold standard operation for PUJA is the Anderson–Hynes pyeloplasty, which allows excision of the fibrotic PUJ segment followed by a funnel-shaped tension-free anastomosis of the ureter to the renal pelvis, enabling dependent drainage. Success rates consistently exceed 95%. Nephrectomy is recommended for those with gross dilatation in a very poorly functioning kidney in the presence of a normal contralateral kidney (**Table 22.1A, B**).

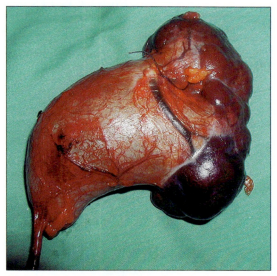

FIGURE 22.4 Pelviureteric junction obstruction: gross pathology.

TABLE 22.1A Indications for close observational management of unilateral PUJA

- Asymptomatic infant
- Stable or decreasing hydronephrosis on serial ultrasound
- Stable or improving differential renal function on MAG3

Many centres recommend antibiotic prophylaxis (e.g. trimethoprim 2 mg/kg at night), although no studies have shown that this prevents urinary tract infection.

TABLE 22.1B Indications for surgery in PUJA

Absolute indications	Relative indications *The recommendations for a 'prophylactic pyeloplasty' vary between unit:*
• Symptoms • Declining function • Increasing hydronephrosis (usually precedes renal deterioration)	• Hydronephrosis >30 mm • Hydronephrosis >20 mm with calyceal dilatation • Hydronephrosis (>20 mm) in a solitary kidney or bilaterally • Intrarenal hydronephrosis (gross calyceal dilatation)

VESICOURETERIC JUNCTION ANOMALY (MEGAURETER)

INCIDENCE/CLASSIFICATION

Congenital vesicoureteric junction anomaly (VUJA) most frequently presents as a result of detection of the associated dilated ureter (primary megaureter), left:right = 1.8:1, male:female = 2:1. Ultrasound, micturating cystourethrogram (MCUG) and diuretic renography assessment allows VUJA and its megaureter to be classified into obstructed, refluxing, non-obstructed and non-refluxing, or both obstructed and refluxing. Coexisting anomalies occur in 16%, including PUJA, multicystic dysplastic kidney (MCDK), renal ectopia and agenesis. It is sometimes difficult to differentiate between a PUJA and VUJA or dual pathology, and an intraoperative contrast antegrade or retrograde pyeloureterogram may be required to clarify the anomaly (**Fig. 22.5**).

TREATMENT

As spontaneous improvement is frequent, close observational management is recommended for the asymptomatic infant with stable or improving dilatation and differential function. Many advocate antibiotic prophylaxis, particularly for refluxing megaureters, and some also advise circumcision. Surgical intervention is indicated in 10–20% of primary megaureters for break-through febrile infection, deteriorating function or dilatation. Ureteric reimplantation after excision of the stenotic VUJ segment, with or without ureteric tapering, is the gold standard, except in those with <10% differential function, for whom nephroureterectomy is advised. In order to avoid extensive dissection in the small infant bladder, temporary placement of a JJ stent across the VUJ for the first year of life is preferred by most. Today, a significant proportion of infants, primarily those with good differential function, have been observed to enjoy good drainage after a period of JJ stenting, thereby escaping ureteric reimplantation.

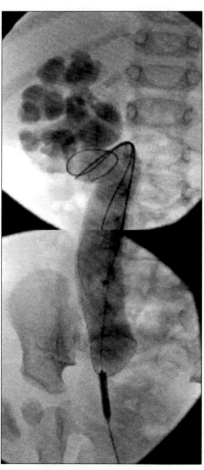

FIGURE 22.5 Intraoperative fluoroscopic image of balloon dilatation of right vesicoureteric junction for the obstructive primary megaureter.

VESICOURETERIC REFLUX

INCIDENCE/CLINICAL PRESENTATION

The retrograde flow of urine from the bladder into the ureters either on bladder filling ('passive' vesicoureteric reflux [VUR]) or on voiding ('active' VUR) accounts for approximately 25% of antenatally diagnosed hydronephrosis. More than 90% of those with antenatally detected reflux are male, whereas those presenting symptomatically with urinary tract infection (UTI) are predominantly female. VUR may be intermittent. Its prevalence is 1–2% of the paediatric population overall, and 30% amongst those with UTI.

AETIOLOGY

VUR may be secondary to urethral obstruction (e.g. PUV), and neuropathic (e.g. spinal dysraphism, following pelvic surgery) or non-neurogenic bladder dysfunction (e.g. detrusor–sphincter dyssynergia). Where there is no underlying aetiology, VUR is described as primary. While this was previously thought to be purely the result of an abnormal VUJ, which is often familial (34% of siblings and 50% of offspring), today VUR is recognised as part of a generalised abnormality of the urinary tract, including renal dysplasia and hypoplasia, bladder dysfunction and a possible predisposition to UTI.

DIAGNOSIS

MCUG is the gold standard and allows the severity of VUR to be graded (see **Table 22.2**). MCUG is an invasive investigation and prophylactic antibiotics must be increased to treatment dose for the subsequent 3 days to reduce the risk of sepsis (**Figs 22.6, 22.7**). For children who present symptomatically later in life or to assess for VUR resolution, an indirect cystogram using MAG3-renography can be obtained once a child has been potty-trained.

Renal dysplasia and scarring is best assessed by a DMSA isotope scan (**Fig. 22.8**). Since the advent of routine antenatal ultrasound scanning it has become clear that about 60% of 'renal scars' in newborns ascertained to have VUR are the result of abnormal kidney development rather than secondary to infection.

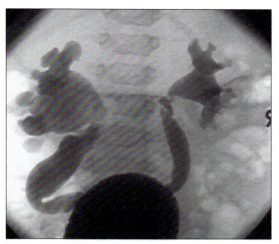

FIGURE 22.6 Bilateral vesicoureteric reflux shown by a micturating cystourethrogram.

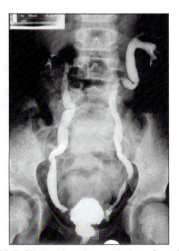

FIGURE 22.7 Bilateral vesicoureteric reflux shown by a micturating cystourethrogram.

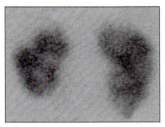

FIGURE 22.8 DMSA scan showing bilateral renal scarring in vesicoureteric reflux.

TABLE 22.2 International reflux study committee classification

- Grade I – reflux into a non-dilated ureter
- Grade II – reflux into a non-dilated renal pelvis and calyces
- Grade III – mild/moderate dilatation of ureter, renal pelvis and calyces
- Grade IV – moderate tortuosity and dilatation of ureter, renal pelvis and calyces with obliteration of angle of fornices but papillary impressions maintained in most calyces
- Grade V – gross tortuosity and dilatation of ureter, renal pelvis and calyces with loss of papillary impressions in most calyces

TREATMENT

Spontaneous improvement is the norm, with persistent VUR more likely with higher grade, bilaterality, older age at presentation and renal dysplasia/scarring.

The goal of treatment is the prevention of renal injury, leading to hypertension and renal failure. The management of VUR is once again intensely debated. Previously, randomised controlled studies centred on surgical versus medical management. Surgical correction of VUR was found to offer no advantage on renal outcome over antibiotic prophylaxis. Today, antibiotic prophylaxis is the focus of randomised controlled trials. No agreement exists on the role of circumcision, endoscopic injection and ureteric reimplantation. In contrast, the importance of optimising bladder and bowel function is beyond doubt and universally accepted.

POSTERIOR URETHRAL VALVE

INCIDENCE/CLINICAL PRESENTATION

A congenital membrane obstructing or partially obstructing the posterior urethra occurs in up to 1 in 4000 male births. Posterior urethral valve (PUV) accounts for almost 10% of antenatally diagnosed uropathies, and can affect the development of the entire urinary tract. An enlarged or thick-walled bladder, bilateral hydronephrosis with or without hyperechogenic renal parenchyma and oligo- or anhydramnios in a male fetus on antenatal ultrasound suggests PUV (**Fig. 22.9**). Oligo- or anhydramnios can have secondary effects on pulmonary and limb development, culminating in Potter syndrome. Antenatal decompression by placement of a JJ stent between the fetal bladder and amniotic cavity may restore an adequate volume of amniotic fluid and hence lung maturation (**Fig. 22.10**). So far, no benefit has been shown for renal and bladder outcomes from *in utero* vesicoamniotic shunting, which tends to be done quite late – during the second half of pregnancy.

The newborn may show signs of chronic kidney disease (CKD), sepsis, or pulmonary hypolasia. While many boys with PUV are detected antenatally, others present in infancy (UTI/sepsis, dysuria, haematuria, CKD) or thereafter (incontinence). The quality of the urinary stream is misleading and voiding pressures in boys with PUV are as high as in normal male infants.

Ultrasound may show a dilated posterior urethra in addition to a thick-walled bladder (keyhole sign), upper tract dilatation and abnormal renal parenchymal morphology. MCUG is still the gold standard for diagnosis, although compared to cystourethroscopy its sensitivity is 80–90% (**Fig. 22.11**).

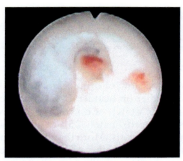

FIGURE 22.9 Endoscopic view of posterior urethral valve filling urethral lumen.

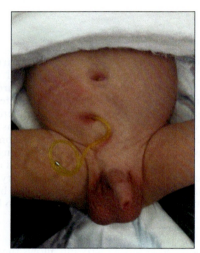

FIGURE 22.10 Newborn boy born with antenatally placed vesicoamniotic shunt *in situ*.

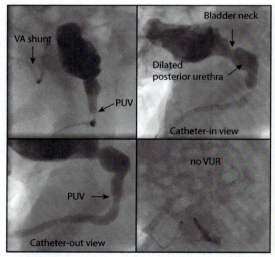

FIGURE 22.11 Micturating cystourethrogram. Note the trabeculated bladder, hypertrophied bladder neck and dilated posterior urethra above the posterior urethral valve (PUV). VA: vesicoamniotic; VUR: vesicoureteric reflux.

TREATMENT/PROGNOSIS

The three initial aims of treatment are to resuscitate the child in renal failure or sepsis, to drain the bladder and then to incise the PUV endoscopically. Subsequent management focuses on the long-term consequences of PUV on the urinary tract. CKD is present in 50%, at the time of diagnosis in most children with PUV. Four factors are associated with poor outcome in the long run: presentation before the age of 1 year, bilateral VUR, proteinuria and daytime incontinence at the age of 5 years. Until recently, antenatal diagnosis appeared to carry a worse prognosis. However, a long-term follow-up study from Leeds, UK observed better renal function in the second decade of life for antenatally detected PUV than for those presenting symptomatically later in childhood. While mortality or stage V CKD in the first 10 years of life appear predetermined by congenital renal dysplasia and the severity of *in utero* obstruction, thereafter, preservation of renal function seems to benefit from early diagnosis and nephrourological care. The association between poor renal outcome and urinary incontinence, present in 14–38% of boys with PUV, points to bladder dysfunction playing a major role in secondary renal damage. Indeed, the need for proactive management of the bladder in boys with PUV is well established today.

MULTI-CYSTIC DYSPLASTIC KIDNEY

INCIDENCE/AETIOLOGY

A faulty interaction between an abnormal ureteric bud and the metanephric mesenchyme may result in a non-functioning kidney consisting of variable-sized cysts and an atretic ureter (**Fig. 22.12**). Today, the majority are detected antenatally, affecting 1 in 4000 live births. Contralateral anomalies, primarily PUJA and VUR, may be present in 20%.

TREATMENT

Serial ultrasounds have shown that these kidneys involute spontaneously: approximately one-third by 2 years of age, one-half by 5 years and two-thirds by 10 years. However, if the kidney fails to decrease in size or enlarges, nephrectomy is indicated (**Fig. 22.13**). Although hypertension and malignant change have been reported, their incidence is similar to the normal population.

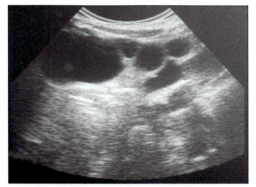

FIGURE 22.12 Multicystic dysplastic kidney: typical ultrasound appearance. No normal renal parenchyma can be found.

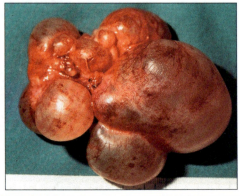

FIGURE 22.13 Multicystic dysplastic kidney: gross specimen. No normal renal parenchyma can be seen.

RENAL AGENESIS, ECTOPIA AND FUSION

The apparent absence of a kidney on ultrasound may reflect a congenital deficiency (agenesis), involution of a MCDK or an ectopic location yet to be identified.

INCIDENCE

- Unilateral agenesis: 1:1000–1500 births, i.e. a solitary kidney; bilateral renal agenesis is incompatible with life (Potter syndrome).
- Horseshoe kidney: 1:400–1800 births; a fibrous band or renal tissue (isthmus) joins the two kidneys across the midline (by the lower poles in 95%).
- Simple ectopia: 1:1000 births, i.e. the kidney is placed on same side as its ureter (60% pelvic, rarely in the thorax, in10% bilateral) (**Figs 22.14–22.16**).
- Crossed ectopia: 1:7000 births, i.e. the kidney lies on the opposite side to the insertion of its ureter into the bladder (usually left kidney crosses to the right, with fusion to the contralateral kidney in 85%).

CLINICAL PRESENTATION/DIAGNOSIS

Most are incidental findings on ultrasound imaging and may be part of multiple congenital anomalies such as the VACTERL association. Other urogenital abnormalities frequently coexist, for instance, contralateral VUR can be detected in one-third of unilateral renal agenesis, a PUJA occurs in 20% of horseshoe kidneys, and renal ectopia is associated with vaginal agenesis, bicornuate uterus or a contralateral ectopic ureter. Renal isotope imaging (DMSA) will reveal all functioning renal tissue. Occasionally, further clarification of the anatomy is required by intravenous urogram (IVU), magnetic resonance urography (MRU) or by intraoperative retrograde studies.

TREATMENT

Treatment is only required for clinically significant consequences, e.g. for VUR or PUJA.

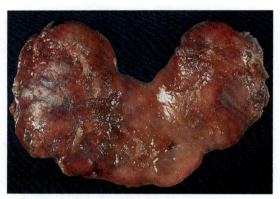

FIGURE 22.14 Horseshoe kidney.

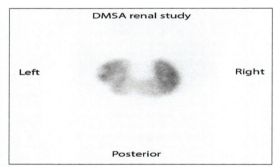

FIGURE 22.15 DMSA isotope study of a horseshoe kidney.

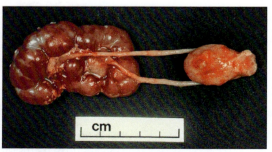

FIGURE 22.16 Fused kidneys with right and left moeity ureters draining to the bladder on their respective sides.

Urology

DUPLEX KIDNEYS

Where a kidney has two parts (moeities) each with their own collecting system it is called a duplex kidney (**Fig. 22.17**). In 60% the ureters join before their insertion into the bladder (incomplete duplex) and in the other 40% the two ureters enter the bladder separately (complete duplex). As a result of the way the ureters are incorporated into the bladder during development, the lower moiety ureter orifice lies above the upper moiety ureteric orifice (Mayer–Weigert Law). The terminal upper moiety ureter is prone to a cystic dilatation (ureterocoele).

INCIDENCE/CLINICAL PRESENTATION

Some degree of duplication is extremely common (approximately 1:100), bilaterally in 40% (**Fig. 22.18**). Complete duplication occurs in 1:1000 and is bilateral in 25%. Where there is a family history the incidence increases to 1:12. Most duplications are an incidental finding. Others are associated with hydronephrosis (**Fig. 22.19**), and today, many of these are detected on antenatal ultrasound screening. An ureterocoele is seen in 1:5000. This may be obstructive to its associated moiety, and if very large the ureterocoele may prolapse into the bladder neck causing obstruction to the entire urinary tract. The lower moiety ureter is ectopic (high and lateral – where it is prone to VUR) in 1:2500 (40% of complete duplex systems). The upper moiety ureter is ectopic in 1:10,000 (10% of duplex systems). While in boys the ectopia of the upper moiety ureter is always above the urinary sphincter, in girls the ectopia may be into the vagina causing dribble incontinence on top of a normal voiding pattern. As a general rule, the more ectopically a ureter inserts, the more dysplastic its associated renal moiety (Stephen hypothesis).

DIAGNOSIS

On ultrasound, the only feature of an uncomplicated duplex kidney may be its greater renal length. Where there is hydronephrosis, this may preferentially affect one moiety of a complete duplex. Providing both moieties have functioning renal tissue, MAG3-renography may show two distinct pelvicalyceal systems (**Fig. 22.20**). A DMSA may be needed to clarify the degree of function in each renal moiety (**Fig. 22.21**). An ureterocoele may be observed on

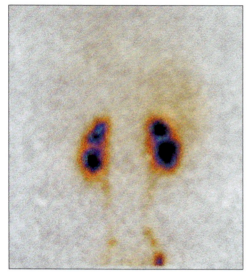

FIGURE 22.18 MAG3 renogram demonstrating bilateral duplex kidneys.

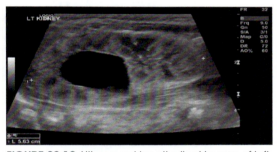

FIGURE 22.19 Ultrasound longitudinal image of left duplex kidney. Note the marked hydronephrosis of the upper moeity.

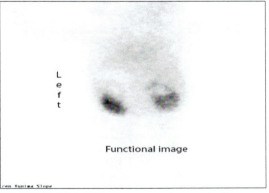

FIGURE 22.17 Ultrasound image of two separate collecting systems in an uncomplicated duplex kidney.

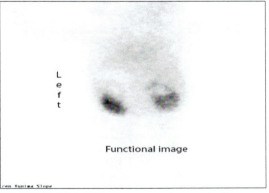

FIGURE 22.20 MAG3 renogram demonstrating very poor function in the upper moeities of bilateral duplex kidneys.

ultrasound or it may show as a filling defect during the early filling phase of a MCUG (**Figs 22.22, 22.23**). During the MCUG, contrast may reflux into the lower moiety pelvicalyceal system, which is orientated lateral and inferior – referred to as the 'drooping lily sign' (**Fig. 22.24**). Rarely, a MRU is needed to demonstrate the very small poorly-functioning upper moiety responsible for the dribble incontinence from its ectopic ureter, known as a 'cryptic upper moiety'.

TREATMENT

No treatment is required in an asymptomatic child with a duplex system not complicated by obstruction, reflux or ectopia. No follow-up is needed for those without hydronephrosis. Endoscopic ureterocoele puncture may be needed to relieve obstruction to its moiety or to the bladder outflow. Where intervention is indicated for VUR to the lower moiety or contralateral ureter, endoscopic injection may be attempted; similar success rates to simplex systems were noted in a recent meta-analysis (64% vs. 68%). As the distal upper and lower moiety ureters share a common blood supply, a combined mobilisation and reimplantation of both ureters is needed during intravesical ureteric reimplantation. Mobilisation of the upper moiety ureter/ureterocoele may leave a defect in the bladder neck that will require repair and risks bladder dysfunction. However, as the renal moieties of the most ectopic ureters typically are very poorly functioning, heminephrectomy allows extensive bladder surgery to be avoided in most.

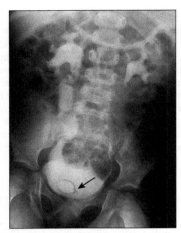

FIGURE 22.22 Intravenous urogram showing ureterocoele in the bladder that contains a stone.

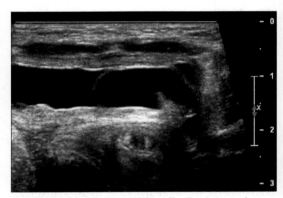

FIGURE 22.23 Ultrasound: longitudinal view of bladder demonstrating a large ureterocoele prolapsing through the bladder neck into the urethra.

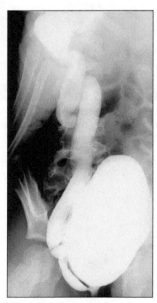

FIGURE 22.21 Micturating cystourethrogram demonstrating the ectopic insertion of the right upper moeity ureter into the urethra.

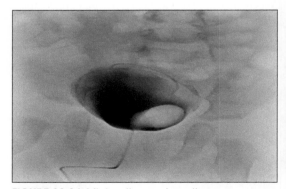

FIGURE 22.24 Micturating cystourethrogram: early filling phase showing a large intravesical ureterocoele.

INCONTINENCE

DEVELOPMENT OF CONTINENCE

In infancy voiding occurs as a result of a reflex coordinated in the brainstem. With increasing age bladder capacity increases and the frequency of voiding reduces. By around 4 years, voluntary inhibition of the voiding reflex has been attained.

Continence requires normal:

- mobility and brain function
- bladder capacity and compliance
- bladder sensation
- voluntary detrusor contraction
- co-ordinated with sphincter control (competence and relaxation).

AETIOLOGY

The key to tackling incontinence is to understand the aetiology, which frequently can be deduced from a careful history and examination followed by basic non-invasive assessments. Structural causes, such as the exstrophy–epispadias complex or an ectopic ureter, and neurogenic pathologies, for example the spinal dysraphisms or secondary to anorectal anomalies, have to be differentiated from the far more common functional causes (see Further reading).

EXSTROPHY–EPISPADIAS COMPLEX

INCIDENCE

Maldevelopment of the cloacal membrane and lower abdominal wall results in a spectrum ranging from epispadias (1 in 120,000), through vesical exstrophy (1 in 50,000) to cloacal exstrophy (1 in 300,000 live births).

EPISPADIAS

Epispadias is the mildest form and generally seen in boys (**Figs 22.25, 22.26**). The bladder is covered but the urethra opens on the dorsum of the penis. The penis is typically wide and short with dorsal curvature. In girls, the urethra is patulous and the clitoris bifid. In addition to reconstructing the genitalia, surgery for continence is also required in the majority of patients as the defect extends through the sphincter and bladder neck.

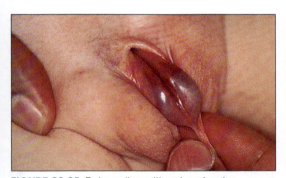

FIGURE 22.25 Epispadias without exstrophy.

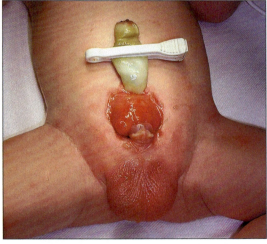

FIGURE 22.26 Classic bladder exstrophy with epispadias in a male.

VESICAL EXSTROPHY

In this anomaly, the bladder opens onto the abdominal wall between split rectus abdominis muscles and separated pubic bones (pubic diastasis) continuing as an open urethral plate on the dorsum of the penis in the male and between divided clitori and labia minora in the female to the anterior edge of the vagina (**Fig. 22.27**). The anus is anteriorly positioned (functionally normal) and the umbilicus is low-lying above the bladder plate. Inguinal herniae are a common association.

The surgical care of these babies has been centralised to a handful of institutions and each have developed their technique for closure of the bladder and abdominal wall, bladder neck repair as well as reconstruction of the penis.

CLOACAL EXSTROPHY

This is the most severe and rarest form of the exstrophy complex (**Fig. 22.28**). Here, the bowel, usually at the ileocaecal valve, opens in the midline between two hemibladders, accompanied by diastasis of the pubis and a small epispadiac penis as well as an exomphalos into the cord. Other anomalies are frequent, such as spinal dysraphism (30%) and Arnold–Chiari malformation, lower limb (25%), renal and cardiac anomalies and a foreshortened intestine. Until 50 years ago, this condition was universally fatal, but since the 1980s survival has been over 90%.

In addition to the above surgery, hindgut reconstruction to a colostomy or ileostomy is required. Pelvic osteotomy is employed to help approximate the pubic diastasis (**Fig. 22.29**) and support the closure.

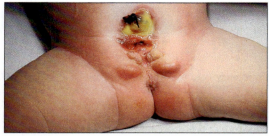

FIGURE 22.27 Classic bladder exstrophy in a female.

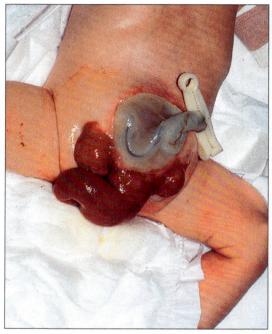

FIGURE 22.28 Cloacal exstrophy.

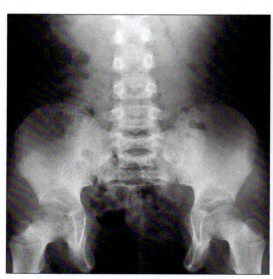

FIGURE 22.29 Widened symphysis pubis.

Urology

NEUROPATHIC BLADDER

INCIDENCE/AETIOLOGY

In most children neuropathic voiding dysfunction is congenital: it must be assessed for in children with spinal dysraphism (1 in 2500) or anorectal anomalies. It is important to consider that this dysfunction can change typically at times of rapid growth such as in the first 2 years of life or in adolescence. Cord trauma or infarction, transverse myelitis, tumours or pelvic surgery may result in acquired neuropathic voiding dysfunction.

CLINICAL FEATURES/DIAGNOSIS

Physical examination may reveal overt lower extremity neurological deficit and/or a hairy patch, dimple or skin tag on the spine may point to spina bifida occulta. Ultrasound will demonstrate upper tract hydronephrosis, bladder wall thickness and volume, and in children less than 3 months the terminal spinal cord. A plain film may show bony spinal abnormalities and constipation; however, for further details of spinal cord abnormalities MRI is required (**Fig. 22.30**). Ultrasound is also used during non-invasive bladder function assessment to ascertain the voiding pattern and efficiency. Urodynamics assess the pressures within the urinary tract during bladder filling and emptying through a small catheter placed into the bladder. MCUG can provide further information during filling and voiding, including secondary VUR, and is combined with urodynamics (videourodynamics) after infancy. DMSA isotope scanning assesses the kidneys for renal damage.

TREATMENT

Regular careful assessment is essential to achieve the treatment aims:

- preservation of renal function
- continence
- sexual function.

Many require frequent bladder catheterisation and daily medication, and a proportion require major surgery to achieve these goals (**Table 22.3**).

PROGNOSIS

With careful monitoring and high levels of compliance renal damage can be minimised. Surgery for continence is required for a significant proportion, with subsequent life-long monitoring for side-effects or late complications.

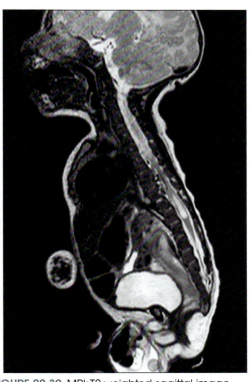

FIGURE 22.30 MRI: T2-weighted sagittal image. Note the hypoplastic spinal cord and segmental anomalies, as well as the large bladder.

TABLE 22.3 Management of neuropathic bladder

Proportion (%)	Bladder detrusor	Sphincter/ bladder neck	Pressures, i.e. risk to kidneys, continence	Management
7	Normal	Normal	Normal	Monitor for change
23	Hyporeflexic	Acontractile	Low pressure incontinence	Catheterisation for emptying Surgery for continence
15	Hyporeflexic	Hypercontractile	Variable pressure	Regular catheterisation, may be continent without major surgery
11	Hyper-reflexic	Acontractile	Variable pressure incontinence	Anticholinergics +/– catheterisation, surgery for continence +/– upper tracts
44	Hyper-reflexic	Hyperreflexic	High pressure, high risk	Anticholinergics and regular catheterisation, may need vesicostomy/augmentation cystoplasty to protect kidneys

DISORDERS OF SEX DEVELOPMENT

Disorders of sex development (DSD) is a complex group of disorders with diverse pathophysiology that affect the internal and/or external genitalia (**Fig. 22.31**). Patients present in the newborn period with atypical genitalia or in adolescence with abnormal sexual development during puberty. Patients with DSD are best managed by a multi-disciplinary team, and where this experience is not available referral to a regional DSD centre is mandatory. For further information on how to evaluate a new patient with DSD the reader is referred to the UK clinical guidelines and Chapter 13 Endocrinology, page 402 for a diagnostic classification of DSD.

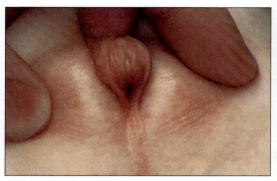

FIGURE 22.31 Ambiguous genitalia.

HYPOSPADIAS

INCIDENCE/CLINICAL PRESENTATION

Hypospadia occurs 1 in 300 live male births. This congenital abnormality is characterised by any combination of the following key features:

- A ventral urethral meatus abnormally positioned anywhere from the glans penis to the perineum (**Fig. 22.32**).
- Chordee forces the penis to point down to the scrotum when erect (**Fig. 22.33**).
- A 'hooded' foreskin present only on the dorsal side.

It is important to distinguish an incompletely virilised hypospadiac penis from a virilised female or other DSD (see below). This is facilitated by the palpation of the testes. Bilaterally descended testes point to a XY karyotype. However, if one or both testes are undescended or impalpable, DSD must be excluded.

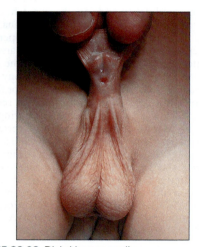

FIGURE 22.32 Distal hypospadias.

TREATMENT

While for the most minor degree of hypospadias no surgery or only excision of the hooded prepuce can be considered, the remainder are likely to require operative correction. The first step of surgery is the correction of the chordee, followed by urethroplasty and skin cover. Depending on the abnormality, the surgeon will advise either a single-stage or two-stage procedure using the prepuce as a graft for the urethroplasty. Therefore, parents must be counselled against circumcision of a newborn baby boy with hypospadias.

PROGNOSIS

A cosmetically acceptable result should be attainable. However, complications are common: 5% meatal or urethral stenosis, 10–15% urethra–cutaneous fistula and 2–5% dehiscence of part of the repair. Voiding difficulties may become apparent only in adolescence.

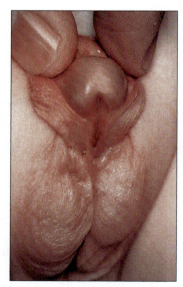

FIGURE 22.33 Severe hypospadias with chordee.

UNDESCENDED TESTIS

INCIDENCE

Testicular descent occurs during the 5th to 7th months of pregnancy, the left descending before the right. An undescended testis is observed in 1 in 50–100 term infants and in up to one-third of premature babies. Descent after birth does occur spontaneously but is rare after the first few months of life.

CLINICAL PRESENTATION/ INVESTIGATION/CLASSIFICATION

A careful history and examination allows the testis palpated outside the scrotum to be categorised into:

- An undescended testis: a testicle that is found in the line of its normal path of descent but outside the scrotum.
- An ectopic testis: a testicle that lies outside the normal path of descent, for instance in the thigh or the perineum.
- An ascended testis: a previously normally descended testis that with growth has failed to retain its scrotal position.
- A retractile testis: a normal testis that on initial examination appears above the scrotum or in the inguinal canal but can be brought to the scrotum without tension once the cremasteric reflex has been overcome.

An impalpable testis requires further assessment under general anaesthesia. If the testis remains impalpable at this point, diagnostic laparoscopy will demonstrate one of three scenarios:

- The vas deferens and testicular vessels run to an intra-abdominal testis.
- The vas deferens and testicular vessels end blindly within the abdomen, pointing to testicular loss before the 5th month of pregnancy.

- The vas deferens and testicular vessels leave the abdomen through the deep inguinal ring. Subsequent groin exploration may reveal a testis within the groin or demonstrate the vas deferens and vessels to be blind-ending, presumably due to torsion or a vascular event during descent. This is known as the 'vanishing testis syndrome'.

TREATMENT

Retractile testes require no intervention. Orchidopexy is performed for palpable testes. If the testicular vessels to an intra-abdominal testis are short, a two-stage Fowler–Stephens procedure is the procedure of choice. Following division of the testicular vessels, the collateral blood supply along the vas deferens is allowed to strengthen before mobilisation of the testis on this second blood supply to the scrotum. Inguinal orchidopexy carries a 5% risk of testicular atrophy, and this increases to 10% for mobilisation of an intra-abdominal testis (**Fig. 22.34**).

PROGNOSIS

Surgery cannot reverse the maturational failure of the undescended testis but it can reduce the impact from further thermal injury. Historical data have documented normal semen analysis in 60% of men with unilateral and 25% of those with bilateral undescended testis, although paternity is achieved by up to 90% and 65%, respectively. Since then, the recommended age for orchidepexy has steadily decreased. So far, improved sperm counts and mobility as well as a reduced malignancy risk have been reported. The risk of malignancy is estimated to be 2–3 times that of the normal population for boys who had an orchidopexy before puberty. Monthly testicular self-examination should commence at puberty.

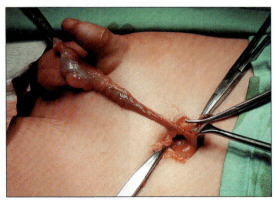

FIGURE 22.34 Undescended testis being brought down into the scrotum at surgery.

ACUTE SCROTUM

CLINICAL PRESENTATION

Sudden onset of scrotal pain, redness and/or erythema warrants emergency review in case of torsion of the testis, whose chance of viability reduces with each hour. In young children the first symptoms are frequently atypical and non-specific, necessitating a high index of suspicion and scrotal examination in all boys presenting with abdominal pain or mere vomiting. The child must refrain from eating and drinking as emergency surgical exploration under general anaesthesia is often the only way to establish the diagnosis.

DIFFERENTIAL DIAGNOSIS

- Torsion of testis: can occur at any age but is more common after 10 years of age and affects 1:4000 males under the age of 25 years each year. A testis torted in the perinatal period is virtually never salvageable; however, the contralateral testis should undergo dartos pouch fixation to prevent contralateral torsion and loss of both testes.
- Torsion of hydatid of Morgagni: twisting of the appendage of the testis classically produces a tender dark spot above a non-tender testis; peak age 11 years,
- Idiopathic scrotal oedema: careful examination will demonstrate the painless, salmon-pink oedema to extend beyond the confines of the scrotum. This condition is self-limiting; peak age 5–6 years.
- Epididymo-orchitis is uncommon in childhood and associated with urinary tract pathology and therefore requires a follow-up ultrasound scan of the urinary tract and pelvis.
- Incarcerated inguinal hernia (see Chapter 18 Neonatal and General Paediatric Surgery, page 562).
- Trauma: rare.
- Testicular tumour: although the vast majority of testicular tumours present as an assiduous painless mass, the sudden detection by a parent may result in an acute presentation (**Fig. 22.35**).

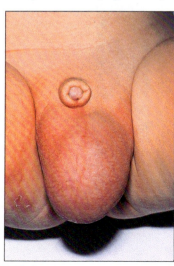

FIGURE 22.35 Scrotal mass caused by a tumour.

UROLITHIASIS

INCIDENCE

Stone formation in the urinary tract affects approximately 5–10% of the population. Children account for just 1–3% of all stone patients. The incidence of urolithiasis shows marked geographical variation: while very rare in Greenland and Japan, a 'stone belt' extends from the Balkans across Turkey, Pakistan and northern India. Overall, boys are twice as often affected as girls and tend to present at a younger age.

AETIOLOGY

Unlike the adult population who have mostly idiopathic stones, most renal calculi in children are either infective, metabolic or are associated with an underlying anatomical abnormality (**Fig. 22.36**). Bladder stones are particularly prevalent in children with bladder augmentation (**Fig. 22.37**).

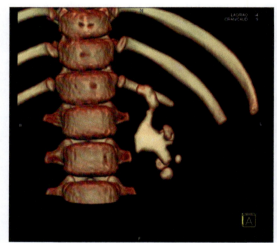

FIGURE 22.36 CT reconstruction of a left staghorn calculus.

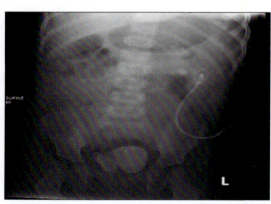

FIGURE 22.37 Plain abdominal radiograph showing two massive bladder stones and a staghorn left renal stone. A perinephric drain has been placed to drain a perinephric abscess.

Urology

The organisms most commonly associated with infective calculi are the urea splitting *Proteus* spp. and *Escherichia coli*. Today, a metabolic abnormality is detected in 44% of children with urolithiasis in the UK. Hypercalciuria (57%) is the most common metabolic abnormality, followed by cystinuria (23%), hyperoxaluria (17%), hyperuricosuria (2%) and unclassified hypercalcemia (2%).

CLINICAL PRESENTATION

Presenting features are macroscopic haematuria, UTI or abdominal pain; however, one in six children appear to be asymptomatic. Obstruction related to calculi may result in pyonephrosis, perinephric abscess, or progressive pyelonephritis and renal loss; emergency admission and relief of obstruction is required.

IMAGING

In contrast to adults, ultrasound combined with a plain abdominal film can accurately determine the stone burden in most children. Occasionally a low-radiation-dose CT or IVU are required. Functional imaging will detect renal damage resulting from the stone and diuretic renography may help identify underlying anatomical abnormalities, such as PUJA, VUJA or VUR.

TREATMENT

Once sepsis/infection has been controlled and obstruction relieved, the first aim of management is to clear all stones. Today, minimally invasive techniques are available even for the youngest of children and, as in adults, have largely replaced open surgery.

- Extracorporal shock wave lithotripsy (ESWL) uses a shockwave generated outside the body and focused through the body tissues onto the stone to break the stone into smaller pieces, which can then be passed out of the body within the urine.
- Ureterorenoscopy (URS) employs tiny telescopes passed though the urethra and bladder to gain access to stones in the ureter and kidney (**Fig. 22.38**).
- Percutaneous nephrolithotomy (PCNL) uses image guidance to gain keyhole access into the kidney. Stones are fragmented using a lithoclast and removed through the keyhole tract (**Fig. 22.39**).
- Bladder stones can be removed by open or keyhole surgery (percutaneous cystolithotomy, PCCL) or cystoscopically.

As a result of the high incidence of underlying metabolic, anatomical or functional causes for stone formation, children are at significant risk of recurrent stone formation. Once stone clearance has been achieved management moves on to the prevention of recurrence. A high fluid intake for urine solute dilution is essential for all. Other treatments will depend on underlying aetiologies.

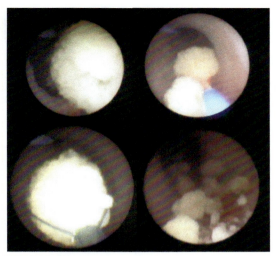

FIGURE 22.38 Intraoperative images of ureterorenoscopic laser stone disintegration and extraction.

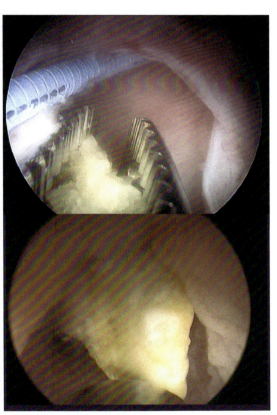

FIGURE 22.39 Intraoperative images of stone fragment extraction and lithoclast stone disintegration via the percutaneous nephrolithotomy tract.

NEOPLASIA

See also Chapter 12 Oncology.

CHILDHOOD RENAL TUMOURS

(Table 22.4)

WILMS TUMOUR (NEPHROBLASTOMA)

Incidence Wilms tumour is named after Dr Max Wilms (1867–1918), who first described this tumour. It is a tumour of early childhood, typically under the age of 5 years, affecting 1 in 125,000. Those with bilateral tumours (approximately 5%) tend to be younger.

AETIOLOGY

The tumour is thought to arise from primitive elements, embryonic metanephric blastema, which has failed to involute. Although mostly sporadic, some children have a predisposing syndrome, such as for instance WAGR (Wilms–Aniridia–Genitourinary malformation–mental Retardation), Beckwith–Wiedemann syndrome or Denys–Drash, and 1% a positive family history of Wilms tumour. Currently, the most common associated mutations identified are on chromosome 11 in the *WT1* and *WT2* genes.

CLINICAL PRESENTATION/DIAGNOSIS

Most present with a painless abdominal mass (**Fig. 22.40**). Others have haematuria, abdominal pain, fever, hypertension or anorexia.

Ultrasound is the first mode of imaging, followed by an MRI (or CT) of the abdomen and a CT of the chest to ascertain the extent of the tumour and presence of metastases (11% at presentation) (**Figs 22.41, 22.42**). In the UK, all renal tumours are biopsied unless they are cystic or the child is less than 6 months of age (see below). A retroperitoneal percutaneous needle biopsy provides histological clarification of the renal mass without altering the tumour stage. Classically, the tumour consists of blastemal, stromal and epithelial

elements (triphasic Wilms). Poor differentiation of these elements is described as anaplasia and confers a worse prognosis (**Fig. 22.43**).

TREATMENT

The treatment of Wilms consists of chemotherapy combined with surgery, and less frequently radiotherapy. Patients are managed by a multi-disciplinary team with detailed protocols tailored to the individual patient. Preoperative chemotherapy has been repeatedly shown to significantly reduce the risk of intraoperative tumour rupture and is routine in Europe. In unilateral disease, nephrectomy is preceded typically by 4 weeks of neo-adjuvant vincristine and actinomycin for stage I–III, and by 6 weeks of vincristine, actinomycin and doxorubicin in stage IV (**Table 22.5**). The exceptions are infants less than 6 months of age, in whom a benign lesion is more common and the risks of chemotherapy increased, and cystic Wilms tumours, which cannot be biopsied and are relatively chemotherapy insensitive. Primary surgery is advised in these situations. Postoperative chemotherapy +/– radiotherapy is dictated by tumour stage, histology (low, intermediate and high risk) and molecular biology (e.g. 1p and or 16q loss).

In bilateral disease, surgery is usually required for both kidneys, aiming to excise the tumours while preserving as much of the normal renal tissues as possible. In addition to the Wilms tumours, multiple foci of primitive elements (nephrogenic rests)

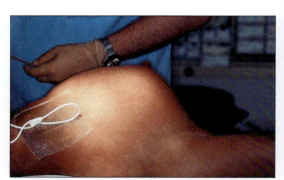

FIGURE 22.40 Wilms tumour causing an abdominal mass.

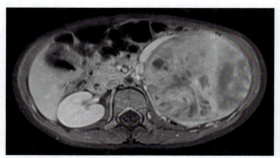

FIGURE 22.41 MRI T2-weighted axial image of left sided Wilms tumour and normal contralateral right kidney.

TABLE 22.4 Benign and malignant renal tumours of childhood

Benign	Malignant
Mesoblastic nephroma	90% Wilms tumour/ nephroblastoma
Cystic nephroma	3% Clear cell sarcoma
Angiomyolipoma	3% Rhabdoid tumour
Haemangioma/ lymphangioma	2% Renal cell carcinoma

Urology

with the potential for future malignant change can be found in all bilateral Wilms tumours. The multidisciplinary team will determine the optimal combination of treatments as well as timing of surgery based on repeat assessments.

PROGNOSIS

Five-year survival is around 90%, but 60% for those with anaplasia and 55% after relapse.

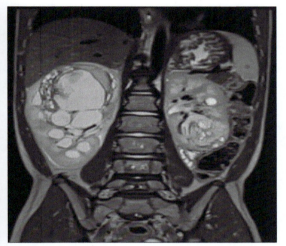

FIGURE 22.42 MRI T2-weighted coronal images of bilateral Wilms tumours.

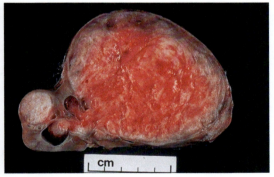

FIGURE 22.43 Wilms tumour showing the cut surface of a specimen.

TABLE 22.5 Wilms tumour staging

Stage I	Confined to kidney, completely excised
Stage II	Extension beyond the confines of the kidney, but completely excised
Stage III	Tumour incompletely excised, pre- or intraoperative tumour rupture, extension to lymph nodes, or open tumour biopsy
Stage IV	Metastases to most commonly lung
Stage V	Bilateral Wilms tumour

GENITOURINARY RHABDOMYOSARCOMA

INCIDENCE/AETIOLOGY

The incidence of this tumour is 1 in 2,000,000. It can occur at any time in childhood, with an early (2–5 years) and late peak (15–19 years). The tumour arises from skeletal muscle precursor embryonal mesenchyme and can occur anywhere except the brain. The most common urogenital sites affected are the prostate/bladder and vagina.

The aetiology is unknown with both genetic (e.g. p53 mutation) and environmental factors implicated.

CLINICAL PRESENTATION/DIAGNOSIS

Depending on the site of origin, children may present with abdominal pain and a mass, difficulty voiding and less commonly haematuria. Tumours arising from the vagina typically grow in an exophytic manner and may present as a 'bunch of grapes' in the introitus. Diagnosis relies on imaging (ultrasound and MRI) and percutaneous or endoscopic biopsy. Tumours frequently are locally invasive and microscopically extend beyond the apparent macroscopic confines. Metastases occur to most frequently to lung, bone, liver and the bone marrow (**Fig. 22.44**).

TREATMENT/PROGNOSIS

The treatment consists of a combination of chemotherapy, surgery and radiotherapy (external beam or brachytherapy) and is based on a complex appraisal of tumour site, size and response to chemotherapy, as well as tumour stage and histology and patient age. In selected cases, brachytherapy may allow less extensive surgical resection with the potential for better functional outcomes.

In those with localised disease, 5-year survival has improved to over 80%, but remains below 30% for those with metastatic disease.

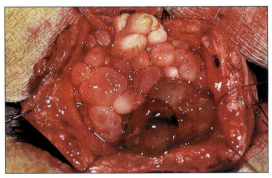

FIGURE 22.44 Opened bladder filled with rhabdomyosarcoma.

FURTHER READING

General

Wilcox D, Godbole P, Cooper C (eds). *Pediatric Urology Book,* http://www.pediatricurologybook.com.

Thomas DFM, Duffy PG, Rickwood AMK (eds). *Essentials of Paediatric Urology*, 2nd edn. London: Informa Healthcare, 2008.

Hydronephrosis

Farrugia MK, Hitchcock R, Radford A, *et al.* British Association of Paediatric Urologists consensus statement on the management of the primary obstructive megaureter. *J Ped Urol* 2013;10:26–33.

Hennus PML, van der Heijden GJ, Bosch JL, *et al.* A systematic review on renal and bladder dysfunction after endoscopic treatment of infravesical obstruction in boys. *PlOS ONE* 2012;7(9):e44663.

Nagler EV, Williams G, Hodson EM, Craig JC. Interventions for primary vesicoureteric reflux (review). *Cochrane Database Syst Rev* 2011;6:CD001532.

Nguyen HT, Herndon CDA, Copper C, *et al.* The Society for Fetal Urology consensus statement on the evaluation and management of antenatal hydronephrosis. *J Ped Urol* 2010;6:212–31.

Routh JC, Bogaert GA, Kaefer M, *et al.* Vesicoureteral reflux: current trends in diagnosis, screening and treatment. *European Urology* 2012;61:773–82.

Thomas DFM. Prenatal diagnosis: what do we know of long-term outcomes? *J Ped Urol* 2010;6:204–11.

Wang HH, Gbadegesin RA, Foreman JW, *et al.* Efficacy of antibiotic prophylaxis in children with vesicoureteral reflux: systematic review and meta-analysis. *J Urol* 2014;4:S0022–5347.

Williams G, Craig JC. Long-term antibioitics for preventing recurrent urinary tract infections in children (review). *Cochrane Database Syst Rev* 2011;3:CD001534.

DSD

Ahmed SF, Achermann JC, Arlt W, *et al.* Society for Endocrinology Clinical Guidance Article: UK guidance on the initial evaluation of an infant or an adolescent with a suspected disorder of sex development. *Clin Endocrinol* 2011;75:12–26.

Mouriquand P, Caldamone A, Malone P, *et al.* The ESPU/SPU standpoint on the surgical management of disorders of sex development (DSD). *J Ped Urol* 2014;10(1):8–10.

Hypospadias

Springer A. Assessment of outcome in hypospadias surgery – a review. *Front Pediatr* 2014;2:1–7.

Fraumann SA, Stephany HA, Clayton DB, *et al.* Long-term follow-up of children who underwent severe hypospadias repair using an online survey with validated questionnaires. *J Ped Urol* 2014;10:446–50.

23 Allergic Diseases

Adam Fox, George Du Toit and Stephan Strobel

INTRODUCTION: CLARIFICATION OF TERMS

Clinical symptoms and signs of adverse reactions to foods and asthma have been described for over thousand years. The term **'allergy'**, derived from the Greek means altered (enhanced) reactivity, has been coined by v. Pirquet in 1906 for the description of symptoms such as fever and rashes after injections of antitoxic serum. A genetic predisposition to allergy was postulated and in 1923, Coca and Cooke chose the term **'atopy'** ('atopos' out of place) to describe hypersensitivity conditions on a genetic background. Today, atopy describes the genetic background of an individual with the ability to respond with increased IgE production to environmental and food allergens (**Fig. 23.1**).

Allergens are antigens that lead to immune responses that cause allergies. They are often proteins although IgE antibodies to carbohydrates and smaller chemical compounds have been described.

Sensitisation describes the state of an immunological encounter and response to an allergen without disease at the time of investigation. Individuals who present with clinical (allergy) symptoms have experienced a varying immunological sensitisation phase during which they did not exhibit clinical symptoms. Often 10–15% of individuals (up to 40% depending on the allergen) who have been sensitised

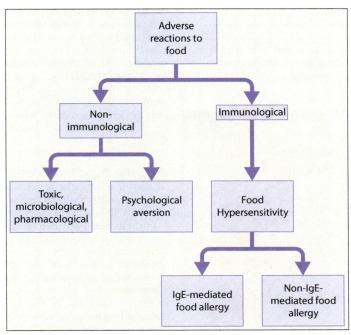

FIGURE 23.1 Classification of adverse reactions to food. The terms food hypersensitivity and adverse reaction to foods are often used interchangeably. In some usage food hypersensitivity indicates the umbrella term for food allergy.

do not develop clinical symptoms on exposure to the sensitising allergen.

Hypersensitivity describes an adverse clinical response where the exact nature of the underlying pathophysiology is unknown.

Allergy describes an immunologically-mediated condition that leads to clinical symptoms and is related to an allergen specific IgE response. The term **'non-IgE-mediated food allergy'** (IUIS2004) is often used to describe a non-IgE related adverse (hypersensitivity) reaction to foods.

THE 'ALLERGIC MARCH'

The term 'allergic march' is used for description of the natural history of atopic manifestations, which develop during the first decade of life (**Fig. 23.2**). Although there exists a great variability, this period is characterised by increasing IgE antibody responses and clinical symptoms that occur in early life and can remit over time. Early eczematous changes and gastrointestinal (GI) symptoms (**Fig. 23.3**) within the first 3 years are

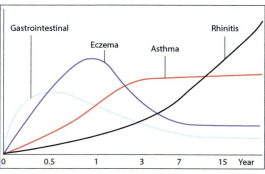

FIGURE 23.2 The relative prevalence of symptoms according to age in atopic children. Symptoms are often exhibited simultaneously.

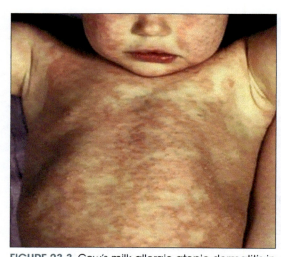

FIGURE 23.3 Cow's milk allergic atopic dermatitis in an 18-month-old toddler covering the entire skin.

followed from around 3–7 years by asthma and later by allergic rhinitis. It has to be noted that many children exhibit multiple symptoms simultaneously. Presence of early eczema in childhood is often associated with the development of IgE-mediated common food allergies. The term 'food allergic march' implies that children typically present with egg or milk allergy or both and then go on to develop additional food allergies followed in adolescence/adulthood by the oral allergy syndrome (OAS). The natural history of these 'atopic marches', including which determinants are modifiable and might become candidates for preventive intervention, is still very poorly understood.

GENETIC FACTORS

Different allergic conditions may exhibit different genetic traits. A child has a 6–7-fold increased chance in developing peanut allergy if he or she has a family member with peanut allergy. A monozygotic twin has an over 65% chance of developing peanut allergy if the twin sibling has peanut allergy, confirming a strong genetic contribution to the development of peanut allergy.

HLA-haplotype associations and interleukin (IL)-4, IL-10 and IL-3 polymorphisms have been associated with allergy manifestations in different populations but their general importance needs to be confirmed.

NON-GENETIC FACTORS: ENVIRONMENTAL AND MODIFIABLE FACTORS

An increase in allergic diseases over the last two decades has been linked to the recognition of new risk factors and the description of protective factors associated with a more 'traditional (rural) lifestyle'. Contributing factors for the development and modification of allergic diseases or symptoms are listed in **Table 23.1**. It has to be born in mind that some of the protective effects may only be short term. However, even if some of these effects may only be experienced for a few years, they may still provide a major health benefit for the child and family.

Hygiene hypothesis and beyond

The hygiene hypothesis describes the epidemiological observation that the exposure to other children and early infections reduces the risk of allergy. This hypothesis has been extended to include evidence that the exposure to certain microbiota at significant stages of development may increase tolerogenic responses and reduce allergies. Clinical observations are inconsistent and a simple shift of T-helper 1 responses to T-helper 2 responses seems unlikely; recent theories favour the idea that outside, e.g. microbial, influences activate regulatory cells that prevent sensitisation. Clinical studies are in progress to assess environmental influences on the genetic background and how to induce a tolerogenic, non-allergic response (**Fig. 23.4**).

TABLE 23.1 Modifiable risk factors affecting the developing of allergic (food) allergic symptoms in childhood

Factor/event	Decreased	Increased	Comments
Caesarian section		+	? Related to delayed microbial colonisation of infant gut
Maternal smoking during and after pregnancy		+	Epidemiological evidence from European study
Vitamin A & D deficiency		+	Emerging supportive evidence
Breastfeeding	+	(+)	Inconsistent evidence related to increased risk
Exposure to endotoxins	+		'Rural lifestyle'
Hydrolysed/amino acid based formulae	+		Only if breastfeeding cannot be maintained for 4 months
Increased consumption in omega-6-fatty acids		+(?)	Inconsistent evidence
Early antigen avoidance	?	?	Inconsistent evidence
Early solid introduction	+(?)	+	Inconsistent evidence
Obesity		+	Emerging evidence
Oral (first) antigen exposure	+?		Experimental evidence, unresolved in humans
Cutaneous (first) antigen exposure		+?	Experimental evidence, unresolved in humans
Vaccinations	–	–	No evidence of adverse effects on development of allergic symptoms (BCG ? reduced risk)
Frequent use of antibiotics in infancy		+?	? Only for eczema
High socio-economic status		+	Results inconsistent and prone to large number of 'lifestyle' confounders

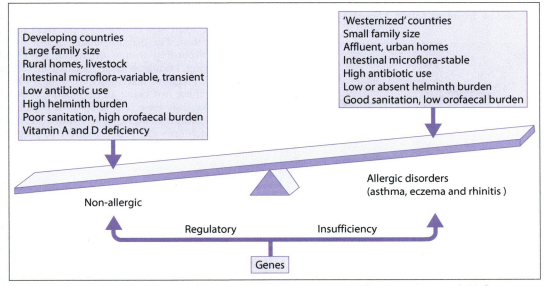

FIGURE 23.4 The hygiene hypothesis balance. The balance depicts different environmental influences on immunoregulatory responses affecting the development of different atopic diseases.

GENERAL DIAGNOSTIC APPROACHES FOR ALLERGIES AND ADVERSE REACTIONS TO FOODS

The mainstay of a clinical diagnosis of an allergy, including a delayed adverse reaction to foods is a careful (family) history and a clinical examination. Only then should further *in vivo* or *in vitro* tests be applied.

Skin testing often correlates with results of intranasal or bronchial antigen challenges taking into account non-specific airway reactivity. In individuals with potential food allergy, the clinical history is the initial screening test, with subsequent skin testing or other *in vitro* blood tests used to support the history (see below). The 'gold standard' for the confirmation of food allergy is a food challenge. These are often performed after a period of elimination of the suspected food. Food challenges can be performed as double-blinded, single-blinded or open challenges. For younger children an open challenge is often adequate – except in a research setting or where equivocal 'open' outcomes occur. In most cases the double blind challenge is the method of choice, especially in the older child. Food challenges carry a risk of adverse reaction to the food and should only be performed under specialist's supervision. In order confirm the results of a challenge and to establish 'clinical tolerance', the food must then be openly introduced into the diet (**Fig. 23.5**).

DIAGNOSIS AND CLINICAL FEATURES OF FOOD ALLERGY

Disease presentation

IgE-mediated, mixed- and cell-mediated food allergic symptoms can affect all organs systems of the body (Table 23.2).

IgE-mediated allergic reactions to food usually occur within minutes of ingestion of the offending food, and by definition within 2 hours. Several organ systems may be involved, including the GI tract, the skin, the cardiovascular system and the respiratory tract. The skin and the GI tract are the most commonly affected systems. It is unusual for respiratory symptoms to be the only manifestations of food allergy. Anaphylaxis is the most severe allergic reaction to food.

Non-IgE-mediated reactions include food-induced enterocolitis and food-induced colitis in young children. They are most commonly caused by reactions to cow's milk and soya proteins. Non-IgE-mediated reactions are not thought to play a role in irritable bowel syndrome, migraine or childhood behavioural problems.

Mixed IgE-/non-IgE-mediated reactions occur hours to days after ingestion, and include atopic dermatitis and the eosinophilic food-induced enteropathies (oesophagitis, gastroenteritis). It is unclear whether coexisting food-specific IgE plays a pathogenetic role in these conditions.

There is no convincing evidence that food allergies play a role in autism, depression, cystitis, enuresis (bed-wetting), chronic otitis media (glue ear), chronic fatigue syndrome, anorexia nervosa, bulimia or epilepsy.

DIAGNOSTIC TESTS

Skin prick (puncture) tests

In cases of suspected IgE-mediated immediate immunological reactions to food, a skin prick test (SPT) can be performed. In it a small amount of an (standardised) allergen in solution is placed on the skin and then introduced into the epidermis by gently puncturing the skin surface to facilitate allergen–IgE interaction. A positive reaction is manifested as the development of a wheal that is larger than the negative control test, which must be included in the assessment. A positive test (**Fig. 23.6**) indicates the likelihood that the patient is atopic and/or allergic and can strengthen suspicions about probable precipitants. An additional advantage of skin testing for food allergies is the ability to perform skin testing with the fresh food, 'prick-prick' test. The diagnostic accuracy of a skin test varies according to the offending food and the underlying immunological mechanism (acute or delayed). Negative reactions have a high (95%) accuracy of there **not** being an IgE-mediated reaction. Positive tests have only a 50–60% predictive accuracy, although at higher levels and for certain allergens, such tests can prove accurate in predicting the likelihood of an allergic reaction.

Specific serum IgE measurements

Specific IgE measurement systems have been developed to measure allergen-specific serum IgE antibodies and these should be used. In individuals with eczema, non-targeted tests correlate only variably with the correct diagnosis of a particular allergy and often indicate a state of immunological sensitisation without clinical reactivity. Overall 10–15% of individuals (up to 40% depending on the allergen) who have been sensitised do not develop clinical symptoms on exposure to the sensitising allergen.

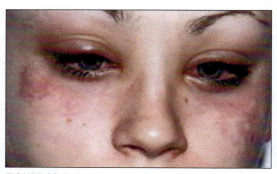

FIGURE 23.5 Acute periorbital swelling and conjunctivitis associated with abdominal discomfort during a low-dose food (peanut) challenge, resulting in systemic anaphylaxis and collapse. The 13-year-old patient also complained of double vision during the onset of the reaction. The reaction followed a low-dose challenge with negative skin test and a specific IgE <2 µg/l.

Atopic eczema ... such as milk, egg and wheat. In order to test for these conditions, an atopy patch test (APT) has been described as a diagnostic tool with a high specificity; however, prospective studies have failed to confirm very specific ...

ORAL FOOD CHALLENGES

Oral food challenges (OFCs) are required when the ... nasal or bronchial antigen challenges taking into account any specific airway reactivity. In individuals suggestive ... tive predictive value (PPV) ... tolerance has been achieved. Screening tests, with subsequent skin testing or other *in vitro* blood tests used to support the history (see below). The 'gold standard' for the confirmation of food allergy is a food challenge. ... nation of the suspected food. Food challenges can ... open challenges. For younger children or ...

to the way in which food challenges can be performed, ... systems may be involved, including the GI tract, the skin, the cardiovascular system and the respiratory ... Additional challenge variables include choice of allergen vehicle, placebo, route of exposure, time allowances between challenges and dose regimens. ... manifestations of food allergy. Anaphylaxis is the most severe allergic reaction to food.

Non-IgE-mediated reactions include food-induced enterocolitis and food-induced colitis in the young, commonly caused by reactions to cow's milk and soya proteins. Non-IgE-mediated ... in irritable bowel syndrome, migraine or childhood behavioural problems ... food allergy, but clinical ... atypical airways and ... and include atopic dermatitis and the eosinophilic food-induced enteropathies (oesophagitis, gastroenteritis). It is unclear whether coexisting food specific IgE plays a patho ...

There is no convincing evidence that food aller ... (bed-wetting), chronic otitis media (glue ear), ... syndrome, anorexia nervosa ...

TABLE 23.2 Symptoms and signs of IgE-mediated food allergic reactions

System	Manifestations
Skin (produced by ingestion or skin contact with the food allergen)	Pruritis, erythema and flushing Immediate worsening of eczema Morbiliform rashes and erythema after skin contact to fruit and vegetables Acute urticaria after contact with food
Gastrointestinal	Swelling, tingling and itching of lips and mouth Nausea and/or vomiting Abdominal pain, cramp, or colic Diarrhoea Oral allergy syndrome
Respiratory (can be produced by ingestion or inhalation of the food allergen)	Rhinitis, conjunctivitis Wheeze or tight cough can be a sign of a severe allergic reaction (anaphylaxis) Swelling of larynx can produce stridor
Multi-system/systemic	Anaphylaxis
Behavioural	Behavioural changes may be noted as the first sign of an allergic reaction
Other/rare	Uterine contractions resulting in severe 'menstruation-like' pains

FIGURE 23.5 Acute periorbital swelling and conjunctivitis associated with abdominal discomfort during a low-dose food (peanut) challenge, resulting in systemic anaphylaxis and ... or double vision during the onset of the reaction. The reaction followed a low-dose challenge with ... solution was negative.

or delayed). Negative reactions have a high (95%) accuracy of there **not** being an IgE-mediated reaction. Positive tests have only a 50–60% predictive accuracy, although at higher levels and for certain allergens, such tests can prove accurate in predicting the likelihood of an allergic reaction.

Specific serum IgE measurements

Specific IgE measurement systems have been developed to measure allergen-specific serum IgE antibodies and these should be used. In individuals with eczema, non-targeted tests correlate only variably with the correct diagnosis of a particular allergy and often indicate a state of immunological sensitisation ... viduals (up to 40% depending on the allergen) who have been sensitised do not develop clinical symp-

Double-blind placebo controlled food challenge

DBPCFC is the gold standard for the diagnosis of food allergies. DBPCFCs are complicated and labour intensive and largely restricted to use in research settings. 'Double-blind' implies that both food and placebo share unidentifiable characteristics to patient, parent and supervising health practitioner. It is sometimes difficult to mask truly the taste, smell and texture of some foods, e.g. crustaceans. Masking the allergen in tablet or capsule form may be dangerous as natural 'early detection' immune mechanisms are bypassed. The DBPCFC may be performed as a **mixed challenge** or a **separate challenge**. The mixed challenge involves giving increments of the food and matching placebos in a random order. The separate DBPCF is when the placebo and the challenge food are eaten in increments on separate occasions, e.g. morning and afternoon, or separate days. After a negative DBPCFC the patient will still need an open food challenge to unequivocally establish tolerance.

Supervised elimination-reintroduction diets

Elimination or exclusion diets can be used in patients with chronic symptoms or when there is a high index of suspicion of a food-related cause. These must be performed with the help of a dietitian to avoid nutritional deficiencies. The content of the elimination diet can be tailored to the patient's symptoms or the suspect foods, and initially excludes as few foods as possible (commonly dairy or egg free).

If this fails to control symptoms, a standard 'few foods' diet (oligoallergenic diet), containing few known food allergens, can be used. In extreme circumstances, an elemental diet (containing basic nutritional necessities without conventional food) may occasionally be needed.

EMERGING DIAGNOSTIC TESTS

Component resolved diagnostics in food allergy

These specialised diagnostic tests measure IgE responses to specific 'components' of the allergen: for example, peanut allergen components can be measured to Ara h1, Ara h2, Ara h3, Ara h8, Ara h9. Specific components may be associated with different clinical expressions and may be becoming helpful in certain clinical scenarios, such as distinguishing allergic sensitisation from clinical allergy and identifying food-allergic patients at risk of more severe reactions (e.g. Ara h2 in peanut allergy and ovomucoid in egg allergy have been associated with more severe reactions).

NON-VALIDATED TESTS FOR THE DIAGNOSIS OF FOOD ALLERGIES

IgG antibodies

Currently the determination of IgG antibodies to food has no or little predictive value for diagnosis and dietary management of patients with food-allergic diseases. Measurement of food-specific IgG_4 alone is not sufficient for a diagnosis of food allergy (Table 23.3).

TABLE 23.3 Examples of unvalidated tests for the diagnosis of (food) allergy

Food-specific IgG and IgG subclass antibody measurements
Cytotoxicity test
Sublingual, subcutaneous and intradermal provocation and neutralisation tests
Immune complex measurements
Electro-acupuncture
'Vega' testing
Applied kinesiology (DRIA) test
Hair and nail analysis

FOOD ALLERGY

Food allergy can be divided into IgE-mediated (immediate-onset) and non-IgE-mediated (delayed), depending on the underlying allergic mechanism. This classification is based on national and international professional body's definitions. IgE-mediated reactions account for a majority of food-induced allergic reactions. There is however, a growing recognition of non-IgE-mediated food-induced allergic reactions, the pathophysiology of which is less well understood.

PREVALENCE/INCIDENCE

Around 1% of adults and 3–5% of children worldwide have food allergy; the prevalence may be even higher in the first year of life, estimated at 6–8% in Western countries. While egg and milk allergy are universally common food allergies, the prevalence of additional food allergies varies, and is influenced by geographic location and distinctive dietary habits.

The higher prevalence of confirmed food hypersensitivity in infants and young children as compared to young adults suggests that much food allergy is a transient phenomenon of early life, and reflects the ability of many food-allergic children to develop immune tolerance.

CLINICAL CONTEXT

Food allergy is thought to be on the increase, possibly in keeping with the increase in other allergic diseases such as asthma and eczema, although there is some epidemiological evidence of a plateau. The prevalence of peanut allergy in the UK has nearly doubled over the past decade, and now approximates 1.8%. An Australian study found a peanut allergy rate of 3% in children at 1 year of age. Emerging new allergens include kiwi, sesame and lupin flour.

RISK FACTORS FOR THE DEVELOPMENT OF FOOD ALLERGY

In over 90% of the population the default state during development is immunological (mucosal) tolerance. The development of food allergy depends on a complex interaction between environmental factors and genetic susceptibility that leads to a failure to develop or to a breakdown in tolerance. The relative importance and effects of prenatal to postnatal allergen exposure is not known, nor is the importance of age, dose, frequency and route of food allergen exposure.

A high proportion of food-induced allergic reactions occur on first known oral exposure, possibly suggesting that sensitisation to foods does not always occur via the oral (GI) route. Atopic eczema is a risk factor for the development of food allergy and early eczema is more strongly associated with the development of food allergy.

PREVENTION STRATEGIES IN INFANCY

Breastfeeding should be encouraged as the infant milk of choice, particularly exclusive breastfeeding for at least 4–6 months. There is inconsistent evidence for use of a hydrolysed infant formula for the prevention of allergic disease (mainly eczema) in high-risk infants who are unable to exclusively breastfeed. New strategies to prevent food allergy through early exposure to one or more common food allergens are currently being investigated in large randomised controlled intervention studies.

AETIOLOGY/PATHOPHYSIOLOGY

Over half of food allergies are **IgE-mediated** and produce immediate symptoms following the release of histamine and other mediators from mast cells and basophils. The reaction can become generalised as the result of the absorption and spread of the allergen and/or as the result of the circulation of the mediators and cells stimulated by the local reaction.

Another recognised mechanism in food allergy is **delayed cell-mediated allergy** (type IV hypersensitivity), developing hours or even days after exposure. **Non-allergic processes** (and toxins) can mimic IgE-mediated allergic reactions through release of mediators or substances that are part of the food, as for example in strawberries, pineapple, cheese and chocolate (**Fig. 23.8**).

COMMON ALLERGENIC FOODS

The most common allergic reactions occur to a relatively small number of foods: cow's milk, hen's egg, peanut, tree nut, wheat, fish, sesame, soya, kiwi, are common causes of food allergy in young children (Table 23.4). Allergic reactions to fruit and vegetables are also commonly reported in infancy, such reactions are often contact reactions, generally mild, and usually transient. They are of greater significance as Oral Allergy Syndrome (OAS) in adolescents.

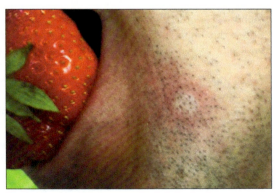

FIGURE 23.8 Acute local reaction during a strawberry challenge.

TABLE 23.4 Common allergenic foods

Food	Typical age of onset	Comment	Persistence likely
Hen's egg	Infancy		No
Cow's milk	Infancy		No
Peanut	Infancy	Usually arises due to sensitivity to the Ara h 1, 2 and 3 proteins. Sensitivity to Ara h 8 and 9 is often due to cross reactivity	Yes
Treenuts	Infancy	Hazelnut, walnut	Yes
Sesame seed	Early childhood	Most reactions occur to sesame concentrates, e.g. in hummus. Reactions to loose seeds are rare	Yes
Other seeds (mustard, poppy, linseed, flaxseed)	Early childhood	Mustard seed allergy often associated with mugwort allergy	Yes
Finfish	Early childhood	Aerosolised fish-induced reactions common.	Yes
Shellfish	Later childhood		Yes
Molluscs	Later childhood		Yes
Kiwi	Early childhood	Cross-reactivity with golden kiwi is high. Cross-reactivity with other tropical fruit unknown	No
Other fruit (pitted fruits, melons)	Common in early infancy as contact allergen, then in older children as part of OAS	e.g. apples, peaches, cherries, avocado	No
Legumes/pulses (soya, pea, lupin, chickpea, bean)	Early childhood	A common allergy in children of South Asian decent	No

TABLE 23.5 Examples of cross-reacting food allergens

Food allergen	Cross-reacting foods
Peanuts	Tree nuts
Select tree nuts	Pistachio and cashew nut, walnut and pecan nut
Peanuts	Legumes, e.g. green peas, lentils, soya, lupin
Sesame	Peanut, possibly other seeds, e.g. poppy
Finfish	Other finfish
Shellfish	Other shellfish
Molluscs	Other molluscs, snails
House dust mite	Crustaceans and molluscs – due to the muscle protein tropomyosin
Wheat	*Poaceae* grains, e.g. barley, oat and rye. Seldom to *Festucoideae* grains, e.g. rice, corn
Cow's milk	Goat's milk and other mammalian milks
Tree pollen, e.g. Birch tree	Fruit and vegetables, e.g. apple, peach, pear, cherry, hazelnut, carrot, raw potato, kiwi, banana, tomato
Grass pollen	Fruit and vegetables, e.g. raw tomato (causing OAS)
Mugwort pollen	Celery, apple, peanut, kiwi fruit, carrot, parsley, spices (fennel, coriander, aniseed, mustard, cumin), causing OAS
Weed pollen, e.g. Ragweed	Fruit and vegetables, e.g. watermelon, honeydew melon, cantaloupe, banana (causing OAS)
Latex products	Banana, kiwi, avocado, chestnut, papaya, pitted fruits. This can cause the 'latex fruit syndrome' due to the shared enzyme chitinase

CROSS-REACTIVITY AND COREACTIVITY

Cross reactivity is the reaction in an individual to a second antigen after sensitisation to the first. This arises due to similar molecular structures and binding epitopes; the closer the resemblance there is between molecules, the more likely a cross-reaction will occur.

An individual may also be independently sensitised to more than one unrelated allergen, known as coreactivity. For example, 20–30% of egg allergic children will also develop (co)reactivity to peanut, whereas 60% of peanut allergic children will develop cross-reactivity to tree nuts.

GENERAL CLINICAL EXAMINATION IN SUSPECTED FOOD ALLERGY

A thorough clinical history should include questions listed below. The physical examination is helpful to determine if the patient appears 'atopic' and to record evidence of concomitant allergic conditions such as asthma/eczema.

1. What food allergen is thought to be causing the reaction?
2. What was the timing of the reaction post-exposure?
3. What were the allergic symptoms?
4. Are there any other foods the patient may be allergic to or tends to 'dislike'?
5. What was the route of allergen exposure?
6. Is there a prior history of tolerance to the food (and to cross-reacting allergens)?
7. Is there a concomitant disease, and in particular, an allergic disease?
8. Are there any associated factors, e.g. asthma, medication use (especially angiotensin converting enzyme inhibitors, β-blockers, salicylates) or exercise.

FOOD-INDUCED ANAPHYLAXIS

Anaphylaxis is an acute life-threatening allergic reaction, which is normally mediated by IgE. It describes a pattern of symptoms that includes constriction of the airways in the lungs, obstruction of the upper airway and mouth (due to oedema of the larynx, pharynx, tongue and lips), a fall in blood pressure and acute swelling of the skin and deeper tissues (urticaria and angioedema). Many other systems may be involved (see **Fig. 23.5**).

Severity of the index reaction or worst past reaction does not always predict for the likely severity of future attacks. Known risk factors for more severe manifestations of food-induced anaphylaxis include:

- previous severe reactions (regardless of aetiology)
- teenage years
- concomitant asthma, especially poorly-controlled asthma
- past reactions to just contact with the allergen.

If a food source is not immediately evident, consider the following alternatives: contamination of the food with a known allergen may have occurred; if latex allergic, consider latex cold adhesives used in some food packaging process, or latex gloves worn by food handlers. Occasionally a modifying factor may be required to induce anaphylaxis; such factors may include exercise (i.e. food-dependent exercise-induced anaphylaxis), emotional or physical stress, food ingestion with alcohol or medications, e.g. salicylates.

PRINCIPLES OF TREATMENT OF ANAPHYLAXIS AND FOOD ALLERGY

Figure **23.9** gives the basic aspects of management (for more details see Chapter 1 Emergency Medicine, page 4).

- Patients with symptoms of anaphylaxis need a prompt dose of intramuscular adrenaline and further treatment in hospital (see Chapter 1 Emergency Medicine, page 4).
- Milder allergic reactions such as urticaria, angioedema and oral allergy syndrome usually respond to a prompt dose of oral antihistamines. Patients should repeat the dose if the initial dose is vomited. Early milder allergic reactions may progress to systemic anaphylaxis. Patients must remain under clinical observation until the reaction has subsided.
- Patients with asthma, rhinitis or eczema in association with food allergy should receive the same drug treatments for these conditions as those who do not have food allergy.
- All food allergic patients should have ready access to an appropriate antihistamine; and those with concomitant asthma should have a salbutamol inhaler and corticosteroids included in their emergency plan.
- Corticosteroids may also provide protection against delayed 'bi-phasic' anaphylactic reactions (which typically occur 4–6 hours postallergen exposure).

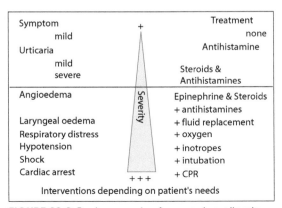

FIGURE 23.9 Basic aspects of managing allergic reactions depending on the individual's clinical needs. CPR: cardiopulmonary resuscitation.

ASTHMA AND ALLERGIC RHINITIS: ASPECTS RELATED TO FOOD ALLERGY

PREVALENCE/INCIDENCE/EPIDEMIOLOGY

The incidence of asthma in childhood is about 10–15% with some European countries reaching rates of about 20%. Although there is a clear comorbid relationship between asthma and food allergy, the reported percentages of children with asthma and clinical symptoms of food allergy vary between 5% and 17%. In the United States, black race, male sex and childhood age have been identified as risk factors for food allergy, asthma prevalence and poor outcomes.

AETIOLOGY/PATHOPHYSIOLOGY

Allergic airways disease encompasses a variety of symptoms and conditions that affect the mucosal lining of the airways, from the nose to the lungs. These symptoms/conditions vary in terms of their site of manifestation and severity. Allergic responses involve a shared mucosal system, and as a result, allergic airways disease is increasingly being viewed as a continuum (see **Fig. 23.2**).

Whereas allergic rhinitis and allergic asthma involve different regions of the respiratory mucosa, both conditions can be triggered by allergen presentation to T-cells, leading to mast cell sensitisation, release of inflammatory mediators and recruitment of leukocytes, which in turn trigger acute, and potentially chronic, allergic airways responses. Given these pathological links, it is unsurprising that allergic airway disorders are often comorbid, e.g. allergic rhinitis being high in patients with allergic asthma.

RISK FACTORS

Children with (poorly controlled) asthma and food allergy have a heightened risk of developing more severe clinical symptoms and anaphylaxis and are at increased risk of fatal anaphylaxis. Virtually all fatal allergic reactions to food occur in children who also have asthma and so it is essential that this group is adequately prepared for severe reactions and carry adrenaline autoinjectors. Food-allergic children are more likely to have more severe asthma, which results in admission to intensive care facilities.

PROGNOSIS

There is some evidence that in those children with allergic rhinitis, desensitising them to the pollen that they are allergic to may reduce the likelihood of them developing asthma. One prospective study shows that only 11% of children with wheezing symptoms and a doctor's diagnosis of asthma at 0–4 years of age had asthma at 7–8 years of age. Children with a history of eczema and food allergy carry a high risk of developing asthma. Around 75% of children with peanut allergy develop asthma.

ALLERGIC ASTHMA

Allergic asthma to environmental allergens is discussed in detail in Chapter 4 Respiratory Medicine. Here we consider the allergic components of asthma.

DIAGNOSIS/TREATMENT

Most preschool children with symptoms suggestive of asthma do not have asthma and are unlikely to respond to asthma treatment. Food allergy does not normally present with isolated or chronic respiratory symptoms. In two large DBPCFC studies in children with a history of food-related wheezing, about 60% had a positive challenge, 40% of those had wheezing as one of several symptoms, while only few patients had isolated wheezing.

Most recent guidelines for the management of asthma recommend allergen avoidance as an important goal of asthma management. Allergen avoidance advice needs to be individually tailored to take into account patient history and evidence of sensitisation. It is unresolved whether allergen reduction or avoidance is an effective treatment for asthma. Clinical trials have also involved allergen immunotherapy, anti-IgE treatment and in severe cases, temperature controlled laminar airflow (**Fig. 23.10**).

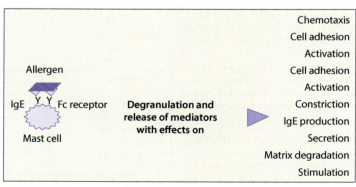

FIGURE 23.10 Schematic representation of the effects of mast cell mediators on different organ systems. Cross-linking of IgE molecules through allergen contact on the mast cell or basophil leads to the release of pharmacologically active mediators including vasoactive amines. These mediators cause smooth muscle contraction, increased vascular permeability, vasodilation and associated effects.

ATOPIC ECZEMA

Atopic eczema (atopic dermatitis) is a chronic inflammatory pruritic skin condition that develops in early childhood in the majority of cases and follows a remitting and relapsing course. Chronic atopic eczema can have a huge impact on the quality of life on both sufferers and their family. It is also often associated with other allergic conditions such as asthma and hayfever as well as having an important overlap with food allergy. Atopic eczema is often the first manifestation of the atopic march and appears to be caused by a combination of genetic and environmental factors. It can be exacerbated by a large number of trigger factors, including irritants and allergens. Although the majority of cases will clear during childhood a minority persist into adulthood.

INCIDENCE/PREVALENCE

The prevalence of atopic eczema has markedly increased in developed countries during the past three decades; 15–30% of children and 2–10% of adults are now affected. Around 45% of atopic eczema begins within the first 6 months of life, 60% begin during the first year, and 85% begin before 5 years of age. 70% of these children have a spontaneous remission before adolescence. There appears to be a lower prevalence in rural areas (see **Fig. 23.4**)

GENETICS/PATHOPHYSIOLOGY

Familial genetic predisposition and other genetic factors relating to the skin barrier and the immune response, play an important part in the underlying mechanism of eczema. Filaggrin (FLG), situated on chromosome 1q21, is an abundantly expressed protein in the outer layers of the epidermis and plays a crucial role in skin barrier formation and protection against ultraviolet radiation. Approximately 10% of Europeans are heterozygous carriers of a loss of function mutation in FLG. Carriers of the FLG mutation are at significantly increased risk of atopic dermatitis, contact allergy, asthma and hayfever and patients with atopic dermatitis who carry the FLG mutation appear to be predisposed to more severe, persistent forms of the disease and possibly to peanut allergy.

CLINICAL PRESENTATION

The clinical manifestations of atopic dermatitis vary with age (see **Fig. 23.2**). In infancy, eczematous lesions usually appear on the cheeks and scalp. Scratching, which often begins a few weeks later, causes crusted erosions. During childhood, lesions involve flexures and the dorsal aspects of the limbs while in teenagers and adults, lichenified plaques affect the flexures, head and neck. In all these stages, itching, particularly at night, causes sleep loss and significantly impairs the patient's quality of life (**Figs 23.11, 23.12**). Food allergy and eczema are closely related, particularly in childhood: they often occur in the same patients and share the same timeline in the allergic march.

DIAGNOSIS

Atopic eczema is a major risk factor for the presence of IgE-mediated food allergies in childhood. Studies reveal that among children with confirmed IgE-mediated food allergies, over 80% will report a clear history of atopic eczema during infancy. Eczema is also more commonly earlier in onset and more severe among children with food allergy compared with the general paediatric population. The earlier the eczema starts and the more severe it is, the more likely the child will have food allergy. The most common food allergens in children with eczema are milk, egg and peanut (although this varies in different geographical regions) and may affect over 60% of infants with severe eczema starting under 3 months of age. In practice, these finding suggest that any infant with significant eczema should have a careful allergy focused history taken and consideration given to allergy testing.

Non-IgE-mediated food allergies, particularly in infants with severe eczema, are unresponsive to conventional first-line treatments. Non-IgE-mediated food allergies can result in significant worsening of eczema, particularly during infancy, while withdrawal of the food can improve the eczema. The most common allergens are milk, soy, wheat and egg. Non-IgE-mediated allergies cannot be diagnosed by SPT or specific IgE testing, and it is important to rely on a careful dietary history before considering exclusion

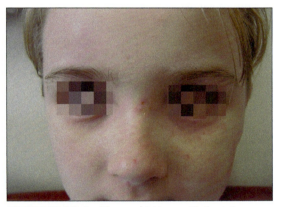

FIGURE 23.11 An 11-year-old boy with facial eczematous changes and allergic conjunctivitis.

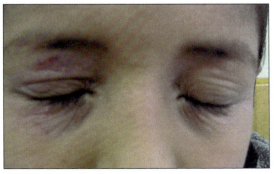

FIGURE 23.12 A girl with Dennie-Morgan creases, particularly on the upper lid, due to chronic moderate to severe eczema.

diets under specialist dietary and medical supervision. It is important to recognise that most parents believe their infant's eczema may be food related and will thus attempt to manipulate their diet. It is therefore important to consider the possibility, particularly in infantile eczema and discuss this with parents. Unless these possibilities are discussed, parents will often attempt unsupervised food exclusions that may result in nutritional deficiencies.

For some children with atopic dermatitis aeroallergens may be relevant contributory factors, particularly in older children, where food allergy becomes less of an issue. While sensitisation to milk and egg most frequently occurs during the first year of life, sensitisation to aeroallergens occurs later in childhood. Sensitisation to indoor airborne allergens (house dust mites [HDMs] and pets) often occurs at an earlier age than sensitisation to pollens (tree and grass).

TREATMENT

(For more detailed description see Chapter 6 Dermatology, page 140.)
First-line treatment:

- Avoidance of recognised aggravating factors such as food allergens and environmental factors.
- Emollients.
- Appropriate topical steroid.
- Antihistamine.

Second-line treatment:

- Assessment of an exclusion diet under supervision.
- Wet dressings with a weak topical steroid and/or moisturising agent.
- Admission to hospital for intensive nursing care.
- Topical immunomodulators such as tacrolimus ointment.

Third-line treatment (see Chapter 6 Dermatology): general measures should include supportive care for the family, ideally with the help of a nurse specialist to liaise between the hospital, the general practitioner and the family. If food allergy is a problem, the involvement of a dietitian is important.

PROGNOSIS

Children with atopic eczema and sensitisation to aeroallergens are likely to progress to rhinoconjunctivitis and/or asthma. The number and type of allergic sensitisations are considered as negative prognostic factors predicting more chronic and recalcitrant course of atopic eczema.

Aeroallergen exposure can impact on the severity of skin symptoms. In children with summer-pattern eczema, an association can be observed between disease severity and outdoor grass pollen counts. HDM allergen reduction is difficult to achieve and maintain due to the near ubiquitous exposure to HDMs. Knowledge of local pollen counts and the flowering seasons of the major allergenic plants is helpful in defining a culprit pollen.

A positive SPT and/or specific IgE test may support a suspected diagnosis but a negative test does not rule it out. Reports on the diagnostic sensitivity and specificity of APTs are inconsistent with proponents suggesting a contribution of enhanced specificity in combination with SPT or specific IgE test. Provocation tests are generally only performed to exclude sensitivities. Optimisation of eczema management will aid restoration of epidermal barrier function and may reduce sensitivity to airborne allergens. There is currently no evidence to suggest that treatment of rhinoconjunctivitis or asthma will improve atopic eczema control, but aeroallergy-associated atopy is in general a systemic disease and controlling its various manifestations will improve a child's overall wellbeing.

CHRONIC URTICARIA

PREVALENCE/INCIDENCE

Chronic urticaria (CU) is rare (0.1–3%) in infancy and childhood. CU is an 'itchy' skin condition (also called hives or wheals) that persist over 6 weeks.

AETIOLOGY/PATHOPHYSIOLOGY

CU is not an allergic condition, although allergies may coexist (like in any other individual patient). The central effector cell is the dermal/mucosal mast cell, which on degranulation releases vasoactive mediators such as histamine, a major mediator of urticaria and angiooedema. CU is in a majority of children strongly associated with circulating 'autoimmune factors', i.e. the immune system wrongly targets skin cells (mast cells). This process results in the itchy skin and mucosal hives and swelling. These IgG autoantibodies can be detected and are usually present in 40–60% of cases; if present, their presence predicts for a more prolonged disease course (**Figs 23.13, 23.14**).

CLINICAL PRESENTATION

CU presents as a skin condition (also called hives or wheals) that persists over some 6 weeks. Angioedema (swellings of the lip and eye lids) is associated in 80% of cases. The condition typically arises in otherwise healthy individuals, often requiring high-dose antihistamines. Associated autoimmune conditions, e.g. thyroid disease, coeliac disease and vasculitis, are occasionally associated with spontaneous CU and must be considered. CU will not result in life-threatening swellings of the throat and self-injectable adrenaline is not required unless patients also exhibit accompanying angioedema (**Fig. 23.15**).

TREATMENT

High-dose non-sedating antihistamines are the medication of choice for prophylaxis, and treatment, of symptoms. The following stepwise approach, for example, has been recommended (BSACI UK):

1 Standard dose non-sedating H1 antihistamine.
2 Alternative H1 antihistamine or higher dose.
3 Add second non-sedating H1 antihistamine or add first generation H1 antihistamine to be taken in the evening.

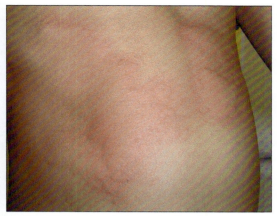

FIGURE 23.13 Chronic truncal urticaria.

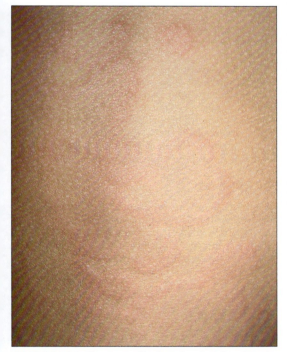

FIGURE 23.14 Close-up of lesions in chronic urticaria.

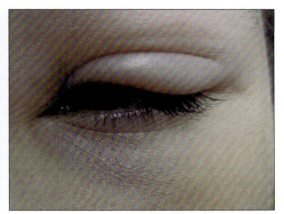

FIGURE 23.15 Chronic urticaria associated with an angioedema of the lid.

4 Consider adding antileukotriene medication.
5 Immune modifiers and other specialist treatments.

Trials off therapy are encouraged during holidays and over weekends (to see if remission has been achieved). Exacerbating 'physical factors' may include: pressure to the skin, e.g. under a tight belt, vibration, ultraviolet, hot temperatures, salicylate medications.

PROGNOSIS

The prognosis is good and CU in childhood is usually outgrown within 3–5 years after onset.

THE ORAL ALLERGY SYNDROME

The OAS is elicited by a variety of plant proteins (Class 2 food allergens) that cross-react with airborne allergens. The onset is typically in the second decade of life although it is becoming increasingly more common in children in their first decade of life. For example, birch pollen cross-reactivity may occur to one or more of hazelnut, apple, peach, pear, apricot, carrot, celery, cherry, kiwifruit and nectarine. Grass pollen cross-reactivity may occur to one or more of melon, tomato, orange. OAS symptoms are most prevalent during the associated pollen season.

Class 2 food allergens are easily digestible, hence allergic symptoms are generally mild and confined to the oral and pharyngeal mucosa, e.g. tingling and a metallic taste. The responsible class 2 proteins are heat labile; most of the troublesome fruits will be tolerated when eaten cooked or peeled.

ALLERGIES/ HYPERSENSITIVITY TO FOOD ADDITIVES

Allergic reactions to food additives are rare. True IgE-mediated food allergy may occur following exposure to enzymes and other proteins of plant or animal origin that are used in food processing (e.g. papain, α-amylase) and possibly to sulphites. There is little evidence that other additives or colourings cause either IgE-mediated or delayed non-IgE-mediated allergy; however, non-allergic mechanisms may be responsible for some of the reported symptoms, for example:

- Tartrazine, other azo dyes and benzoic acid may lead to the direct release of histamine and other mediators that mimic an allergic reaction in their effect.
- Some additives may occasionally lead to worsening of pre-existing allergic conditions such as urticaria, asthma or rhinitis, but the mechanism of this action is unclear.
- Sulphur dioxide and related compounds in food and drinks can act as an irritant to the airways and thus precipitate an asthma attack in susceptible patients.

DRUG HYPERSENSITIVITY AND ADVERSE REACTIONS TO DRUGS

PREVALENCE/INCIDENCE

Drug hypersensitivity reactions represent adverse effects of drugs taken at a dose that is tolerated by normal subjects and that clinically resemble allergy. Prevalence rates are around 5 (–10)% with higher rates in hospitalised patients.

AETIOLOGY/PATHOPHYSIOLOGY

Adverse drug reactions (ADR) can be divided into type A and type B reactions; type A reactions are more common (85–90% of all ADR), are often dose dependent and can be anticipated. Type B reactions, which arise due to allergies, are less common and cannot be anticipated. Drug reactions of an allergic nature can further be subclassified as immediate (at around an hour after exposure) or delayed (which occur beyond an hour) in onset (**Fig. 23.16**).

Drug-induced allergic reactions may arise due to IgE and /or T-cell-mediated reactions or unknown, idiosyncratic reaction. There are many reactions to drugs for which an allergy-like aetiology is suspected but for which no such mechanism can be firmly established.

CLINICAL CONTEXT

Drugs that more commonly result in allergic reactions include medications belonging to the following classes: antibiotics, antihypertensives, anticonvulsants, local anaesthetics agents and agents associated with general anaesthesia. Latex allergy is often (inappropriately) considered a drug allergy. Drug allergies can result in significant morbidity and mortality. It is for this reason that a detailed allergy assessment should be made in patients who are likely to require repeat exposure to the drug or to a medication belonging to the class of drug (**Fig. 23.17**).

Antibiotic allergies

It is the large group of beta-lactam antibiotics that are commonly used to treat bacterial infections and are most commonly associated with allergic reactions. In 80–90% adverse drug reactions affect the skin. Cutaneus presentations classically occur at the time of viral infections and so it can be very difficult to determine whether associated rashes (drug allergies usually present with cutaneous manifestations) arise due to the index infection for which the antibiotic was administrated or due to the antibiotic itself. If such a diagnosis is not taken forward this may cause unnecessary patient anxiety and compromise health care in the future.

DIAGNOSIS

Diagnostic tests currently available for the diagnosis of drug allergy are limited but include specific IgE and skin testing (SPT and/or intradermal tests) and basophil activation test, which is largely restricted to research settings. The sensitivity and specificity of these tests are highly variable; sensitivities are generally low but specificities high. Allergy testing can however prove highly predictive for some drugs, e.g. allergic reactions to neuromuscular blocking agents (these drugs are the most common cause of allergic reactions during the onset of general anaesthesia).

PROGNOSIS

The natural history of drug allergy varies according to the underlying immunological mechanism of the hypersensitivity. It has been described that penicillin allergy can be outgrown and that individuals can rarely become resensitised to it.

MANAGEMENT PRINCIPLES OF COW'S MILK AND OTHER FOOD ALLERGIES

In infants and children with presumed allergic GI symptoms, a duodenal biopsy is occasionally indicated and may demonstrate symptomatic eosinophilic infiltration. (See Chapter 9 Gastroenterology, page 262 and **Figs 23.18A, B**.)

The mainstay of treatment for all food allergies in infants and children is the avoidance of specific allergens, which often includes cow's milk protein (CMP)-derived infant formulas and other dairy products.

In formula fed infants, an appropriate hypoallergenic infant formula will need to be selected. If CMP allergy symptoms persist in the breastfed infant, a strict maternal CMP exclusion diet as supervised by a dietitian may be required, with appropriate maternal calcium supplementation. A dietician should be involved in advising on nutritional supplementation and adequacy during a food allergen/CMP avoidance diet.

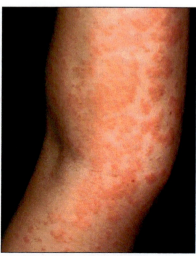

FIGURE 23.16 Urticarial drug eruption in a teenage boy with an upper respiratory infection during antibiotic therapy with amoxicillin.

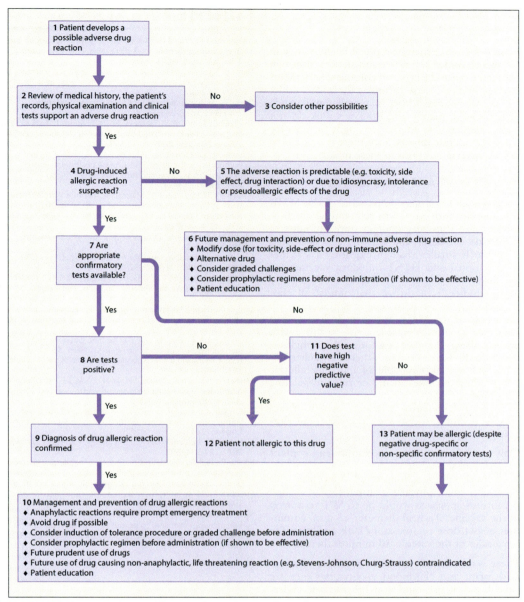

FIGURE 23.17 Drug allergic reactions and syndromes (From Smolensky R, Khan DA [eds]. Drug allergy: an updated practice parameter. *Ann Allergy, Asthma Immunol* 2010;105:259–73, with permission.)

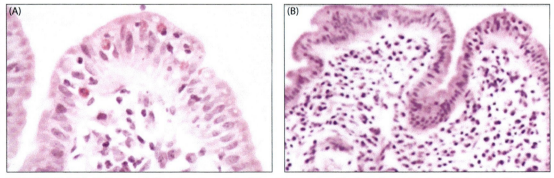

FIGURES 23.18A, B Eosinophilic infiltration (A) of the mucosal epithelium in a duodenal biopsy with mild atrophy (B) in a child with gastrointestinal food allergy.

SOY-BASED FORMULAE AND USE OF OTHER MAMMALIAN MILKS

Soy-based formulae may be a possible alternative in CMP allergy under certain circumstances although North American and European consensus statements do not recommend these formulae for infants under 6 (12) months of age. Other mammalian milks such as goat's, ewe's, mare's and donkey's milk do not provide an acceptable alternative infant formula for use in CMP allergic infants since there is a potential to induce adverse reactions in these infants.

LIVE VACCINES AND EGG ALLERGY

The measles and mumps components of the MMR vaccine are currently grown in cell cultures of chick fibroblasts and thus may contain trace amounts of egg proteins. However, the quantity and associated risk are much smaller than in egg-grown vaccines such as seasonal and H1N1 influenza vaccines, or yellow fever.

Many studies have shown that almost all children, including those with severe egg allergy, will tolerate measles or MMR vaccines. Influenza and yellow fever vaccines represent a risk to those with severe egg allergy, i.e. past egg-induced anaphylaxis. Vaccines do, however, contain other allergenic components that are also capable of inducing allergic reactions; these include bovine or porcine gelatine and antibiotics.

In higher-risk scenarios, when the benefit of vaccination is deemed to outweigh the risk in an egg-allergic patient, then:

- Only vaccines with stated maximum egg content <1.2 μg/ml should be used.
- Vaccines should be administered in a centre with experience in anaphylaxis treatment.
- A cautious approach would be to SPT to a drop of the vaccine, if wheal diameter <3 mm, administer a split dose regime as 1/10th and then the remainder of the vaccine 30 minutes thereafter.

There is no scientific evidence that normally prescribed infant and childhood vaccinations increase the likelihood of IgE- and non-IgE-mediated allergic diseases.

PROGNOSIS OF FOOD ALLERGIES

The chance of outgrowing food allergy is allergen specific. Egg and CMP allergy are outgrown in the majority of children by the age of 5–7 years but it may take up to 16 years. Allergies to wheat, soya, vegetables and fruit are also commonly outgrown. Coeliac disease is the exception (not a food allergy in the strict sense of the definition). Peanut, tree nut, sesame and fish allergies are infrequently outgrown (in about 20% of children).

FURTHER READING

Anagnostou K, Stiefel G, Brough HE, Du Toit G, Lack G, Fox AT. Active management of food allergy – an emerging concept. *Arch Dis Child* 2015;100(4):386–90.

Barbi E. Specific oral tolerance induction increased tolerance to milk in children with severe cow's milk allergy. *Evid Based Med* 2009;14:2–50.

Burks W. Skin manifestations of food allergy. *Pediatrics* 2003;111:1617–24.

Du Toit G, Santos A, Roberts G, Fox AT, Smith P, Lack G. The diagnosis of IgE-mediated food allergy in childhood. *Pediatr Allergy Immunol* 2009;20(4):309–31.

Johansson SG, Hourihane JO, Bousquet J, *et al*. A revised nomenclature for allergy. An EAACI position statement from the EAACI nomenclature task force. *Allergy* 2001;56(9):813–24.

Katelaris CH Linneberg A, Magnan A, Thomas WR, Wardlaw AJ, Wark P. Developments in the field of allergy in 2010 through the eyes of Clinical and Experimental Allergy. *Clin Exp Allergy* 2011;41:1690–710.

Khan DA, Solensky R. Drug allergy. *J Allergy Clin Immunol* 2010;125:S126–37.

Lack G. Epidemiologic risks for food allergy. *J Allergy Clin Immunol* 2008;121(6):1331–36.

Leung DYM, Sampson HA, Geha R, Szefler SJ (eds). *Pediatric Allergy: Principles and Practice*, 2nd edn. Philadelphia: Mosby, 2010.

Longo G, Barbi E, Berti I, *et al*. Specific oral tolerance induction in children with very severe cow's milk-induced reactions. *J Allergy Clin Immunol* 2008;121(2):343–7.

Marrs T, Lack G, Fox AT, du Toit G. The diagnosis and management of antibiotic allergy in children: Systematic review to inform a contemporary approach. *Arch Dis Child* 2015;100(6):583–8.

Muraro A, Halken S, Arshad SH, *et al*. EAACI Food Allergy and Anaphylaxis Guidelines. Primary prevention of food allergy. *Allergy* 2014;69(5):590–601.

NICE Clinical Guideline 116, Food allergy in children and young people. Developed by the Centre for Clinical Practice, London, 2011.

Sicherer SH. Epidemiology of food allergy. *J Allergy Clin Immunol* 2011;127:594–602.

Sporik R, Hill DJ, Hosking CS. Specificity of allergen skin testing in predicting positive open food challenges to milk, egg and peanut in children. *Clin Exp Allergy* 2000;30(11):1540–6.

Strachan DP. Hay fever, hygiene, and household size. *Br Med J* 1989;299(6710):1259–60.

Strid J, Hourihane J, Kimber I, Callard R, Strobel S. Epicutaneous exposure to peanut protein prevents oral tolerance and enhances allergic sensitization. *Clin Exp Allergy* 2005;35(6):757–66.

Index

Index

Index

Index

For Product Safety Concerns and Information please contact our EU representative GPSR@taylorandfrancis.com Taylor & Francis Verlag GmbH, Kaufingerstraße 24, 80331 München, Germany

T - #0144 - 090625 - C736 - 254/178/34 - PB - 9781482222791 - Gloss Lamination